PSYCHIATRY UPDATE

The American Psychiatric Association Annual Review

VOL. II

Edited by Lester Grinspoon, M.D.

American
Psychiatric
Press, Inc.

Washington, D.C. 1983

American
Psychiatric
Press, Inc.

1400 K Street, N.W.
Washington, D.C. 20005

Psychiatry Update: Volume II
ISSN 0736-1866
ISBN 0-88048-007-6

Printed and bound in the United States of America.

CONTENTS

Part

III

Family Psychiatry

Introduction

Psychiatry Update:
Volume II

Psychiatry Update:
Volume II

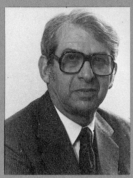

Lester Grinspoon, M.D.,
Editor

Associate Professor of Psychiatry
Harvard Medical School
Massachusetts Mental Health Center

Introduction

by Lester Grinspoon, M.D., Editor

This second volume of the *Annual Review* embodies the same spirit that animated the 1982 volume; it is a fresh and consolidated view of what we have learned and are still learning about several major topics in psychiatry. Like Volume I, Volume II addresses the need of mental health professionals for comprehensive and current knowledge in a complex and rapidly changing field. Again, the volume covers five major topics, each developed by a Preceptor and faculty members who are known for their contributions in the field. And again, the 1983 *Annual Review* is designed to mirror and magnify the Annual Review program of the Annual Meeting of the American Psychiatric Association.

We have changed the title this year to reflect more clearly the place intended for these volumes in the growing body of psychiatric knowledge. The title *Psychiatry 1982* misleadingly suggested that the series would be useful for only a short time. We actually intend each volume to encompass a knowledge base that will serve mental health professionals for some years. The Parts of Volume I—"The Psychiatric Aspects of Sexuality," "The Schizophrenic Disorders," "Depression in Childhood and Adolescence," "Law and Psychiatry," and "Borderline and Narcissistic Personality Disorders"—will be relevant and current until new theoretical developments, research findings, or clinical techniques demand another review. The same is true of this year's volume. Therefore we have given it the title *Psychiatry Update: The American Psychiatric Association Annual Review, Volume II.* Last year's volume will be referred to as *Psychiatry 1982* (*Psychiatry Update: Volume I*), and next year's volume will be *Psychiatry Update: Volume III.*

Several other formal changes should make both Volume II and the series as a whole more useful. Since material in Volume II is often related to material in Volume I, Volume II contains a detailed cumulative index covering the subjects of both volumes. The style of references has been simplified, and the reference lists themselves are keyed to the titles, as well as to the numbers of the chapters. Several of the Preceptors and faculty members have prepared annotated bibliographies or appendices which add to the practical value of the volume. Finally, I have included Editor's Notes telling the reader where to find further information on a given topic in Volume I or in Volume II.

This year's topics should interest a wide range of mental health professionals: "New Issues in Psychoanalysis," with Dr. Arnold M. Cooper as Preceptor; "Geriatric Psychiatry," with Dr. Ewald W. Busse as Preceptor; "Family Psychiatry," with Dr. Henry Grunebaum as Preceptor; "Bipolar Illness," with Dr. Paula J. Clayton as Preceptor; and "Depressive Disorders," with Dr. Gerald L. Klerman as Preceptor.

The Parts on bipolar illness and depressive disorders are intended to be used together to correspond with our current concept of the affective disorders. The Preceptors of these two Parts and I worked to guard against redundancy while ensuring that the main common issues would be covered in one or the other of the two Parts. The Part, "Geriatric Psychiatry," will also interest those concerned with affective disorders and the special diagnostic and therapeutic issues with elderly people. Of related interest is last year's treatment of "Depression in Childhood and Adolescence."

Producing a volume of this scope and depth in just one year requires the attention and cooperation of many people. In putting together their topics, the Preceptors have in effect served as associate editors. The faculty members have worked hard to prepare material that will be useful to the whole spectrum of mental health practitioners and researchers. This volume is the fruition of much work on the part of the Preceptors and their faculties. Their only reward is the pleasure they take in sharing knowledge with their colleagues. All of us who learn from what they have written are indebted to them.

There are others to whom I should like to express gratitude for the help they have given in launching this idea and producing the first two volumes. Dr. Melvin Sabshin supported the idea wholeheartedly and contributed to the solution of many of the problems that any new project of this magnitude is bound to encounter. The members of the Scientific Program Committee, and particularly the members of the Long-Range Planning Subcommittee, were most generous in sharing their thoughts and suggestions with me. Ron McMillen and the staff at the American Psychiatric Press (APPI) played a key role, attending to many details of copy editing, as well as to the numerous managerial responsibilities involved in design and production. Hermine Dlesk has diligently and ably borne much of the technical responsibility, while APPI's new in-house editor David Andrews has provided valuable expertise. Given APPI's extensive list of books in production and its recent loss of proximity to the APA reference library, the APPI staff deserves particular notice for its effort.

I especially appreciate the contribution of a new member of our team, Ms. Ruth Cross. Ms. Cross is responsible for the expertly conceived and executed index which appears at the end of this volume.

Nancy Palmer, my assistant, has served not only as an invaluable aid to me in the coordination of the scientific program, but also as an essential and highly effective liaison between the production of the book and the development of the program.

I am most indebted to my editorial assistant, Carolyn Mercer-McFadden. If this volume enjoys the same success as its predecessor, much of the credit will belong to her. Again, she has examined every sentence of the manuscript with exceptional intelligence and caring attention.

Planning for next year's *Annual Review* is already under way. Again, there will be five Parts: "Brief Psychotherapies," with Dr. Toksoz Byram Karasu as Preceptor; "Consultation-Liaison Psychiatry," with Dr. Zbigniew J. Lipowski as Preceptor; "Children at Risk," with Dr. Irving Philips as Preceptor; "Anxiety Disorders," with Dr. Donald F. Klein as Preceptor; and "Alcoholism" with Dr. George E. Vaillant as Preceptor.

It is my pleasure to introduce *Psychiatry Update: Volume II*, the second of the *Annual Review* series from the American Psychiatric Association.

November 1982
Boston, Massachusetts

I

New Issues in Psychoanalysis

Part I

New Issues in Psychoanalysis

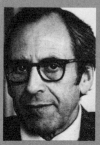

Arnold M. Cooper, M.D.,
Preceptor

Professor of Psychiatry
Cornell University
   Medical College
Director of Education
The New York Hospital-
   Cornell Medical Center
Department of Psychiatry
Training and Supervising Analyst
Columbia University

Authors for Part I

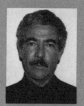

Daniel N. Stern, M.D.
Associate Professor
   of Psychiatry
Cornell University
   Medical Center

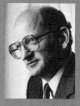

Otto F. Kernberg, M.D.
Medical Director
The New York Hospital-
   Cornell Medical Center
Professor of Psychiatry
Cornell University Medical College
Training and Supervising Analyst
Columbia University

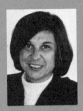

Ethel S. Person, M.D.

Director and Training and
   Supervising Analyst
Columbia University
Clinical Professor of Psychiatry
Department of Psychiatry
Columbia University College
   of Physicians and Surgeons

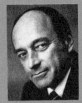

Leon N. Shapiro, M.D.

Training and Supervising Analyst
Boston Psychoanalytic Institute
Associate Clinical Professor
Harvard Medical School
Massachusetts Mental Health Center

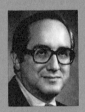

Robert Michels, M.D.

Professor and Chairman
Department of Psychiatry
Cornell University
   Medical College
Psychiatrist-in-Chief
The New York Hospital
Training and Supervising Analyst
Columbia University

New
Issues in
Psychoanalysis

Introduction
by Arnold M. Cooper, M.D.

During the past decade in America, traditional psychoanalytic attitudes and ideas have been closely reexamined and vigorously debated. The most prominent immediate sources of this internal scrutiny were the rapid development of and growing interest in self psychology and object-relations theory and the challenge that these developments posed to the predominant ego-psychological model of psychoanalysis. More distantly, this reexamination can be traced to a number of broader developments in psychoanalysis and related fields. Growing knowledge of early development through direct child observation, changes in the philosophy of science away from logical positivism, deeper clinical experience with the more severe character disorders, closer observation of the psychoanalytic situation and the analyst's role, and a climate of psychoanalytic maturity which permitted easier challenge to some of Freud's ideas—these and other factors have all had an impact on psychoanalytic theory and practice. The result is an extraordinary new excitement in psychoanalysis, a flourishing of ideas, and the production of new clinical data for discussion.

In developing this Part on new issues in psychoanalysis, the Preceptor decided to focus on a few areas where our ideas are changing rapidly and where new knowledge is being accumulated, rather than to review the major debates involving self psychology and object-relations theory. These debates have already been set forth in great detail in the literature. The five chapters presented are intended to give the reader a clear idea of the broad changes in theory and technique which are in process or being debated, as well as a sampling of some newer areas of psychoanalytic interest. As will be apparent, the authors of these chapters are not always in accord with each other in all areas.

In the first chapter, Dr. Daniel N. Stern describes some of the startling infancy-research findings that indicate a degree of predesign or "prewiring" of behaviors which few had foreseen. Infancy research has revealed that the infant has a much greater capacity than previously believed for early complex experience in the perceptual, affective, interpersonal, subjective, conceptual, and learning domains. This discovery has deep implications for psychoanalytic techniques and theories of development. Some of the findings directly challenge current psychoanalytic beliefs, while others suggest important new possibilities for understanding psychoanalytic data. Dr. Stern also highlights an issue that is addressed somewhat differently in the later chapters by Drs. Person and Michels, the lack of concordance in the views of development derived from infant observation and from reconstruction in psychoanalysis.

Dr. Otto F. Kernberg presents a condensed but comprehensive review of the status of efforts to apply psychoanalytic concepts to behavior in groups and societies. While many psychoanalysts maintain that psychoanalytic theory cannot be relevant to groups since the theory has developed from experience with individuals, individual behavior clearly is altered by group processes. Furthermore, as Dr.

Kernberg illustrates, important aspects of the group can be profitably elucidated by a sophisticated understanding of the nature of psychological regression. Since one of the major threats to human existence today is posed by the irrational behavior of people in groups, large and small, it is no exaggeration to suggest that this is currently one of the most important areas of investigation to pursue.

Dr. Ethel S. Person, in her careful analysis of changing psychoanalytic ideas of female sexuality, demonstrates the many hidden sources of value judgments in any scientific enterprise, their effects on scientific ideas, and the conditions for their change. Her views, beautifully documented, are at the farthest distance from the claims once made that psychoanalysis is value free.

Dr. Leon N. Shapiro takes up the topic of the alleged widening scope of psychoanalysis and concludes that its purview is still smaller than many would prefer. Those who oppose his view of the range of analyzability will point to his chapter's vividly described cases. They could suggest that the resistances of the patient in the second case went unanalyzed because of the analyst's preconceived ideas about the limits of analyzability and not, as Dr. Shapiro claims, because of the inherent nature of the resistance. Dr. Shapiro clinically illustrates much of the current debate concerning the analysis of narcissistic resistances and transferences and the various alterations of theory or technique which have been urged.

In the final chapter, Dr. Robert Michels discusses the value of genetic reconstruction versus here-and-now interpretation and presents a sharply etched overview of the philosophical issues which color this debate. In some ways, Dr. Michels's wide-ranging chapter is a summary of the issues which are brought up in the earlier chapters. In the context of his particular topic, interpretation, he touches on psychoanalysis as causal or hermeneutical and as science or art. He explores interpretation as specific in meaning or as a general mode of communication. He also considers whether the effective factor in analysis is the relationship of therapist and patient, or the production of new knowledge (insight), and he examines whether the relationship of therapist to patient is objective or intersubjective.

It is now a century since the birth of psychoanalysis and almost half a century since Freud's death. The best tributes to the basic health of psychoanalysis are that the field continues to generate new knowledge and ideas and that the challenges to the older ideas are more vigorous than ever.

Chapter 1

Implications of Infancy Research for Psychoanalytic Theory and Practice
by Daniel N. Stern, M.D.

INTRODUCTION

This chapter presents some of the recent findings in infancy research with the particular purpose of discussing their potential implications for clinical theory and practice. Since much of the interesting infancy research is conducted by experimentalists and developmentalists whose interest in clinical issues is not central or sometimes even peripheral, this research does not readily come to the attention of those for whom clinical issues occupy center stage. This review therefore attempts to serve a cross-disciplinary bridging function. It aims once again to update the necessary dialogue between the biobehavioral sciences and the clinical domain.

The chapter is ultimately most concerned with affective experience, but it is difficult to address affect alone, especially in infants. Indeed, since the relations between perception, cognition, drive, and affect are so intertwined, the author has not chosen to focus the review on issues that are exclusively in the affective domain. Rather, he discusses six areas in which the newly accumulated findings about infancy are such that a renewed dialogue is generally needed, trusting that the implications for affective development will be obvious when not overt. In a sense, the most urgent need at present is to alter our overall view of the infant. With such an overall alteration in view, the perspective on affects and affect development will fall into place.

STIMULUS SEEKING, THE STIMULUS BARRIER, AND THE NORMAL AUTISTIC PHASE

Our traditional clinical notion was that during the first months of life, if not the first weeks, the infant was protected from external stimuli by a stimulus barrier, or what Freud called a protective shield against stimuli (Freud, 1920). As Freud described it, this barrier was of intrinsic biological origin and took the form of sensory thresholds which were very much heightened except in relation to internal stimuli. Theoretically, the infant was considered unable to handle stimulation that broke through the shield. More recently, an active dialogue has focused on whether and when the stimulus barrier comes under some active control of the infant, as an anlage of ego-defensive operations, or whether the barrier remains essentially a passive mechanism (see reviews by Benjamin, 1965; Gediman, 1971; Esman, 1982).

The full and irrevocable opening of this door came with Wolff's description (1966) of the recurring states of consciousness that infants go through, beginning at the neonatal stage. For the present discussion, the most important state of consciousness is that of alert inactivity. In this state the infant is quiet and unmoving but has all eyes and ears trained on the external world. He or she is not just passively receptive, but is actively, in fact avidly, taking it all in. The infant not only looks receptive and is receptive, but will even work to get stimulated from the outside. Witness the infant who has an electronically bugged pacifier that will respond to sucking by operating a slide carousel and projector. Even when the infant is not hungry, he or she will suck long and vigorously enough to make the carousel present new and different slides. Clearly the stimulus barrier is not simply permeable. At times the infant is actually reaching through it. Furthermore, this responsiveness and active reach are not limited to the inanimate. Indeed, the infant is exquisitely tuned to things human, to those external physical stimuli which happen to be most likely performed by the human voice, face, and body. Brazelton (1980) has described beautifully the many ways that the newborn actively seeks out selected features of the caregiver's behavior, and experimental laboratories have supported such naturalistic observations. They have demonstrated that infants show preferences (implying stimulus-seeking and stimulus-maintaining behaviors) for certain features of the human voice or face (Cohen and Salapatek, 1975; Lamb and Sherrod, 1981). And these features are only part of the repertoire of external stimuli that the infant will seek and select.

It is still true that the young infant's tolerance for stimulation, even during alert inactivity, is far less at one week or one month of age than it will be several months or years later. But even the very young infant generally acts like a person at any other age in having optimal levels of stimulation below which more stimulation is sought and above which stimulation is avoided (Brazelton et al., 1974; Stechler and Carpenter, 1967; Stern, 1974; 1977). Mahler and her colleagues (1975) hinted at this idea in their conceptualization of the stimulus barrier in its active form. What remains, then, to distinguish a stimulus-barrier period are only the levels of stimulation and the acceptable or tolerable durations of engagement. But there is no basic difference in the active regulatory engagement that the infant makes with the external environment.

While the issue of the stimulus barrier is important in conceptualizing an early "autistic" phase and in speculating about the possibility of earliest infant memories of external events, its greatest clinical relevance may lie in the general problem of instincts and the drive to develop. Before grappling with this latter topic, however, let us deal with the notion of a primary autistic phase, since it also has considerable clinical relevance. Does the fact that the infant engages actively and regulates incoming stimulation for short periods during the first months require that we abandon the notion of the stimulus barrier and of a normal autistic phase? The author believes that it does.

The weight of new evidence suggests that the infant is only quantitatively different during the first weeks and months. It is true that somewhere around two to three months the infant undergoes a general biobehavioral shift (Emde et al., 1976). The shift ushers in a change in EEG patterns, an emerging social and instrumental usage of behaviors such as smiling, babbling, and the like, a greater ability to tolerate more stimulation for longer durations, and overall a more social "feel." Generally, this shift coincides in time with the infant's leaving an "autistic" phase. These two coinciding events are, in the author's opinion, too often used erroneously to describe and explain one another. Although the infant does become more social, this is not the same as becoming less autistic. If *autistic* means uninterested and unregistering of external stimuli, particularly human stimuli, then the infant never was autistic and cannot become less so. Rather, the infant's intrinsically determined social nature simply continues to unfold.

Moreover, it is not simply a matter of making a judgment about how much quantitative change must occur to constitute a qualitative change. The crucial idea behind the notion of a stimulus barrier and a normal autistic phase was that a qualitative difference arose at that point in life from quantitative differences in relative cathexis, responsiveness, or the capacity to handle internal vs. external stimuli. These were considered to be of such magnitude that the infant then occupied a qualitatively different position with regard to the world of stimulation, a position that could clinically be described as autistic. The recent data fail to find a great difference between infants, children, and adults in the generally active manner in which they regulate the level of external stimulation when they attend to it and, when engaged, the intensity of their engagement with the external world.

In summary, the concept of a stimulus barrier and the related idea of an autistic phase of development are no longer tenable as such and require reconceptualization along different lines. We can no longer, with any surety, speak clinically of regressions to such a phase.

When we abandon the concept of a stimulus barrier and view the infant as an active seeker and regulator of stimulation, a new set of problems arises. How then do we conceptualize the stimulus-seeking act? What drives it? Do we require that curiosity be established as a separate and third drive? The stimulus-seeking act is clearly not a derivative of libido that emerges during the oedipal period. It works, if it exists, from the first moment after birth. Lichtenberg has argued the implications of this issue well (1981), and the discussion will return to it after the next area has been discussed.

LEARNING AND KNOWLEDGE

Since learning is one of the major ways that the past can come to influence the present, it is a cardinal concern in clinical theory and practice. In spite of this, our focus has been mainly on what may be learned and unlearned, not on the learning process itself. The learning theories behind clinical practice are generally implicit, and they rest principally on associational learning as understood in classical and operant-conditioning paradigms. Do recent infancy studies shed any new light on this issue?

One of the first realizations from the explosion of infancy studies during the past two decades is that the infant begins to learn much earlier and faster than expected. Historically, the problem was that while we have always been asking the right questions of infants, only recently have we learned what might constitute the right answers on the infant's part. Beginning in the newborn period, the infant can answer with those sensorimotor systems which are relatively precocious and under voluntary control. The infant answers by looking, sucking, and head turning. Three examples will suffice. (1) When two breast pads that cover the nipples and collect excess breast milk between feedings are placed on either side of a week-old infant's head, one from his or her mother and one from another woman on the ward, the infant will reliably smell the difference and turn toward his or her mother's pad. Within one week, then, the infant has learned to discriminate the smell of his or her own mother's milk. Are we talking about cognition or affect here? (2) By one month of age, an infant will show a different nonnutritive sucking pattern when hearing a tape recording of mother's voice compared with that of another woman reciting the same material. Within one month, then, the infant has learned to discriminate the voice quality characteristic of his or her own mother's speech. (3) If an infant is simultaneously shown two faces side by side, differential looking times demonstrate that by a month or so he or she can discriminate the features of the mother's face from those of another woman.

These three examples were chosen for three reasons. First, each illustrates a different possible answer by the infant: a head turn, a sucking pattern, a gazing pattern. Second, they give evidence that the infant has learned very early during the "autistic phase" to discriminate the mother as a recognizable, specific object in a world of many such potential objects. Third, they demonstrate that the infant is a very fast learner indeed. These findings are entirely compatible with our view of the infant as a classical learner and are even compatible with our earlier view that the infant arrives in the world as a *tabula rasa*. The only revision required in traditional views is that the infant be seen as a fast rather than a slow learner.

Reviewing a second great advance, we come to even more intriguing findings. This advance in our view of the infant concerns the extent of the infant's prewired "knowledge." The more the infant is constitutionally given in terms of cognitive and emotional processes, the more early learning processes become fine-tuning and enabling mechanisms. This does not reduce the importance of learning, rather how its role is viewed. Again three examples will suffice. (1) Infants appear to be born with prewired "knowledge" of colors. As physical phenomena, colors of the same brightness and saturation differ only in hue, i.e., in wavelength emitted. Physically, a continuous spectrum of wavelengths makes up the spectrum of colors, but neither adults nor one-month-old infants see this continuous physical spectrum continuously. We and they perceive it discontinuously, such that the difference between two blues that are x wavelengths apart is seen as smaller than the difference between a greenish blue and bluish green that are also x wavelengths apart. In other words, naturally given, innate perceptual boundaries exist, lying between what we call major color categories. Cultural variations are likely to occur at the boundary areas, not in the central zones. Also the infant will tend to prefer the modal representative of each color. That is to say, the infant will choose to look longer at the color that an adult will judge to be the best exemplar of that color category e.g., the "reddest" red (Bornstein, 1975). The task of teaching color names to children would in fact be extremely difficult without the predesigned perceptual bias of discontinuous hue perception.

(2) The same applies to speech sounds. The infant is predesigned to perceive boundaries between the phonemes that make up the building blocks of speech. For instance, if one varied the sound from a "ba" to a "pa" by making smooth gradations from one to the other with a sound synthesizer (a shift in voice-onset time), one would hear "ba" until some point of discontinuity was passed, and then one would hear "pa." No humanly audible sound exists in the middle. The auditory system processes this domain discontinuously just as the visual system does with blue and green. Once again, without this predesigned feature the infant's task of learning the basic speech sounds that will ultimately constitute words, syntax, and meaning would be staggering (Eimas, 1975; Eimas et al., 1971).

(3) These two predesigned features, wonderful as they are, concern only perceptual biases. The infant is also predesigned with certain kinds of abstract "knowledge" about the world. Again, three examples of this third phenomenon will suffice. First, infants show the ability to transfer knowledge from one modality to another. They apperceive that something presented in one modality, such as vision, is the same thing as when it is presented in another modality, such as in its auditory form. Thus, infants are intermodally fluent. Meltzoff and Borton (1979) placed one of two nipples into the mouths of blindfolded infants, a normal rounded nipple and a nipple with many nubs sticking out from its surface. The infants were permitted to feel the round or the nubbed nipple with their mouths and tongues. The nipple was then removed and the blindfold taken away. Next each infant was shown the two different nipples, only one of which he or she had mouthed. Three-week-old infants looked more at the nipple they had mouthed. They had some-

how transferred the information from the haptic (touch) mode to the visual mode. Our previous learning theories would have required that the infants first establish a schema of what each nipple felt like in the mouth and then establish a second schema of what the two looked like. And finally, we would have expected, the infant would have to learn that the visual and the haptic schema of the same object were associated, resulting in a unified visual-haptic schema (Piaget, 1937; 1952). For some basic pieces of world knowledge, no such learning is necessary. The abstract knowledge is inherent in how the organism perceives. Spelke (1979) and MacKain et al. (1982) have provided some different examples of infants' capacity for perceiving cross-modal equivalences between the auditory and visual domains. Recent experiments on early imitation in the newborn period suggest that certain visual-proprioceptive equivalences may also be abstracted (Meltzoff and Moore, 1977; Field, 1981). An exploration of this phenomenon is outside the scope of this paper.

A second predesigned bit of inherent abstract knowledge is the apperception that sounds belong in synchrony with the visual events that cause them (Spelke, 1976). This very fundamental bit of world knowledge need not be learned. A reason for considering these first two predesigned capacities as forms of abstract knowledge is that they not only apply to specific examples, but actually constitute generic information-acquiring operations.

A third form of abstract knowledge relates to the nature of the cognitive apparatus. From the beginning of life, the cognitive apparatus functions with a central tendency to make and test hypotheses (Bruner, 1975). A recent experiment by DeLoache et al. (1979) is illustrative. Infants were shown many variants of a face. Each variant differed in length of nose or placement of eyes or ears on the face. All infants were "asked" which of all the variants best represented the entire set of faces. They chose a face that they had never been shown but which represented the mathematical average of all the variants they had seen. The infants had to have abstracted this averaged face from the set, since they had never seen it before. It was a hypothetical face which the infants constructed as the schema that best represented the set. Like the other two examples, this one represents an inherent tendency or process for generating world knowledge, a generative process which itself does not have to be learned but is built into the way cognition and perception work.

Implications

The implications of such findings as these are threefold. The findings first suggest that constitutional differences in this newfound set of capacities could elucidate individual differences within and beyond the normal range. Second, they shed light on the nature of the normal symbiotic phase. And third, they relate to the larger issue of drive.

Regarding the first implication, the findings are still too new for us to have any normative information about the range of individual differences or even any longitudinal assessments of the stability of these capacities. Nonetheless, some speculations can be offered. If an infant were constitutionally defective or simply poor at abstracting intermodal equivalences or at perceiving, preferring, and expecting synchrony between the multimodal manifestations of a single event, he or she would be at an enormous disadvantage in constructing a cohesive, unified picture of the world of human behavior and of his or her own behavior. Such abstract knowledge and generative perceptual operations are essential for comprehending not only the basic fabric of the human behaviors that constitute emotional expressions and verbal meanings, but also the material that makes up school learning. Suppose, further, that deviant functioning in these areas could be selective, either to certain types of events such as human but not inanimate events or vice versa, or to certain states of consciousness. Without further evidence, it is pointless to go on, except to alert clinicians to such etiologic possibilities and to see what unfolds over time.

The second implication bears on the status of the so-called normal symbiotic phase of life (Mahler and Furer, 1968; Mahler et al., 1975). This concept has been of great importance in conceptualizing many clinical issues ranging from childhood psychoses to borderline personality to regressive phenomena in general. The infant capacities discussed above have implications for the notion of a normal symbiotic phase for one simple reason. Normal symbiosis is among other things an important statement about what the infant perceives about his or her world and what abstract knowledge or knowledge-acquiring procedures the infant has available. The author has previously argued (Stern, 1980) that the infant's capacities for making cross-modal transformations and for perceiving synchrony between different manifestations of the same event, along with his or her ability to recognize causal relationships (Watson, 1979), would make the infant very unlikely on cognitive grounds to confuse self and other consistently. Given these capacities, which are functioning well shortly after birth, it is difficult to imagine the infant lingering in a long phase of undifferentiation.

The counterargument that normal symbiosis concerns only the emotional apperception of experience leads to the idea of a baby with antithetical cognitive and affective experiences. In the view of Heinz Werner, it is likely that everything in the infant's experience is affectively perceived (Werner, 1948; Werner and Kaplan, 1964). In fact, the distinctions between cognitive and affective knowing may have little substance until a language-based semantic system emerges (see discussion below on memory). Furthermore, there is no reason to assert that the apperception of a distressed causal self acting distinctly from a causal other is a less affective apperception than the apperception of a moment of merging. Both apperceptions are both cognitive and affective. And it appears that the infant simultaneously forms schemata of self with other, self alone in the presence of other (see Winnicott, 1971), and self alone (Sander, 1980b). The central point is that once the assumed "cognitive" incapacity and the assumed "emotional" need to see self and other as a dual unity have been deeply mitigated, then the central tenet of a normal symbiotic phase has been removed. The infant need not individuate from an initial symbiotic position. From nondifferentiated experiences, the infant can form in parallel various schemata of self and of self fused with other.

A period of cognitive-affective self-other fusion no longer dominates the landscape during this life phase. Such a point of view, initially given momentum by new findings in infants, forces a reconsideration of the normal symbiotic phase and the extent of its clinical explanatory power. An alternative point of view has now become possible. The states, schemata, or representations of self-other fusion are not primarily the hallmarks of a developmental epoch from which one emerges in part and to which one may regress. Rather, they are the continually forming, continually evolving, positive and adaptive organizations of self experience with another.

The third and final implication concerns the matter of drives and autonomous ego functions. Here the discussion returns to material that was only partially explored in the discussion of the stimulus barrier, the normal autistic phase, and stimulus seeking. From what we are learning about infant perception, cognition, memory, and affectivity in the early months of life, several points are of particular relevance. The course of development and the functional specifics of various ego capacities are greatly determined by the orderly unfolding of specific pre-adapted capacities. This predesign of separate functions thus partially obviates the need to talk in terms of larger drive systems that operate either locally or generally, such as libido or its neutralization. It was one thing to think of libido as investing one major anatomical locus, the mouth, during a developmental stage or as one modality of inter-activity with the world à la Erikson which then influenced or even organized all other functionings. Now, however, our infant does not appear to be particularly mouth dominated or anything dominated. Vision, audition, smell, touch, memory, hunger feeding, feeling, schema formation, and so on—each appears to be a separate and thought-related area of furious functioning. Furthermore, none of these is a mechanism which is brought to functioning when some local or generalized energy activates it. Indeed, it is impossible to separate passive mechanism from activating energy. Each function itself consists insepa-rably of both. Moreover, the specifics both of the mechanisms and of the triggering and threshold phenomena that activate the function are largely biologically determined. Freud clearly saw libido as a predes-igned aspect of human psychobiology with a predetermined schedule of unfolding and so forth. In that sense, Freud's view of libido and our current views of, say, visual perception, have great similarities. The author does not intend to argue libido theory, but rather to point out that, for those who wish to retain it, the new evidence would picture libido as extremely fragmented both anatomically and functionally from the very first minutes of life. In this light, it would be almost impossible to determine what constituted a drive derivative. To consider each infant function as a drive derivative is not parsimonious and adds little to our understanding of the infant.

MEMORY

The major issue involved with early memory concerns the nature and onset of recall memory, more often called evocative memory in the psychoanalytic literature (Fraiberg, 1969). Recall or evocative memory, in contrast to recognition memory, involves remembering in the absence of the to-be-remembered person, thing, or event. Long-term recognition memory, which only requires recognition when the to-be-remembered stimulus is present again, can be demonstrated quite early. Fagan (1973) has shown convincingly that five- to seven-month-old infants have recognition memory for pictures of the faces of strangers seen more than a day or even a week previously. The earlier cited abilities of infants to discriminate the mother's voice pattern and facial configuration during the first few months of life also require that recog-nition memory be operating. But these phenomena of recognition are less crucial to clinical theory than are the phenomena of recall memory.

Only recall memory permits free associations, creative fantasy, dream work, or the "suffering from remembrances."

The traditional psychoanalytic position on recall memory, perhaps best explicated by Fraiberg (1969), is very close to that of the dominant cognitive psychologies exemplified by the work of Piaget (1937). For both, recall memory is only possible when adequate language or some other cognitive code (e.g., mental imagery) is available to facilitate storage and retrieval operations, and this in turn is possible only toward the middle or end of the second year when language competence is considerable. This view of a language-based recall memory continues unchallenged. However, it is now clear that the recall-memory story does not end here. Rather, there now appear to be recall-memory systems which are not language based. Rovée-Collier and her colleagues have demonstrated long-term cued recall for motor memories (Rovée-Collier et al., 1980; Rovée-Collier and Lepsitt, 1981). Parenthetically, cued recall and recall memory are the same, and a kind of memory that is spontaneously evoked *in vacuo* probably does not exist. Some association or cue is responsible for the evocations, and a continuum of cues exists, from far-flung, slight cues to cues that are very close but not identical to the to-be-remembered original. In this sense, recognition memory and recall memory are at opposite ends of a dimension defined by gradations of similarity to the original.

Motor memory has been demonstrated in infants by placing three-month-old infants in cribs with attractive overhead mobiles. Strings were tied to the infants' feet so that each time they kicked, the mobiles would move. The infants quickly learned to kick to make the mobiles move. Several days after this training session, the infants were brought back to the laboratory and placed in the same cribs with overhead mobiles. The context of lab, crib, mobile, and so forth recalled the motor act, and the infants began to kick at a high rate, even though the strings were absent and the mobile did not move. If a different-looking mobile was used during the memory-test session, the kicking was less than with the original mobile. The different mobile was a poorer cue for retrieving the motor act. These experiments documented what was suspected or even obvious for a long time: infants go about acquiring a huge repertoire of motor skills, including the articulation of speech, during the first months and year of life. The flexible use of such a repertoire requires some kind of motor memory.

Affect Memory

More recent evidence suggests the existence of a third type of memory system beyond semantic and motor memory, an affect memory (Bower, 1981; Zajonc, 1980). Affect memory may be present early in infancy (Nachman, 1982; Nachman and Stern, 1982). Six- to seven-month-old infants were first shown two hand puppets, a frog and a rabbit, and their time spent looking toward each was recorded. No infants smiled during this pretest. Then came a game of peekaboo in which one of the puppets disappeared and then reappeared and said, "Peekaboo." Many of the infants smiled at the game puppet during the peekaboo procedure. One week later, the infants came back and were again shown the two puppets as they had been for the pretest. This time, if they had smiled during the peekaboo game the week before, they now smiled when they looked at the game puppet they had played with, even though it was motionless. They also looked longer at the one they had played with. The infants who did not smile during the peekaboo game did not smile at the game puppet one week later, and they tended to look more at the puppet that they had not played with. The authors concluded that the sight of the game puppet one week later evoked the memory of the affective experience. The fact that the smiling infants and the nonsmiling infants both had their looking preferences altered by the game experience, albeit in opposite directions, indicates that while both groups did have recognition memory for the game puppet, the smiling act could not be attributed to recognition memory alone, since both groups recognized the game puppet. What they remembered included the affective experience.

The implication is that affects can serve as a nonlinguistically based encoding vehicle. It remains to be seen how closely related are the motor and affect memory systems. For now, the major relevance of the finding is that it permits us to conceive of long-term storage and retrieval of affective experience in the preverbal child. Further, it gives us a mechanism whereby various environmental cues could remind the infant of prior and even somewhat removed affective events. In other words, we can now readily conceive of the infant having evocative memories for a variety of experiences long before the advent of a language-based memorial code. Since our major theoretical and clinical concern has always been with emotional experience in comparison with semantic knowledge, for all important purposes the infant does have recall or evocative memory by at least the age of seven months.

What happens to affect memories when a language-based code arrives on the scene? Here two further questions arise. First, what happens to affect memories laid down prior to language acquisition? Do they ever gain access to the linguistic encoding system, and if they do not, is this the major locus for discontinuity in reconstructive analytic work? Second, what happens to affect experiences that occur after the language-based memorial system is in place? Are they encoded in two parallel memorial systems, a semantic system and an affect system? Recent research in memory suggests that most experience is encoded dually in parallel systems which communicate readily with important mutuality of influences (Zajonc, 1980; Bower, 1981). For affect memories laid down prior to a language-based code, when they get retrieved after the language-based code is established, which involves some dose of reexperiencing, they should at that point establish connections with the language-based code. In this fashion, the active memories of affective experience from early preverbal infancy should become partially accessible to linguistic rendering. It is important to note that even current affect memories are only roughly translatable into a language code. No immediate reason suggests that reexperiencing preverbal affect memories that arise from a verbal phase should be handled any differently from reexperiencing affect events that occur during the verbal phase. In summary, our inability to establish greater continuity between pre- and postverbal periods may stem largely from our failures to be imaginative in technique and from the presence of a discouraging theory.

The issue of amnesia for infantile events may thus have little to do with a memorial discontinuity brought about by the acquisition of language. Yet this has too often been assumed to be the obstacle to reconstructions reaching back into the preverbal period. Two alternate explanations of infantile amnesia now offer themselves. The long-held notion that repression is brought about during and because of oedipal-period conflicts remains viable. It is compatible with the fact that no infantile amnesia exists for motor memories. Infants do not forget how to walk, throw, pull, and so forth. Infants' motor skills, also memory based, simply continue to accrue. And it is also compatible with the fact that no infantile amnesia exists for semantic memory. Infants do not forget how to talk syntactically or lose vocabulary. Their linguistic competence also continues to grow uninterruptedly. Only their episodic memory for affect-laden experiences suffers from this infantile amnesia. But the repression theory in itself does not explain why the memory for affective experiences should get wiped clean going all the way back. If repression alone were operating, one might expect more selectivity. Very likely, during the oedipal years when dramatic growth and change occur in almost all mental functions, various psychobiological reorganizations also occur, including the restructuring of prior infantile experiences which do not depend to any considerable extent on the earlier landmark of language acquisition (Hofer, 1980). These considerations reduce the importance of language per se in our considerations of emotional memories, and they strengthen the view that nonverbal techniques may permit continuous reconstructions proceeding backward well into the preverbal period of life.

One final intriguing datum bears on early memory and dreams, or at least on sleep. Rovée-Collier has reported that motor memories shown by three-month-olds are considerably enhanced or consolidated by sleep (Carolyn Rovée-Collier, 1982, personal communication). For instance, some hours after a foot-kicking training session, the infant will recall the motor act better if he or she has been able to "sleep on it." Appropriately controlled experiments indicate that something occurs during sleep that consolidates the memory. Dreaming is the favored candidate, but further research is in order.

One final implication of these reflections on memory concerns the repetition compulsion. Sander provocatively stated, "One of the effects of the unique strategies by which regulation of the infant-caregiver system is established is that from these strategies we *construct a perceptual world* towards which we then behave in such a way as to validate [it]" (Sander, 1980a, 198, emphasis added). This is an interesting flip-around of the relationship of perception to behavior, but as therapists, we are constantly trying to undo this process, what we call repetition compulsion. The construction of a "perceptual world," in the sense Sander used it, is the task of an affect-based recall-memory system. If the preverbal infant has an affect-based memory system which operates well before the advent of language, then he or she will be able to construct a perceptual world of likely affective, interactive sequences and of dyad-specific or standard events which will in turn guide behavior. And this means that by about the sixth month of life, the essential relationships between memory, perception, and behavior which may describe the anlage of the repetition compulsion are present and operating.

INTERSUBJECTIVITY

A growing number of infant researchers have recently converged on the idea that sometime between the seventh and the ninth month or so the infant comes upon a momentous discovery, namely, that he or she can share with another a state of mind such as an intention (Bates,

1976; Bretherton, 1981; Newson, 1977; Trevarthan, 1979; 1980). In other words, the infant develops a "theory of interfaceable minds" (Bretherton, 1981). This has several implications: that the infant has the ability to impute, unawares, an internal mental state to another; that he or she has some apperception, at the moment, of a particular internal mental state; and that the interfacing, in the sense of sharing or reciprocally manifesting, these two states, is not only possible, but a goal to be sought. All of this assumes some apperception of a framework of meaning, assumes the availability of an interfaceable medium such as language or gesture, and assumes some apperception of the existence of two separate but interfaceable minds.

The observable phenomena on which these conclusions are based can be summarized in three examples. (1) When an infant begins to point at an object and at the same time to alternate his or her gaze back and forth between the caregiver's face and the object, we can posit that the infant is entertaining the notion of the existence of joint attention. (2) When an infant reaches toward an object being held by another and opens and closes his or her outstretched hand toward the object, grunting "Eh! Eh!" while looking eagerly from the object to the person's face, we can posit that the infant anticipates that the other can read, share, and act upon his or her intention and that interintentionality can occur between him- or herself and another. (3) When an infant reacts to a mother's misreading and her consequent mismatching or misattuning of behaviors to his or her own state of arousal or level of affect, we can speak of interaffectivity.

We may accept these phenomena as evidence of intersubjectivity on the infant's part, an inference which seems to cause philosophers no trouble. If we do so, we may find we must shift our emphasis on developmental timetable and our theoretical perspective. As stated earlier, we have good reason to believe that a state of undifferentiation of self and other never does exist (as compared with nondifferentiation) and that a steadily growing sense of self and other as separate *physical* entities exists early. The above data suggest that at around seven months the infant comes to sense self and other as separate *mental* entities. We would then date at seven months a fairly advanced and cardinal feature of individuation. The developmental timetable for individuation would be set back in time, and this leap in individuation would be seen as a consequence of an early cognitive jump forward that is not directly related to the later motor milestones which permit the advance of separation.

EMPATHY

Along with the increased interest in the psychology of the self, the role of empathy as a mode of understanding, and even perhaps as a therapeutic function, has received more and more attention. Until recently, most infancy research that examined interactions or relationships was concerned largely with communication. Communication, as it is usually defined, concerns the exchange of information and the intention to alter someone else's belief or action systems. More recently, studies have emphasized the extent to which mothers and fathers attune with their infants' affect states and levels of arousal (Stern et al., 1982). The important part of these attunements is that they are generally not intended to convey information nor to alter the babies' motor or mental states. Rather, they are intended to align the adult with the infant, to "be with" the baby and to share in his or her experience. In this sense, the attunements are more in the nature of communion than communication. The more we look, the more pervasively and frequently appear the attuning process and the establishment of moments of communion. In the study cited, attunements occurred in mother-infant play sessions at the rate of about one per minute. The exciting part of such moments is that they seem to establish a springboard from which the mother and the baby can expand their interactive repertoire. It is a different kind of mental "fueling." In this respect, the early attunements act quite similarly to the empathic attunements in therapy as described in the work of Kohut (1982) and many others (for example, Schwaber, 1980).

The early appearance and apparent importance of this phenomenon during the first year of life argues for paying even more attention to empathic phenomena. Empathy appears to have strong effects on the interpersonal climate, from the earliest months throughout the life span.

ALIGNMENT WITH THE POSSIBLE AND THE PROBABLE

Empathy is an alignment with currently felt internal states. One can also make an alignment with potential states of being. Friedman has pointed this out in an intriguing paper where he stated, "It is not necessary for the analyst to know the exact nature of the development he is encouraging. It is sufficient that he treats the patient as though he were roughly the person he is about to become. The patient will explore being treated that way, and fill in the personal details" (Friedman, 1982, 12). In a discussion of Friedman's paper, Knapp (1982) urged that this notion be extended to include the emotional domain. Friedman made no special claims for the therapeutic or change-effecting nature of this alignment in comparison with interpretation and the like. However, he did make the important distinction between interpretations or empathic maneuvers and this potential therapeutic phenomenon.

A fascinating aspect of alignments with future states of being is that mothers with their infants are perhaps the ultimate experts on this perspective. A closer view of how a mother performs to effect change (development) in her baby may be instructive clinically. Much of the time, a mother is in a dialogue with her infant as she imagines, guesses, and wishes what he or she will soon become. Let us call this imagined infant the potential infant. Maternal speech to infants is a clear case in point. The mother characteristically targets her linguistic repertoire so that it is exactly several months ahead of the infant's productive competence (Bloom, 1973; Snow, 1972). The more effective mothers stay just far enough ahead, months not weeks or years, to facilitate the infants' language acquisition. In this way, they are helping the infants to become the persons they are likely to become. This same dialogue with the potential infant is seen in a mother's open-ended attribution of intention, not her specific intention, but her state of being a declared intender. Similarly, the affective dialogue between mother and infant shows this same general feature: the attribution of affect states and ranges of intensity or arousal which are still in formation. In fact, the art of mothering is often characterized by how the mother times her switches between the actual and the potential infant as her partner. Addressing the potential infant is more than teaching and more than providing expansions or elaborations of the infant's behavior for the purpose of teaching or changing. Such teaching behavior is addressed to the actual infant. Address to the potential infant is more generic. The mother holds in her mind no specific change or thing to be learned. Rather, she treats the infant "as though he were roughly the person he is about to become." The infant provides the specifics.

In summary, studies on infancy may prove helpful to our clinical science in two very different ways. The first way is the more traditional and obvious: the studies increase our knowledge of the developmental course of human behavior. The second way comes from our observation of the mother as an agent for change and has less obvious implications for clinical science. To the extent that normal development and therapeutic change are comparable, the caregiver-infant dyad offers us a partial model for the therapist-patient relationship, and vice versa.

Chapter 2

Psychoanalytic Studies of Group Processes: Theory and Applications
by Otto F. Kernberg, M.D.

PSYCHOANALYTIC THEORIES OF GROUP PSYCHOLOGY

The Psychology of Large and Small Groups

Freud (1921) initiated the psychoanalytic study of group processes and explained them in terms of his then newly developed ego psychology. As Freud explained group processes, individuals in mobs had an immediate sense of intimacy with each other which derived from the projection of their ego ideal onto the leader and from their identification with the leader as well as with each other. The projection of the ego ideal onto the idealized leader would eliminate moral constraints as well as the superego-mediated functions of self-criticism and responsibility. While the sense of unity and belonging would protect the members of the mob from losing their sense of identity, it would be accompanied by a severe reduction in ego functioning. As a result, primitive, ordinarily unconscious needs would take over, and the mob would function under the sway of drives and affects, excitement and rage, stimulated and directed by the leader.

In works written in the 1940s and early 1950s, Bion (1961) described the regressive processes that occur in small groups of 7 to 12 members. He based his observations on the fantasies, fears, and behavior that members of small unstructured groups evidenced when the leader consistently refused to participate in any group decision making or structuring. The leader would only observe and comment on the group's behavior. Bion described the regressive processes in terms of three basic emotional assumptions which are the foundation for group reactions that potentially exist at all times, but which are particularly activated when the task structure or "work group" breaks down.

The first "basic-assumptions group" operates under a "dependency" assumption. Members perceive the leader as omnipotent and omniscient and themselves as inadequate, immature, and incompetent. They match their idealization of the leader with desperate efforts to extract knowledge, power, and goodness from the leader. The group members are thus both greedy and forever dissatisfied. When the leader fails to live up to their ideal of perfection, they first react with denial and then react by rapidly and completely devaluing the leader and searching for a substitute. Thus, primitive idealization, projected omnipotence, denial, envy, and greed, together with their accompanying defenses, characterize the dependency group.

The second group operates under a "fight-flight" assumption, united against what it vaguely perceives to be external enemies. This group expects the leader to direct the fight against such enemies and also to protect the group from infighting. Since this group cannot tolerate any opposition to the ideology shared by the majority of its members, it easily splits into subgroups which fight with each other. Frequently, one subgroup becomes subservient to the idealized leader, while another subgroup attacks the subservient one or goes into flight from it. Prevalent features include the group's tendencies to control or to experience itself as being controlled by the leader, to experience closeness through shared denial of intragroup hostility, and to project aggression onto an out-group. In short, splitting, projection of aggression, and projective identification prevail. In the fight-flight group, the search for nurture and dependency that characterizes the dependency group is replaced by conflicts around aggressive control, along with suspiciousness, fighting, and dread of annihilation.

The third group operates under a "pairing" assumption. Members tend to focus on a couple within the group, usually but not necessarily heterosexual. The focal couple symbolizes the group's hopeful expectation that it will in effect reproduce itself and thus preserve the group's threatened identity and survival. The pairing group experiences general intimacy and sexual developments as potential protections against the dangerous conflicts around dependency and aggression that characterize the dependency and the fight-flight groups. While the latter two groups have a pregenital character, the pairing group has a genital character.

Both Le Bon (1895) and Freud (1921) referred to the direct manifestations of violent aggression in mobs. In contrast, the potential for violence is still generally under control in small groups. Not only do small groups make use of the mechanisms just described, but the context of eye-to-eye contact and mutual acquaintance helps small groups to maintain a certain civilized attitude. Occasionally, however, the external enemy is absent, and this raises the small group's tensions to a high pitch. An external enemy serves to absorb the aggression generated within the group, and this aggression threatens the basic-assumptions group which cannot define or locate an enemy on the outside.

Rice (1965) and Turquet (1975) studied the behavior of large unstructured groups of 40 to 120 persons and used methods similar to those Bion had used in his study of smaller group processes. Turquet described how the individual member of a large group felt a total loss of identity. Concomitantly, the individual's capacity for realistically evaluating the effects of his or her words and actions decreased dramatically within the large-group setting. In a large group, the ordinary social feedback to the individual member's verbal communications disappears. Nobody seems to be able to listen to anybody else, all dialogue is drowned by the discontinuity of communication that evolves, and efforts to establish small subgroups usually fail. The individual is thrown into a void. Even projective mechanisms fail, because no one can evaluate realistically the behavior of anyone else. In this context, projections become multiple and unstable, and the individual has the urgent task of finding some kind of "skin" that will differentiate him or her from the others.

Turquet also described fears of aggression, of loss of control, and of the violent behavior which could emerge at any time in the large group. Fear is the counterpart to provocative behaviors among the group's members, behaviors that they partly express at random but mostly direct at the leader. Gradually, it becomes evident that those individuals who try to stand up to this atmosphere and maintain some semblance of individuality are the ones who are most attacked. At the same time, efforts at homogenization are prevalent, and any simplistic generalization or ideology that permeates the group may be easily picked up and transformed into an experience of absolute truth. In contrast to the simple rationalization of the violence that permeates the mob, however, the large group has a vulgar or commonsense philosophy which functions as a calming, reassuring doctrine and which reduces all thinking to obvious clichés. One cannot escape the impression that aggression in the large group for the most part takes the form of envy of thinking, individuality, and rationality.

Anzieu (1971) proposed that under conditions of regression in the unstructured group, the relationship of individuals to the group as an entity would acquire the characteristics of fusion. In Anzieu's view, individual instinctual needs would be fused with a fantastic conception of the group as a primitive ego ideal, equated with an all-gratifying primary object, the mother of the earliest stages of development. The psychology of the group, then, reflects three sets of shared illusions. (1) The group is constituted of individuals who are all equal, thus denying sexual differences and castration anxiety. (2) The group is self-engendered, that is, a powerful mother of itself. (3) The group itself might then repair all narcissistic lesions, since it becomes an idealized "breast-mother".

Chasseguet-Smirgel (1975) expanded on Anzieu's observations, suggesting that under such conditions any group, small or large, tends to select leadership that represents not the paternal aspects of the prohibitive superego, but a pseudopaternal "merchant of illusions." Such a leader provides the group with an ideology, a shared system of ideas which serves to unify the group, and in this case, the ideology is an illusion that confirms the individual's narcissistic aspirations of fusing with the group as a primitive ego ideal—the all-powerful and all-gratifying preoedipal mother. Basically, the small- or large-group members' identification with each other permits them to experience a primitive narcissistic gratification of greatness and power. When groups are violent and are operating under the influence of ideologies that have been adopted under such psychological conditions, their violence reflects their need to destroy any external reality that interferes with the group's illusionary ideology. The losses of personal identity, cognitive discrimination, and any differentiating individuality within the group are compensated for by the sense of omnipotence that all its members share. In this conceptualization, the regressed ego, the id, and the primitive (preoedipal) ego ideal of each individual are seen as being fused in the group illusion.

An Object-Relations Approach to Group Psychology

In earlier works, the author has proposed that the strikingly regressive features of small groups, large groups, and mobs may be even better understood using our present concept of the internalized object relations that predate object constancy and the consolidation of the ego, superego, and id (Kernberg, 1976; 1980). From this viewpoint, one might consider two levels of internalized object relations. A basic level would be characterized by multiple self- and object-representations that correspond to primitive fantasy formations linked with primitive impulse derivatives. The second and higher level would be characterized by sophisticated, integrated self- and object-representations linked with higher levels of affect dispositions. These higher-level object relations reflect more accurately than the basic-level object relations the early childhood experiences and conflicts between the individual and his or her real parental figures and siblings. At the higher level, the integrated self-concept, together with integrated, realistically invested object-representations that are related, constitute ego identity. When an integrated concept of the self and integrated concepts of others are lacking, the syndrome of identity diffusion develops.

Impressive clinical evidence indicates that regardless of the individual's maturity and psychological integration, certain group conditions tend to bring on regression and activate primitive psychological levels. Groups that are small, closed, and unstructured, as well as groups that are large, minimally structured, and lacking clearly defined tasks to relate them to their environment, tend to bring about an immediate regression in the individual. This regression consists in the activation of defensive operations and interpersonal processes that reflect primitive object relations. The potential for this exists within all of us. When we lose our ordinary social structure, when our ordinary social roles are suspended, and when multiple objects are present simultaneously in an unstructured relationship, reproducing in the interpersonal field a multiplicity of primitive intrapsychic object relations, under such circumstances primitive levels of psychological functioning may be activated.

Combining the observations made of mobs, large groups, and small groups, the author has proposed that group processes in general pose a basic threat to personal identity (Kernberg, 1980). This threat is linked to the proclivity in group situations for primitive psychological levels to be activated, including primitive object relations, primitive defensive operations, and primitive aggression with predominantly pregenital features. Turquet's description of what happens in large groups constitutes the basic situation for the activation of defenses in a group of any size. The horde's idealization of the leader as described by Freud, the group's idealization of group ideology and of leadership that promotes the group's narcissistic self-aggrandizement as described by Anzieu and Chasseguet-Smirgel, and the small-group processes described by Bion—all are ways of defending against the situation Turquet described. Obviously, large-group processes can be obscured or controlled by rigid social structuring. Bureaucratization, ritualization, and well-organized task performance are different methods with similar immediate effects.

Large-group processes also highlight the intimate connection between threats to retaining one's identity and the fear that primitive aggression and aggressively infiltrated sexuality will emerge. Throughout group and organizational processes, an important part of nonintegrated and unsublimated aggression is expressed in vicarious ways. In the group processes of organizations and institutions, for example, the exercise of power constitutes an important channel for expressing the aggression that would ordinarily be under control in the smaller settings of dyads and triads. Aggression emerges more directly and much more intensely when group processes are relatively unstructured.

Narcissistic personalities, as the author has pointed out elsewhere (Kernberg, 1980), are ideally constituted for assuming leadership under the conditions of large-group processes. Their lack of deep conviction regarding their own values makes it easy for them to swim with the currents of a group. Given that the particular narcissistic personality has the requisite communication talents, he or she may be able to provide the large group with an acceptable ideology and to convey a sense of certainty without triggering the group's envy against individualized thinking. All of these abilities make such a leader the grand leveler of the large group's tensions. By the same token, the large-group members' identification with the narcissistic leader reinforces some of the pathologically narcissistic characteristics of "static" crowds (Canetti, 1980). They are conventional, ideologically simplistic, conforming, and able to indulge themselves without guilt or gratitude, and they lack a sense of personal responsibility and any deep investment in others.

Another striking characteristic of group life is the activation of infantile sexual features. In the small group, sexuality emerges when the basic assumption of pairing serves as one defense against primitive aggression. In the large group, sexuality is either denied or expressed in sadistically infiltrated sexual allusions. Usually sexuality goes underground in the large group, and couples form secretly as a direct reaction to and defense against large-group processes. In the horde, the unchallenged idealization of the leader has a counterpart in the group's intolerance of any couple that attempts to preserve its identity as such. Freud (1913) saw crowds' intolerance of sexuality as a derivative of the original danger that faces the primitive horde, namely, the sons' rivalry in competition for their mothers and sisters. He proposed that totemic exogamy protected the social structure at the cost of repressing sexual urges within it. Anzieu (1971) and Chasseguet-Smirgel (1975) both stressed the denial of oedipal sexuality in unstructured group processes.

The projection of superego functions onto the group and its leader and the related submission to authoritarian leadership does protect against both violence and the destruction of couples within the group. It is condensed, however, with the prohibition against incest and the most infantile aspects of sexuality. Thus, group morality veers toward a conventionalized desexualization of heterosexual relations, toward the suppression of erotic fantasy insofar as it involves infantile polymorphous trends, and toward acknowledging and sanctioning only the more permissible love relations. In large groups, the alternative to these defensive efforts—and to their miscarriage in repressive ideologies—is the eruption of a crude and particularly anally tinged sexuality which is very reminiscent of the sexualized group formations of latency and early adolescence.

APPLICATIONS TO GROUP PSYCHOTHERAPY

The following summary is significantly influenced by several overviews of the psychoanalytic group-psychotherapy literature (Foulkes and Anthony, 1957; de Mare, 1972; Whiteley and Gordon, 1979; Scheidlinger, 1980).

The Psychoanalytic Psychotherapy of Individuals in Groups

Slavson (1959; 1962; 1964) pioneered psychoanalytic group psycho-therapy in the 1930s. He attempted to stimulate individual patients in the group to free associate, and he interpreted resistances and trans-ferences directed toward both the group leader and the other members of the group. Slavson believed that the multiple expression of trans-ferences toward other group members would cause a dilution or a decrease of transference intensity and that this might facilitate working with it. In fact, since Slavson considered group processes to be poten-tially detrimental to the therapeutic use of groups, he came to place his emphasis on working with individuals within the group. Similarly, Wolf and Schwartz (1962) stressed the psychoanalytically based treatment of the individual in the group, but they gradually paid more attention to the group process itself, focusing on the interacting patterns of the group members.

Expanding upon the contributions of these pioneers, an entire school of psychoanalytic group psychotherapy developed in the United States. These developments were first based upon applying psychoanalytic theory and technique to individual psychotherapy and then on carrying out individual psychoanalytic psychotherapy in the setting of a group. Gradually, other theoretical and technical principles were incorporated from sociological analyses of small-group processes. In particular, sys-tems theory was applied to the interrelationships between the indi-vidual, the group, and the social environment. Finally, psychoanalytic theories of group processes proper were developed and incorporated. Bach (1954), Durkin (1964), and Scheidlinger (1982) offer outstanding examples which, in varying degrees, synthesize psychoanalytic con-cepts, systems theory, and Kurt Lewin's (1951) contributions to the social dynamics of small groups.

The Psychoanalytically Oriented Treatment of the Whole Group

Group therapists in Britain developed a theoretical and technical ap-proach that focused on the psychoanalytic meaning of group processes, rather than on the psychopathology of any individual patient within it. Their psychoanalytic frame of reference stemmed from the British psychoanalytic schools of Fairbairn and Melanie Klein and particularly from the works which Bion wrote in the 1940s and early 1950s (Bion, 1961). The most radical of the British theoretical and technical ap-proaches is reflected in Bion's own technique. Here, the group psycho-therapist interprets the dominant basic assumptions of dependency, fight-flight, and pairing as shared aspirations, fantasies, and behaviors of the entire group. The defensive functions of these basic assumptions are interpreted as protections against the experienced danger that "psychotic anxieties" could erupt, anxieties which are related to primi-tive levels of aggression and to the corresponding threats to the self and internalized objects.

Bion assumed that each patient has a particular "valency" toward the conflicts and fantasies of these basic-assumptions groups and that the dominant group mentality at any time is a consequence of the moment-to-moment summation of the individuals' valencies. Implicitly, the indi-vidual patient's psychopathology would be explored at points when his or her valencies are dominant in the atmosphere of the entire group.

Working through is therefore carried out in terms of the repetitive activation of alternating basic-assumptions phenomena, rather than in terms of the intrapsychic structures of individual patients.

Ezriel (1950) and Sutherland (1952) modified Bion's approach to small groups by focusing more on the individual patient's particular reactions to the predominant group tension. Accordingly, they expanded on the interpretation of the dominant group mentality to include the individual patient's specific ways of expressing or reacting to the group mentality. Ezriel's concept of the "common group tension" corresponds roughly to Bion's dominant group mentality. This common group tension expresses the moment-to-moment summation of each individual's predisposition to participate in a certain group theme. In Ezriel's view, this theme can be interpreted as a dominant "required relationship," which is established as a defense against another "avoided relationship." The avoided relationship, in turn, is feared because of the fantasied disastrous consequences of yet another relationship, a "calamitous relationship."

In common, the approaches of Bion, Ezriel, and Sutherland call for the therapist to maintain a basic distance. The therapist interprets all communications, even those directed by individual patients to him or her, in terms of common group features. The group therapist's role is exclusively interpretive, and the interpretations are focused on the meaning of the group situation as a whole and on transferences. Moreover, whether these transferences are individual or group transferences, they are interpreted only in terms of the here and now, not in terms of an individual patient's past or any genetic reconstructions. The free-floating verbal communications within the group are used as primary data, similar but not equivalent to the free associations of an individual patient. The effect of this particular technique, maximally in the case of Bion, and significantly less so with Ezriel and Sutherland, is to reduce the ordinary role relationships between patients and therapist. And this prevents the ordinary group structuring that develops through socially acceptable and reassuring roles and interactions.

This technique has both advantages and dangers. Among the advantages are the sharp highlighting of primitive modes of mental operations and the possibility of examining the unconscious processes that influence group behavior. On the negative side, a number of questions have been raised (Scheidlinger, 1960; Malan et al., 1976). The concerns pertain to the artificial distance of the group leader, the elimination of the ordinary supportive features of group interactions, and the fact that cognitive instruments for self-understanding are not offered to individual patients regarding their particular psychopathology. These features of the technique may be too demanding on the individual patient and thus be therapeutically counterproductive.

The Psychoanalytic Psychotherapy of Individuals through the Analysis of Group Processes

Foulkes and Anthony (1957) developed a technique of group psychotherapy based upon the promotion of a group culture characterized by free-floating discussions. They considered these discussions to be analogous to free association, offering the raw material used for the interpretive work. Within the group culture, a network of interpersonal communication or "group matrix" develops.

Foulkes's approach is less centered on the group leader than that of Bion, Ezriel, and Sutherland, but his approach does use an understanding of group processes derived from their work. Technically, though, his use and stimulation of individual patients' observing ego functions and the growth-promoting and supportive potential of the group process more closely resembles the ego-psychological approach characteristic of American psychoanalytic group psychotherapy. Other features of Foulkes's techniques are closer to the Bion, Ezriel, and Sutherland models: he focuses on the transferences in the here and now only, and on group process at large.

Summary

Thus, when the psychoanalytic theory of group processes is applied to group psychotherapy, it seems that the more the technique focuses on the analysis of group processes per se, the more it approaches a purely Bionian model. Consequently, primitive group phenomena and transferences may emerge more dramatically, giving rise to the possibility of concrete learning about deep anxieties and fantasies that are close to what dominates in the psychopathology of borderline conditions.* Clearly, all of this has enormous heuristic value for the study of regressive processes in groups. The risks, however, are relative neglect of the individual nature of each patient's psychopathology and a minimizing of ego-supportive group processes. Furthermore, the individual patient's responsibility for his or her own participation in the psychotherapeutic process may not receive sufficient attention. To highlight primitive transferences is not to guarantee that they will be resolved.

On the other hand, bypassing the analysis of group processes and focusing on individualized psychoanalytic exploration within the group also has its advantages and disadvantages. Among the apparent advantages, the individually oriented application may maximize the supportive aspect of group functioning and minimize the activation of the phenomena of basic-assumptions groups. This application may also highlight dominant pathological character traits in the context of activating triadic, "high-level" transferences. Finally, it may have the advantage of facilitating what may in practice resemble most closely a supportive-expressive psychotherapy, making full use of group socialization for reeducative purposes. The risks of the individually oriented application include intellectualizing the understandings of intrapsychic dynamics, underutilizing the psychoanalytic understanding of deeper aspects of unconscious intrapsychic conflicts, and having a supportive-reeducative effect on character pathology without facilitating its deep resolution.

HOSPITAL-TREATMENT AND THERAPEUTIC-COMMUNITY MODELS

Main (1957) studied the group reactions of nursing staff who were treating predominantly borderline and some psychotic patients ("special" cases) in the hospital and found that these patients managed to activate in the nurses phenomena similar to those Bion observed in the

*Editor's note: Part V of *Psychiatry 1982* (*Psychiatry Update: Volume I*) discusses in detail the psychopathology, diagnosis, and treatment of borderline and narcissistic conditions. Dr. Kernberg served as the Preceptor for that Part.

basic-assumptions groups. He suggested that regressed patients, and borderline patients in particular, may under certain conditions activate their own intrapsychic object relations in the interpersonal relations of the hospital staff. In effect, these patients induce in their social fields a reenactment of the conflicts within their intrapsychic worlds. The massive projection, omnipotent control, denial, primitive idealization, and, above all, the splitting observed in staff reflect both their own intrapsychic mechanisms and the behavioral means by which the patients' intrapsychic worlds distort the staff relationships. Stanton and Schwartz (1954) demonstrated the corollary—how splits and covert conflicts in the interpersonal and social fields of the hospital may intensify the intrapsychic conflict and disorganization of "special patients" (borderline and in some cases psychotic patients). The pathology that the patient induces in the social field naturally utilizes preexisting cleavages in that field, cleavages that reflect conflicts in the administrative structure of the social organization. Intrapsychic conflict and social conflict thus reinforce each other.

If channels of communication within the staff group and between the staff and patient are kept sufficiently open, interpersonal conflicts generated around each patient can be explored, and immediate knowledge may be gained about the individual patient's psychopathology. The hospital therapist can explore psychoanalytically the patient's evolving deployment of primitive object relations in the hospital's social field by systematically examining with the patient his or her interpersonal experiences in the hospital.

To strengthen the diagnosis and therapeutic utilization of the patient's interactions within the immediate social field, the techniques of therapeutic-community approaches may be useful. Although various authors describe the essential aspects of this approach in somewhat different ways, the basic orientation stems from Jones (1953) and Main (1946) and emphasizes the following features. A community-treatment feature requires that staff and patients function jointly as an organized community to carry out the treatment of the patient population. A second feature is the concept of therapeutic culture, which requires that all activities and interactions relate to the goal of reeducation and socially rehabilitating the patients. Finally, the living-learning-confrontation feature opens the flow of communication between patients and staff and provides immediate feedback regarding observed behaviors and reactions.

Three particular types of meetings facilitate the therapeutic community and are common to all models. This typology of meetings is different from the small, large, and task-group types of meetings, but principles from the latter typology may apply as well. The community meeting includes all patients and the entire staff. With a free flow of communication, this meeting aims to examine the total staff and patient social environment, the distortions and interferences from whatever source, and the development of antidemocratic or authoritarian processes and their possible resolution. Patient-government meetings are a second common type. Regardless of the specific form that patient government takes, therapeutic-community models tend to foster patients' organization in order that the patients can participate in the social and decision-making processes. The third type of meeting is the staff meeting. Complementing patient government, this meeting expresses the concept of democratic decision making among staff. It allows staff members to study how they are influenced by administrative and other pressures, as well as by their interactions with the patients.

The most important precondition for the development of a therapeutic community is that it be functionally integrated with the administrative structure of the psychiatric or general hospital within which it operates. If the therapeutic community is to explore openly the social system actualized by the patient-staff community, it will of necessity also activate all the stress and latent conflicts in the system. Obviously, then, it will influence the political dimensions of the institutional decision-making process.

Therapeutic communities can powerfully reinforce the therapeutic utilization of the hospital's social milieu. They can also become a real or experienced threat to the patient's treatment. Patient meetings, staff meetings, and particularly the community meeting itself easily acquire the characteristics of large-group processes. The regressive effects of large-group processes can in turn affect the individual patient's development in the community in antitherapeutic ways.

The author has previously pointed to the dangers when patients as a group regress to the functioning of a basic-assumptions group (Kernberg, 1976, chapter 9; 1980, chapter 11). Under such regressive circumstances, patient groups may become intolerant of individuals, establish a group dictatorship that acquires the characteristics of a primitive morality, and foster the ascendance to leadership positions of personalities with narcissistic and antisocial features. Staff may contribute to this regression with their ideologically determined denial of differences between individual patients, with their implicit expectation that all patients have the same needs, and with their consequent expectation that all patients will react or participate in similar ways. The most regressed patients, including chronic monopolizers, highly effective manipulators, or simply the most violent ones, gain control of unstructured group processes and significantly distort first the content of meetings and later the total allocation of resources, thus reducing many patients' treatment time. Elsewhere (Kernberg, 1981; 1982) the author has proposed a model that attempts to maximize the advantages and to control the potential liabilities of the therapeutic community.

APPLICATIONS TO GROUP AND ORGANIZATIONAL DYNAMICS

Underlying this discussion of the broader area of applications to group and organizational dynamics are the contributions of Jaques (1955; 1976; 1982), Menzies (1967), Rioch (1970a; 1970b), and very fundamentally, Rice (1963; 1965; 1969; Miller and Rice, 1967). Parenthetically, Bion (1970) has also explored the area of relationships among individuals, groups, and institutions, but his work will not be a focus of this discussion. Some other recent contributions to this expanding field can be found in the works of Colman and Bexton (1975), Kreeger (1975), Miller (1976), and Lawrence (1979) and in the overview by De Board (1978).

Rice's work employs a systems theory of organizations, in which the individual, the group, and the social organization are seen as a continuum of open systems. Along with the open-systems theory of organizations, Rice (1965) integrates with his own theory Bion's theories of small-group functioning and Turquet's understanding of large-group functioning. His perspective represents the core set of concepts that circumscribe organizational applications of psychoanalytic thinking. From Rice's theoretical perspective, all open systems carry out their tasks in exchange with the environment. A task that the system must carry out in order to survive is called a primary task. Each system must include a control function which will permit analyzing the environment, the internal reality of the system, and the executive organization of task performance within this reality. Because open systems must by definition carry out exchanges with their environments in order to survive, this control function must be at the boundary between the system and its environment. Breakdown of system boundaries implies a breakdown of the open system's control, and this in turn brings about a breakdown in carrying out the primary task and threatens the survival of the system. In the field of clinical psychiatry, this open-systems theory may be applied to individual patients, to groups, and to the hospital as a social system.*

In the psychic life of an individual, the ego may be conceived as the control function, ego boundaries as the system boundaries defined and protected by the ego functions, and the person's intrapsychic world of object relations as the inner space or inner world of the system. The individual's primary task is to satisfy the instinctual and object-oriented needs of his or her internal world by means of interactions with the social environment. In the course of this task, the individual adapts to and creatively modifies his or her interpersonal world in terms of intrapsychic needs and in turn elaborates intrapsychic needs in terms of external realities.

In the life of the group, the group leader may be seen as the control function, and the primary task of the group is whatever determined its existence in the first place. The activation of primitive object relations within the group structure (Bion's "basic-assumptions group") represents the group's internal world of object relations (Rice, 1969). The equilibrium between the group focusing on the task (task group) and the group focusing on the activation of primitive object relations in its social field (basic-assumptions group) depends on several factors. The extent to which the task is clear and defined, the adequacy of task leadership, and the examination of the basic assumptions within the task or considered as task constraints will all influence the group's equilibrium.

In a social organization, such as an industry, an educational establishment, or a hospital, the administration represents the leadership or the manager of system control functions. The purposes for which the organization has been established represent the primary tasks of the system. For example, the primary tasks of a psychiatric teaching hospital are patient care, education, and research. The organization must create and protect within it an optimal social atmosphere so it can carry out its primary tasks. This requirement reflects a basic constraint of organizational functioning, namely, that human needs must be gratified in the course of carrying out the specific tasks of the organization. A further constraint of organizational systems is that they must organize task systems so that intragroup and intergroup processes will facilitate rather than interfere with task performance. Group processes reflect the inner space or inner world of the organization as an open system.

*Editor's note: In Part III of this volume, Family Psychiatry, Bloch discusses the application of systems theory to families and the treatment of individual patients within a family context.

Effective organizational management requires that the administrators define adequately the primary organizational task or tasks and constraints and that they establish priorities and constraints on a functional basis. Management needs adequate control over organization boundaries, and this implies stable, fully delegated authority regarding all organizational functions from the managing board to the director or managing team.

Within this model, psychopathology may be conceptualized as breakdown of the control function, a failure to carry out the primary task, and a threat to the survival of the system. In the case of the individual, we see breakdown of the ego and emotional regression; in the group, breakdown of group leadership and paralysis in basic assumptions; in the institution, breakdown of the administration, failure to carry out the institutional tasks, and loss of morale. Breakdown of boundary control is the principal manifestation of breakdown in the control function.

Group-Relations Conferences

Rice's theories have served as the basis for the group-relations conferences sponsored by the Tavistock Clinic in Leicester, England, and their offshoots in the United States, the A. K. Rice Group Relations Conferences organized by the Washington School of Psychiatry. These conferences are time-limited organizational structures designed for learning group, organizational, administrative, and leadership functions. They usually last a few days to two weeks and are organized around specific events. Small-group meetings ("study groups") of 7 to 12 members are conducted with a strictly Bionian technique, and large-group meetings of 30 to 80 members apply this same technique with their corresponding leadership functions as described by Rice and Turquet. "Intergroup exercises" bring together the entire conference membership or students to organize ad hoc tasks, to interact with other groups, and to relate spontaneously with the management or staff as a group. In addition, theoretical conferences or lectures expand on the experiential learning, offering brief overviews of key concepts. Finally, "application groups" give individual members or students the opportunity to discuss problems of their home organizations and to apply their learning to problems at home.

The author has participated in these conferences as both member and staff. Several processes have emerged in these conferences with impressive regularity and intensity. First, intense anxieties and primitive fantasies are activated in the small study groups. Second, a primitiveness of group functioning and of potential individual aggression is activated in the large-group experiences, dramatically illustrating Bion's, Rice's, and Turquet's observations regarding large groups. Ad hoc myths about the conference or its leadership and the search for a comprehensive, simplistic ideology develop rapidly and contrast with discriminating reason, illustrating in one stroke what happens during a breakdown of organizational functioning. The crucial functions of boundaries in task performance and of task-oriented leadership become apparent as groups confront the dramatic temptation, at points of regression, to select the most dysfunctional members of subgroups to become leaders of basic-assumptions groups.

One important drawback to the temporary group-relations conferences is their relative neglect of the functions that time and personality issues have in stable social organizations. Katz and Kahn (1966) pointed out that the staffs of social and industrial organizations frequently fail to learn new attitudes in the context of exploring the irrational aspects of group processes in an experiential setting. This failure results from neglecting to analyze the stable features of organizational structures and the relationships between those structures and the real (in contrast to fantasied or irrational) conflicts of interests that such organizational structures mediate.

Short-term learning experiences in groups also may not allow for studying the impact of the organizational members' personality structures, particularly the personalities of key leaders. Distortions in the organization's administrative structure may be derived from the leader's personality structure and can be compensated for by structural rearrangements in the organization. These rearrangements may not seem functional in a short-term, cross-sectional analysis. In the long run, however, they may be a most functional compromise between an optimal organizational use of the leader's personality, on the one hand, and an effort to reduce or control the leader's distortion of administrative structures, on the other.

Recent Developments

Several specific areas are currently being explored within the general framework of psychoanalytic approaches to organization and leadership. Knowledge of the efforts on the part of large groups to develop organizing myths and ideologies stimulated Arlow (1979) to study the characteristic contents of ideology as a group process. Similarly, Kaes (1980) and Anzieu (1981) have applied Bion's, Rice's, and Turquet's techniques of exploring small and large groups in studies of ideology. Their original studies highlight the formation of group ideologies and ways of understanding ideologies in terms of the dominant unconscious themes that emerge in small and large groups.

Braunschweig and Fain (1971) have explored typical group-formation processes in terms of the relationships of male and female members from earliest childhood on through adulthood. Using socially prevalent myths regarding various age groups, they have illustrated a developmental sequence of culturally framed relationships between the sexes.

Levinson (1972) and Zaleznik (1979) have used psychoanalytic theory to analyze organizational conflicts. Levinson has focused on how transference phenomena influence the relationships between hierarchical superiors and subordinates as well as the peer relationships within organizations, and he has examined the nature of the drive gratifications and superego controls that are expressed in the context of work and organizational structures. Zaleznik has focused on the distribution of power and the function of organizational ideology in protecting the stability of the institution.

In the author's own earlier work (Kernberg, 1980), he attempted to analyze the relationships between particular personality types as organization leaders and the regressive processes within their organizations.

Roger Shapiro (1979) has applied the psychoanalytic theories of group processes to the study of family processes and family therapy. Robin Skynner (1976) in England has used a systems approach to relate the psychoanalytic understanding of group processes to the analysis of family dynamics and family therapy.

APPLICATIONS TO LEADERSHIP, CULTURE, AND SOCIETY

As mentioned earlier, Freud (1921) explained that the emotional climate of hordes or mobs, their sense of immediate closeness and their impulse-ridden behavior, was derived from the projection of their ego ideal onto the leader and their identification with the leader as well as with each other. Freud linked these concepts with his hypotheses regarding the historical origin of the primal horde (1913). He suggested that the totemic law that regulates the life of the horde and that protects it from both self-destructive rivalry and incestuous endogamy derives from the alliance of sons who have killed their father. Because of their unconscious guilt, the sons have replaced the father's living laws with the totemic law that nonetheless symbolizes the father's law. The leader who is idealized therefore both represents the oedipal hero who killed his father and symbolizes the alliance of all the sons. Ultimately, he also symbolizes the father and his law, which the horde obeys out of unconscious guilt over the patricide.

This concept, as Lasch (1981) pointed out, has provided a theoretical underpinning for generations of Marxists and other socialist philosophers from Wilhelm Reich (1935) to Althusser (1976). The patriarchal bourgeois family was seen as the locus of introjection for the repressive ideology of capitalism, linked with the sexual prohibitions of the oedipal father. Where Freud thought that the repression of sexuality was the price paid for cultural evolution, Reich thought that the repression of sexuality represented the effects of a pathological superego determined by the social structure of capitalism. Soviet Russia's sexual repressiveness, he proposed, reflected the development of a Soviet authoritarian power structure. Robinson (1969) pointed out that Marcuse (1955) agreed with Reich that the excessive repression of sexuality created the danger of a predominance of aggression in human affairs. Marcuse differed from Reich, however, in other respects. It was not genital sexuality, but pregenital polymorphous infantile sexuality, that the capitalist system repressed. As Marcuse saw it, the system aimed its repression at restricting sexual functions to the genital zone so it could use man's unsatisfied broader eroticism in the service of social production.

More recently, Foucault (1978) criticized the idea that the capitalist state and bourgeois society foster the repression of sexuality. To the contrary, he suggested, the bourgeois society has never had a keener interest in studying sexual phenomena and in transforming sexual phenomena from moral into scientific and medical issues. Foucault added, however, that this keen interest has been accompanied by an interest in controlling sexual behavior, thereby controlling the family structure, and in manipulating sexual behavior to suit the state's requirements.

A final application of Freud's formulations about the oedipal father is that of Althusser (1976). As Anderson (1976) points out, Althusser used Freud's concept of the unconscious to construct a new theory of ideology. Ideology, for Althusser, is a system of unconsciously determined illusory representations of reality. Specifically, the ideological system derives from the internalization of the dominant illusion that a social class harbors about the conditions of its own existence. This dominant illusion stems from the internalization of the paternal law, which in turn is part of the internalization of the superego.

The foregoing applications or extrapolations from the psychoanalytic theory of group processes all made use of Freud's concept of the leader as the symbolic oedipal father. But the theories offered by Bion, Rice, Turquet, Anzieu, and Chasseguet-Smirgel have focused rather on the infiltration of preoedipal conflicts in regressive group formation and a more primitive nature of leadership as well. In contrast to their predecessors, these theorists focused specifically on the psychology of regression in groups. That regression, as they saw it, reflected the fantasies of merger that are linked to the preoedipal conflicts of the separation-individuation stage or even of the symbiotic merger of earliest infancy.

Mitscherlich (1963) pointed to the cultural consequences of the absence of the father at the social and familial level. He described the rejection of the father in contemporary society as part of the rejection of traditional cultural values, and he pointed to the intoxicating effects of mass production. Mass production promises immediate gratification and consequently fosters a psychology of demand for immediate gratification, and it contributes to the lack of a sense of individual responsibility. Mitscherlich described the new "mass person" as classless, stressed the real absence of the father in the contemporary family due to the industrial revolution, and pointed out that individualized functions of the father were lost in the large contemporary institution.

Writing under the pseudonym André Stéphane, Chasseguet- Smirgel and Grunberger in L'Univers Contestationnaire (1969) analyzed the social psychology of both French fascism and the "new left" in light of the 1968 student rebellion. They described several characteristics that the left and right movements have in common. Both left and right reject traditional society's values of the nuclear family and of individual responsibility for one's action. Chasseguet-Smirgel and Grunberger interpret this as a symbolic rejection of both paternal and maternal principles and as a search for gratification in a primary, diffuse, maternal group. The group, left or right, symbolizes a preoedipal mother who provides love and diffuses sexual gratifications without demands for either individual differentiation or commitment within couples. The destruction both of authority and of highly individualized and exclusive forms of sexuality reflects not only a rejection of the oedipal couple, but also reflects a denial of the oedipal stage of development and a regression to an early form of narcissism.

Several years ago, Lasch described the correspondence between characteristics of the narcissistic personality and characteristics of current society. The author suggests that large-group processes can help explain these correspondences. Lasch suggested (1977; 1978) that the family no longer serves as a source of moral guidance. Instead of demanding that children accept responsibility for their behavior, parents try to avoid conflict by compromising and offering instinctual gratification, and this attitude serves to corrode the development of a mature superego in the child. When the child's superego development is faulty, the child depends internally on sadistic and primitive superego forerunners and overindulges in impulse gratification. This dynamic entails not only the lack of superego restrictions, but also the lack of internal superego approval, and it leads to a secondary overdependence on external sources for the gratification of self-esteem. The corrosion of authority within the family is amplified by the general societal shift from a traditional mode of social leadership that derived from ethical principles and intellectual consistency to a mode of leadership that has abandoned its moral justification and basis of control. Now dangerously frail, the new mode of control is based primarily on power, and controlling techniques take the form of manipulation and pseudohumanization of the interpersonal and working conditions within the social organizations.

More recently, Lasch (1981) has expanded his ideas with some of Chasseguet-Smirgel's theory of group processes. He particularly draws from her image of the preoedipal mother to symbolize large-group psychology. The all-embracing and inexhaustible breast-mother gratifies the voracious, greedy, and totally self-centered infant, symbolizing the basic psychological characteristics of crowds. With Lasch, the author finds that Chasseguet-Smirgel and Grunberger are convincing in their explanation of regressive phenomena in crowds (phenomena which Ortega y Gasset described so beautifully in 1929). This symbolic preoedipal mother image is very different from that of the reasonable, differentiated oedipal mother who is separate from the child and in a private union with the oedipal father. That is a condition which regressive groups cannot tolerate.

A curious circumstance emerges here. Under conditions of large-group functioning, the dominant sexual ideology tends, on the one hand, to be marked by an excessive projection of superego function onto the authoritarian leadership of the group, thus inducing a conventional ideology that is sexually repressive. On the other hand, it can be marked by "preoedipal" ideology which is expressed in the condensation of a random aggressive propensity with preoedipal forms of sexuality, manifesting trends toward polymorphous perverse infantile sexuality. Either extreme, however, produces a similar outcome, a conventional morality that is directed against the private sexual fulfillment of the autonomous couple.

Chapter 3

The Influence of Values in Psychoanalysis: The Case of Female Psychology
by Ethel S. Person, M.D.

INTRODUCTION

At the heart of the psychoanalytic enterprise is the purpose of examining the ways in which thoughts and behaviors, beliefs, preferences, and values are influenced by unconscious mental processes. Psychoanalysis is a discipline that fosters skepticism about the apparent and self-evident meaning of surface phenomena, thereby challenging the certainty of either revealed or objective truth, the first (religion) explicitly and the second (science) implicitly. Like philosophy, psychoanalysis alerts us to the fact that we must look for the values and ideology underlying any body of knowledge, including psychoanalysis itself.

No cultural enterprise is value free, including science. Science values objective knowledge. Objectivity is fundamental to the pursuit of science, as is evident in the historical fact that science is an achievement of Western culture, not an autonomous development in every culture. Yet as Kuhn (1962) has pointed out, scientific research is based on beliefs about the nature of the world. While these beliefs appear to be objective and truthful, they may be superceded when new findings or anomalies arise to contradict the existing set of beliefs, assumptions, or traditions. Thus, despite its objectivity, science is both the product of cultural values and a contributor to the cultural evolution of values. According to Hogan and Emler, "Science supports the myth of developmental progress. Innovation, experiment, the rebuilding of theory, all these are justified because they will make things better . . . the extraordinary success of science in the modern era has contributed to the influential position of individualism and rationalism" (Hogan and Emler, 1978, 486).

A similarly complex relationship exists between cultural values and psychoanalysis. Psychoanalysis, beginning with Freud's assumptions, embodies values central to Western culture. Chief among these are an interest in the individual and his or her welfare and a commitment to self-knowledge as an end unto itself. Rieff claimed that "Freud created the masterwork of the century, a psychology that . . . unriddled—to use Emerson's prophetic catalogue of subjects considered inexplicable in his day—'language, sleep, madness, dreams, beasts, sex'" (Rieff, 1961, xx). In insisting that nothing human was alien to him, Freud revealed a commitment to the worth of the individual, no matter how marginal or mad. Freud's work is thus an integral part of an intellectual tradition that elevates individualism to an ideology.

In turn, psychoanalysis has given a distinctive shape to intellectual life in the twentieth century. According to Rieff, "Freud's doctrine, created piecemeal and fortunately never integrated into one systematic statement, has changed the course of Western intellectual history; moreover, it has contributed as much as doctrine possibly can to the correction of our standards of conduct" (Rieff, 1961, xx). Indeed, some psychiatrists and critics of culture have raised the objection that individuals living in an era of declining objective moral authority attempt to substitute the goals of mental health and normalcy for a comprehensive moral system (Rieff, 1966; Morgenthau and Person, 1978; Gross, 1978). Psychoanalysis and values, then, like science and values, ply a two-way street.

This discussion is meant to emphasize the fact that no *cultural* enterprise can be value free. A cultural enterprise must, by definition, be value laden and embody a set of beliefs. Values are not always easily separated from prejudice and bias. Values may be generally defined as highly abstracted ideas about what is good or bad, right or wrong, desirable or undesirable. Prejudice and bias carry a particularly pejorative connotation. To be prejudiced or biased means to judge without adequate knowledge or examination and to come to a premature conclusion, usually unfavorable. Therefore, it is important to distinguish values that are implicit in the context and framework of any cultural enterprise from values and prejudices that contaminate either the application or the theoretical assumptions of an enterprise.

In psychoanalysis, as in the other behavioral sciences, observations and hypotheses are inevitably distorted by historical bias and sometimes, more pervasively, by values buried in major theoretical assumptions. As Macklin (1973) has pointed out, values are implicit in psychoanalysis in at least three ways. Values are held by the patient.

Values are held by the therapist. And values are implicit or explicit in the theory. As long as those values coincide, they go virtually unnoticed. Cultural biases become most apparent during times of social change, times when they no longer coincide.

Freud sincerely but mistakenly believed that analysts were ethically neutral and that the observations of analysis were value free. Freud himself, however, offers an example of the influence of bias in his own beliefs about the nature of femininity.

Under the impact of changing cultural norms, we have become aware of the presence of sexism in all of the psychotherapies, including psychoanalysis, and of the theoretical justifications for sexism in fundamental psychoanalytic assumptions. Changing prescriptions and changing concepts of the female role(s), as well as the persistence of outdated theories, have led us to scrutinize value biases implicit in practice and theory.

This chapter describes changes in the definition of normative femininity and in psychoanalytic formulations of female psychology. Reformulations of female development seem to have lagged unduly, given the considerable countervailing data and the serious critiques of early formulations. As the chapter demonstrates, the reasons for this lag illustrate the methodological problems and value biases in psychoanalytic theory making that transcend the special case. The chapter employs a dual concept of values, examining some of the perversions of values (biases, prejudices) that have developed and also exploring the beliefs and commitments (general values) that underlie psychoanalytic formulations. By focusing on one example, the author intends to demonstrate how new data, both from psychoanalysis and from other fields, have forced a reexamination of its methodology and of the values embedded in its major theoretical assumptions.

SEXISM AND CHANGING GOALS IN THERAPY

Many feminist scholars and mental health professionals have used the theme of sexism in psychotherapy to illustrate value bias underlying therapeutic decisions, practices, and theoretical formulations. The concept of "normalcy" or appropriate femininity necessarily colors the assessment of both pathology and treatment goals. According to Broverman et al. (1970), mental health professionals, rather than challenging gender stereotypes, shared popular biases. Dependency and passivity were seen as normal female qualities and assertiveness and independence as normal male qualities. Accordingly, mental health professionals attributed role dissatisfaction in women to psychopathology. The debate about normal female development and femininity relates to the more general debate in psychiatry about the distinction between difference (or deviation) and mental illness. Arguments about "what women want" and whether these goals reflect health or neurosis are analogous in form to arguments about homosexuality or political dissidence.

Because psychoanalytic theory proposes mental health norms, it also implies therapeutic goals. This is true regardless of what one proposes should be the primary mental health objective—genital maturity, motherhood as the ultimate resolution of penis envy, the cult of true feminity, mature object relations, or generativity. For clinicians, knowledge of this existential dilemma, what has been called the dual descriptive-normative role of theory (Macklin, 1973), translates into vexing clinical problems. Clinicians no longer have the certainty of fixed, external definitions of abnormality and mental health, previously conceptualized as mature genitality or as the achievement of gender-appropriate behavior. And the therapeutic community stands charged "with fostering traditional gender roles, stereotyping of women, biased expectations and devaluation of women, sexist use of theoretical constructs, and responding to women as sex objects, including seduction" (Vaughter, 1976, 140).

What Women Want: Changing Treatment Goals

Analysts disagree strongly about whether the nature of psychological illness has changed or whether a new language has simply developed for describing old problems. Some classes of clinical problems do seem virtually unchanged, such as the biologically derived mental illnesses. But a decisive shift has occurred in the problems of living that patients predominantly complain about and in the goals they seek.

Attitudinal changes towards sex, gender, and pair-bonding implicit in the sexual revolution, the women's movement, and the crisis of the family have complex and contradictory implications for opportunity and security in women's lives. With the changing definitions of femininity, women have assumed greater latitude in their lives, and the modern woman does not entirely resemble her more traditional counterpart. Many goals have changed radically, while some remain the same. In any case, we can no longer be dogmatic about what are the appropriate choices in women's life trajectories. A greater range of plausible and acceptable adaptations exists, stemming from the dramatic changes that have taken place in the cultural milieu. Whatever the major presenting symptom, newer treatment goals, insofar as they are articulated, are cast in terms of enabling a woman's individual enhancement in the professional, sexual, or relational sphere. The emerging pattern is one of activity and achievement, not one of passive acceptance, and while underlying conflicts may be the same, different adaptive resolutions are sought.

Increasingly, women are seeking treatment as an explicit aid to their search for autonomy and self-realization, and they believe that the vehicle for this is their professional or creative achievement. This stands in marked contrast to goals commonly stated twenty years ago. At that time, such ambitions were often believed to represent masculine aspirations and hence to be misguided. Penis envy and its attendant anxieties were considered to lie at the heart of a woman's work problems. Today, the goal is to work through any inhibition of assertion or achievement motivation.

Women today are also seeking greater sexual fulfillment. They are looking for new modes of interpersonal relationships, different from the more traditional role in which submissiveness and ingratiation were deemed so integral to their "femininity." Today, women place increasing value on egalitarian relations, and this new bias extends to the therapy situation. Many more women seek female therapists in order to avoid a stereotypical relationship in which a young and helpless female patient is dependent on an older and authoritative male.

Some goals, of course, are not at all new. Women are still motivated toward stable affiliative relations, as are men. Many seek treatment because they are unable to form permanent relationships, while others seek it to help them through the breakup of a marriage, a deteriorating relationship, or the stresses that accrue from the breakdown of the family.

Shifting goals highlight the intrinsic problem in the dual descriptive and normative roles of theory. The serious potential for therapeutic bias in goal setting is sometimes underestimated. Take, for example, Barglow and Schaefer's (1976) response to a question raised by Marmor (1973). Marmor had posed a hypothetical question about treating Ibsen's Nora. Should an analyst interpret her penis envy and rejection of a normal female role, or should he foster her healthy rebellion? Barglow and Schaefer disavow the dilemma. They ask, "Are these really psycho-analytic problems? Psychoanalysis, after all, is not an ideology (the critics to the contrary), but professes to be a science" (Barglow and Schaefer, 1976, 322). In the author's opinion, Marmor was right, and Barglow and Schaefer have missed the point: an analyst's response (countertransference) must be permeated by his or her world view. Preferences and beliefs influence the therapist's judgment and may thereby slant interpretations or therapeutic emphasis.

Therapists communicate their values not primarily with directives, but with silences, questions, and the very rhythms and cadences of the therapeutic hour. Sometimes, though, their directives are explicit. The author has seen this in consultation and treatment with any number of women, particularly those now in their fifties and sixties. Many of these women were directly advised by analysts and psychiatrists that their feminine obligation, destiny, or duty lay in preserving the marriage, in not threatening their husbands, in modulating their own sexuality, and so forth. Parenthetically, this age group of former patients bears the most hostility to psychiatry. While such inappropriate direct interventions are manifestations of countertransference reactions, the underlying theory has enabled clinicians to remain blind to them. In other words, although such countertransference reactions were individually derived and not theoretically mandated, they were culturally and theoretically reinforced. Furthermore, psychoanalysts may have tended to be more prescriptive with women than with men because of their shared counter-transference response toward women. For example, Chodorow (1978) has pointed out the prescriptive quality in Freud's discussion of female psychology: the little girl "must," "has to," and so on. Finally, at a time when dependency was more consonant with the female role, women may have sought such interventions transferentially with more insistence than male patients.

AN OVERVIEW OF CHANGING THEORIES

Freud essentially used only a single concept, that of penis envy, to explain the development of sexuality, normal gender development, and neurotic conflict in women. By ascribing femininity solely to the outcome of thwarted masculinity, his theory doomed women to infantilism and immaturity relative to men. Contemporary psychoanalysis, in contrast, takes a systems approach. Most important, theories of normal sexual development, of the acquisition of femininity (gender), and of the predominant neurotic conflicts have now been revised.

The following sections discuss the changing theories of sexuality, gender identity, and penis envy in some detail, since dramatic theoretical revisions have taken place in these areas. A review of changes in these formulations highlights the faulty methodology and the underlying ideology that for so long locked the old ideas into place. Many other aspects of female psychology must be omitted here because of limitations in the length of the discussion. Despite the importance of changes in conceptions about conscience and morality (Schafer, 1974; Gilligan, 1982) and about early object relations (Chodorow, 1978), for instance, the review cannot extend to these areas.

Changing Theories of Sexuality

It was a tenet of Freudian theory that female sexuality must necessarily be somewhat debilitated or hyposexual, given the need to switch both object and organ. According to Freud, penis envy was decisive in sexual development, as well as in neurotic conflict and the development of femininity. Penis envy was responsible for the girl's turn away from her mother (renouncing the clitoris) and toward her father (to get a penis from him). Such a double switch was believed to result necessarily in a diminished libido. This theory appeared to be substantiated by the inability of many women patients to achieve orgasm. Clara Thompson (1950) was among the first to readdress the apparent problem of female sexuality. She believed that the major sexual dilemma for women was not penis envy, but acknowledging their own sexuality in this culture. Her insight proved prophetic.

It is in the area of sexuality that the most radical changes have occurred, both in women's expectations and in psychoanalytic theory. The continuing role of clitoral eroticism in adult women, as demonstrated by Masters and Johnson (1966) and others, has led to a repudiation of Freud's theory of a clitoral-vaginal transfer, hypothetically triggered by the young girl's sense of clitoral inferiority. No one today holds that true femininity depends on achieving vaginal orgasms. Female sexuality is no longer viewed as intrinsically debilitated: it is now viewed as actively robust.

Along with rhetoric, actual sexual practices have also changed. Female sexuality has been liberated in two ways. First, it has been freed from ignorance. The recognition that maximum sexual pleasure in orgasm depends on adequate clitoral stimulation and that it is not an automatic outcome of heterosexual coitus was a crucial insight. Coupled with significant changes in sexual behavior, this knowledge has permitted more women to find sexual fulfillment than ever before, a major benefit of the scientific studies of sex.

Second, sexuality has been freed from an exclusive focus on male preferences and from the traditional idea of female submissiveness in relationships. Female sexual inhibition was often based on deference to the male and fear of him. It included a repertoire of behaviors such as faking orgasm, not insisting on adequate stimulation, assuming that male orgasm terminated the sexual encounter, and paying excessive attention to pleasing rather than receiving pleasure. In many women, these sexual inhibitions begin to resolve themselves when women achieve greater assertiveness and a sense of autonomy. This would not be possible, however, without a significant redefinition of the female-male bond. In fact, many so-called frigid women have no substantive problems with achievement of either arousal or orgasm. They suffer instead from ignorance about what constitutes appropriate stimulation or from interpersonal intimidation.

Somewhat surprisingly, many psychiatrists persist in minimizing the effect of the sexual revolution on women. Frequently, they argue that we only see changes in behavior and that unconscious wishes and conflicts remain unchanged. Such an argument utterly neglects the psychological function of orgasm per se, the power of orgasm to reaffirm the "incontrovertible truth" of the reality of personal existence (Lichtenstein, 1961; see also Eissler, 1958; and Person, 1980). The liberated sexual behavior among women thus may open new potentialities which, while sexual in nature, transcend the sexual. Sexual achievement has almost unequivocally benefited women, not only proffering sexual gratification, but often serving as a cornerstone for increased self-esteem.

It would, however, be erroneous to dismiss the suppression or expression of female sexuality as merely cultural in its origin. The critical developmental and psychoanalytic question is why the female erotic impulse is vulnerable to suppression across so many different historical and cultural circumstances (Person, 1980). For example, the inhibited sexuality of many Victorian women has had a permanent validity that poses a theoretical problem to be addressed.

Changing Theories of Gender Identity

Gender identity has also been systematically reevaluated. There is a growing psychoanalytic consensus that classical formulations fail to theorize acquisition of core gender identity ("I am female/male") and gender identity (femininity/masculinity) in accordance with the facts of development. Anatomical differences, while important, are no longer seen as determining per se. According to Howell, "It is the study of gender identity that has offered the most important correction to Freud's theory of feminine development" (Howell, 1981, 16).

Freud (1925; 1931; 1933) believed that prephallic development was essentially congruent for both sexes. Development diverged only with the child's discovery of the anatomical distinction that boys have penises while girls do not. Freud derived his theory of masculinity and femininity, what we now call gender role identity, from the contrast between the behavior of the two sexes after that discovery. In Freud's psychology, penis envy or the masculinity complex was at the center of the female psyche, whereas castration anxiety was central in the male. Freud thus postulated that femininity grew out of thwarted masculinity. He suggested that on discovering the sexual distinction, the little girl was overcome by clitoral inferiority and penis envy and hence developed the compensatory characteristics of passivity, masochism, narcissism, and dependency. These characteristics represented her adaptation to a profound narcissistic wound. Since Freud believed that the problems he saw clinically in women could be traced to the penis envy, he also believed that their treatment was inherently limited: the cause of their problems, genital inferiority, was essentially incurable.

Such a theory is intrinsically odd, because it should be apparent to even a casual observer that girls and boys begin to diverge in behavior, mannerisms, and interests by 12 to 18 months of age. Freud's formulation underscores the danger of deriving developmental theories from adult analyses without validation from child observations. Horney (1924; 1926; 1932; 1933) and Jones (1927; 1933) strongly challenged Freud's theories, noting that the masculine-feminine divergence occurred early in childhood, before the discovery of the anatomic distinction. In contrast to Freud, they proposed that femininity was primary, not derivative, that it antedated the phallic phase and was innate. Horney attributed heterosexual object choice to innate femininity, itself grounded in female biology and awareness of the vagina, not in disappointment over lacking a penis. Jones supported Horney's contention. As he put it, "The ultimate question is whether a woman is born or made" (Jones, 1935, 273). Thus, in the opinions of both Jones and Horney, heterosexual desire was innate. The girl desired the penis libidinally, not narcissistically.

Contemporary theorists confirm Horney's and Jones's observations but have held their explanations to be narrowly derived. Their formulations, like Freud's, gave too much exclusive priority to perceptions of genitals and of genital sensations. Blind children, boys with congenital absence of the penis (Stoller, 1968), and girls with congenital absence of the vagina (Stoller, 1968) have all been observed to differentiate along gender lines corresponding to their biological sex. Furthermore, current research reveals that sexual object choice is acquired, not innate. These observations prove that gender differentiation cannot be primarily derivative from body awareness, from perception of the sexual distinction, or from innate heterosexuality.

Money and his colleagues (1955a; 1955b; 1956) demonstrated that the first and crucial step in gender differentiation is the child's self-designation as male or female. This self-designation evolves according to the sex of assignment and has unconscious as well as conscious components. Core gender arises out of the very early self-identification as male or female, later symbolized in terms of the external genitals, and is therefore for the most part cognitively and socially constructed. Core gender derives from nonconflictual learning experience, not from conflict. The distinction between gender and biological sex is central to current formulations. Most theorists now believe that the developmental lines of gender precede those of sexuality, a complete reversal of Freud's original formulation.*

This change in theoretical formulation has manifold implications for therapy, and many of these have been achieved without being made explicit. The concept of normative femininity is freed from the stereotypes of passivity, masochism, dependency, and narcissism. The content of femininity is now regarded as being multidetermined, with significant input from cultural prescriptions. Femininity and masculinity are seen as parallel constructs, removing any theoretical reason to posit inherent restrictions on women's creativity and autonomy. Consequently, modern theory does not view female prospects as being intrinsically dim.

However, as in the case of sexuality, a critical developmental and psychoanalytic question remains, one that cannot be reduced to a simple cultural perspective. The question remains regarding the universal polarity of gender role(s) that exists despite the plasticity of the content of those roles. One requires a theory that integrates object relations, the symbolic investment of the genitals, and sexual differences, along with the cultural perspective.

Differences in gender role are now attributed to diverse antecedents that include biological differences, learning, power relations, scripting,

*Editor's note: In Part I of *Psychiatry 1982* (*Psychiatry Update: Volume I*), Dr. Jon K. Meyer uses this current formulation of gender and sexual identity in his chapter on gender disturbance at various life stages.

socialization, sex-discrepant expectations that shape fantasies, and guiding myths, in addition to the standard psychoanalytic emphasis on body awareness, sexual distinction, and the vagaries of the Oedipus complex.

Changing Views on the Centrality of Penis Envy

Feminists have complained bitterly about the damage done by the propagation of the penis-envy doctrine as the irreducible dynamic in female mental life. They have raised the suspicion that it is not women who are fixated on penis envy, but psychoanalysis. While analysts of different theoretical persuasions ascribe varying significance to penis envy as an operative dynamic, few stress it to the same degree as Freud or Deutsch. Many analysts have since reevaluated the data and come to different conclusions.

According to Blum, "Though very important and ubiquitous, penis envy can no longer be regarded, if it ever was, as the major organizer of femininity . . . To derive femininity mainly from penis envy would be developmental distortion and reductionism" (Blum, 1976, 186). Although Tyson believes that the awareness of anatomical differences may function as a "psychic organizer," she has echoed Blum, arguing that "we must look to the early identifications with the idealized mother-ego ideal in order to understand the greater portion of the feminine personality organization" (Tyson, 1982, 77). And Lerner has written, "Today's analyst is less quick to label women's aggressive, ambitious, and competitive strivings as 'masculine' or to interpret them a priori as a manifestation of penis envy" (Lerner, 1980, 39).

While Freud put penis envy at the center of the female's neurotic conflicts, different conflicts are seen as predominant today. One hears much more today, and much more to the point, about conflicts over the fear of loss of love or over excessive dependency needs than about conflicts over penis envy. First alluded to by Freud (1924), the fear of loss of love belongs with a cluster of traits that are particularly characteristic of women in Western cultures: dependency needs, fear of independence, fear of abandonment, unreconstructed longing for love relationships with a man, and fear of being alone. These problems are viewed not as bedrock, replacing penis envy as a core, but as preoccupations in the minds of contemporary women. They may, however, be rooted in early female object relations, socialization, or a combination of factors. And to some degree, they may reflect the individual's response to the external situation. Many analysts and psychologists have come to recognize the need to distinguish contextual responses from internalized stable personality traits.

VALUES AND THEORY MAKING

Recent changes in practice and theory are of inestimable practical benefit to women. From the vantage point of psychoanalysis as an intellectual and scientific discipline, however, we would risk trivializing the theoretical failures of Freud and his followers if we were to restrict our interests solely to correcting the inaccuracies and misperceptions related to the special case of female development. Thus, while we may applaud various corrections in our theories of female psychology, we must also confront the reasons why penis envy for so long retained its power as a monolithic explanation and why sexuality and femininity were essentially seen as meagre and distorted. Some have insisted that these early formulations reveal the severe limitations of psychoanalytic theorizing. The emphasis here is on *theorizing* rather than on *theory*, because the whole psychoanalytic enterprise has been challenged, not just one tenet of psychoanalytic theory. The specific questions concern how these theories have persisted for so long and what their persistence reveals both of faulty methodology and of value biases. As the following discussion illustrates, they have persisted so long for at least three reasons: misogyny, the lack of a requirement for verification in psychoanalytic theorizing, and the underlying biological assumptions in psychoanalysis.

Freud's Patriarchal Bias

Feminist scholars and analysts, under the impact of changing social values, have correctly insisted that Freud wrote from the patriarchal stance typical of his cultural milieu. Because he viewed female development simply as a variant of the male counterpart, he failed to achieve a comprehensive or accurate description and theory. Furthermore, they argue, his theoretical biases were automatically translated into therapeutic biases and had profound negative impacts on women patients. Freud not only viewed women as powerless, but also saw them as lacking essential special capacities and a powerful unique sexuality. Penis envy, as doctrine, focusing as it does on female inadequacy, coincided with this traditional perception of the woman as powerless, inferior, and subordinate. A number of feminist writers have eloquently pointed this out, challenging the analytic formulation of the origins of "femininity." In fact, theories of female psychosexual development have, in the past, been misused as theoretical justifications for women's subordinate positions in society.

Horney (1926) literally charted Freud's bias. She drew a close parallel between a small boy's ideas about the sexual difference and psychoanalytic ideas about feminine development. Doing so, Horney was among the first to raise the possibility that Freud's insistence on the centrality of penis envy was related to the male's own envy of the female and particularly of her capacity for motherhood. In a remark which Rohrbaugh (1979) has also quoted, Millett made an interesting and relevant observation. "Freudian logic has succeeded in converting childbirth, an impressive female accomplishment, and the only function its rationale permits her, into nothing more than a hunt for a male organ" (Millett, 1970, 185).

The charge that Freud's psychology of women is infused by patriarchal values has not been restricted to feminists. Consider, for example, Schafer's objection. "Freud's ideas on the development and psychological characteristics of girls and women, though laden with rich clinical and theoretical discoveries and achievements, appeared to have been significantly flawed by the influence of traditional patriarchal and evolutionary values. This influence is evident in certain questionable presuppositions, logical errors and inconsistencies, suspensions of intensive inquiry, underemphasis on certain developmental variables, and confusions between observations, definitions, and value preferences" (Schafer, 1974, 483). Freud's beliefs mirrored those of his culture. His systematic distortion alerts us to the danger of using common sense corroborated by cultural consensus to confirm scientific theory. Value bias lulls us into theoretical complacency.

The Lack of Systematic Verification in Psychoanalytic Theory

Psychoanalytic data are subject to a variety of interpretations. Analysts and therapists of different persuasions encounter the same underlying data from the couch: symbols, dream content, fantasies, and so forth. Yet Freudians, Jungians, culturists, and others use these data to verify their theories, thereby revealing the inadequacy of the couch as the sole source of data for verifying theory.

Biases in perception and interpretation occur all the time. The fact that they persist and become codified in psychoanalytic theory reflects a methodological problem in psychoanalytic theorizing. Misperception does not usually or necessarily take the form of distorting the symbols of conflict. Nor is it based on thin air. Misperception can occur from selective inattention to data or from incorrectly weighing their significance. A random fantasy is different from an organizing fantasy. Most commonly, bias is reflected in a misinterpretation of the meaning of the data. On the one hand, the analyst may view attempted conflict resolution as symptomatic rather than adaptive, in accordance with his or her subjective values. On the other hand, the analyst may interpret certain symbols as being causal, irradicable, or intrinsic rather than as being secondary, maladaptive attempts at conflict resolution.

Grossman and Stewart (1976) have illustrated the latter distortion in their paper, "Penis envy: from childhood wish to developmental metaphor." They presented two clinical examples of analyses in which the interpretation of penis envy, apparently grounded in clinical data, *"had an organizing effect, but not a therapeutic one"* (Grossman and Stewart, 1976, 194). In both examples, the interpretation of penis envy was close enough to the data of the analyses that the women accepted the interpretation and used it to rationalize and consolidate their real pathological constellations. Thus, penis envy is often a symbolic condensation that conceals significant underlying conflicts. As Blum stated, "It is necessary to theoretically distinguish between penis envy as a dynamic issue and as a developmental influence" (Blum, 1976, 186). Freud himself made a peculiar jump from patients' clinical fantasies about castration to his developmental hypothesis about the little girl's discovery of "the fact of her castration." His confusion between fantasy and reality precluded his investigation of the meaning of castration fantasies.

One must distinguish between the meaning of clinical themes and developmental causality (Person, 1974).* Meaning can be separated from assumptions of continuity insofar as the latter imply a causal chain. Many analysts have criticized certain of the assumptions of continuity and causality that are routinely made in psychoanalysis, along with those made in the other historical sciences such as history, evolution, or developmental psychology. However, it would be inaccurate to claim that psychoanalysis is simply a science of meaning and that it therefore does not belong to the natural sciences. Psychoanalysis is a natural science insofar as it deals with the composition of self-sustaining characteristics of current mental organization. Thus it addresses the schemata of meaning and their association with affect in a horizontal segment of time (see Modell, 1978). It is out of the

*Preceptor's note: For an extensive discussion of the cause-effect issue and the role of the past in psychoanalysis, see the chapter by Michels.

correspondence between meaning sets and affects that we generate psychoanalytic hypotheses.

Klerman (1982) made an apt observation that is worth echoing here. Psychoanalysis has been rich in generating hypotheses, but has not been sufficiently committed to their verification. This case study regarding the psychology of women clearly illustrates the dangers of theorizing developmental processes without seeking validation from nonanalytic data. To hold to theories without such validation is to invite contamination by value biases.

The Biological Assumptions of Psychoanalysis

While misogyny has been posited as the culprit responsible for certain inaccuracies in the early psychoanalytic theories about women, misogyny alone does not account adequately for their persistence in the presence of countervailing data. An explanation based on Freud's misogyny is too narrow if his misogyny is seen as emanating solely from simple historical bias. The question really is whether his misogyny is incidental to the basic assumptions of psychoanalysis or whether it is intimately related to the structure of the ideas Freud generated. To the degree that we raise this question, we must move beyond an examination of susceptibility to a particular value bias in psychoanalysis and consider that biases may be even more broadly based in their underlying assumptions.

In 1961, Rieff raised exactly this point. "A denial of the Freudian psychology of women cannot depend on historical reductions of Freud's own psychology . . . His misogyny, like that of his predecessors, is more than prejudice; it has a vital intellectual function in his system . . . And just as sympathetic expositors of Schopenhauer and Nietzsche want to dismiss these philosophers' views on women as idiosyncratic and philosophically irrelevant, so the neo-Freudians (led by eminent women analysts like Karen Horney) would like to omit that part of Freud's work as mere culture-prejudice, maintaining that much of the remaining doctrine can be realigned without damage" (Rieff, 1961, 199–200).

In general, Freud was able to use criticism from both his followers and his defectors by integrating it into his theories. For example, Adler's concepts of masculine protest and power strivings are regarded as having been catalytic in Freud's consideration of aggression. On the other hand, despite cogent contemporary criticisms about his theories of female development (for example, Horney, 1924; 1926; 1932; 1933; Jones, 1927; 1933; 1935), Freud never revised these theories. Later criticisms met the same fate at the hands of Freud's followers. Although Clara Thompson (1943) clearly stated that women envy men at least in part because of women's subordinate position in culture, she had no impact on mainstream psychoanalytic theories about women. Ovesey's observations on the devaluation of women (1956), Moulton's work on primary and secondary penis envy (1973), as well as the work of others, all now well regarded, were originally viewed as merely culturist. Thus, Freud and his followers never really confronted or resolved Freud's schema of female development, and the argument about the critical factors in female development remained dormant until the 1970s.

During the past decade, women's expectations were radically altered, and feminists were extremely vocal in their protests against psychoanalytic theories about women. Parallel with changing cultural directives about appropriate goals and the content of "femininity," psychoanalytic theories about the development of women were fundamentally revised. This is not to say, however, that psychoanalytic theory changed in direct response to the women's movement. Indeed, many of the criticisms leveled against psychoanalysis in the 1970s were the same as those raised by an earlier generation of feminists and dissident analysts. The pertinent question, then, is why psychoanalysis became more receptive to the same critiques.

The delay in incorporating such critiques can only indicate the vital function of misogyny underlying the psychoanalytic theories. Alluding to Freud's problem in theorizing the psychology of women, Schafer has stated that "it . . . was introduced into Freud's theorizing, and thus his comparative view of men and women, by his adhering to a biological, evolutionary model for his psychology . . . This model requires a teleological view of the propagation of the species . . . One observes in this entire line of thought the operation of an implicit but powerful *evolutionary value system*. According to this value system, nature has its procreative plan, and it is better for people to be 'natural' and not defy 'natural order'" (Schafer, 1974, 468–469). Rohrbaugh (1979) has raised the same question about Freud's theory, provocatively asking whether psychoanalysis can exist without penis envy. She believes that the concept of penis envy is embedded in Freud's insistence on a framework of biologically unfolding psychosexual stages and that his theory cannot account adequately for input from the familial, social, or cultural context.

Although Freud's clinical studies reveal a broad perspective, what has been referred to as his psychological theory or his metapsychology rested on reducing mental processes to biology and on minimizing the influences of experience and learning. By adhering to a strictly instinctual frame of reference, his theory could not offer an adequate means for understanding the influences on female development of early object relations, the prephallic development of personality, or the subordinate societal role of women. In effect, Freud was unable to theorize adequately the interface between individual psychology and cultural injunction.

Toward a Paradigm Shift

Retrospectively, it appears that psychoanalysis was unable to encompass early criticisms about theories of female development until it had developed the ability to theorize the intersection between individual psychology and the cultural milieu. Analysts had objected to the theories of the interpersonal school because they implied that subjectivity simply mirrored the external world. Thus, they viewed the critiques of classical formulations of female development as largely culturist. These analysts were unwilling to embrace a perspective that seemed to undermine their hard-won recognition of the importance of intrapsychic and unconscious factors. Only recently have the theoretical assumptions of psychoanalysis been enlarged to the point that the earlier criticisms could be assimilated. Before this could happen, the question of whether "the unconscious has a history" had to be addressed (the phrase is Marcus's, 1982). More narrowly, this question relates to the way in which external reality is internalized and so organizes individual psychology. What was required, then, was a shift away from a theory which posited that development was exclusively the preordained outcome of libidinal development, that is, a shift away from reducing mental processes to biology, and a shift toward a theory that focused on object relations and internalization as the major psychic organizers. Bias regarding women could apparently not be fully recognized or acknowledged before a more general paradigm shift had occurred.

There is today a growing consensus that libido theory, taken alone, provides an inadequate explanation of human development. While the basic constructs of psychoanalysis (motivation, the importance of childhood experiences, unconscious mental processes, and so forth) are still viable and are almost universally accepted, some tenets of metapsychology have been challenged. Given the studies of ego psychology, Ross (1970) and Lichtenstein (1970) have suggested that personality maturation can no longer be seen as the sole dependent variable and sexuality as the sole independent one. Sexuality is considered one independent variable among others, although it is still regarded as the leading one by some theorists. Object-relations theory attempts to formulate those ways in which the experience of the external world is internalized, not just in the organization of perception and affective relationships, but in the very creation of subjectivity. While all psychoanalytic theory acknowledges the internalization of external values and prohibitions in the formation of ego ideal and superego, object-relations theory places more emphasis on the way subjectivity (fantasies, wishes) and the formation of ego are influenced by the experiential. Even sexuality, so clearly grounded in biology, is embedded in meaning and cannot be understood without reference to culture. Individuals internalize aspects of their interpersonal world, albeit in a way that is distorted by infantile mental processes and fantasies. This internalization shapes both their experience of desire and their expression of sexuality (Person, 1980).

These evolutions in psychoanalytic thinking did not occur primarily in response to social movements but in response to new data and the systematic critique of its metapsychological assumptions. The new data were accumulated from the direct observation of children, from studies of intersex patients, from the study of psychoanalytic treatment failures, and from the psychoanalytic therapy of new types of patients (the widening scope). These new data have led to a paradigm shift in psychoanalysis, a shift which in turn can more adequately confront the many apt criticisms raised against Freudian theories about women.

SUMMARY

The case of female psychology stands as a cautionary tale. Not only does it reveal the impact of historical bias on scientific assumptions, but more important, it lays bare some underlying assumptions in early psychoanalytic theories. This special case, in which theories appeared to be verified by clinical data, reveals methodological problems specific to the field of psychoanalysis. The temptation to confuse the symbols and meanings uncovered in analysis with developmental causality is readily apparent. Such confusion causes us to risk mistaking the accidents of historical contingency for eternal underlying truths. Consequently, the case of female psychology encourages us to distinguish systematically between the contingent and the universal. It reveals the impact of beliefs and value biases on both patients and analysts. It forces us to refine our scientific paradigms, first to acknowledge the inevitable dual descriptive-normative role of any psychoanalytic theory (Macklin, 1973), and second to separate hypothesis generating from hypothesis testing (Klerman, 1982).

Finally, the case of female psychology leads us to reexamine certain underlying psychoanalytic assumptions. As the author has argued here, misogyny may be too narrow an explanation for Freud's misunderstanding of women. Freud's misunderstanding and misogyny have broader meaning than simple cultural prejudice. His scheme of female psychosexual development betrays a biological bias that leads to an overemphasis on genitals and reproduction and that lacks an appropriate theoretical scaffolding to support a full understanding of the manifold influences in personality development. It is indeed ironic that in attempting to avoid culturist reductionism, Freud mistook Victorian femininity for eternal femininity.

Given its recent theoretical developments, psychoanalysis can now encompass the issues raised by the study of female psychology. We have made significant revisions in theory. We will no doubt revise the revisions. We will base these on insights into our current blind spots. The acknowledgment that values are pervasive in psychoanalysis, as in other scientific disciplines, ought not to discourage us. Psychoanalysis as a theory and methodology is constantly evolving, and this, indeed, is what distinguishes it from blind ideology.

Chapter 4

Has the Scope of Psychoanalysis Changed?
by Leon N. Shapiro, M.D.

INTRODUCTION

Arguing in 1954 that we ought to widen the scope of indications for psychoanalysis, Stone put forth an optimistic viewpoint that is still appealing. Rather than limiting psychoanalysis to the classical indications and techniques, many analysts prefer to take a more optimistic view, both of the range of patients who can benefit from psychoanalysis and of the range of techniques which may be used. The optimism regarding the range of patients is rooted not only in some success with more difficult patients, but also in some of the newer insights into early development which have come from the growing body of child observation studies.

This chapter explores the viability of suggestions for altering analytic technique and for widening the scope of indications for psychoanalysis. It begins with a necessarily cursory review of the rigors of the classical method, emphasizing the regression in the transference during the long middle game. The chapter then examines requisite qualities of patients who can enter into and sustain analytic work. As an organizing device, the author evaluates the suggested changes in the scope of psychoanalysis through the lenses of two clinical examples. The first case is one in which the patient was, by all conventional standards, a suitable candidate for a classical psychoanalysis. The analyst used a conventional technical approach in this case and considered the treatment outcome favorable.

As a background to the second case, the author describes some representative contributions to the more commonly suggested modifications in technique. The patient in the second case seemed unable to tolerate the deprivations which the classical analytic method entails, and the analyst modified the technique. In retrospect, this analyst felt that while the psychotherapeutic outcome of the case had been favorable, the modification in technique had compromised the psychoanalysis. The author then evaluates this case and suggests alternatives the analyst might have considered. The chapter concludes by discussing the implications of the two cases for the integrity of the psychoanalytic and psychotherapeutic disciplines.

TECHNIQUES AND PREREQUISITES FOR THE MIDDLE GAME

Freud's (1913; 1923) image of analysis as a chess game is still serviceable. During the long middle game, the analytic process unfolds in a matrix of a more or less organized transference. *The middle game* here refers to that long period in analysis after a relatively stable transference has been established and during which the analyst and patient are engaged primarily in interpretative work. The middle game is unique for each analysis, and it is that aspect of the work which most sharply distinguishes psychoanalysis from the analytically derived psychotherapies. While the opening and end games of analysis may involve more clarifications, supportive maneuvers, and educational devices, once the process of the middle game has started, the technique is essentially neutral, interpretive, and focused on intrapsychic processes. The interpretive technique and the neutral stance are intended to bring about the patient's regression and to facilitate the analysis of instinctual vicissitudes.

Three key elements in the formal analytic technique are designed to facilitate the regression. First, the relatively silent, out-of-sight analyst tends to block out the usual confirmations and supports of face-to-face encounters. Second, particularly during the middle game, the analyst maintains a steady emphasis away from the ordinary concerns of reality and assumes a neutral position with regard to drives, superego, and ego functions. Where the analyst does take an interest in the patient's reality, he or she emphasizes reality in terms of defenses and adaptive ego functions. Third, the systematic analysis of resistances disrupts defensive operations.

Freud's statements about who could benefit from psychoanalysis were very cautious. "To be quite safe, one should limit one's choice of patients to those who possess a normal mental condition" (Freud, 1905, 264). However, Freud in truth worked with extremely difficult cases. Most of our cases today are other than ideal, and certainly none are easy. Nonetheless, we generally do have in mind certain criteria when we consider a patient for analysis.

The fact that Eskimos have fifteen different names for snow reflects the importance of that element in their lives. Psychoanalysts probably have at least as many names for that solid sense of self and others which can allow integrative work to continue in the face of the intense affects and the regressive pull of the middle-game transference. A partial list would include a sense of autonomy (Erikson, 1950), a cohesive self (Kohut, 1977), a stable sense of separation and individuation (Mahler, 1971), object constancy (Kernberg, 1967), and most important, a normal ego (Freud, 1905, 264). A patient will probably fulfill the criteria for middle-game analysis if four conditions are met. (1) The important people in the patient's life stand out sharply as human and multidimensional, in spite of ambivalent feelings. (2) These others are well differentiated from the patient and from each other. (3) The patient's sense of him- or herself, however conflicted, overburdened, or in pain, remains well defined. (4) The patient is generally able to locate affects appropriately, i.e., is relatively free of projection.

Recent theoretical developments, derived both from clinical observations on less-than-ideal cases and from direct child observations, have given us the courage to take into treatment patients with other than normal egos. These are patients whom we earlier would not have considered to be analyzable, since they would not have seemed to meet the above-listed criteria. Most patients entering psychoanalysis today have had rather extensive diagnostic interviews, if not extensive psychotherapy, prior to analysis, and the test of whether the patient can use the process may continue on the couch. Parenthetically, as we evaluate the various suggestions for broadening the scope of indications for psychoanalysis, we must confront the problem that the methods suggested to prepare the broader group of patients for the middle game may end up compromising the analytic procedure.

An Example of the Middle Game

The patient was a 29-year-old lawyer who entered analysis because of her persistent performance anxiety in work and in personal relationships. Although outwardly successful in both areas, she was constantly critical of herself, to the point where she worried that she would withdraw both from her career and from her marriage, if only to be rid of the anxiety.

Developmentally significant for this patient were the following. Her presenting dissatisfaction with herself seemed to have its major roots in relation to what she perceived as her ambitious mother. She always felt pushed to perform, and the mother of the rapprochement appeared particularly unwelcoming of any of her wishes to regress. As the only girl in a family of boys, however, she clearly felt herself to be the vehicle of her mother's ambitions. Her basic self-confidence and almost grandiose expectations of admiration from the significant and well-defined people in her life seemed to reflect the quality of her earliest acceptance in her family: she always felt she was the favorite. There was little question of her capacity for basic trust: the world always contained a core of responsiveness for her.

By the end of the second year of analysis, her symptoms had disappeared, and she was involved in a classical oedipal transference with warm, romantic feelings, sometimes overtly sexual, in which the analyst seemed to be an idealized father, lover, brother, and friend. This alternated and sometimes coexisted with angry, competitive feelings in which she seemed to experience the analyst as a withholding, critical mother.

The hour discussed below followed a four-day interruption. The patient began the hour by describing a professional meeting in which she felt she had been unnecessarily caustic and outspoken. She left the meeting feeling that people would be critical of her. She then described a "stupid" professional mistake that she had made, in which she had temporarily misjudged the relative importance of an issue. Several times during this hour, she reached down to replace the fold of a wraparound skirt which repeatedly fell and revealed her knee. After several other indications of her concern about revealing too much of herself, she complained that she was feeling somewhat disconnected from the analysis.

The analyst commented on her concern about revealing too much of herself. She responded angrily that she could not understand how the analyst would come to such a conclusion, and she was silent for a few moments. She then flushed and said that there were things that she was too anxious to say. She mentioned that during the hours before the four-day interruption she had felt very gassy but had not mentioned her concerns about it during those hours. She then proceeded to describe a series of inhibitions and worries about her sloppiness, her dirty underwear, and vaginal smells during sex. With this came references to earlier episodes of sexual investigation during latency and their secret quality.

The resistance analysis led to a deepening of material and a regressive deepening of the transference. The following hour she felt very "connected" to the analyst, described a recent trip home, and associated to early struggles with both parents.

THE TRANSFERENCE CONTEXT   Several months earlier the patient had asked to change an appointment time, which the analyst was able to do. At the time of the changed appointment, she was clearly anxious, could not get comfortable on the couch, would say only a few words, and would then break off into silence. She then angrily demanded that the analyst tell her whether he had changed the hour because he cared about her, or whether he would have done this for any patient.

She had made many direct demands before, particularly in the opening phase. At those times, the analyst would usually acknowledge the urgency of her feelings and simply encourage her to try to describe what she was experiencing. This time, the analyst remained silent, and so did she. She folded her arms on her chest and said, "I won't say another fucking word until you answer me." She remained silent for the rest of the hour and left angrily.

The next day she arrived promptly, lay down, and folded her arms, clearly prepared to continue her boycott. The analyst offered her the following interpretation. "It's as if you don't dare to bring in the feelings about me until I first tell you I love you." She flushed immediately, remained silent for a moment, then unfolded her arms, and began to describe a series of highly romantic fantasies, which were both tender and erotic. She had been consciously and secretly involved with these fantasies for weeks and had found it too humiliating to reveal them.

In the next hour, she said, "I feel a lot better since yesterday. Once I got started, it didn't seem so frightening. I was so uncomfortable with two days of anxiety, not understanding, not getting beyond it. I felt out of control, being difficult, giving you a hard time. It's a relief to talk again. You were right. I was afraid that if I told you, you would say, 'Who do you think you are?' It's so narcissistic to think that I am irresistibly seductive. It's embarrassing to admit. Figuring that out made me feel better. You don't have the awful responses I was afraid of. If I admit I love you, it threatens my marriage (she was crying during most of this). I never wanted to have these feelings unless I knew you cared about me."

During that hour and for a period of about a week following, a storm of feelings came up for her. In effect, these feelings summarized the major conflictual issues which constantly colored her experience: a pervasive sense of deprivation, the feeling that the world was unfair, intense romantic fantasies, a sense of unlimited entitlement, and terror that her grandiose expectations would be rebuffed. The feelings were in turn accompanied by an almost paranoid, argumentative sensitivity.

Implications of the Case

The details in this example are less startling than the consuming quality of the experience, for both the patient and the analyst. Also remarkable is the fact that such intense affect in the analysis was accompanied by unusual tranquillity in the rest of the patient's life. This patient's experience in the middle phase of the analysis differed quite clearly from her experience of the beginning and end phases. During the middle phase with this patient, as with others, the figure of the analyst was suffused with the complex images of the oedipal period. During the introductory and termination phases, the experience tends to be much less primary-process dominated and much more sensitive to the analyst as an actual person. While tactlessness and unempathic responses can be highly disruptive during the opening and end games, the analyst will be forgiven almost any "error" during the middle game. Although the patient showed many narcissistic phenomena, she could in no way be considered a narcissistic character. To enter into and sustain the effort throughout the middle game, this patient had to exercise a number of requisite capacities.

First, she had to be able to maintain consciously (or preconsciously in readily available form) two strongly different affective attachments in the transference, the positively toned father transference and the aggressively toned mother transference.

Second, in the face of these feelings, she had to be able to tolerate and to be guided by the neutral comments of the analyst. Generally, his comments required that she take her attention away from what appeared to be the pressing and real need for some response to the wishes aroused in the process and that she refocus her attention on examining her own fantasy life. The entire thrust of the analyst's interventions, whether he was actively interpreting or not, said to her, "You must not expect me to respond to the wishes you have about me. You must bear that frustration and continue to trust that I am on your side."

Third, she had to both trust the analyst's benign intentions and allow herself to regress. Occasionally, she had to overcome a loss of trust, such as when she became angry when the analyst picked up some resistance. The regression, then, would bring in even more of her wishes, fantasies, secrets, and memories, threatening to make her transference longings even more unrealizable.

Finally, she had to be able to keep the regressive wishes in the analysis and, for the most part, not act them out in her life.

The crucial question of scope revolves around the issue of what the analyst can do if the patient does not have these capacities. In this case, for example, the question could have arisen if the patient had experienced her wish for the analyst's love less as a wish to be understood and more as a need to be fulfilled. In an effort to address such problems, a number of technical suggestions have been made throughout the history of psychoanalysis. Generally, these suggestions focus on ways of dealing with patients who seem unable to cooperate in the psychoanalytic process.

TECHNICAL MODIFICATIONS

Thirty years ago, Kurt Eissler (1952) defined the heart of the classical psychoanalytic technique as its neutral interpretive stance. Eissler called the deviations from this stance parameters, any interventions other than interpretation which might be necessary to initiate or to maintain the analytic process. To the extent that these noninterpretive interventions were unanalyzed, or were not interpreted in their full developmental meaning in the transference, Eissler believed the analysis might be compromised.

Over the years, insights into preoedipal developmental deficits or distortions have accumulated to suggest that certain modifications might restore or in some way substitute for the ego capacities necessary for middle-game analytic work. Compiling a list of contributors to highlight the persistence of the issues over the analytic generations, one would include at least Ferenczi (Ferenczi and Rank, 1924), Alexander (1956), and Kohut (1977). The insights that these and other analysts have contributed are twofold. They have added to our understanding, and this has been of widespread and continuing use. And they have contributed to technique, but the usefulness and applications here are more controversial.

For instance, Ferenczi's emphasis on the affective side of the analytic experience has become a permanent part of our way of thinking about the therapeutic aspects of psychoanalysis (Ferenczi and Rank, 1924). His suggestions about active technique, however, have not been found useful to the analytic experience per se. On the other hand, Ferenczi's technical suggestions have survived in the analytically informed treatment of hospitalized patients and children, witness the fairly standard practice of using a therapist as a substitute primary object in the treatment of young children.

Similarly, while Alexander's (1956) suggestions that the analyst deliberately act in ways to distinguish him- or herself from primary objects has found little acceptance in analytic work, his thinking has been useful at a conceptual level. There is no doubt that the analyst provides the matrix for a "corrective emotional experience" by being (rather than acting) different from the parents, by simply doing the work of the analyst, by being committed to the patient, and by trying to understand.

Just as Ferenczi and Alexander suggested that the analyst could in some way make up for a missing or defective developmental experience, a similar notion runs through Kohut's work (see, for example, Kohut, 1977). Again, while Kohut's theory of the effects of early empathic failures may help our understanding of narcissistic phenomena, the jury is still out on the question of technique. Whether the finely tuned empathic responses of the analyst can actually repair defects resulting from empathic failures of early development is still not certain (Arnold Cooper, personal communication, 1982).

In his last talk at Berkeley, Kohut (1982) insisted that he had never stated that empathic responses repair deficits, but rather that empathic responses are essential to the setting for the analytic understanding which will in turn permit correct interpretation. Kohut was also explicit in his writing about the preconditions for analyzing narcissistic character traits. "The observing segment of the personality of the analysand, which, in cooperation with the analyst, has actively shouldered the task of analyzing, is not, in essence, different in analyzable narcissistic disorders from that found in analyzable transference neuroses" (Kohut, 1971, 207). Goldberg has characterized Kohut's approach as follows. "The analyst does not actively soothe: he interprets the analysand's yearning to be soothed . . . Of course the analyst's mere presence, or the fact that he talks or, especially the fact that he understands, all have soothing and self-confirming effects on the patient *and they are so interpreted*. Thus the analytic experience that makes analytic work possible becomes an object for analytic interpretation" (Goldberg, 1978, 447–448).

Although the foregoing quotations do clarify the roles of empathy and interpretation somewhat, the actual case examples cited in Kohut's own work (1971; 1977) and in Goldberg's casebook (1978) still seem to this author to lean toward the idea that the soothing function itself produces structure, and they seem to give insight and interpretation relatively less emphasis.

The contributions of some others have also been more helpful to our understanding than to our technique. Zetzel's (1956) idea of the therapeutic alliance, Modell's (1976) adaptation of Winnicott's notion of the holding environment, and Balint's (1968) suggestions for healing the "basic fault" have helped us to understand the ways in which preoedipal pathology may limit a patient's participation in the middle game. They have thereby suggested ways of improving our sensitivity, our timing, and our patience. But they have left the technically neutral stance of the middle game fundamentally unchanged. Any insight into early developmental process has limited applicability to an adult. Whatever has occurred in early experience in any of the developmental lines (the self, the libido, reality sense, and so forth) is constantly reworked with each new push of development.

Essentially, all of the contributors cited argue that aspects of the analyst's presence, his or her holding function, or the fine tuning of empathy will not only have a therapeutic function, but will lead to the kind of structural change that makes middle-game work possible. The following case illustrates how these technical modifications do make people feel better and can be therapeutic. It also shows, however, that introducing them into a psychoanalysis risks compromising the very elements that distinguish psychoanalysis from all other forms of treatment.

An Example of Technical Modifications

In the following case, the analyst modified the technique because of the patient's exquisite sensitivity to humiliation, his persistent object hunger, and evidence that the transient regression of the rapprochement period was rejected by his mother. These characteristics suggested that the patient could not tolerate the middle-game work in its purely classical form (Myerson, 1981).

> A 30-year-old man reported a transient writing block when he wanted to send a letter consoling his mother about the discovery that she had diabetes. He felt overcome with a "maudlin sentimentality," felt anxious, and he was unable to write. All were unusual symptoms for him. He wanted to "connect" with his mother, to let her know that he shared her anxiety, and to comfort her. He associated to an earlier fantasy of his father's incompetence. The preconscious oedipal fantasy was immediately apparent to him with minimal clarification, and the symptom disappeared.
>
> The last of six children, the patient was "an accident." He was born to an angry, depressed woman four years after she thought she was through with childbearing. The mother's "accident" actually appeared to be her (partially successful) attempt to hold on to her husband, who was having an affair with another woman.
>
> In the analysis of this very bright young man, the writing block episode was typical. The patient always understood things quickly, both in and out of the analysis, and would proceed to master "the problem." His inclination to interpret the world of his experience in competitive oedipal terms was, to be sure, a major piece of baggage that he carried around from childhood, and repetitive examination of this theme freed him from some conflict in his personal and professional life.
>
> In the first few months, the patient was often silent. He posed carefully stated intellectual formulations and desperately searched for a way to please the analyst.

He wanted to be "pushed" in the analysis, just as he had always wanted to be pushed. If you pushed him, it meant you cared about him, and his side of the bargain was to perform.

Short term successes, as in the above episode, led to the patient's idealizing the analyst and to his profound gratitude for the symptomatic improvement. They did not lead, however, to the development of a deepening transference or to therapeutic regression in the analysis.

Where the patient was able to examine his homosexual longings and his wishes to be cared for and adopted (in transference), as each new issue arose, he would apply the insight gained and quickly modify his behavior so that the crescendo of feeling would be cut off by his new sense of competence. The analysis was thus an uninterrupted progression to new forms of mastery, and the patient interpreted any effort to call his attention to the meaning of this need to master things as criticism.

While his life and loves were changed by the process, real intimacy continued to elude him. His work and marriage, while more successful, had the quality of projects to be completed (like the analysis). The transient sense of merger and the capacity to let things be, rather than control or solve them, still seemed beyond him. He could not let go long enough to experience and share the nature of his wishes.

For example, an episode from his fifth year came up repeatedly. He had gone to a friend's house to play. At lunchtime, when he brought his friend home, his mother sent him back to his friend's house for lunch. Even as an adult, the patient was humiliated when he thought about the episode. After six children, his mother must have wished desperately for him, the youngest, to grow up. It seemed clear that the patient's need to be a good, compliant boy was embedded in his pervasive fear of being either unwelcome or barely tolerable.

While the patient would gain some insight, it was never sufficient for him to risk the rapprochement regression again. As one might expect, even though the patient was much improved at the end of treatment, a sense of underlying sadness remained beneath his successful competence.

The "analysis" lasted for four years. Rarely if ever did the kind of middle-game regression described in the first case develop. The end game was formal, with some sadness at separation for both the patient and the analyst. The patient felt he had been analyzed, and certainly he did feel better. But the analyst felt that he had simply done psychotherapy with the patient on the couch, and that if he had taken more risks with the patient's sense of sadness and fears of humiliation, he could have done better for this patient.

An Assessment of the Approach

A review of this rather limited outcome reveals that the analyst's empathic, interventive activity was crucial. The situation was complex, but the patient's compliance and wish to please seduced the analyst into an active style. If the analyst did not push him, which the patient seemed to need, he would feel ignored and abandoned. On the other hand, the patient tended to experience as critical any comments that pushed him to look at himself. The statement, "You seem to be very careful about the way you phrase that," he heard as a demand to be more forthcoming. When the analyst would point this out to him, he would then hear this comment as yet another demand. And so it would go.

Similarly, when the analyst responded with clarification or an attempt to convey empathic understanding, the patient might on one level be transiently gratified. At another level, though, he would also turn this intervention into an implied criticism or a demand that he perform, or both. But, then again, if the analyst was less active, the patient would feel abandoned. In response to this patient's increasing sense of abandonment and depression, the analyst tended to intervene.

The patient himself acted as if he could make no demands, rarely showed dissatisfaction, anger, or frustration, and always had to be quick and insightful, lest the analyst give up on him. For example, the analyst once said to him, "You feel that you must understand and change your behavior as quickly as possible, that if you linger over it, associate to it, or play with it, I will be impatient with you." In response to this, the patient heard, "You have again failed to meet my standards of performance." He believed that he had misunderstood once again what he was supposed to do in order to be the good boy who does the right thing.

The analysis of this patient seems ultimately to have been compromised by the analyst's overemphasis on the patient's early environmental deprivation. The analyst felt that by being unresponsive he would be recreating the unwelcoming mother of the rapprochement. Feeling thus, the analyst tended to accept the apparent reality of the unwelcoming mother, and he felt that he had to do something about this reality lest the patient experience again the empathic unresponsiveness of his childhood.

The emphasis of the analyst's interventions was also influenced by the direction of his environmental interpretation of the patient's screen memories of the rapprochement. For example, in the patient's screen memory of the humiliation at age five, the analyst understood the memory as representing an experience in which the patient's wish to regress was actually rebuffed by the "mother of separation." Alternatively, he could have interpreted such screen memories as statements of the patient's then current anxieties in the transference, namely, the patient's feeling that the analyst would not tolerate his regression.

With such an alternate interpretation, the analyst might then have chosen another, more classical analytic technique. He might not have intervened so sympathetically in the patient's deepening depression. And for this, he would have to have made a different clinical judgment. He would have needed to believe that the patient could tolerate and use effectively the potentially disrupting and disorganizing aspects of intense affects, which in turn might have been examined as drive and defense constellations.

Instead, the analyst allowed this patient's object-relations style to be recreated in the transference. He was, in effect, seduced into responsiveness by the patient's profound sadness and sense of humiliation. Because of his judgment that the patient could not bear his feelings, the analyst attempted to convey his empathic understanding of the patient's affective predicament.

As a result, the patient was never able to tolerate the feelings of humiliation and deepening depression long enough to examine their meanings. The effect of the analyst's empathic responsiveness was to prolong the opening game, and this may have put the recreation of the patient's inner experience beyond the reach of the transference. The middle game, with its regression and interpretations, never did develop.

DISCUSSION

Psychoanalysis advances by a slow accretion of insights. The past decade has led us to a better understanding of the ways in which early preoedipal experience may manifest itself in the analytic process. The contributions in this area have come from child development researchers and from clinical work with patients who show both borderline and narcissistic phenomena. As a result of these insights, many analyses which might earlier have foundered have the potential of coming to more satisfactory conclusions. There has also been an increased interest in and understanding of the noninterpretative elements in analyses. Perhaps inevitably, this had led some analysts to neglect some aspects of the fundamental role of interpretation.

Kohut himself seemed acutely aware that his work might be misinterpreted in this way. In *The Analysis of the Self* (1971), he made a considerable effort to differentiate from psychotherapeutic or educational intervention his proposals regarding the activation and interpretation of emerging primitive transferences. If he has been misinterpreted, the roots of that misinterpretation seem to lie in his theoretical presentation of two issues. The first concerns how narcissistic pathology develops, in his view through unempathic parental behavior. The second issue relates to how the therapeutic process proceeds with these disorders. In Kohut's view, the therapeutic process entails microinternalizations of aspects of the analyst, a process that depends on the patient's having new empathic experiences in the analysis.

Kohut's work is careful, scholarly, and above all helpful. The problem of misinterpretation of his work seems to lie in the environmental tilt. A first problem that arises in this approach is the difficulty of identifying actual environmental deficit. While useful as a rough guide to technique, the developmental history can be misleading. The recollected history changes over the course of the analysis. In the course of treatment, patients encounter what seems like a discovery of new facets of the past in their current work or love relationships. Whether the patient chooses to emphasize what was or is there, or what was or is missing, is a function of mood and the intensity of wishes. If we are thirsty, the glass appears half empty. If we are not, it seems half full.

It matters little whether the analyst does or does not believe the patient's interpretation of current or past events (especially current or past deprivations). A major analytic task is to help the patient take increasing responsibility for his or her current and past reality. For this kind of work, a theory in which reality is an aspect of inner experience is useful. Adopting such a theoretical position and implied technical stance need not require the analyst to be either tactless or witless. The analyst need not ignore the fact that both the analyst and the patient live in the real world. But when analyst and patient are doing analytic work, the real world, past and present, fades.

The analyst must provide an adequate matrix of support to allow the analysis to proceed, yet maintain sufficient nonresponsiveness and barriers to intimacy to allow examination of the patient's developmental lineage. For many patients, we may provide a variable period of empathic holding (Modell, 1976) to develop a safe atmosphere for middle-game analytic work. This certainly requires patience, respect for the patient's defensive needs, and an empathic stance which is curious yet nonintrusive. But if this is all we do, we may sacrifice major opportunities to develop effective insight.

In every case, we face decisions about whether to encourage the elaboration of regressive fantasy or to attend to the patient's discomfort, anxiety, or depression. We may postpone the examination of certain issues or simply acknowledge to the patient how difficult it must be for him or her. This holding presence can let the patient know that difficulties need not be experienced alone. Such efforts to be empathic, however, often misfire by being misinterpreted in the distortions of the transference. Our decisions to intervene on the side of developing more fantasy material therefore depend on our moment-to-moment assessment of what the patient in the analytic relationship can bear.

This assessment rests first of all on the analyst's immediate sense of the patient's affects in the transference and, in particular, on the analyst's appraisal of the patient's liability to be hurt, frightened, or simply insulted by the analyst's activity (or inactivity). The analyst must also judge the patient's capacity to tolerate and integrate the analyst's help and to use the painful affect productively by placing it in a developmental context.

CONCLUSIONS

Holding to a distinction between psychotherapy and psychoanalysis proper is important, especially in the training of candidates, who come with broad psychotherapeutic backgrounds informed by many of the current developmental theories. Those candidates who are still struggling with the "deprivations" of their own analyses may be particularly inclined to blur the distinctions.

If, as Loewald (1981) has suggested, the analyst's view of the patient encompasses not only what the patient is now, but what the patient can become, then the technique will always lean in the direction of respecting the patient's capacity to interpret the analyst's stance as an effort to be helpful. If, on the other hand, the analyst accepts too readily the patient's complaints of actual past deprivation and current needs for a soothing or confirming relationship, he or she may place unnecessary limits on the insight that the patient can achieve.

Thirty years later, Eissler's (1952) paradigm concerning psychoanalysis remains essentially correct. The recent advances have had a major impact on psychotherapy. It is also true that the new theoretical insights into early development have increased our understanding of those who can be treated with psychoanalysis and that they have clarified the effects of noninterpretive interventions.*

The implications for selecting patients for analysis are several. Under most circumstances, the patient should be able to recognize, tolerate, and use productively the analyst's steady de-emphasis of the real world of interactions and also be able to appreciate the analyst's focus on the meaning of inner experience. If the patient is for the most part unable to tolerate this peculiar process, with its accompanying regression, and if the patient seems to need consistent "reparative" responsiveness, then psychoanalysis would not seem to be the best mode of intervention. If the nature of the patient's apparent reality is so overwhelming and the wishes or needs are such that he or she cannot bear the emphasis of analytic work, most analysts would probably opt for a psychotherapeutic approach. The analyst might more helpfully and easily give such a patient mirroring, confirmation, and empathic responsive signals, with the patient sitting up and interactive.

*Preceptor's note: In her chapter, Person illustrates several other significant benefits of recent advances in psychoanalytic theory and practice, namely, the accommodations which they have facilitated in underlying theoretical difficulties and the particular benefits they have had in the psychoanalytic theorizing about women.

Chapter 5

Contemporary Psychoanalytic Views of Interpretation
by Robert Michels, M.D.

INTRODUCTION

Interpretation is the major activity of the psychoanalyst and is one of the essential ingredients of psychoanalytic psychotherapy. *Interpretation* has been defined in various ways. For some, any intervention that aims to increase the patient's insight and understanding or to expand his or her awareness is an interpretation. For others, interpretations must be differentiated from the preliminary steps of clarification and confrontation (Greenson, 1967) or from the more comprehensive process of reconstruction and construction. The term may refer to the process of discovery, decoding, and translation of latent or concealed meaning, or it may refer to communicating the results of that process to the patient. This chapter begins by discussing the functions of interpretation and the content or focus of interpretation. It then explores the role of theory or strategy in guiding interpretation, the role of interpretation in alternate theoretical models of psychoanalysis, and the issue of cause and meaning. Finally, the chapter examines the special significance of interpretations that refer to the past, the relationship between interpretation and the therapeutic process, and the relevance of these issues to the controversy regarding the place of interpretations of the past in comparison with interpretations of the here and now.

THE FUNCTIONS OF INTERPRETATION

Interpretations serve multiple functions. They are generally intended to provide the patient with insight and understanding, to increase the patient's awareness of his or her mental life, to make unconscious aspects of experience conscious, to undo repression, and to construct or reconstruct memories of critical and possibly pathogenic early experiences (Sandler et al., 1973). The knowledge that follows from interpretations is considered central in the therapeutic action of psychoanalysis and essential if the patient is to change (Friedman, 1978; Valenstein, 1981). Interpretations may also have results beyond providing knowledge about the patient. Whether or not these other results are intended, interpretations contain information about the analyst as well as about the patient. The communication of this information is rarely the analyst's primary intention, but it is often the patient's primary interest. Furthermore, the information about the analyst that is implicit in an interpretation is consistently valid, while an interpretation's explicit information about the patient may often be in error.

Interpretations also have nonspecific effects on the therapeutic process. They have an impact on the relationship between the patient and the analyst, communicating understanding and "empathy" (or the opposite) and conveying the atmosphere of emotional acceptance and psychological resonance that is so essential for psychoanalysis (Stone, 1981a). In fact, the negative therapeutic responses seen with overly silent analysts early in the course of treatment more often stem from the lack of this resonant atmosphere than from the analyst's failure to provide insight. Conversely, the most important therapeutic effect of early interpretations may be their positive effect on this atmosphere.

Many theorists of psychotherapy believe that these nonspecific effects of interpretations are far more important than their specific content. Some theorists go so far as to suggest that the quest for insight and understanding is therapeutic primarily as a sort of occupational therapy in which the patient and the therapist share the experience of pursuing together a difficult and important task, along with the inevitable frustrations and accomplishments that are associated.

Interpretations also serve technical functions within the therapy itself. They educate patients about what treatment is and how it works, and they serve as rewards and punishments, shaping the patient's behavior in the therapy. As in most other activities, one learns best by participating, and the patient learns about treatment, as well as about him- or herself and the analyst, by receiving and responding to the analyst's interpretations. This form of instruction is generally more important and more effective than any attempt at overt indoctrination. Many analysts do instruct patients overtly about "the basic rule" and about how treatment is to be conducted, but patients learn these things primarily from their personal participation in the treatment.

THE CONTENT OF INTERPRETATION

Psychopathology

Interpretations can be about a variety of different subjects. The oldest and perhaps the most obvious area for interpretation is the patient's pathology, the symptoms or other pathological constellations that led the patient to become a patient and that provide the immediate context of the treatment. Early in the history of psychoanalysis, however, it became apparent that exploring the meaning of a patient's psychopathology most often involves a complex, tortuous path which veers quickly away from the symptoms without directly disclosing their hidden meaning. Today, the interpretation of the meaning of symptoms occupies a relatively minor role in psychoanalysis, just as general psychoanalytic concern with symptoms has receded in importance. In psychoanalysis, the analysis of symptoms is now seen primarily as a tool in the analysis of character. In psychoanalytic psychotherapy, there is generally a greater interest in symptoms themselves, but the interpretation of symptoms has become less central as a therapeutic technique. While the psychoanalytic psychotherapist's understanding of the meaning of the patient's psychopathology does continue to be essential, the communication of that meaning to the patient is less consistent and more variable.

The Past

The psychoanalytic exploration of symptoms and psychopathology quickly led to an interest in exploring the patient's memories of past experiences or sequences of similar experiences stemming from childhood. These memories were frequently fragmentary, distorted, or difficult to recover consciously, and interpretive work was required to assist the patient in reconstructing them (Blum, 1980). Recent psychoanalytic theorists have suggested that the reconstruction of a personal life history in psychoanalysis is similar to other historical reconstructions. Actually, they suggest, this reconstruction is a construction, a process of creating a new structure which integrates the known data, but which also reflects the setting, themes, choices, and strategies of those who are constructing it. Thus, they emphasize, it is not the unveiling of a preexisting concealed reality, but rather the creation of a new reality (Schafer, 1982; Leavy, 1973).

Freud initially believed that the patient's memories of childhood experiences were related to events that had occurred during the child's life. Freud radically revised this view when it became clear that many such memories pertained to events that could not possibly have occurred in reality and that the phenomenological characteristics of these memories were indistinguishable from those that might actually have occurred. Freud then hypothesized that all memories were valid, but valid in terms of a "psychical" rather than a material reality. They were valid in terms of the subjective world of the child's experience, a world that persisted unconsciously into adult life, rather than in terms of the objective and externally apparent world of the child's behavior and interaction with others. With this dramatic shift in focus, the goal of interpretation shifted again. Interpretation was now directed at reconstructing the psychic reality of the child, rather than the material reality or the events that had transpired in the child's life. This removed any possibility of external validation of the construction that resulted. It was a difficult enough task to test a version of the overt events of a distant past or the conscious subjective experience of the present; to evaluate a version of the largely unconscious subjective experience of the distant past was insurmountable. The role of the interpreter and the theories, attitudes, beliefs, and strategies that he or she brought to the task became all the more important (Leavy, 1980).

The shift of attention from the externally apparent facts of childhood to the inner experience of the child naturally led to an interest in those factors that determine that inner experience. The mental life of the child is of course responsive to the external events of the child's life, but it is also determined by the unfolding of the child's innate drives, predispositions, and capacities. Psychoanalysis turned its attention from the external events to the nature of the child's mental development, the major themes that influence it, and the regular and characteristic patterns of wishes, fears, and fantasies that determine the subjective meaning of all human events. In this context, interpretations were not simply reconstructions of the events of the child's life. They were speculations regarding the developmentally phase-determined meanings that the child had constructed in response to those events (Greenacre, 1980; 1979; 1981). The clinical data that relate to these issues in a single patient are at best hazy, partial, and confusing. As a result, the theories of mental development that the analyst brings to the patient are of considerable significance in shaping the analytic understanding of the patient's past experience and in formulating the interpretations that stem from that understanding (Schafer, 1982).

Associations

Much of the time in psychoanalysis is spent discussing neither the patient's symptoms nor the patient's memories of childhood, but rather the immediate content of the patient's mental life, the stream of associations including fantasies, dreams, parapraxes, jokes, metaphors, and thoughts that occur to him or her during the analytic process. Freud's first use of the term interpretation was in relation to unraveling the hidden meaning of dreams and communicating that meaning to the patient. Some would say that all analytic interpretation is the interpretation of the flow of free associations and that analytic discussion of symptoms, childhood, or anything else has importance only insofar as it occurs in the context of the patient's spontaneous associations (Kris, 1982). Since the patient's associations may seem relatively distant from his or her psychological problems or early life, the patient may be less guarded or wary in discussing this superficially "neutral" material. Most analysts, however, believe that the insights and understandings that stem from exploring the patient's dreams, fantasies, or associations must eventually be related to his or her pathology and persistent childhood structures, if in fact these understandings are to be integrated into the treatment and lead to a therapeutic effect. Otherwise, the treatment is marked by independent investigations of the meanings of specific symbols or events, investigations that do not lead to an understanding of the meaning of the patient's problems in relation to his or her life.

Transference

As psychoanalysts studied their patients' symptoms, memories, dreams, fantasies, and associations, they discovered that patients were often preoccupied with something that at first seemed unobjectionable because it seemed to facilitate the therapeutic process; at the same time, patients were hiding these preoccupations because of their social embarrassment. Rapidly, however, this seemingly unobjectionable phenomenon would become a major area of concern as it began to interfere with the treatment, often in an insistent and intrusive way. It was, of course, the patient's thoughts and feelings about the analyst. Psychoanalytic interest in the transference aspects of the patient-analyst relationship thus originated in the need to understand and analyze the transference because of its prominence as a resistance. The transference was to be interpreted not because of its inherent therapeutic interest, but rather because the analysis of symptoms and memories could not continue unless transference resistances were first explored. These transferences might be positive or negative, affectionate or hostile, but they shared one critical characteristic: they interfered with the patient's experience and disclosure of his or her mental life.

The study of transference experiences soon revealed that they not only explained important resistances to disclosing information, but that they also provided a vital source of information. The patient's characteristic patterns of relationships with significant others were displayed in the transference relationship with exceptional clarity and intensity. The transference relationship could therefore serve as a valuable laboratory for therapeutic study, combining an immediacy of the psychological data with the controlled participation of the therapist. Furthermore, the transference reenacted the critical developmental experiences in a way that was perhaps even more faithful to psychic reality than the objective account of the original events. There was less contamination in the therapeutic situation by material reality or by the specific character of other figures in the patient's life, and there was a greater likelihood that an undisguised representation of the patient's subjective experience would develop in his or her conscious awareness and that this experience would be enacted in the relationship with the analyst. The interpretation of the transference thus became more than a means of removing resistances. It was also a means of exploring the patient's pathology and his or her memories of the past and, of particular value, the links between them. The analysis of the transference could encompass the analysis of resistances, psychopathology, and persistent childhood fantasies.

The Totality of Experience

Perhaps the simplest way of stating a modern view of psychoanalysis is to say that everything is to be interpreted—the patient's symptoms and his or her memories of the past, the patient's fantasies, dreams, parapraxes, jokes, metaphors, and pattern of associations, as well as the evolving pattern of his or her transference response, in other words, the patient's entire life. There is nothing that the patient thinks, says, or does that does not serve as a basis for interpretation. This, however, creates a new problem for the analyst, that of selecting what to interpret (Glover, 1958). When the business of interpretation was believed to be that of explaining the patient's symptoms or recovering repressed childhood memories, the analyst might then have had difficulty knowing the correct interpretation, but he or she had little doubt about the correct focus of interpretation. Since then, as each new area of interpretive focus has been added, the problem has grown more complex. This is the context within which the apparent dispute between different general strategies of interpretation has emerged, such as whether to focus on the genetic origins of behavior or on the here and now (Gill, 1979; Stone, 1981b; Simons, 1981).

THE ROLE OF THEORY IN PSYCHOANALYSIS

The question of strategies for selecting among alternate interpretations raises a more basic one, the question of the role of strategy in psychoanalysis in general (Michels, 1983). Freud's instructions to psychoanalysts advised an attitude of evenly hovering attention with a suspension of specific focused intention. This is not the mental state of someone deductively applying a general theory to an array of specific facts. Psychoanalysis or psychotherapy should not be conducted with the analyst trying to apply a theoretical scheme to the patient. When this does occur, the patient tends to experience the process as one in which he or she is the object to which the method of analysis is being applied, rather than one in which he or she is a participant in a conjoint inquiry. However, if the analyst is not applying a strategy that determines which interpretive theme to pursue, what does guide the analyst's determination? And what sense can we make of the arguments concerning the relative importance of the past and the here and now in the interpretive process?

An alternate view would have the analyst or therapist work spontaneously, freely, and creatively, interpreting what feels most meaningful rather than applying a theory that determines which interpretive path to follow. But this does not mean that the analyst's approach is inconsistent, chaotic, or atheoretical. It does mean that good psychoanalytic work is informed by theory, not determined or dictated by it. The psychoanalyst studies theory and absorbs and internalizes it. Theory thus becomes a part of the equipment that the analyst brings to the analysis, shaping his or her perception of the patient and the situation and influencing his or her understanding and interpretive choices. Theories should function for the analyst as interpretations do for the patient; they should not dictate truths, but they should enhance and expand the meaning of the analytic experience.

Although the analyst should not try to follow a set of rules about interpreting the present or the past, the psychopathology, or the transference, the analyst should be influenced by an understanding of these issues, and his or her free, spontaneous interpretive behavior in the analysis will reflect this influence. The analyst's work here is analogous to the patient's experience in living his or her life. The patient has created a psychic reality that is one version of the multiple possible meanings of the material reality that has transpired and has then responded to that psychic reality. Similarly, the analyst will create a psychoanalytic reality that is one version of the multiple possible constructions of the patient's experience in the psychoanalytic situation and of the patient's psychic reality, a version informed by the analyst's theoretical understanding as well as his or her empathic experience of the patient and knowledge of the patient's life. This psychoanalytic reality that the analyst has constructed will then organize his or her perceptions and shape his or her responses, and discordant perceptions or responses will lead to refinements and revisions of the reality. Our discussion of the relative importance of genetic interpretations and those in the here and now should not dictate what the analyst ought to do, but it should have some influence on what the analyst spontaneously and freely chooses to do, and therefore on the reality that he or she constructs.

CAUSE AND MEANING

Psychoanalysis initially focused attention on the past as the cause of the present. At first, this cause-effect relationship was quite straightforward: traumatic events in the past led to problems in the present. In his earliest clinical writing, Freud repeatedly emphasized that his patients were essentially normal individuals suffering from the sequelae of pathogenic occurrences. Later, in spite of the shift in emphasis from childhood events to childhood experiences, from the occurrences themselves to the child's experience of them and the meanings attached to them, Freud still maintained his basic cause-effect framework. This shift in emphasis has nonetheless had an influence on psychoanalytic theory. Moving the focus from the world of at least potentially verifiable facts to the world of reconstructed subjective experiences, it provided the basis for an alternate psychoanalytic framework that has recently grown in popularity.

This newer model would emphasize that the primary data of psychoanalysis are neither what happens in childhood nor what happens in adult life, and not even the cause-effect relationships between them. The primary data in this model are what the patient says in the analyst's consultation room, how the analyst responds, and the impact of those responses on the patient's psychological functioning, both within and outside of analysis. In this framework, the question about an interpretive intervention is not whether it explains the cause of the patient's behavior or even whether it is valid or "true," but rather whether that intervention leads to change in the behavior, whether it is effective or "works."

Interpretations, whether of the present or the past or both, are evaluated by their results. Clearly, a statement may be viewed as an accurate description of a present or past, material or psychic reality that was indeed an important causal determinant of a patient's behavior, and yet when offered as an interpretation, this statement may have little impact on that behavior. A great deal of the theory of psychoanalytic technique is designed to explain why such correct statements have no effect as interpretations. Tact, timing, phrasing, resistance, psychological mindedness, and many other reasons are invoked. Those interpretations that do have results, those that put the patient's experience in a new context, that give it new meaning, and that integrate it in a new way, may have important meaning in the patient's life, although they may have no relationship to the cause of the patient's behavior. More precisely, these interpretations may be irrelevant to considerations of cause and effect. This is the mechanism of many religious and political conversion experiences, as well as of many therapies. In this framework, psychoanalytic interpretation is seen as facilitating a new developmental progression in psychic integration, rather than the reworking of a previously unsuccessful developmental process that has been regressively revived in the treatment. This newer model would therefore see interpretation as providing a new meaning for the patient's experience and thereby changing that experience, not as explaining the cause of that experience in terms of its necessary antecedents. These alternatives are not mutually exclusive, but they are far from synonymous, and they stem from quite different intellectual traditions.

Interpretations are composed of symbols, language that crystallizes and organizes otherwise inchoate and amorphous experience. The process of interpretation, viewed from this perspective, has been described as being more like a mother teaching the meaning of words to her child than a scientist explaining the cause of a phenomenon to a student (Shapiro, 1970). As in the psychoanalytic interpretive process, the child's experience must be sufficiently differentiated and articulated to be organized by the symbol. You cannot teach a two-year-old the meaning of an abstract noun, but the process of hearing a word does more than provide a label to a preexisting category or set. It helps to create the category, to provide the organizing framework and mental structures that order the experiential world. Interpretations, like language, cannot be true or false, but they can be better or worse for certain purposes, organizing experience in ways that are more or less adaptive.

An immediate danger is apparent with this newer approach. There are well-known and effective scientific rules for deciding whether or not one event caused another. While it is true that psychoanalysis has never progressed very far in applying these rules, the complexities of the data and the difficulties of both the method and the subject matter might explain this as a practical delay rather than a theoretical impossibility. Currently, however, the criteria and rules do not exist for selecting among alternate meanings. If historical validity and scientific truth are not to be used as the criteria, how is it possible to distinguish a good interpretation from a bad one, or indeed does this distinction have any significance? One answer, discussed above, is that interpretations may be judged by their effects, but there is a disturbing circularity to the view that good interpretations should have therapeutic effects and that those interpretations that do have therapeutic effects are therefore good interpretations. In spite of this circularity, such an approach to judgment does allow the psychoanalyst to work within the realm of psychoanalytic data, the words and events of the consultation room, rather than with conjectures derived from theoretical biology or from studies of the behavior of young children.

The evaluation of a psychoanalytic interpretation will be psychoanalytic. The content of interpretations may be enriched by the analyst's understanding of biology or child development. Conversely, the interpretation may be of interest to experts in these fields, but the status of the interpretation in these other disciplines will not alter its psychoanalytic value. It may even be "wrong" by the standards of other sciences and yet be effective from the point of view of psychoanalysis.

PSYCHOANALYSIS AND THE PAST

The special role of the past in psychoanalytic theory stems from the etiologic cause-effect model. If this model is challenged, what then is the role of the past in clinical interpretations? A psychoanalytic model that disavows interest in the causes of behavior does not necessarily disavow interest in the past (Michels, 1981). The past is a primary source of meaning as well as a location of cause. Even before psychoanalysis, our interest in the past involved a search for meanings that would provide context and understanding to the present. This is a theme in both religion and history, and in the universal interest in familial origins and personal biography. We experience our personal identity in terms of our history, not because our history caused that identity, but because it is synonymous with it. The question of interpretation shifts from what are the causal determinants of adult behavior to what are the special characteristics of psychoanalytic meanings as opposed to other meanings. The question becomes, What differentiates psychoanalytic interpretations from interpretations made by the many others who attempt to suggest meanings for experience, whether religious, political, or magical? The further question is, What is the role of the past in these psychoanalytic interpretations?

The original discovery of psychoanalysis was that the hidden meaning of psychopathological symptoms was embedded in unconscious, but intensely emotionally charged memories and that the exploration of these memories, together with the disclosure of the symptoms' hidden meaning, had a therapeutic effect. This in turn was understood as suggesting that the memories were of events with etiologic significance, a plausible, but not logically necessary inference. And while such an inferred understanding may indeed be open to logical questioning, the observation upon which it is based has been replicated many times. The psychological past is important in psychoanalysis because it provides meaning to the present, regardless of cause and effect. One of the tenets of psychoanalysis is that only the living past is relevant, those memories that are active in the patient's contemporary experience and that are part of his or her current mental life, both conscious and unconscious. The past as the cause of behavior is not important therapeutically because psychoanalysis is not an etiologic treatment. But the living past that persists in active unconscious fantasies is important therapeutically because it is one of the most important determinants of present meaning, and psychoanalysis is about the present and about meaning. The past is important because it is part of the present, and particularly because it is that part most likely to be enmeshed in maladaptive patterns of conflict resolution.

Psychoanalytic interpretations have to do with the unique meanings that individuals develop in relation to their experiences of self and others, and they therefore pay close attention to the unique characteristics of individual histories. Political and religious interpretations tend to ignore individual characteristics and to seek meaning by studying the general characteristics of people's relationships with each other, with the social order, or with the future.

INTERPRETATIONS AND THE THERAPEUTIC PROCESS

Psychoanalysis discovered that the meanings that individuals create from events can be far more significant than the events that serve as stimuli for those meanings. This is also true of interpretations as events. The analyst may believe that he or she is interpreting the here and now or the past, but the patient will hear the analyst's interpretations in terms of the psychological complexes that are active at that time in his or her own mental life and in terms of the phase of the treatment and the nature of the transference. As a result, if we wish to know what an interpretation is about, it may be more important to know what was going on in the analysis and in the patient's mind at the time that the interpretation was made than to know what words the analyst said. Most of the time in a successful analytic process, the patient is involved in a complex mixture of concerns: concerns with his or her current relationship with the analyst, concerns with memories of earlier relationships reactivated by the current one, concerns with the impact of those earlier memories on the current relationship and with the impact of the current relationship on the memories, and so on in a never-ending process of reverberating resonance.

Individual interpretations may be aimed at one or another concern, at the past, at the here and now, or at the interaction between them. If they are successful, though, it is because they become part of the reverberating process and because they in turn influence it. An interpretation directed to the here and now must therefore be related to or at least open to the patient's memories and fantasies of the past if it is to have the possibility of enlarging the patient's experience of the here and now, of providing it with new meanings. Similarly, an interpretation directed to the past must be about that living past that is shaping and forming the patient's present if it is to have a therapeutic impact and alter the present. Some interpretations do both at once. Some poor interpretations may be "true," but they are truths which have no psychic relevance. Such statements about the patient's mental development or mental functioning may be of interest to a psychodynamicist or a psychogeneticist, but they will have no impact on the patient's inner world. The question is not whether a specific interpretation is directed at the present or at the past, but whether it is part of an interpretive net, a therapeutic process that involves both. It is the nature of this process, rather than the focus of a specific interpretation, that defines psychoanalysis.

The special role of transference in the therapeutic and interpretive process may be easier to understand in these terms. Transference refers to the blending of past and present in the patient's relationship with the analyst, and transference interpretations therefore combine past and present in an immediate and intimate human context. For interpretations to be heard, they must be related to issues that are on the patient's mind, and in most psychoanalyses, these issues are more often transference issues than anything else. In other forms of treatment, and even in psychoanalysis at times of dramatic life events, transference themes may be displaced from the center of the patient's attention. At such times, the interpretive process either should be suspended or should be shifted to the area of psychological concern, to the "now" that is not "here" but is outside the transference. It is less common for the patient to be preoccupied with the past without obvious relation to the present, and if the patient is truly preoccupied, it is always with a past that is really present. The past also may appear as a defensive avoidance of the present or as a transferential compliance with what the patient believes the analyst wants. Sometimes, too, a contact with someone who was significant in the patient's childhood, the discovery of a critical fact about the past, an anniversary or symbolic reminder, or some similar event may command the patient's attention to the past. Still, the general principle of interpreting what is on the patient's mind applies, along with the corollary of interpreting in a way that expands what is on his mind, that emphasizes linkages and relationships, and that facilitates the integration of past and present.

INTERPRETATION OF THE PAST AND THE HERE AND NOW

Our question about the current role of the past in psychoanalytic interpretations may be answered by the following suggestions. Psychoanalysis is about the meaningful (not causal) relationship of present and past, the way in which childhood fantasies and memories persist unconsciously and shape the present, interacting with the present external reality. Psychoanalytic interpretations are about the patient's experience of that process, and they may be directed at any aspect of that experience, at childhood fantasy, at present reality, or at the interaction between them. In turn, these interpretations become a part of the process and influence it. This is what psychoanalytic treatment is about. Furthermore, since interpretations are couched in language, they always mean that this memory or this experience is related to all of the memories and experiences that have been described with the same language in the past. Thus, the use of language, after the very first introduction to it, always involves a genetic interpretation.

The dichotomies of past and present, childhood and transference, memory and desire, genetic and dynamic, id and ego, content and resistance, reconstruction and interpretation, all refer to themes or components of a dialectical process. That process must include both members of each dichotomy if it is to lead to a psychoanalytic integration. Therapeutically effective communications in an analysis must be concrete, specific, and brief, and so any given interpretation is only about a small piece of this totality. In time, however, this piece must be brought together with the others. Only then is the process psychoanalytic.

References for Chapter 1

Implications of Infancy Research for Psychoanalytic Theory and Practice

Bates E.: Language and Context: The Acquisition of Pragmatics. New York and London, Academic Press, 1976.

Benjamin J.D.: Developmental biology and psychoanalysis, in Psychoanalysis and Current Biological Thought. Edited by Greasfield N.S., Lewis W.C. Madison and Milwaukee, University of Wisconsin Press, 1965.

Bloom L.: One Word at a Time. The Hague, Mouton, 1933.

Bornstein M.H.: Qualities of color vision in infancy. J. Exptl. Child Psychol. 19:401–419, 1975.

Bower G.: Mood and memory. Am. Psychologist 36:129–148, 1981.

Brazelton T.B.: New knowledge about the infant from current research: implications for psychoanalysis. Paper presented at the American Psychoanalytic Association Meeting, San Francisco, May 1980.

Brazelton T.B., Yogman M., Als H., et al.: The infant as a focus for family reciprocity, in The Child and Its Family. Edited by Lewis M., Rosenblum L.A. New York, Plenum Press, 1974.

Bretherton I.: Early person knowledge as expressed in gestural and verbal communication, in Infant Social Cognition. Edited by Lamb M.E., Sherrod L.R. Hillsdale, N.J., Lawrence Erlbaum Associates, 1981.

Bruner J.S.: The ontogenesis of speech acts. J. Child Language 2:1–19, 1975.

Cohen L.B., Salapatek P. (eds.): Perception of Speech and Sound, in Infant Perception: From Sensation to Cognition, vol. 2. New York, Academic Press, 1975.

DeLoache J.S., Strauss M.S., Maynard J.: Picture perception in infancy. Infant Behavior and Development 2:77–89, 1979.

Eimas P.D.: Speech perception in early infancy, in Infant Perception: From Sensation to Cognition, vol. 2. Edited by Cohen L.B., Salapatek P. New York, Academic Press, 1975.

Eimas P.D., Siqueland E.R., Jusczyk P., et al.: Speech perception in infants. Science 171:303–306, 1971.

Emde R., Gaensbauer T., Harmon R.: Emotional expression in infancy: a biobehavioral study. Psychol. Issues 10:1–200, 1976.

Esman A.H.: "The stimulus barrier"—a review and reconsideration. Unpublished paper submitted for publication, 1982.

Fagan J.F.: Infants' delayed recognition memory and forgetting. J. Exptl. Child Psychol. 16:424–450, 1973.

Field T.: Imitation by neonates. Paper presented at the New York Infancy Group, New York, May 1981.

Fraiberg S.: Libidinal constancy and mental representation. Psychoanal. Study Child 24:9–47, 1969.

Friedman L.: The interplay of evocation. Paper presented at the Postgraduate Center for Mental Health, New York, May 1982.

Freud S.: Beyond the pleasure principle (1920), in Complete Psychological Works, standard ed. vol. 18. London, Hogarth Press, 1955.

Gediman H.: The concept of stimulus barrier: its review and reformulation as an adaptive ego function. Int. J. Psychoanal. 52:243–257, 1971.

Gibson E.J.: Principles of Perceptual Learning and Development. New York, Appleton-Century-Crofts, 1969.

Hofer M.: The Roots of Human Behavior. San Francisco, W.H. Freeman & Co., 1980.

Hoffman M.L.: Toward a theory of empathic arousal and development, in The Development of Affect. Edited by Lewis M., Rosenblum L.A. New York, Plenum Press, 1978.

Kagan J., Kearsley R.B., Zelano P.R.: Infancy: Its Place in Human Development. Cambridge, Harvard University Press, 1978.

Knapp S.: Discussion of "The Interplay of Evocation" by L. Friedman. Paper presented at the Postgraduate Center for Mental Health, New York, May 1982.

Kohut H.: Intraspection, empathy, and the semicircle of mental health. Int. J. Psychoanal. in press, 1982.

Lamb M.E., Sherrod L.R., (eds.): Infant Social Cognition. Hillsdale, N.J., Lawrence Erlbaum Associates, 1981.

Lichtenberg J.: Implications for psychoanalytic theory of research on the neonate. Int. Rev. Psychoanal. 8:35–52, 1981.

MacKain K., Studdert-Kennedy M., Spieker S., et al.: Infant perception of auditory-visual relations for speech. Science 1982, in press.

Mahler M., Furer M.: On Human Symbiosis and the Vicissitudes of Individuation. New York, International Universities Press, 1968.

Mahler M., Pine F., Bergman A.: The Psychological Birth of the Human Infant. New York, Basic Books, 1975.

Meltzoff A.N., Borton R.W.: Intermodal matching by human neonates. Nature 282:403–404, 1979.

Meltzoff A.N., Moore M.K.: Imitation of facial and manual gestures by human neonates. Science 198:75–78, 1977.

Nachman P.: Memory for stimuli reacted to with positive and neutral affect in seven-month-old infants. Doctoral Dissertation, Graduate School of Arts and Sciences, Columbia University, 1982.

Nachman P., Stern D.N.: Recall memory for emotional experience in pre-linguistic infants. Paper presented at the National Clinical Infancy Conference, Yale University, New Haven, CT., January 1982.

Newson J.: A general approach to the systematic description of mother-infant interaction, in Studies on Interaction in Infancy. Edited by Schaffer H.R. London, Academic Press, 1977.

Papousek H.: A method of studying conditioned foot reflexes in young children up to the age of six months. Parlor J. of Higher Nervous Activity 9:136–140, 1959.

Piaget J.: The Construction of Reality in the Child (1937). Translated by Cook M. New York, Basic Books, 1954.

Piaget J.: The Origins of Intelligence in Children. New York, International Universities Press, 1952.

Rovée-Collier C.K., Lepsitt L.P.: Learning, adaptation, and memory, in Psychobiology of the Human Newborn. Edited by Stratton P.M. New York, John Wiley & Sons, 1981.

Rovée-Collier C.K., Sullivan M.W., Enright M., et al.: Reactivation of infant memory. Science 208:1159–1161, 1980.

Sander L.: New knowledge about the infant from current research: implications for psychoanalysis. J. Am. Psychoanal. Assoc. 28:181–198, 1980a.

Sander L.: Polarity, paradox, and the organizing process in development. Paper presented at the First World Congress of Infant Psychiatry. Cascais, Portugal, March 1980b.

Schwaber E.: Self psychology and the concept of psychopathology: a case presentation, in Advances in Self Psychology. Edited by Goldberg A. New York, International Universities Press, 1980.

Snow C.: Mothers' speech to children learning language. Child Development 43:549–565, 1972.

Spelke E.S.: Infants' intermodal perception of events. Cognitive Psychology 8:553–560, 1976.

Spelke E.S.: Perceiving bimodally specified events in infancy. Developmental Psychology 15:626–636, 1979.

Stechler G., Carpenter G.: A viewpoint on early affective development, in The Exceptional Infant, vol. 2. Edited by Hellmuth J. Seattle, Special Child Publications, 1967.

Stern D.N.: Mother and infant at play: the dyadic interaction involving facial, vocal, and gaze behaviors, in The Effect of the Infant on Its Caregiver. Edited by Lewis M., Rosenblum L. New York, John Wiley & Sons, 1974.

Stern D.N.: The early development of schemas of self, of other, and of various experiences of "self with other." Paper presented at the Symposium on Reflections on Self Psychology. Boston Psychoanalytic Society and Institute, Boston, October 1980.

Stern D.N.: The First Relationship: Infant and Mother. Cambridge, Harvard University Press, 1977.

Stern D.N., Hofer L., Haft W., et al.: The attunement of affect states. Paper presented at the Thirteenth Annual Margaret S. Mahler Symposium Series, Symposium on Child Development. Philadelphia, May 1982.

Trevarthan C.: The foundations of intersubjectivity: development of interpersonal and cooperative understanding in infants, in The Social Foundation of Language and Thought, Essays in Honor of Jerome S. Bruner. Edited by Olson D.R. New York, W.W. Norton & Co., 1980.

Trevarthan C.: Communication and cooperation in early infancy: a description of primary intersubjectivity, in Before Speech. Edited by Bullowa M. Cambridge, Harvard University Press, 1979.

Watson J.S.: Perception of contingency as a determinant of social responsiveness, in The Origins of Social Responsiveness. Edited by Thoman E. Hillsdale, N.J., Lawrence Erlbaum Associates, 1979.

Werner H.: The Comparative Psychology of Mental Development. New York, International Universities Press, 1948.

Werner H., Kaplan B.: Symbol Formation. New York, John Wiley & Sons, 1964.

Winnicott D.W.: Playing and Reality. New York, Basic Books, 1971.

Wolff P.: The causes, controls and organization of behavior in the neonate. Psychol. Issues 5:17, 1966.

Zajonc R.B.: Feeling and thinking: preferences need no inferences. Am. Psychol. 35:151–175, 1980.

References for Chapter 2

Psychoanalytic Studies of Group Processes: Theory and Applications

Anderson P.: Considerations on Western Marxism. London, NLB, 1976.

Althusser L.: Positions. Paris, Editions Sociales, 1976.

Anzieu D.: L'illusion groupale. Nouvelle Revue de Psychanalyse 4:73–93, 1971.

Anzieu D.: Le groupe et L'inconscient: L'imaginaire groupal. Paris, Dunod, 1981.

Arlow J.A.: Psychoanalytic knowledge of group processes. Panel Report. J. Am. Psychoanal. Assoc. 27:147–149, 1979.

Bach G.R.: Intensive Group Psychotherapy. New York, Ronald Press, 1954.

Bion W.R.: Experiences in Groups. New York, Basic Books, 1961.

Bion W.R.: Attention and Interpretation. London, Heineman, 1970.

Braunschweig D., Fain M.: Eros et Anteros. Paris, Petite Bibliotheque Payot, 1971.

Canetti E.: Masse und Macht. Frankfurt/Main, Fischer Taschenbuch Verlag, 1980.

Chasseguet-Smirgel J.: L'Idéal du Moi. Paris, Claude Tchou, 1975.

Colman A.D., Bexton W.H. (eds.): Group Relations Reader. Sausalito, CA, Grex, 1975.

De Board R.: The Psychoanalysis of Organizations. London, Tavistock Publications, 1978.

de Mare P.B.: Perspectives in Group Psychotherapy: A Theoretical Background. New York, Science House, 1972.

Durkin H.E.: The Group in Depth. New York, International Universities Press, 1964.

Ezriel H.: A psychoanalytic approach to the treatment of patients in groups. J. Ment. Science 96:774–779, 1950.

Foucault M.: History of Sexuality: An Introduction. New York, Pantheon, 1978.

Foulkes S.H., Anthony E.J.: Group Psychotherapy: The Psychoanalytic Approach. Baltimore, Penguin Books, 1957.

Freud S.: Totem and taboo (1913), in Complete Psychological Works, standard ed., vol. 13. London, Hogarth Press, 1953.

Freud S.: Group psychology and the analysis of the ego (1921), in Complete Psychological Works, standard ed., vol. 18. London, Hogarth Press, 1955.

Jaques E.: Social systems as a defense against persecutory and depressive anxiety, in New Directions in Psychoanalysis. New York, Basic Books, 1955.

Jaques E.: A General Theory of Bureaucracy. New York, Halsted, 1976.

Jaques E.: The Form of Time. New York, Crane-Russak, 1982.

Jones M.: Therapeutic Community: A New Treatment Method in Psychiatry. New York, Basic Books, 1953.

Kaes R.: L'idéologie: études Psychanalytiques. Paris, Dunod, 1980.

Katz D., Kahn R.L.: The Social Psychology of Organizations. New York, John Wiley & Sons, 1966.

Kernberg O.F.: Advantages and liabilities of therapeutic community models, in The Individual and the Group, vol. 1. Edited by Pine M., Rafaelsen L. London, Plenum Publishing Corp, 1982.

Kernberg O.F.: A systems approach to priority setting of interventions in groups. Int. J. Group Psychother. 25:251–275, 1975.

Kernberg O.F.: Internal World and External Reality: Object Relations Theory Applied. New York, Jason Aronson, 1980.

Kernberg O.F.: Object Relations Theory and Clinical Psychoanalysis. New York, Jason Aronson, 1976.

Kernberg O.F.: Some issues in the theory of hospital treatment. Soertrykk av Tidsskrift for den norske loegeforening 14:837–843, 1981.

Lasch C.: Haven in a Heartless World. New York, Basic Books, 1977.

Lasch C.: The Culture of Narcissism. New York, W.W. Norton & Co., 1978.

Lasch C.: The Freudian left and cultural revolution. New Left Review 129:23−34, 1981.

Lawrence W.G. (ed.): Exploring Individual and Organizational Boundaries. New York, John Wiley & Sons, 1979.

Le Bon G.: The Crowd (1895). New York, Ballantine, 1969.

Levinson H.: Organizational Diagnosis. Cambridge, Harvard University Press, 1972.

Lewin K.: Field Theory in Social Science. New York, Harper & Row, 1951.

Main T.F.: The ailment. Br. J. Med. Psychology 30:129−145, 1957.

Main T.F.: The hospital as a therapeutic institution. Bull. Menninger Clinic, 10:66−70, 1946.

Malan D.H., Balfor F.H.G., Hood V.G., et al.: Group psychotherapy: a long-term follow-up study. Arch. Gen. Psychiatry 33:1303−1315, 1976.

Marcuse H.: Eros and Civilization: A Philosophical Inquiry Into Freud. Boston, Beacon Press, 1955.

Menzies I.E.P.: The functioning of social systems as defense against anxiety. A report on the study of a nursing service of a general hospital. Tavistock Pamphlet No. 3, 1967.

Miller E.J.: Task and Organization. New York, John Wiley & Sons, 1976.

Miller E.J., Rice A.K.: Systems of Organization. London, Tavistock Publications, 1967.

Mitscherlich A.: Auf dem Weg zur vaterlosen Gesellschaft: Ideen zur Sozial-Psychologie. Muenchen, R. Piper & Co., Verlag 1963.

Ortega y Gasset J.: La Rebelión de las Masas (1929). Madrid, Expasa-Calpe, SA, 1976.

Reich W.: The Sexual Revolution: Toward a Self-Governing Character Structure (1935). New York, The Noonday Press, 1962.

Rice A.K.: The Enterprise and Its Environment. London, Tavistock Publications, 1963.

Rice A.K.: Learning for Leadership. London, Tavistock Publications, 1965.

Rice A.K.: Individual, group, and intergroup processes. Human Relations 22:565−584, 1969.

Rioch M.: Group relations: rationale and techniques. Int. J. Group Psychother. 10:340−355, 1970a.

Rioch M.: The work of Wilfred Bion on groups. Psychiatry 33:56−66, 1970b.

Robinson P.A.: The Freudian Left. New York, Harper Colophon Books, 1969.

Scheidlinger S.: Focus on Group Psychotherapy: Clinical Essays. New York, International Universities Press, 1982.

Scheidlinger S.: Group process in group psychotherapy. Am. J. Psychother. 14:104−120, 1960.

Scheidlinger S. (ed.): Psychoanalytic Group Dynamics. New York, International Universities Press, 1980.

Shapiro R.: Psychoanalytic knowledge of group processes. Panel Report. J. Am. Psychoanal. Assoc. 27:150−152, 1979.

Skynner A.C.R.: Systems of Family and Marital Psychotherapy. New York, Brunner/Mazel, 1976.

Slavson S.R.: A critique of the group therapy literature. Acta Psychother. 10:62−73, 1962.

Slavson S.R.: The era of group psychotherapy. Acta Psychother. 7:167−196, 1959.

Slavson S.R.: A Textbook in Analytic Group Psychotherapy. New York, International Universities Press, 1964.

Stanton A.M., Schwartz M.: The Mental Hospital. New York, Basic Books, 1954.

Stéphane A.: L'Univers Contestationnaire. Paris, Petite Bibliotheque Payot, 1969.

Sutherland J.D.: Notes on psychoanalytic group therapy. I: Therapy and training. Psychiatry 15:111−117, 1952.

Turquet P.: Threats to identity in the large group, in The Large Group: Dynamics and Therapy. Edited by Kreeger L. London, Constable, 1975.

Whiteley J.S., Gordon J.: Group Approaches in Psychiatry. Boston, Routledge & Kegan Paul, 1979.

Wolf A., Schwartz M.: Psychoanalysis in Groups. New York, Grune & Stratton, 1962.

Zaleznik A.: Psychoanalytic knowledge of group processes. Panel Report. J. Am. Psychoanalytic Assoc. 27:149−150, 1979.

References for Chapter 3

The Influence of Values in Psychoanalysis: The Case of Female Psychology

Barglow P., Schaefer M.: A new female psychology? J. Am. Psychoanal. Assoc. 24:305−350, 1976.

Blum H.P.: Masochism, the ego ideal, and the psychology of women. J. Am. Psychoanal. Assoc. 24:157−191, 1976.

Broverman I.K., Broverman D.M., Clarkson F.E., et al.: Sex-role stereotypes and clinical judgments of mental health. J. Consult Clin. Psychol. 34:1−7, 1970.

Chodorow N.: The Reproduction of Mothering: Psychoanalysis and the Sociology of Gender. Berkeley, CA, University of California Press, 1978.

Ehrenreich B., Hess E., Jacobs G.: A report on the sex crisis. Ms Magazine, 61−88, March 1982.

Eissler K.: Notes on problems of technique in the psychoanalytic treatment of adolescents: with some remarks on perversions. Psychoanal. Study Child 13:223−254, 1958.

Freud S.: The dissolution of the oedipus complex (1924), in Complete Psychological Works, standard ed., vol. 19. London, Hogarth Press, 1961.

Freud S.: Some psychical consequences of the anatomical distinction between the sexes (1925), in Complete Psychological Works, standard ed., vol. 19. London, Hogarth Press, 1961.

Freud S.: Female sexuality (1931), in Complete Psychological Works, standard ed., vol. 21. London, Hogarth Press, 1961.

Freud S.: Femininity (1933), in Complete Psychological Works, standard ed., vol. 22. London, Hogarth Press, 1964.

Gilligan C.: In a Different Voice: Psychological Theory and Women's Development. Cambridge, Harvard University Press, 1982.

Gross M.: The Psychological Society. New York, Random House, 1978.

Grossman W.I., Stewart W.A.: Penis envy: from childhood wish to developmental metaphor. J. Am. Psychoanal. Assoc. 24:193−212, 1976.

Hare R.: The philosophical basis of psychiatric ethics, in Psychiatric Ethics. Edited by Block S., Chodoff P. New York, Oxford University Press, 1981.

Hogan R.T., Emler N.T.: The biases in contemporary social psychology, in Social Research: An International Quarterly in the Social Sciences 45:(3) 478−534, 1978.

Horney K.: On the genesis of the castration complex in women. Int. J. Psychoanal. 5:50–65, 1924.

Horney K.: The flight from womanhood; the masculinity-complex in women, as viewed by men and by women. Int. J. Psychoanal. 7:324–339, 1926.

Horney K.: The dread of women, observations on a specific difference in the dread felt by men and by women respectively for the opposite sex. Int. J. Psychoanal. 13:348–360, 1932.

Horney K.: The denial of the vagina, a contribution to the problem of the genital anxieties specific to women. Int. J. Psychoanal. 14:57–70, 1933.

Howell E.: Women: from Freud to the present, in Women and Mental Health. Edited by Howell E., Bayes M. New York, Basic Books, 1981.

Jones E.: The early development of female sexuality. Int. J. Psychoanal. 8:459–472, 1927.

Jones E.: Early female sexuality. Int. J. Psychoanal. 16:263–275, 1935.

Jones E.: The phallic phase. Int. J. Psychoanal. 14:1–33, 1933.

Klerman G.L.: Testing analytic hypotheses: are personality attributes predisposed to depression? in. Psychoanalysis: Critical Explorations in Contemporary Theory and Practice. Edited by Jacobson A.M., Parmalee D.X. New York, Brunner/Mazel, 1982.

Kuhn T.S.: The Structure of Scientific Revolutions. Chicago, University of Chicago Press, 1962.

Lerner H.: Penis envy: alternatives in conceptualization. Bull Menninger Clin. 44:39–48, 1980.

Lichtenstein H.: The changing concept of psychosexual development. J. Am. Psychoanal. Assoc. 18:300–318, 1970.

Lichtenstein H.: Identity and sexuality. J. Am. Psychoanal. Assoc. 9:179–260, 1961.

Macklin R.: Values in psychoanalysis and psychotherapy: a survey and analysis. J. Am. Psychoanal. Assoc. 33:133–150, 1973.

Marcus S.: Culture and psychoanalysis. Partisan Review 2:224–252, 1982.

Marmor J.: Changing patterns of femininity: psychoanalytic implications, in Psychoanalysis and Women. Edited by Miller J.B. New York, Brunner/Mazel, 1973.

Masters W.H., Johnson V.E.: Human Sexual Response. Boston, Little, Brown, & Co., 1966.

Millett K.: Sexual Politics. New York, Doubleday, 1970.

Modell A.H.: Affects and the complementarity of biologic and historical meaning, in The Annual of Psychoanalysis vol. 6. New York, International Universities Press, 1978.

Money J., Hampson J.G., Hampson J.L.: An examination of some basic sexual concepts: the evidence of human hermaphroditism. Bull. Johns Hopkins Hosp. 97:301–310, 1955a.

Money J., Hampson J.G., Hampson J.L.: Hermaphroditism: recommendations concerning assignment of sex, change of sex, and psychologic management. Bull. Johns Hopkins Hosp. 97:284–300, 1955b.

Money J., Hampson J.G., Hampson J.L.: Sexual incongruities and psychopathology: the evidence of human hermaphroditism. Bull. Johns Hopkins Hosp. 98:43–57, 1956.

Morgenthau H., Person E.: The roots of narcissism. Partisan Review 3:337–347, 1978.

Moulton R.: A survey and re-evaluation of the concept of penis envy, in Psychoanalysis and Women. Edited by Miller J.B., New York, Brunner/Mazel, 1973.

Ovesey L.: Masculine aspirations in women: an adaptational analysis in psychiatry. J. Study Interpersonal Processes 19:341–351, 1956.

Person E.S.: Sexuality as the mainstay of identity: psychoanalytic perspectives. Signs: J. of Women in Culture and Society 5:605–630, 1980.

Person E.S.: Some observations on femininity, in Women and Analysis: Dialogues on Psychoanalytic Views of Femininity. Edited by Strouse E. New York, Grossman, 1974.

Person E.S.: Women working: fears of failure, deviance and success. J. Am. Acad. Psychoanal. 10:67–84, 1982.

Rieff P.: Freud: The Mind of the Moralist. New York, Anchor Edition, Doubleday, 1961.

Rieff P.: The Triumph of the Therapeutic: Uses of Faith After Freud. New York, Harper & Row, 1966.

Rohrbaugh J.B.: Women: Psychology's Puzzle. New York, Basic Books/Harper Colophon Books, 1979.

Ross N.: The primacy of genitality in the light of ego psychology. J. Am. Psychoanal. Assoc. 18:267–284, 1970.

Schafer R.: Problems in Freud's psychology of women. J. Am. Psychoanal. Assoc. 22:459–489, 1974.

Stoller R.: Sex and Gender. New York, Science House, 1968.

Thompson C.: Penis envy in women (1943), in Psychoanalysis and Women. Edited by Miller J.B. New York, Brunner/Mazel, 1973.

Thompson C.: Some effects of the derogatory attitude towards female sexuality. Psychiatry 13:349–354, 1950.

Tyson P.: A developmental line of gender identity, gender role, and choice of love object. J. Am. Psychoanal. Assoc. 30:61–86, 1982.

Vaughter R.M.: Review essay on psychology. Signs: J. of Women in Culture and Society 2:120–146, 1976.

References for Chapter 4

Has the Scope of Psychoanalysis Changed?

Alexander F.: Two forms of regression and their therapeutic implications. Psychoanal. Q. 25:178–196, 1956.

Balint M.: The Basic Fault. London, Tavistock Publications, 1968.

Eissler K.: The effect of the structure of the ego on psychoanalytic technique. J. Am. Psychoanal. Assoc. 1:104–143, 1952.

Erikson E.: Childhood and Society. New York, W.W. Norton & Co., 1950.

Ferenczi S., Rank O.: The Development of Psychoanalysis. New York/Washington, Nervous & Mental Disease Publishing Co., 1924.

Freud S.: The ego and the id (1923), in Complete Psychological Works, standard ed., vol. 19. London, Hogarth Press, 1961.

Freud S.: On beginning the treatment (1913), in Complete Psychological Works, standard ed., vol. 12. London, Hogarth Press, 1958.

Freud S.: On psychotherapy (1905), in Complete Psychological Works, standard ed., vol. 7. London, Hogarth Press, 1953.

Goldberg A. (ed.): The Psychology of the Self: A Casebook. New York, International Universities Press, 1978.

Kernberg O.F.: Borderline personality organization. J. Am. Psychoanal. Assoc. 15:641–685, 1967.

Kohut H.: The Analysis of the Self. New York, International Universities Press, 1971.

Kohut H.: The Restoration of the Self. New York, International Universities Press, 1977.

Loewald H.: Regression: some general considerations. Psychoanal. Q. 50:22–43, 1981.

Mahler M.S.: A study of the separation-individuation process. Psychoanal. Study Child 26:403–424, 1971.

Modell A.H.: "The holding environment" and the therapeutic action of psychoanalysis. J. Am. Psychoanal. Assoc. 24:285–307, 1976.

Myerson P.: The nature of transactions that occur in other than classical analysis. Int. Rev. Psychoanal. 8:173–189, 1981.

Stone L.: The widening scope of indications for psychoanalysis. J. Am. Psychoanal. Assoc. 2:567–594, 1954.

Zetzel E.R.: Current concepts of transference. Int. J. Psychoanal. 37:369–376, 1956.

References for Chapter 5

Contemporary Psychoanalytic Views of Interpretation

Blum H.P.: The value of reconstruction in adult psychoanalysis. Int. J. Psychoanal. 61:39–52, 1980.

Friedman L.: Trends in the psychoanalytic theory of treatment. Psychoanal. Q. 47:524–567, 1978.

Gill M.M.: The analysis of the transference. J. Am. Psychoanal. Assoc. 27:263–288, 1979.

Glover E.: The Technique of Psychoanalysis. New York, International Universities Press, 1958.

Greenacre P.: Reconstruction and the process of individuation. Psychoanal. Study Child 34:121–144, 1979.

Greenacre P.: A historical sketch of the use and disuse of reconstruction. Psychoanal. Study Child 35:35–40, 1980.

Greenacre P.: Reconstruction: its nature and therapeutic value. J. Am. Psychoanal. Assoc. 29:27–46, 1981.

Greenson R.R.: The Technique and Practice of Psychoanalysis. New York, International Universities Press, 1967.

Kris A.O.: Free Association: Method and Process. New Haven, Yale University Press, 1982.

Leavy S.A.: Psychoanalytic interpretation. Psychoanal. Study Child 28:305–330, 1973.

Leavy S.A.: The Psychoanalytic Dialogue. New Haven, Yale University Press, 1980.

Michels R.: The present and the past. Bull. Assoc. Psychoanal. Med. 20:49–56, 1981.

Michels R.: The scientific and clinical functions of psychoanalytic theory, in The Future of Psychoanalysis. Edited by Goldberg A., Wolf E. New York, International Universities Press, in press, 1983.

Sandler J., Dare C., Holder A.: The Patient and the Analyst. The Basis of the Psychoanalytic Process. New York, International Universities Press, 1973.

Schafer R.: The relevance of the "here and now" transference interpretation to the reconstruction of early development. Int. J. Psychoanal. 63:77–82, 1982.

Shapiro T.: Interpretation and naming. J. Am. Psychoanal. Assoc. 18:399–421, 1970.

Simons R.: Contemporary problems of psychoanalytic technique. J. Am. Psychoanal. Assoc. 29:643–658, 1981.

Stone L.: Notes on the noninterpretive elements in the psychoanalytic situation and process. J. Am. Psychoanal. Assoc. 29:89–118, 1981a.

Stone L.: Some thoughts on the "here and now" in psychoanalytic technique and process. Psychoanal. Q. 50:709–733, 1981b.

Valenstein A.F.: Insight as an embedded concept in the early historical phase of psychoanalysis. Psychoanal. Study Child 36:307–315, 1981.

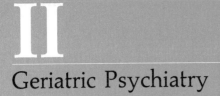

II
Geriatric Psychiatry

Part II

Geriatric Psychiatry

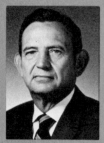

Ewald W. Busse, M.D.,
Preceptor

J.P. Gibbons Professor of Psychiatry
Department of Psychiatry
Duke University Medical Center

Authors for Part II

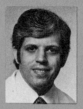

Dan Blazer, M.D., Ph.D.
Associate Professor of Psychiatry
Head, Division of Social and
   Community Psychiatry
Department of Psychiatry
Duke University Medical Center

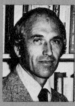

R. Bruce Sloane, M.D.
Franz Alexander Professor of
   Psychiatry
Chairman, Department of Psychiatry
   and the Behavioral Sciences
University of Southern California
   School of Medicine

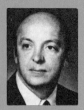

Robert O. Friedel, M.D.

Professor and Chairman
Department of Psychiatry
Medical College of Virginia
   Campus
Virginia Commonwealth University

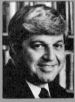

Carl Eisdorfer, Ph.D., M.D.

Departments of Psychiatry
   and Neurosciences
Montefiore Medical Center
Albert Einstein College
   of Medicine

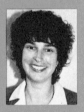

Donna Cohen, Ph.D.

Departments of Psychiatry
   and Neurosciences
Montefiore Medical Center
Albert Einstein College
   of Medicine

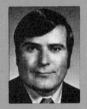

Eric Pfeiffer, M.D.

Professor of Psychiatry
   and Director
Suncoast Gerontology Center
University of South Florida
   Medical Center

Geriatric
Psychiatry

Introduction
by Ewald W. Busse, M.D.

Over centuries of recorded human existence, people have persisted in hoping that death was not certain, that immortality or resurrection by divine fiat was possible, and that the adverse changes associated with aging would be eliminated. One of the earliest legends linked with avoiding death is found in the Babylonian poem, "The Epic of Gilagmesh," which is believed to have originated about 3000 B.C. (Gruman, 1966). On the bottom of the sea, Gilagmesh finds a thorny plant which possesses the power of rejuvenation. But he subsequently loses the plant when it is eaten by a serpent. In the modern era, death is usually accepted as inevitable. The emphasis has shifted to the possibility of extending the human life span, and life has indeed been prolonged throughout the world. Today's hope focuses on understanding the aging processes and developing preventive measures. Enmeshed within this broader hope are the specific goals of prolonging sexual activity, avoiding the loss of mental capacity, and maintaining the physical ability to pursue an active and satisfying life.

The mere prolongation of life could bring more detriments than assets, as we are currently witnessing in the apparent increase in the numbers of persons with dementia of late life. Life is being prolonged, but we are unable to avoid many of the incapacities of aging. Mythology and literature foretold our predicament. The Greek goddess Aurora with great effort persuaded Zeus to grant her husband Tithonus immortality. Unfortunately, Aurora did not ask and Zeus did not grant eternal youth for Tithonus. He became more and more mentally disabled and frequently prayed for death. In one version of the myth Tithonus escaped his misery by turning into a cicada. The male of this insect produces a shrill sound similar to the voice of an old demented person (Kerenyi, 1974). In *Gulliver's Travels*, Swift's hero encountered the pathetic Struldbrugs. These unfortunate persons could not die, but had every physical and mental disability gradually increasing.

Attempts to prolong youth have existed for centuries. One of the best known was the determined but misinformed effort by medieval European adventurers to find the fountain of youth. The second-century writer and geographer Pausanias created mystical stories about the search for a fountain of youth, and his works were revived and popularized centuries later to inspire new quests. Ponce de Leon's 1512 expedition was organized and financed for such a quest, but he found instead what is now the state of Florida.

Rejuvenation efforts were abundant in the Near and Far East centuries ago. One which persisted in many societies is called gerocomy. Gerocomy is the belief and practice that a man, particularly an older man, absorbs virtue and youth from women, particularly younger women. King David in the Old Testament believed in gerocomy and practiced it accordingly. There is clear evidence that the Romans had a similar view. In recent times gerocomy is believed to have been associated with the downfall of Mahatma Gandhi. In his extensive review of Gandhi's life, Erik Erikson (1969) indicates that in spite of Gandhi's expressed preference for celibacy, he was accused of gerocomy, and that this contributed to his political demise.

The search for a method of rejuvenation has led to some bizarre approaches in our modern society. Medvedev, a respected Russian geneticist now living in London, has published an account of a rejuvenation technique that was advocated by a woman named O.B. Lepeshinskaya, a disciple of the pseudoscientist Lysenko. She first advocated the use of soda baths in 1949, claiming that they would prolong life and restore youth. Lysenko supported this practice, and it became widespread in the USSR. Within a short time, the soda baths were replaced by the drinking of soda water and finally by the introduction of soda into the body by enema. Medvedev explains that the latter two techniques were used as substitutes for the baths by those who were unable to take frequent soda baths. Lepeshinskaya also claimed that she could make living from nonliving material (Busse, 1981).

Interest has not faded in reaching the age of one hundred years or more while maintaining a vigorous life. In recent years, the media have periodically given attention to several small groups which are reportedly particularly long-lived. These are the Abkhasians of the Republic of Georgia in the USSR, the inhabitants of Vilcabamba, a small village in Ecuador, and a third group in the Karakoram Range in Kashmir. These groups have all been studied by competent scientists, and claims of their being especially long-lived have been proven invalid (Busse, 1981).

Geriatric psychiatrists and mental health workers associated with the care of the elderly are aware of prejudice, bias, and numerous misunderstandings that impair the quality of care for the elderly. The possibility that this social phenomenon may be more prevalent in the United States than elsewhere is debatable, however. Elderly people maintain positions of leadership in the United States and in other modern societies. This is evident in the age of the national leaders in the USSR, China, and to a lesser extent the United States. The existence of gerontophobia (Comfort, 1967) and the prejudice and bias affecting elderly people have been reviewed in some detail (Busse, 1968; 1977), and these issues have also been highlighted by Butler (1975).

During the last several decades, professional concern about the conditions that elderly people confront in themselves and in their environments has led to a number of public and private organizational efforts to understand and mitigate these conditions.

Authorized by the constitution of the American Psychiatric Association, the APA Council on Aging was established in 1979 with the following rationale:

> The APA represents a body of knowledge, experience, and skills indispensable to the identification, treatment, relief, and prevention of mental disorders in the aging population. The APA identified six specific areas of activity including evaluation and diagnosis, training, interface problems between psychiatry and other disciplines in geriatric care, design of services and third party payment for psychiatric treatment of the elderly, decisions made by government that influence the mental health of the aged, and lastly identifying and implementing research into the problems of geriatric psychiatry (American Psychiatric Association, 1981, 71–72).

The Council on Aging is composed of nine psychiatrists and is responsible for developing and maintaining liaison with the appropriate non-APA organizations involved in the mental health care of aging Americans, with federal agencies similarly involved, and with other APA components so involved. Between May 1981 and May 1982, three council task forces were operating. These included a Task Force on Fellowships and Career Development in Geriatric Psychiatry, a Task Force on the White House Conference on Aging, and a Task Force on Psychiatric Services for the Elderly. In addition, the APA Council on Research in 1979 established the Task Force on the Treatment of the Dying Patient and Family. The Council on Research of the APA also has had a Task Force on Research on Aging since 1974. The American Psychiatric Association can take pride in the roles its members have played in the development of geriatrics.

The Group for the Advancement of Psychiatry (GAP) was organized in 1946. By 1950 its membership was composed of approximately 150 psychiatrists divided into 17 working groups. In 1950 the Committee on Hospitals published *The Problem of the Aged Patient in the Public Psychiatric Hospital*, GAP's Report No. 14. In 1966 GAP established the Committee on Aging, and this committee has been active ever since, publishing a number of reports.

Psychiatrists have played leadership roles in the activities of two major United States societies concerned with aging—the Gerontological Society of America and the American Geriatrics Society. The Gerontological Society of America, founded in 1945, is a multidisciplinary organization with four distinct sections. In recent years, three psychiatrists have served as president of this important organization. The American Geriatrics Society, established in 1942, is composed largely of physicians and members of the health care professions. Psychiatrists have also led this medical society, which for over the last twenty years has given the Edward B. Allen Award for contributions to geriatric psychiatry.

The impacts of the National Institute on Aging, the National Institute of Mental Health, and the Administration on Aging upon gerontology in the United States cannot be overestimated. The Administration on Aging was created in 1965 to develop and coordinate research and service programs for the elderly. The administration was originally a component of the Department of Health, Education, and Welfare. Its mission was and is in many respects quite different from those of the National Institute on Aging and the National Institute of Mental Health.

The Center for Studies of the Mental Health of the Aging was established at the National Institute of Mental Health in 1975. In 1977 it received funds to support and coordinate research, research training, and clinical training projects. Its efforts in the area of geriatric psychiatry have been focused on two general areas. Clinical training has focused on developing specialty-training fellowship programs, of which there are presently six, on establishing a faculty development program, as yet unfunded, and on continuing education, in-service training, and demonstration training and curriculum projects. The second area of focus is research training. A new research career program (Geriatric Mental Health Academic Award) has just been announced in this area. While the future of the training projects supported by clinical training funds is highly uncertain, training initiatives from research and research training funds are likely to increase (G.D. Cohen, personal communication, 14 May 1982).

The National Institute on Aging (NIA) was established in May 1974 as part of the National Institutes of Health. NIA's first director was a psychiatrist, Robert N. Butler. The establishment of NIA represented the culmination of twenty years of effort to gain government recognition and support for research on aging. Enabling legislation designated NIA as the chief federal agency responsible for promoting, coordinating, and supporting basic research and training relevant to the aging process and to the diseases and problems of the elderly. A unique aspect of NIA's mandate was that it was the first component of the National Institutes of Health to be formally charged by Congress with conducting research in the biological, biomedical, behavioral, and social sciences. This broad research mandate has resulted in activities which are different from those of the other national health research institutes. Since 1974 NIA basic research funding has tripled, grant applications have more than doubled, and over one hundred new researchers have been in training (Kawecky, C.A., "Legislative and Administrative History, NIA," draft document not for circulation).

For many years, medical and health care education related to geriatrics received little attention. The first training program in geriatric psychiatry supported by the National Institute of Mental Health was established at Duke University Medical Center in 1965 and was the only such program for almost a decade. There are now six geriatric psychiatry fellowship programs. In the last few years, federal and state agencies have provided financial support for training in geriatrics in the medical fields of internal medicine, family practice, psychiatry, and neurology. While the American Board of Medical Specialties has discouraged the formation of separate subspecialty boards such as geriatric psychiatry, it does favor certification in subspecialties by primary specialty boards. The American Board of Psychiatry and Neurology, for instance, certifies diplomates who obtain and can demonstrate special competence or special qualifications in a subspecialty, e.g., child psychiatry and child neurology.

Some people today advocate developing a specialty of geriatrics, pointing to Great Britain where a more or less distinct hospital-based specialty of geriatrics has emerged. Although there have admittedly been some gains in Britain, there have also been some losses, particularly because the specialty is hospital-based. Moreover, the emergence of the geriatrics specialty in the United Kingdom has spanned a period of 25 years and is tied to a system of health insurance and social assistance that has not been acceptable in the United States.

Geriatric psychiatry is thus a relatively new area of concentration. Its clinical and scientific development has not been clearly traced or documented, and its future as an area of specialization is not yet entirely certain. Personality and developmental theories of aging are complicated by the fact that as human beings pass through life experiences, they become increasingly different rather than increasingly similar. This life-span divergence is largely related to the wide array of possible learning and life experiences and, to an unknown degree, to late-onset genetic influences (Busse, 1981). Psychiatrists with a strong commitment to geriatrics and gerontology have been in the forefront of those whose efforts are directed toward improving the health and care of the elderly and toward maintaining and increasing their life satisfaction. The late Jack Weinberg and Alvin Goldfarb are both remembered for their important contributions to geriatric psychiatry. Both were psychoanalytically trained, and both made contributions to psychotherapeutic techniques and theory. Goldfarb developed an effective brief therapeutic approach that was particularly applicable to the elderly in homes for the aged. Weinberg conveyed a deep compassion for the elderly and a conviction that the elderly needed to be maintained in the community as long as possible. Geriatric psychiatry is indebted to Jack Weinberg and Alvin Goldfarb (Weinberg, 1975; Goldfarb, 1955; 1959).

Each of the chapters in this Part comes from a recognized authority in the area of geriatric psychiatry. All of the authors have made significant contributions to the medical and psychiatric literature, including a number of important books concerned with the psychological, social, and psychiatric aspects of late life. So that the chapters would have very little overlap, the Preceptor and faculty developed and adhered to outlines which would capitalize on their familiarity with the biologic and behavioral aspects of aging in general and with specific psychiatric disorders of the elderly in particular. Dr. Dan Blazer begins the Part with a survey of the demography of aging and the epidemiology of psychiatric disorders among the elderly. The Preceptor then reviews a number of biologic and psychosocial theories of aging as they relate to geriatric psychiatry, pointing out that there is no unified theory of aging. The four remaining chapters deal with particular classes of psychiatric disorders which affect the elderly patient. In his chapter, Dr. R. Bruce Sloane presents a review of the etiology, diagnosis, and treatment of the organic mental disorders. Dr. Robert O. Friedel discusses the diagnosis and treatment of the affective disorders in elderly patients. Drs. Carl Eisdorfer and Donna Cohen review late-onset schizophrenia and paranoia in the aged. In the final chapter, Dr. Eric Pfeiffer discusses a number of psychiatric disorders related to physiological changes—anxiety reactions, somatoform disorders, sleep disturbances, and problems associated with psychosexual changes.

Chapter 6

The Epidemiology of Psychiatric Disorder in the Elderly Population
by Dan Blazer, M.D., Ph.D.

INTRODUCTION

The management of psychiatric disorder in the community requires data that parallel the data required in clinical practice. Decisions on the clinical management of an individual psychiatric patient in late life require a clinical diagnosis based on history, mental status, and appropriate laboratory procedures. Similarly, the community management of psychiatric disorders among elderly people requires a community diagnosis based on epidemiologic methods. These disorders can be described and classified according to clinical diagnostic criteria (Barker and Rose, 1979). In addition, the epidemiology of mental disorders in late life entails studying both the distribution of mental disorders among the elderly and the factors that influence that distribution (MacMahon and Pugh, 1970, 1). Thus, epidemiologic methods are valuable to clinicians and mental health planners alike, and they focus on five areas: (1) the identification of cases; (2) the distribution of psychiatric disorder in the population; (3) historical trends of psychiatric disorder; (4) etiologic studies; and (5) the utilization of mental health and general health facilities. This chapter reviews each of these areas of inquiry and illustrates them with representative studies of elderly populations. First, however, since community diagnosis is grounded in a thorough understanding of the basic demography of the population being studied (Morris, 1975), the chapter begins with a brief review of the demography of the elderly population.

DEMOGRAPHIC CHARACTERISTICS OF THE ELDERLY POPULATION

The absolute number and percentage of persons who are 65 and older continue to increase in developed countries, highlighting the need for an increase in the quantity and effectiveness of psychiatric services to the elderly. The 1980 census counted 25.5 million over 65, amounting to 11.3 percent of the U.S. population. In absolute numbers, this represents an increase of over 5 million persons in this age group since the 1970 census. Forty percent of the elderly population are male, and 8 percent are over the age of 85. Compared with 12.2 percent of whites, only 7.3 percent of blacks and 4.9 percent of Hispanics are over the age of 65. Females predominate in these two ethnic minority groups in a proportion similar to that found in the white population. In the group that is 85 or older, the predominance of females is even greater, for 70 percent of those over the age of 85 are female (Bureau of the Census, 1981).

In 1976, eight out of every ten older men lived in family settings, compared with only six out of every ten older women. Three fourths of the men 65 and older lived in a family setting that included the wife, whereas only one third of older women lived in a family that included the husband. Seventy-seven percent of older men were married, compared with only 47 percent of older women. More than one third of all older women lived alone. In 1977, it was estimated that 1,126,000 older adults were living in nursing home facilities, slightly over 4 percent of the total population (Sourcebook on Aging, 1977).

The elderly tend to be distributed geographically in the same pattern as the total population, except that the proportion of older persons is somewhat greater in most of the larger states. For example, 17 percent of the population of Florida are 65 or older, compared with 7.9 percent of the population of Wyoming. In 1974, fewer older than younger persons lived in metropolitan areas (64 percent versus 69 percent). Within the metropolitan area, most older persons (51 percent) lived in the central city, while most of those under 65 (57 percent) lived in the suburbs (Sourcebook on Aging, 1977).

What accounts for the progressive increase in the population that is 65 and older? Some population theorists have argued that the increase is largely determined by the greater birth rate that existed in those birth cohorts represented in the group that is now 65 or older (Manton, in press). Projections based on cohort size with a stable mortality rate, however, cast doubt on this argument. The projections consistently underestimated the number of older adults counted in the 1980 census, because the mortality rates had actually decreased.

After rapid declines in mortality rates during the 1940s and 1950s, little change occurred in the early 1960s. At the time, theorists argued that the increase in life expectancy would cease because of biological constraints on the length of the human life span. In effect, they accepted the leveling in the early 1960s as evidence that the potential for extended life expectancy had been largely exhausted. Contrary to these arguments, life expectancy has increased rather dramatically over the past ten years, due primarily to a decreased mortality rate among the elderly. For example, the decreased mortality rate for females since 1900 is demonstrated in Table 1. The rate is nearly double the rate for males and has been for every twenty-year period since 1900. At the same time, the rate for both males and females over the age of 85 has continued to decrease, so neither sex group appears to be near its biological limits. At the present time, the life expectancy for men who are 65 averages 15 more years, while the average life expectancy for women at age 65 is approaching 20 more years.

Table 1. Death Rates for Older U.S. White Females (1950–1979)

Age	Death Rate per Thousand by Year			
	1950	1960	1970	1979
55–64	12.9	10.8	10.1	8.8
65–74	32.4	27.8	24.7	20.1
75–84	84.8	77.0	67.0	56.6
85 +	194.8	194.8	159.8	133.7

Source: Manton (1982). Data derived from *Vital Statistics of the United States*, published periodically by the National Center for Health Statistics.

THE IDENTIFICATION OF SPECIFIC PSYCHIATRIC DISORDERS

Grouping individuals into classes for comparison is essential to the epidemiologic method. The process of classifying mental disorders may take two different orientations. A first approach groups persons according to the presence or absence of mental health impairment or psychiatric disorder (Schwab and Schwab, 1978). A second approach groups mentally ill persons into categories such that the characteristics of the members of one category permit them to be distinguished from the members of another. Such categories are then viewed as disease entities (MacMahon and Pugh, 1970, 47). Psychiatric epidemiologists were previously unable to study the epidemiology of specific disorders with confidence, but recent diagnostic methods have significantly increased the ability to define a number of psychiatric syndromes reliably (Goodwin and Guze, 1979; American Psychiatric Association, 1980).

The increased frequency of certain symptoms in elderly populations does not necessarily signify an increased frequency of specific psychiatric disorders. Diagnostic categories are clusters of symptoms and signs which derive their validity from regularities of natural history and outcome, a common morbid anatomy, and common biochemical disturbances. As new laboratory diagnostic techniques become available, such as the dexamethasone suppression test, new categories of symptoms may be lumped together to define a particular syndrome. Each succeeding generation will in turn split and lump groups of symptoms and signs to suit its own purposes (Morris, 1975). Analysis of population data may demonstrate that what has previously been lumped together needs taking apart because its components are differently distributed in the population. For example, depressive symptoms are known to be more frequent in elderly populations. Yet when strict operational criteria are applied, as required in DSM-III, the actual rate of depressive disorders in the elderly population is found to be no greater than in populations at other stages of the life cycle (American Psychiatric Association, 1980; Blazer and Williams, 1980).

Are there unique late-life symptom presentations which would render our present diagnostic categories inadequate? DSM-III has age-specific diagnostic categories for children, but not for older people. However, clinicians who work with the elderly have frequently commented that their symptom presentations seem unique to late life. They cite, for example, the frequent occurrence of apparent cognitive impairment or pseudodementia in older persons suffering from such psychiatric disorders as depression (Wells, 1979). Despite these observations, there is still no compelling evidence for developing diagnostic classifications specific to older adults. Actually the DSM-III criteria have been demonstrated in some studies to be quite adequate for case identification in the elderly (Blazer, 1980a). The Diagnostic Interview Schedule (DIS), an instrument designed to elicit DSM-III diagnoses through a survey, is presently being used in a large-scale cooperative epidemiologic study (Robins et al., 1981; Eaton et al., 1981). Over 4,000 persons 60 years old and older will be assessed, providing significantly improved estimates of the rates of psychiatric disorder among the elderly.

RATES AND DISTRIBUTION OF LATE-LIFE PSYCHIATRIC DISORDERS

Studies of the epidemiology of psychiatric disorders have until now concentrated almost exclusively on the distribution in the population of symptoms indicative of these disorders. Table 2 displays findings on the prevalence of four common symptoms or symptom clusters which are well recognized as the common complaints of older outpatients. As noted above, however, equating these symptoms with the presence of psychiatric disorders would lead to overestimating the prevalence of such disorders. Each symptom may derive from a number of sources and be a part of more than one diagnostic complex. On the other hand, the symptom may not be associated with any specific disorder.

The common depressive symptoms may result from a number of etiologies. At a given point in time, grief reactions, which are more

Table 2. The Prevalence of Selected Symptoms in Community Populations of Older Adults

Source	Symptoms	Prevalence	Sex Distribution
Blazer and Williams (1980)	Depression	15%	M = F
Blazer and Houpt (1979)	Hypochondriasis	14%	M = F
Lowenthal and Berkman (1962)	Suspicion	17%	F > M
McGhie and Russell (1962)	Sleep Difficulties	25–40%	F > M

frequent in late life than in any other stage of the life cycle, are virtually indistinguishable from major depressive episodes. They can be distinguished from depressive episodes only when a loss of significance is identified. Depressive symptoms may also accompany major life adjustments such as a forced change of residence, retirement, decline in economic resources, and so forth.

Physicians caring for older adults frequently note their perception of poor health and increased complaints of symptoms. Yet healthy elders who perceive their health as poor do not generally frequent physicians' offices excessively. One study found that they maintained their usual activities of daily living, that they did not overuse medications, and that the majority did not score out of the normal range on the hypochondriasis scale of the MMPI (Blazer and Houpt, 1979).

Symptoms of suspiciousness are frequently associated with living alone or with living in environments where persons must relinquish control over their financial resources and personal possessions. Older adults who appear suspicious may also be suffering from organic mental disorders which decrease their ability to assess the social environment.

Sleep difficulties are among the most common of complaints that older adults bring to primary care physicians. Older persons do experience an increased incidence of real and significant sleep disorders. Sleep in general becomes less efficient with the aging process. For example, older adults have an increased sleep latency, awaken more during the night, and are more likely to suffer from the adverse consequences of inadequate sleep (Dement et al., 1982).

Except for chronic organic mental disorders, the most frequent psychiatric disorders of late life are no more common than at any other stage of the life cycle (Table 3). In fact, early-onset "neuroses" (anxiety states and dysthymic disorders) and schizophrenic disorders probably decrease in *incidence* with increased age, although these conditions once established do persist into late life. Because of this persistence, the *prevalence* of these disorders may not change significantly with advancing years. With other disorders, such as depressive disorders, the

Table 3. The Prevalence of Psychiatric Disorders in Community Populations of Older Adults

Source	Disorder	Overall Rate	Population Characteristics		
			Sex	Race	Age[1]
Kay et al. (1964); Nielsen (1963)	Senile Dementia (Chronic Organic Brain Syndrome)	3–6%	M = F	B = W	↑
Weissman and Myers (1978); Blazer and Williams (1980)	Major Depression	3–5%	M = F	B = W	→
Kay et al. (1964); Leighton et al. (1963)	Schizophrenia and Paranoid Psychoses	1–2%	F > M	?	↓
Kay et al. (1964); Sheldon (1948)	"Neuroses"[2]	5–10%	F > M	B = W	↓

[1] ↑ = increase with age; → = no change with age; ↓ = decrease with age
[2] Anxiety states and dysthymic disorders

prevalence may actually decrease slightly. This decrease can be partially explained by a somewhat higher mortality rate in persons suffering from psychiatric disorders in general (Tsuang et al., 1980), while a gradual cessation of symptomatology over time may explain the remainder. New-onset cases of major depression, schizophrenia, paranoid psychoses, anxiety states, and dysthymic disorders are not rare in late life, however. Overall, major depressive episodes and senile dementia are by far the most serious psychiatric disorders in the elderly, and their relatively high prevalence underlines the importance of treating these disorders in late life.

HISTORICAL TRENDS IN THE RATES

Although historical studies of the frequency of disease among populations are essential to a complete clinical understanding, they have been rare in psychiatric epidemiology. Despite inherent methodological difficulties, one study illustrates the value of longitudinal follow-up (Srole and Fischer, 1980). Subjects who had participated in the Midtown Manhattan Study were interviewed in 1974, twenty years after the initial 1954 survey, and the presence or absence of mental health impairment was assessed in 695 of the original group of 1,660. Table 4 abstracts some illustrative results from this study. In both 1954 and 1974, rates of mental impairment were highest for the older subjects. For all but the youngest birth cohort (born about 1920), the rates within cohorts declined between 1954 and 1974. Comparing people of similar age in the two survey years, those who were about 54 in 1954 had a far higher rate of mental impairment (22 percent) than those who were about 54 in 1974 (8 percent).

Table 4.   Mental Health Impairment Rates in 1954 and 1974 Midtown Manhattan Surveys

Birth Cohort	1954 Survey		1974 Survey	
	Age	Rate	Age	Rate
±1900	±54	22%	±74	18%
±1910	±44	16%	±64	12%
±1915	±39	14%	±59	10%
±1920	±34	7%	±54	8%

±54 years old

Source: Srole and Fischer (1980).

A striking finding was the decline of mental health impairment among women in the age range of 40 to 60 years. While the rates for mental health impairment declined slightly for most individual cohorts, they declined markedly for this particular age and sex group. The advent of women's liberation occurred between the initial and follow-up studies, and Weissman and Klerman (1977) have suggested that the decline may be the result of an appreciable drop in the rate of depression among women in this age group. "Involutional melancholia" among women may thus have been decreasing. DSM-III contains no diagnostic classification for this entity. Some clinicians have noted that the entity is not seen as frequently as it was 25 to 30 years ago. Others have suggested, based on improved diagnostic techniques, that the entity never actually existed, but was a variant of unipolar affective disorder. Regardless of the interpretation in this case, it does illustrate how historical data can provide clinicians with useful perspectives which would be unavailable within the confines of an office or hospital practice.

ETIOLOGIC STUDIES

The most prevalent hypothesis concerning the etiology of psychiatric disorder throughout adulthood is that social stress in some way causes mental illness. Many epidemiologic studies have established a relationship between social stress and mental disorder (Langer and Michael, 1963; Leighton et al., 1963; Hollingshead and Redlich, 1958). A particular interest in social stress as a contributing factor in late life stems from certain characteristics of late life. First, most psychiatric disorders in late life are first-time events, and late onset discourages the assumption that genetic factors play a major role. Second, both clinicians and researchers have noted that social and economic pressures accompany the transition into late life, such as prejudice, declining income, and declining physical health (Blazer, 1981).

Unfortunately, the relationship between social stress and psychiatric disorders is not a simple one, since conceptual issues and research design decisions can introduce bias. Figure 1 illustrates the various etiologic models relating stress to psychiatric disorder in late life, beginning with the general model which holds that social stress leads to psychiatric disorder (model 1). Four examples of the potential for bias in this general model are then presented (models 2 through 5). In model 2, age confounds the relationship of social stress and psychiatric disorder, since increased age theoretically may contribute to both increased social stress and increased psychiatric disorder. Present knowledge of the relationship of age to both social stress and psychiatric disorder does suggest, however, that age may not be a significant confounding variable. Intervening variables can also confound the relationship, as demonstrated in model 3. Social stress, such as the fear of walking to the local grocery, may lead to changes in dietary habits and to malnutrition,

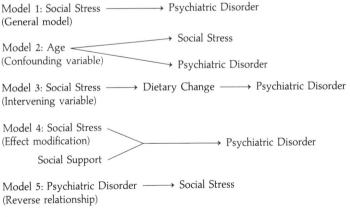

Figure 1. Etiologic models for the study of psychiatric disorders in late life: the problem of bias.

and these in turn may be the key factors in the development of the psychiatric disorder. The effect of social stress on psychiatric disorder may be modified, as diagramed in model 4, by an intervening variable such as social support (MacMahon and Pugh, 1970). George Brown and his colleagues, for example, have demonstrated the importance of social support as an effect modifier in the relationship between stressful life events and psychiatric disorders in women (Brown and Harris, 1978). Finally, as shown in model 5, psychiatric disorders may precipitate changes in the social network, and these changes may increase social stress on an already disturbed subject. Miles, among others, has studied the burden of mental illness upon the family (Miles, 1981).*

Despite the potential for bias, evidence does suggest that certain types of social stress contribute to the etiology of mental disorders in older people (Blazer, 1980c). Better-designed studies, with more rigorous definitions of independent and dependent variables, can contribute to our understanding of the exact nature of the association between social stress and psychiatric disorder.

THE USE OF HEALTH SERVICES BY THE ELDERLY WITH PSYCHIATRIC DISORDERS

According to the National Nursing Home Survey (1979), 20.4 percent of the nursing home population have a primary diagnosis of a psychiatric disorder. However, only 12.4 percent of cases indicated that a mental or behavioral problem was the principal reason for admission. The prevalence of chronic brain syndromes was estimated to be 24.9 percent and the prevalence of "senility" 32 percent. The lack of uniformity in record keeping across nursing homes makes it difficult to deduce specific diagnoses from these categories, but the overall rate of slightly over 50 percent with some type of organic mental disorder is similar to that found in other studies (Blazer, 1980b). In the national survey, 11.4 percent of patients were diagnosed as suffering from mental illnesses other than the organic mental disorders and 2.8 percent as suffering from alcoholism.

In 1970, 15 percent of the institutionalized elderly population were residents of psychiatric facilities (Redick et al., 1973), and the great majority of these were in state and county mental hospitals. Most of those 65 and older admitted to these facilities were admitted because of organic mental disorders. While patients suffering from schizophrenic disorders made up one third of the residents over the age of 65, schizophrenic disorders accounted for less than 5 percent of the admissions. Over the past 12 years, the number of older persons in state mental hospitals has declined significantly. On the other hand, between 1969 and 1973 the number of elderly nursing home residents with a chronic mental disorder increased more than 100 percent. During the same period, people over age 65 residing in all types of psychiatric hospitals decreased by 37 percent (Regier and Taube, 1981).

Organic mental disorders are the main reason that elderly people seek outpatient services at community mental health centers and other

*Editor's note: This view of the role of mental illness in the family and alternate views are explored further in the chapter which Bloch has prepared for Part III, Family Psychiatry.

psychiatric outpatient facilities (Blazer, 1980b; Redick et al., 1973). Anxiety states and dysthymic disorders, especially the depressive disorders, constitute the second most common reason for consultation, whereas schizophrenia and paranoid disorders account for only 5 to 10 percent of those patients seeking such services. Clinics designed specifically to reach community-based elderly with general problems of adaptation attract a disproportionate number of older adults suffering from adjustment disorders (Blazer, 1980b).

Most older persons who are suffering from psychiatric disorders and living in the community do not seek outpatient mental health services. In 1969, the 65-and-older group accounted for only 4 percent of the total patient care episodes in mental health centers, and there is no evidence that this percentage has increased in recent years (Redick et al., 1973). Many of those elderly who seek care for psychiatric problems go to a general practitioner. Shephard et al. (1966) estimated conservatively that the psychiatric morbidity rate among persons 65 and older who consulted a general practitioner during a year's period was 11 percent for males and 15 percent for females.

The management of psychiatric disorder among the elderly appears heavily oriented to pharmacotherapy. Older persons consume more psychotropic medications than any other age group. In a national study, 24 percent of those who were 60 or older had used at least one prescription psychotropic drug during a one-year period (Mellinger et al., 1971). Another study showed a gradual increase in the use of sedative hypnotics and tranquilizers with increased age and a corresponding decrease in the use of over-the-counter sleep preparations (Balter and Bauer, 1975). As documented for the entire U.S. population by Regier and Taube (1981), most persons with psychiatric disorders receive care from the general health care system, not from the mental health service system. Psychotropic medications are a significant component of the therapeutic approach by the primary care physician to the psychiatrically ill elder. In fact, evidence is now emerging that psychotropic medications are significantly overused in the treatment of the elderly (Ray et al., 1980).

CONCLUSION

Epidemiologic data can be of value in at least three areas of planning for psychiatric services for the elderly. First, prevalence rates and projections can facilitate the prediction of future levels of psychiatric disorder among the elderly in community and institutional populations. These data may then be translated both into predictions of how older persons may use mental health services and into identification of barriers to their using such services. Second, epidemiologic studies can generate survey data which can guide the staffing of clinics designed to serve the older population. Given that a number of surveys suggest that older persons who seek mental health services have multiple impairments (Blazer and Maddox, 1982), a multidisciplinary staff may be indicated. Such a staff could meet the need for comprehensive assessment and respond to people's interacting impairments in social, economic, psychological, and biological functioning. Third, epidemiologic data can provide the baseline for studies of treatment outcomes among the elderly. If funds are to be allocated for serving older persons, we must address the question, What is the value of the service?

Chapter 7

Biologic and Psychosocial Bases of Behavioral Changes in Aging

by Ewald W. Busse, M.D.

DEFINITION AND OVERVIEW OF BIOLOGIC AGING

The term *aging* is commonly used in biology to designate those decremental physical changes that usually develop with the passage of time and eventually end with death. The process of aging is not confined to the end phase of the life span. The consequences of aging are accumulative. For operational purposes biologic age changes can be separated into primary and secondary processes. *Primary aging* (senescence) is usually intrinsic to the organism and is consequently determined by inherent or hereditary factors. *Secondary aging* (senility) refers to defects and disability caused by hostile factors in the environment, particularly trauma and disease. This operational separation of the aging processes has limitations. For example, it does not adequately distinguish the so-called normal age changes from the late-onset diagnostic entities that are related to inborn defects and that are also often precipitated by adverse events, such as maturity-onset diabetes.

With the passage of time numerous biologic changes occur in the human body and brain. Aging is accompanied by gradual loss of muscle cells and neurons within the brain and nervous system. Physiological changes transpire throughout the body and alter how the brain functions while awake or asleep. While such changes obviously have an impact on how the nervous system responds, the older person who is physically healthy and mentally active does not appear to progress inevitably to intellectual loss and mental incapacity. When serious losses of intellectual capacity do develop, and when disruptive patterns of behavior appear, they result from one of several diseases which are referred to as organic brain disorders.*

The loss of irreplaceable cells plays an important role in aging physiological changes. The loss of brain cells may not only alter important aspects of body metabolism but may also make the brain more sensitive to certain drugs.

Striated musculature diminishes to about one half by approximately 80 years of age. As these muscle cells disappear, they are replaced by fat cells in fibrous connective tissue. Hence, the storage capacity of those drugs that are stored in fat cells will clearly be increased.

Aging also produces a decrease in heart cells, resulting in a decline in cardiac output. Thus, drugs given orally may be absorbed at a reduced rate, as the blood flow to the upper gastrointestinal tract is decreased. In some elderly people the loss of P-cells of the heart results in a dysrhythmia or other conductive disturbance of the cardiac rhythm.

The aging changes that affect neural transmitters contribute to placing the elderly patient at risk for a number of mental disorders. Certain substances decline in concentration and decrease within the brain, including dopamine, norepinephrine, serotonin, tyrosine hydroxylase, and cholinesterase (Meier-Ruge, 1975). The activity of monoamine

*Preceptor's note: See the discussion by Sloane in his chapter on organic mental disorders.

oxidase increases with age (Nies, 1973), which would in turn contribute to a decline in norepinephrine, dopamine, and serotonin.

The metabolic dimensions that are affected by age include absorption, distribution, destruction, excretion, the kinetics of drug binding, and alterations in biologic rhythms (Reinberg, 1974). Drugs are therefore metabolized differently in old people than they are in younger adults.

BIOLOGIC CHANGES AND BIOLOGIC THEORIES

Among the many theories of biologic aging, none are satisfactorily unified. In part, this stems from the fact that the body is composed of three major components—cells that are capable of dividing, cells that are not able to undergo mitosis, and interstitial noncellular material. Age changes can often be recognized in one or even two of the three body components, but rarely in all three.

One early biologic explanation of aging rested on the assumption that a living organism contained a fixed store of energy, diffusely or strategically located, not unlike a coiled watch spring. At some time the energy would be unwound, and life would end. This is a type of *watch-spring theory*. Another simple theory of aging related to the *accumulation of deleterious material* such as lipofuscin.

The *theory of deliberate biologic programming* holds that within a normal cell are stored the memory and the capability of ending the life of the cell. Beginning in 1961, Hayflick and Moorhead reported that, when cultured, normal human fibroblasts underwent a finite number of population doublings and then died (Hayflick and Moorhead, 1961). A number of years later Hayflick and his coworkers reported that human fibroblast cultures derived from embryo donors as a group underwent significantly more population doublings (forty to sixty) than those derived from adults as a group (ten to thirty).

Genetic Theories

Certain individuals seem to age prematurely or rapidly. Their accelerated changes are considered to be inherited and/or acquired through disease, trauma, or social stress. A number of the theories of aging and diseases of late life are related to genetic determinants. Some relate to alterations of genes and others to chromosome loss or damage. Chromosome loss is likely to be linked to the aging process and senile dementia (Jarvik, 1975), while chromosome damage tends to be associated with the causes of cancer and birth defects and with exposure to toxic agents. Gene (DNA) repair can be completely or partially successful, or it can be a misrepair. In the latter instance, the repairing mechanism results in an abnormal type of DNA which can initiate defective and dangerous processes.

The *theory of genetic redundancy* holds that the amount of DNA reserve within the genome that can be called upon to initiate and maintain vital functions plays an important role in determining life span.

The Free Radical Theory

Free radicals are molecular entities that have an unpaired electron. Often considered molecular fragments, free radicals are highly reactive and destructive, but they are produced by normal metabolic processes and are ubiquitous in living substances. They can also be produced by ionizing radiation, ozone, and chemical toxins such as insecticides. Free radicals have been linked to DNA damage, the cross-linkage of collagens, and the accumulation of aging pigments, and they have their highest concentration in mitochondria. The ability of free radicals to generate potent oxidants when they interact with peroxides is a constant threat to cellular integrity.

In recent years, scientific inquiry has focused on normal metabolic processes, free radicals as intermediate by-products, and the defenses within the cell against this destructive molecular fragment. Several enzymes have been identified as catalytic scavengers of the free radical 0_2-. The first of these to be recognized was superoxide dismutase (Fridovich, 1979). Superoxide dismutase has a higher activity in long-lived than in short-lived primates. Other enzymes contribute to cellular defense mechanisms. Paradoxically, it has been demonstrated that normal human phagocytes intentionally make a free radical (0_2-) and use the free radical to kill ingested invading microorganisms (Hart, 1981). It is possible that some aging phagocytes lose this capacity.

The Immune System and Aging

The immune system performs both surveillance and protective tasks. An effective immune system is essential for the preservation of life. Consequently it is a complex and widespread bodily function. Traditionally the immune system is considered to have two major components. One is the humoral (or chemical) immune response, characterized by the production of antibody molecules which specifically bind the introduced foreign substance. The second is the cellular immune response. Cells are mobilized which can specifically react with and destroy the invader. Considerable evidence indicates that with aging immune competence decreases and the regulation of the immune system is altered. With aging, surveillance is impaired, and the efficiency of the protective mechanism declines. Furthermore, a loss of control causes the immune functions to become so distorted that they are self-destructive.

Autoantibodies increase with the passage of time, and the presence of autoantibodies identifies subpopulations at high risk of early death. The older body has an increased susceptibility to infection, and in general effective immunization cannot be induced in late life (Suskind, 1981). The progressive failure and perversion of the immune system with advancing age are believed to increase the incidence of maturity-onset diabetes, emphysema, amyloidosis, and Alzheimer's dementia. The specific defect is probably one of autoimmunity.

The Cross-Linkage Theory

The cross-linkage or *eversion theory* was originally based upon the changes in collagen structure that occur with age. The most important protein in the human body, collagen is one of the four major constituents of connective tissue and constitutes 30 to 40 percent of body protein. Collagen serves to strengthen and maintain the structural integrity of tissue and organs. There are two general types of collagen, interstitial and basement-membrane. Interstitial collagens predominate and are responsible for the great tensile strength of connective tissue. Basement-membrane collagen is also noncellular. It is a delicate layer of variable thickness interposed between the epithelium and adjacent connective tissue of the intestinal tract, blood vessels, renal glomeruli and tubules, and most other tubular and glandular structures. All collagen molecules are composed of polypeptide strands. Each interstitial collagen molecule contains four units that are held together by pairs of ester bonds. With the passage of time, the ester bonds switch from within to between the individual collagen molecules, binding the molecules together. This aging change alters the characteristics of connective tissue, particularly its elasticity.

The Hypothalamus and Homeostasis

One currently important theory of aging holds that the hypothalamus plays a significant role in the loss of homeostasis mechanisms in the body (Samorajski and Hartford, 1980). Some believe the hypothalamus is the location of an "aging clock." The hypothalamus has numerous roles, including the regulation of the pituitary gland. While the cells within the hypothalamus certainly have their own internal controls, many of their actions are clearly responsive. With a feedback mechanism they respond to body changes that are stimulated by the environment. The hypothalamus accomplishes its task by neuroendocrines (hormones) and neurotransmitters.

Cell loss, a common event in late life, has been observed in the hypothalamus. The disappearance of a few critical cells in the hypothalamus may have far-reaching consequences. The death of these critical cells may be genetically determined or may be the result of acquired disease or trauma.

Endocrine Changes with Aging

The endocrine changes associated with aging are not simply due to system imbalance produced by an overall reduction in hormones or a decrease in selected hormones. In fact, most individuals who develop late-onset diabetes have normal or even elevated levels of insulin production. It appears, however, that reduced sensitivity accounts for their impaired ability to use glucose. The search for a specific defect revealed that the cells of late-onset diabetes patients have fewer receptors for binding insulin than do normal cells. This phenomenon may be comparable to the finding that a reduction of cell receptors permits the fat cells of aging rats to bind the adrenal steroid hormone cortisol.

In addition to the alterations in hormone levels and receptor concentrations, other age-related cell changes seem to play a role. Within the cell itself, defects in the messenger or signal cell may alert the interior of the cell to initiate the production of enzymes that are intimately associated with the activity of hormones (Marx, 1979).

Musculoskeletal Changes

The cells that make up voluntary muscles diminish in number with age, and approximately one half are left at the age of 80 years. As muscle cells disappear, they are replaced by fat and fibrous connective tissues. Despite continuing physical exercise, muscle strength is reduced as a person gets older.

Morphology and Physiology of the Aging Brain

The functions of the brain are obviously complex. They interact with and are influenced by many body processes through a multitude of reciprocal neural and humoral mechanisms. Neural and humoral functions are often altered by age changes, and many of these changes seem to start within a cell. When an aging defect emerges within the cell, it begins a chain of events that is often primarily manifest by changes in mechanisms and processes external to the cell. Obviously, no cell is autonomous from its milieu. Brain activity normally varies from moment to moment. Feedback mechanisms influence this rapid alteration, and each change may produce a cascading effect. The complexity of these events is evident and presents a formidable challenge to the scientist and to the clinician.

THE LOSS OF NEURONS   In the aged brain are many morphological and physiological changes. One of the changes most frequently mentioned is the gradual loss of neurons. The type of cell plays a role in the rate of cell death. In the cerebral cortex, smaller-sized cells decrease in greater numbers than do larger cells. It is assumed that the larger cells represent earlier development along the phylogenetic scale, while the smaller cells are much younger in developmental sequence. In general, the sequence of neuronal cell death is consistent with the rule: First in, last out (Brody, 1981).

The loss of neurons is not uniform throughout the brain, and selected areas appear to be more vulnerable (Brody, 1980). Vulnerable areas of the brain stem include the locus coeruleus and the substantia nigra. The locus coeruleus, an area involved in sleep and other functions, declines from 18,000 cells in youth to 12,000 in old age. These two areas of the brain stem both contain pigmented cells. Consequently the question arises, Does the presence of melanin pigment interfere with cell metabolism and survival? The presence of the pigment lipofuscin, which is associated with aging in a number of cells and particularly those in the brain and heart, has not been shown clearly to disrupt cell metabolism.

In addition to gradual cell loss, there are age-related alterations of neuronal synapses and networks. With aging occurs a selective loss of horizontal dendritic components. If information is actually stored within these dendrites, the loss would be even more severe. These dendritic losses may well be associated with declines in cognitive performance, ability to recall, and other mental symptoms associated with aging (Scheibel and Scheibel, 1975).

Within the cell body of the neuron occur neurofibrillary degeneration, granulovacular degeneration, lipofuscin accumulation, Lewy bodies, and Hirano bodies. Changes in the neuropile include senile plaques, amyloid deposits, shrinkage of the dendritic arbor, and a decrease of extracellular space. Glial changes include corpora amylacea and myelin remodeling. Furthermore, there are arteriosclerotic and other vascular lesions (Wisniewski and Terry, 1976).

The two age-related lesions most frequently assumed to be causative in senile dementia are neurofibrillary changes and senile plaques. Very little more is known about neurofibrillary degeneration except that it is common in Alzheimer's disease and senile dementia, that it is found in lesser degree in the normal aged brain, and that it is also excessive in such conditions as Down's syndrome, "punch-drunk" boxers, postencephalitic parkinsonism, and the amyotrophic lateral sclerosis-parkinsonism-dementia complex found in the indigenous population of Guam.

As to senile plaques, also called neuritic plaques, they are composed of three elements: degenerative neuronal processes, nonneuronal cells, and amyloid. In the body there are three types of amyloid: A, B, and C. Amyloid B found in the senile plaque is the result of a complex of light chains of immunoglobulins. This is the basis for the theory that the immune system is involved in senile dementia. The occurrence of neurofibrillary tangles and senile plaques in other disorders such as Down's syndrome resulted in the study which found a correlation within families between Alzheimer's disease, Down's syndrome, and hematologic malignancies (Heston and Mastri, 1977).

Also important and relatively new is the observation of a sevenfold increase in aluminum in the brains of patients with Alzheimer's disease. Whether the large amount of aluminum is a primary contributing factor or whether it accumulates as a secondary phenomenon is at this point unknown.

NEUROTRANSMITTERS   At least 35 different substances are known to be or are suspected to be neurotransmitters in the brain, and additional neurotransmitters will undoubtedly be identified. Each of these substances has a characteristic excitatory or inhibitory effect on neurons. Neurotransmitter substances and the cells that generate them are not randomly distributed throughout the brain. Clusters of neurons produce or respond to certain neurotransmitters, and the neurons of these clusters have axonal projections to other highly specific brain regions. Progress has been made in mapping the distribution of the substances in the brain and in elucidating the molecular events of synaptic transmission.

The brain is the most active energy consumer of any organ of the body. The brain represents 2 percent of the total body weight, yet at rest it consumes at least 20 percent of the oxygen used by the entire body. This enormous expenditure of energy appears to be related to maintaining the ionic gradient across the neuronal membrane on which the conduction of impulses depends. There are billions of neurons in the brain demanding this large amount of oxygen. Neurons use only glucose and adjust their metabolic rate according to their need.

According to Snyder, transmitters are "those peptides localized in specified neuronal systems and released on depolarization which produce changes in neuronal activity" (Snyder, 1980, 976). Snyder believes that the known peptide transmitters represent 10 percent or less of the total that will be identified. The rapidly expanding knowledge about peptide neurotransmitters will undoubtedly result in important advances in knowledge and therapeutic applications.

For many years, it has been recognized that the right and left halves of the cerebrum function differently. Now added to the traditional neurological observations related to cerebral dominance is the knowledge that the right hemisphere is likely to be involved with spatial relations and with artistic and holistic thought processes, while the left hemisphere is usually involved with speech and with logical and analytical thinking. The mapping of neurotransmitters in various areas of the human brain emphasizes this difference. In the thalamus, for instance, the left side is especially rich in norepinephrine as compared with the right side. Similarly, a patient with Parkinson's disease was shown to have an asymmetry of the neurotransmitter dopamine. These differences parallel other observations such as the left anterior temporal foci frequently encountered in the EEGs of elderly people (Busse and Wang, 1979).

NEUROHORMONES   The proliferating knowledge of the brain and its various processes has led inevitably to some difficulty in the classification of certain substances. Confusion seems to arise at times over whether a messenger is a neurotransmitter, a neurohormone, a neuroregulator, or a neuromodulator (Barchas, 1978).

Hormones (from the Greek word meaning to set in motion) are "chemical messengers" produced by tissues or organs to regulate or modulate effects on other tissues or organs. Since the action of hormones includes alteration of mood and behavior, and the excretion of a number of hormones follows circadian rhythms, their role in many affective disorders is of considerable importance, particularly in the elderly population where both suicide and depressive episodes increase. While many hormones are produced by nonneuronal cells, the neurons called neuroendocrine transducers produce substances called neurohormones. Most neuroendocrine transducers are located in the hypothalamus. The hormones produced in the hypothalamus are carried to the anterior pituitary via a fine capillary system, the hypophyseal portal system, and move along axons to the posterior pituitary. Parts of the brain are affected in other ways, including a pathway through the cerebral spinal fluid.

The neurohormones resemble neurotransmitters in that they first bind to specific receptor sites on the plasma membrane of the cell. After binding at the receptor site, they then affect activity within the cell. Steroid and thyroid hormones are quite different in that they freely permeate the cell membrane and interact within the cell with proteins and receptors in the cytoplasm and nucleus. Generally speaking, neurotransmitters interact with other neurons, while neurohormones interact with a variety of cells.

PERCEPTUAL CHANGES

Visual Changes

Age-related visual changes involve several parts of the eye. Over the life span, the lens increases in both size and thickness due to the continual proliferation of new cells at the periphery. Lens fibers develop and migrate to the central region of the lens where they become compressed and more rigid, reducing the transparency of the lens nucleus and the overall elasticity of the lens. In addition, the capsule of the lens becomes thicker and less permeable. These changes in the lens alter the absolute threshold for vision such that the amount of light which can be detected by the eye decreases. In addition, yellow or yellow-brown substances accumulate over time and interfere with the blue-light spectrum. Thus, to some older people a true blue light appears to be greenish blue.

The pupil size also diminishes with age and is another factor in reducing the amount of light that reaches the retina. At age 60 the amount of white light that reaches the retina is reduced to one third of the amount at age 20, and as noted the blue-light decrement is much more pronounced (Sandoz Pharmaceuticals, 1980a).

Light-dark adaptation is another visual problem in late life. When an older person emerges from a dark room into a brightly lighted area, the recovery period is prolonged. Similarly, an older person has difficulty when driving at night and meeting a car with very bright headlights. The slower responses can be quite dangerous.

Visual acuity is usually defined as the ability of the eye to detect a separation between two points. The decline in visual acuity with aging is probably due to the decreased amount of light reaching the retina as well as to changes in the vitreous humor. Furthermore, with aging the numerous reflexes that are important for normal functioning of the visual system appear impaired in varying degrees. A longitudinal study conducted at Duke University Center for the Study of Aging and Human Development found that a best-corrected vision of 20/50 or worse occurred in 8 percent of those aged 60 to 69, 14 percent of those 70 to 79, and 36 percent of those 80 and over (Anderson and Palmore, 1974). In an examination of the possible relationship of visual loss to social and emotional changes, the study found that patients with significant visual impairment were rated poor on their participation in leisure, work, and group activities, but were not significantly different from others on the happiness ratings.

Presbyopia is the most commonly recognized visual change that appears with aging. It generally appears at age 45 or shortly thereafter with the symptomatic inability to see near objects clearly. Among several possible causes are the compression of the older lens fibers toward the central region and the lessened ability of the ciliary muscles to change the lens. Another factor is the loss of elasticity of the lens. Fortunately presbyopia is easily corrected by glasses.

Pathological conditions that are common in late life include cataracts, glaucoma, and senile macular degeneration. Some cataracts can be treated by surgical intervention. Glaucoma can be treated by appropriate medications and if necessary by surgery. Unfortunately no good method is available for treating senile macular degeneration.

Loss of Hearing

Presbycusis is the term applied to the most common type of hearing loss in the elderly. It refers to a slowly progressive bilaterally symmetrical type of sensory-neural hearing loss that often involves poor speech discrimination. Presbycusis does not lead to total deafness. Although presbycusis is usually considered to be a part of the "normal" aging process, it does vary from one individual to another. Inherent biologic individual differences and differences in exposure and sensitivity to certain types of noise, disease, drugs, trauma, and so forth may interact with the aging process to contribute to this particular type of hearing loss. As is so often true of the aging process, the exact underlying pathological changes are unknown.

Typically, persons with presbycusis complain that while they can hear they cannot understand speech. This inability to comprehend speech is best explained by examining the frequencies of sound that are important for understanding speech. Vowels are low-frequency sounds within the range of 250 to 270 cps, while consonants are high-frequency sounds above 2,000 cps and up to 4,000 cps. Those with presbycusis have difficulty hearing consonants, particularly s, z, t, f, and g, which have high-frequency components. Consequently the person with presbycusis often has difficulty following a normal conversation and may have particular difficulty hearing at a cocktail party where so many speech sounds are covered by the so-called background noises or room noises. A complicating factor is that older people require more time than younger ones to process messages in their higher auditory centers (Sandoz Pharmaceuticals, 1980b).

Some older people have a deafness up to a certain volume threshold. When that is exceeded, the person hears reasonably well. This is the type of person who first says, "I am sorry I did not hear you," and then when the other person speaks louder, says, "You don't have to shout."

A second type of hearing loss that older people experience is conduction deafness. Among the several causes are wax in the ear canal, adhesion of the ossicles to the bony walls, new growths of bone that bind the stapes, and thickening of the tympanic membrane. Patients with conduction deafness often obtain good results with hearing aids.

Central deafness, a third type of hearing loss, is relatively rare. People with this disorder hear but do not properly interpret speech.*

Loss of Taste and Smell

Taste and smell are often altered by age. Taste buds are lost from middle adulthood on. By the time of old age, people have lost approximately 50 percent of their taste buds (Busse, 1980). Taste buds, which are primarily located on the tongue, atrophy from the front of the tongue posteriorly. The first to go are the taste buds that detect sweet and salty, leaving those devoted to the detection of bitter and sour tastes. As a result, some older people complain that all food tastes bitter or sour. Food preference is a very complex matter, involving not only smell and taste, but also temperature, consistency, texture, and appearance. The ability to identify foods declines significantly with advancing age.

Forty percent of old people have markedly diminished capacity to detect odors (Busse, 1980). Schiffman (1979) investigated how amplifying odor would affect elderly people's appreciation of food. Young and old subjects were required to taste and smell blended foods both in their natural forms and in an amplified form in which the characteristic odor was added to the food. The amplification of the gustatory sensation increased appreciation ratings for elderly subjects (ages 77 to 84) but lowered the ratings for young subjects (ages 17 to 25). Clearly the amplification of foods with artificial flavors, particularly odors, increases the appreciation of food for the elderly but does not do the same for younger subjects.

The same investigator has studied elderly perfumers between the ages of 70 and 78 (Schiffman, 1979). Elderly perfumers did not show anywhere near the decline in olfactory thresholds that the matched normal controls did. Schiffman interprets this finding as a suggestion that the use of smell over the life span may delay its decline. Quite possibly, this interpretation could explain why elderly wine tasters seem to maintain their efficiency.

*Preceptor's note: The effects of visual and hearing losses on the development of paranoia in the elderly have been the subject of several studies. Eisdorfer and Cohen review the findings of these studies in their chapter.

PSYCHOSOCIAL THEORIES AND APPROACHES

Currently several theories and issues frequent the discussions of social and behavioral scientists who are interested in aging. These include the disengagement theory, the activity theory, and the continuity theory. Advanced by Cumming and Henry (1961), *the disengagement theory* maintains that high satisfaction in old age is usually present in those individuals who accept the inevitability of reduced social and personal interactions. *The activity theory* is the opposite of the disengagement theory and holds that continued activity is important to most individuals as a basis for obtaining and maintaining satisfaction, self-esteem, and health (Havighurst, 1963).

The continuity theory holds that the majority of aging people retain certain psychosocial patterns throughout the life span and that the person's lifelong experiences create predispositions that will, under ordinary circumstances, be maintained. The predispositions are influenced by both biologic and psychological factors and by socioeconomic opportunities. Whether a person disengages or remains active is determined by the complex interaction among predispositions. Related to the continuity theory is the hypothesis that most old people tend to maintain similar attitudes, levels of functions, and activities relative to their age cohort, despite overall age changes. This hypothesis contrasts with the life-event stress theory which holds that major life events are inevitable and result in marked changes in attitudes and activities (Palmore, 1982).

Beyond these theories, several other psychosocial approaches are gaining importance, among them the influence of period and cohort effects. While age changes are believed to be caused by "normal" biologic aging, normal aging does not appear to be free of the cohort and the period effects. Basically, the cohort approach hypothesizes that the index of the date of birth differentiates one cohort from another with respect to broad classes of behavior. For example, changes in the environment experienced by a 65-year-old in 1965 are likely to be quite different from those that are experienced by a 65-year-old in 1975. Furthermore, the response to a given environmental stimulus in 1965 may be quite different from the response in 1975 because the options for response may be quite different. The period effect is related to the tendency for behavior once established to persist over time. Consequently behavior acquired in early childhood will continue despite environmental changes.

Social Value Changes

Over the last decade sharp changes in public priorities have had a direct impact upon the life-style of the elderly person. In 1965 the Medicare and Medicaid programs were signed into law and were believed to be of considerable importance to the public. At the time no one realized that by 1980 these two programs would cost the government $60 billion a year. In the early 1970s national public opinion polls showed that the public was quite concerned with social issues such as better health care, education, and welfare. Those polls also indicated a high level of confidence in the government's ability to manage these problems. But the polls in 1981 and 1982 are quite different. Attention to certain social problems is no longer high on the public agenda, and priorities have shifted to solving the problems of inflation, a stalled economy, and mounting unemployment (Rogers et al., 1982).

Attitudes toward retirement are also changing. In 1978 Congress amended The Age Discrimination Act in Employment of 1967 and made it unlawful to retire forcibly most nonmilitary federal workers at any age and most other public or private workers under age 70. As of 1 July 1982, the Act prohibits mandatory retirement under age 70 for tenured employees of colleges and universities.

From an individual perspective, the relative merits of voluntary versus mandatory retirement will vary, because people attach varied values to work. For some, work is the major source of self-esteem. It provides an opportunity for new and exciting experiences, and for some it offers the satisfaction of rendering needed services to others. For many, work means financial security. Work can also be a locus of social participation, a means of escape from an unhappy family life or social group, and simply a way of consuming time and energy. Unfortunately many individuals in our modern society perform very repetitive work. For these individuals, work per se is an unlikely source of self-esteem, and employers often attempt to correct this defect by providing other sources of self-esteem associated with the place of work. To those whose occupations are at best a minor source of personal worth, the major loss at retirement is the decline in income. In recent years, Social Security has become the principal if not the only source of financial security, despite the growth of private pension plans. Now the life-style that has become part of many retired persons' lives is threatened by the financial instability of the Social Security program.

Adjustment to retirement is related to both personal and socioeconomic factors. Mandatory retirement does not generally seem to have a negative impact on health status, nor does it increase mortality rates. Many individuals who enter retirement reduce and then replace sources of life satisfaction and opportunities for maintaining self-esteem. A few adjust quite well to a type of social isolation. But most individuals need to feel needed and to feel that they can contribute to the well-being of others. For the sake of many elderly people's mental health, more emphasis should be placed on providing older persons the means to evolve fulfilling roles in the retirement years.

Chapter 8

Organic Mental Disorders
by R. Bruce Sloane, M.D.

INTRODUCTION

This review is selective and somewhat personal.

Cognition has been rediscovered by American psychiatry in the last decade and even stands in danger of being adopted as the new fair-haired child. In the disorders of the senium, one can only welcome its advent. Dementia and delirium are heterogeneous, and their clinical presentation, description, and assessment are important to their distinction and treatment.

Using DSM-III (American Psychiatric Association, 1980), Barnes and Raskind (1981) were able to classify almost all of 64 patients in a nursing home, the majority of whom had nonspecific or inaccurate chart diagnoses. With Roth's classification (Roth and Morrissey, 1952), Christie (1982) found that there were many fewer depressed inpatients and that the late paraphrenics stayed a shorter time. Demented patients, however, were much older and more demented, illustrating their longer survival in the 1970s.

Wells (1982) pointed to twin errors in the diagnosis of dementia: first, the failure to recognize it (Kiloh, 1961; Liston, 1977), and second, the tendency to confuse it with a primary functional disease (Nott and Fleminger, 1975; Ron et al., 1979; Good, 1981). Reifler et al. (1982) diagnosed depression in 20 (23 percent) of 88 cognitively impaired geriatric outpatients. Seventeen had depression superimposed on an underlying dementia, illustrating once again the coexistence of the two diagnoses. Snowdon, a decade ago, suggested that all demented patients be given a therapeutic trial of antidepressants (Snowdon, 1972). McAllister and Price (1982) pointed to the profound cognitive impairment that can occur in depressive illness. Wells emphasizes that cognitive loss is in fact a frequent feature of many functional psychiatric disorders (Folstein and McHugh, 1978; Weingartner et al., 1981; Wells, 1979b). Although cognitive impairment is the hallmark of the organic brain syndromes, it is not diagnostic of them. Wells calls for the evaluation and characterization of changes in cognition, behavior, and affect in every patient suspected of having dementia. A primary diagnosis of dementia will be justified only if changes in each of these three spheres are roughly congruent.

Prevalence rates for dementia do not vary greatly throughout the world. Approximately 4 percent of the population over 65 years of age have the malignant form of senile dementia, and about 20 percent have mild forms (Kral, 1978). The prevalence rises sharply with age, approaching 20 percent for severe forms at age 80 (Mortimer, 1980). Clinicians believe that more women than men have senile dementia, but this has not been adequately documented (Kay and Bergmann, 1980). No patterns for race and geographic distribution have been detected. Senile dementia of the Alzheimer type may shorten life. More frequently, age, male sex, and poor general physical condition are associated with early death, suggesting that Alzheimer's disease is not fatal in itself.

DELIRIUM

Delirium and dementia are often intertwined. Not infrequently, a delirium ushers in dementia in an older person. Most elderly delirious patients lack many of the positive features found in younger ones (Roth, 1976). Older patients show disorientation for time and place, impaired consciousness, retardation, and exhaustion. Involuntary movements, especially coarse tremors or choreiform ones, may occur. Lipowski (1980) stresses disorders of cognition, wakefulness, and psychomotor behavior. A global disorder of cognition leads to impaired perception and memory and to thinking which is invariably disorganized to some extent (American Psychiatric Association, 1980).

Engel and Romano (1959) found slowing of EEG background activity, a finding which has withstood the test of time. Rabins and Folstein (1982) showed a highly significant incidence of diffusely slowed EEGs in 48 (81 percent) delirious patients, compared with 25 (33 percent) of the demented. Such slowing may be absent if the delirium is predominantly hyperactive (Pro and Wells, 1977). Rabins and Folstein deprecate the lack of interest in the clinical divisions of cognitive disorder. The brain is not a jelly bag, and the lumpers risk the loss of valuable heuristic distinctions.

Etiology and Treatment

Ten common causes of delirium are (1) overmedication, (2) metabolic imbalance, (3) malnutritional states, (4) intercranial tumors, (5) cirrhosis of liver or hepatitis, (6) cardiovascular disease, (7) cerebrovascular accidents, (8) any fever, (9) pulmonary disease, and (10) acute alcoholic intoxication. Although depression may be sudden in onset, it is more likely to mimic dementia and seldom shows sensorial clouding (Libow, 1973; Habot and Libow, 1980). Rarely is there a single cause for delirium in the aged. Multiple defects are usually present. A common example is the elderly patient who has mild congestive heart failure, anemia, and hypoxia and who is given diuretics and sedative drugs for agitation, thus causing an electrolyte imbalance. When patients have symptoms of relatively short duration, or when a minor head injury is involved, suspect a subdural hematoma.

First rule out hypoxia, hypoglycemia, and metabolic acidosis. Several treatment measures are generally applicable to all. Ensure oxygenation, maintain circulation, give blood glucose, restore acid-base balance, treat infection, control body temperature, and stop seizures (Posner, 1975). A quiet, well-lit single room with one sitter, who may be a relative or a friend, helps delirious patients to orient themselves. Staff can reassure the patient by introducing themselves and by telling the patient the time and where he or she is.

DEMENTIA

To distinguish the treatable causes of dementia from the untreatable ones is of great importance. Here early diagnosis is both critical and difficult. Kiloh (1961) points out that any suggestion that the illness is of short duration virtually eliminates the possibility of dementia. Early subtle changes in mental function can be detected only by those who know the patient best. Occasional spots of soup on the tie of the previously immaculate businessman may be more revealing than a careful clinical examination. Denial mechanisms may be evident, as they are so necessary to the patient whose mind is disintegrating (Wells, 1977; Post, 1965). Wells (1979b) urges us to be generally suspicious about the presence of dementia, especially when the complaints remain vague and difficult to categorize.

Diagnosis

To the DSM-III diagnostic criteria can be added a rich fabric of clinical description (American Psychiatric Association, 1980; Wells, 1977; 1978a; 1979b; Birren and Sloane, 1980; Slater and Roth, 1977; Schneck et al., 1982). Fatigue and lassitude are often early signs and are sometimes noticed more by relatives than the patient. Delirium, which in itself may usher in a dementia, must be differentiated, and some of its causes overlap those of various types of dementia.

Depressive disorders have in the past been overlooked, but more so in the United States than in Canada or Britain (Duckworth and Ross, 1975). It is also important to remember that some 10 percent of the cases of depression in old age present with a short-lived delirious phase (Slater and Roth, 1977). McAllister and Price (1982) found depressive illnesses in older patients to be brief, with rapid progression and without pervasive affective changes. The patients tended to give "don't know" answers despite intact attention spans and were variable in their performance. Complaints of memory loss almost invariably point to a depressive illness rather than a dementia (Kahn et al., 1975).

Physical illness is frequent in all psychiatric disabilities in the aged (Kay and Roth, 1955; Roth and Kay, 1956). Inconspicuous and muted symptoms may make the physical illness difficult to diagnose and thus can be attributed to the mental disturbance.

The *specificity* of the diagnosis is paramount. Wells (1979a) reports the diagnoses of 417 patients from six studies (Smith et al., 1976; Marsden and Harrison, 1972; Katzman and Karasu, 1975; Freemon, 1976; Harrison and Marsden, 1977; Victoratos et al., 1977). Dementia of unknown cause is commonest and is mostly Alzheimer's disease, either senile or presenile. Vascular disease is much rarer, varying from perhaps 8 percent (Wells, 1978a; 1978b) to 18 percent (Tomlinson et al., 1970). The 10 to 15 percent of potentially reversible disorders in these studies include normal-pressure hydrocephalus, benign intracranial masses, drug toxicity, epilepsy, pernicious anemia, hypo- or hyperthyroidism, liver disease, and pseudodementias (depression, mania, hysteria). An additional 25 to 30 percent of patients have disorders that call for a specific therapy, although the particular therapy may not reverse the symptoms of the dementia itself and lead to full recovery from it. These include multiinfarct dementia, malignant brain tumor, alcoholism, neurosyphilis, Huntington's chorea, Parkinson's disease, herpes simplex encephalitis, and the irreversible cases of pseudodementia and normal-pressure hydrocephalus. Seltzer and Sherwin (1978) report similar results.

PRIMARY DEGENERATIVE DEMENTIA

In the past, the illnesses which DSM-III calls Primary Degenerative Dementia were often categorized as diffuse parenchymatous disease, Alzheimer's disease, and Pick's disease. Katzman (1976) argues that both Alzheimer's disease and senile dementia are progressive dementias, with similar mental and neurological changes and with pathological signs that are indistinguishable. Terry (1976) points out that most American neurologists do not differentiate clinically or pathologically between Alzheimer's and Pick's disease. For practical purposes, the two can best be lumped together. The diagnosis of Alzheimer's disease is established by autopsy. As Alzheimer's disease progresses, the intellectual deterioration is often accompanied by a variety of neurological changes such as gait disturbances, incontinence, focal weakness, abnormal reflexes, dysphasia, dyspraxia, seizures, myoclonic jerks, and rarely, blindness (Coblentz et al., 1973).

Neurochemical Pathology

Consistent demonstrations have shown that in Alzheimer's disease choline acetyltransferase (CAT) and acetylcholinesterase (AChE) activity is reduced, especially in biopsy and autopsy specimens of the hippocampus and in CSF (Bowen and Davison, 1980; Bowen et al., 1976a; 1976b; 1979; Davies and Maloney, 1976; Perry et al., 1977; Reisine et al., 1978; Soininen et al., 1981; Terry and Davies, 1980; White et al., 1977). The small decrease in neurons might indicate loss of a critical class of cells, small in number and above 40.0 μm^2 in size. This loss might correspond to the loss of CAT (Terry and Davies, 1980; Rossor et al., 1981).

Increasing intellectual deterioration is correlated with an increasing number of senile plaques (Farmer et al., 1976; Kurucz et al., 1981; Tomlinson et al., 1970). Moreover, CAT and AChE activity is decreased significantly as the mean plaque count rises, and in depressed and demented subjects the reduction in CAT correlates with the extent of intellectual impairment (Perry et al., 1978). There are losses of γ-aminobutyric acid (GABA), 5-hydroxytryptamine (serotonin), and dopamine receptors, but it is not known if these relate to cholinergic losses (Bowen et al., 1979; Reisine et al., 1978; Rossor et al., 1981).

Mann and Yates (1981) found severe loss of nerve cells from the locus coeruleus. While this finding may apply to a subtype of Alzheimer's disease, characterized by a high dementia score and a preponderance of women (Bondareff et al., 1981b; 1982), it illustrates a more specific noradrenergic deficit than has been demonstrated in the cholinergic system (Perry et al., 1981; Tomlinson et al., 1981). Perry et al. report that the cholinergic defect is common in cases of Alzheimer's with or without extensive neuronal loss in the locus coeruleus. Norepinephrine is important in processes relating to memory, such as arousal, attention, and neuroplasticity (Kubanis and Zornetzer, 1981).

Etiology

Alzheimer's disease is presently of unknown etiology, but a number of intriguing hypotheses are currently being investigated.

GENETIC FACTORS   Although Kay et al. (1964) found advanced age to be the main causal factor in senile dementia, a hereditary factor is strongly suggested (Larsson et al., 1963).

Heston and his colleagues showed that the relatives of probands in whom Alzheimer's disease was established by autopsy had an excess of dementing illness, Down's syndrome, lymphoma, and immune diatheses (Heston and Mastri, 1977; Heston et al., 1981). There is also a twenty-fold increase of the incidence of leukemia in Down's syndrome. Heston suggests a unitary genetic etiology, possibly expressed through disorganization of the microtubules.

Salk (1982) suggests that Werner's syndrome, possibly due to a rare single-gene defect, has many features of rapid premature aging. Identification of the defective protein might illuminate the findings of Crapper et al. (1979). In subjects with Alzheimer's disease they found heterochromatization in both neuron- and glia-enriched fractions with a reduced amount of euchromatin, suggesting a major alteration of protein metabolism.

Chromosomal studies of patients with familial and nonfamilial Alzheimer's disease, both presenile and senile, have yielded inconsistent results. The most persistent abnormality encountered is aneuploidy (Ward et al., 1979). Both White et al. (1981) and Snowden et al. (1981) failed to confirm aneuploidy or chromosome aberrations in Alzheimer's patients, their relatives, or normals.

Stam (Op Den Velde and Stam, 1973) points to a significant increase in the frequency of haptoglobin gene Hp^1 in patients with Alzheimer's disease.

INFECTION   The possibility that Alzheimer's disease is a slow infection, in which a conventional virus plays a major role, is an attractive but unlikely theory.

Alzheimer's disease shares several clinical and pathological features with the transmissible subacute spongiform encephalopathy, Creutzfeldt-Jakob disease (CJD). Traub et al. (1977) believe that the CJD agent may affect a brain already damaged by Alzheimer's. The CJD agent has been accidentally transmitted by surgical procedures (Baringer et al., 1980).

Although a very few (3 of 61) inocula from brains of two patients with familial Alzheimer's disease have induced spongiform encephalopathies in monkeys, there has been no *consistent* reproducibility of transmission either from the original tissue or from that of many other patients with familial and nonfamilial, presenile or senile Alzheimer's disease. Thus, the group who originally demonstrated this have concluded that a relationship between Alzheimer's disease and a spongiform encephalopathic agent is *unproven* at present (Goudsmit et al., 1980).

Antibody levels for a range of classical viruses have not yet been shown to have any abnormality in Alzheimer's disease (Whalley et al., 1980). Nonetheless the nagging question of the relationship of the two diseases remains, and Mayer et al. (1978) report an intriguing cluster of CJD and other organic presenile dementias in a small rural area of Czechoslovakia.

IMMUNOLOGICAL FACTORS   Wilcox et al. (1980) found an association of antigen human leukocyte antibody (HLA-A2) with Alzheimer's disease. Henschke et al. (1978), Snowden et al. (1981), and Walford and Hodge (1980) failed to confirm this. Walford and Hodge (1980) did find a positive association with HLA-B7. Miller et al. (1981) pointed to exaggerated concanavalin A (Con A) suppression and reduced lymphocyte proliferation in Alzheimer's, suggesting impaired immunity regulatory mechanisms.

Taken together, the viral and immunological evidence allows the possibility of an unconventional virus only weakly exciting an immune response (Crapper et al., 1978).

METAL   Both zinc (Burnet, 1981; Constantinidis, 1979; Constantinidis and Tissot, 1981) and aluminum (Shore et al., 1980; Yates, 1979) have been indicted as possible causes of Alzheimer's disease. The role of aluminum, which is found in Alzheimer's, remains controversial (McLaughlin et al., 1962; Alfrey et al., 1976; Dunea et al., 1978; McDermott et al., 1979; Crapper et al., 1976). Aluminum may be merely age correlated but not dementia correlated (McDermott et al., 1977).

CHOLINERGIC DEFECT   This is presently the most exciting if controversial area.

Treatment

The putative etiologic factors have spawned a ferment of interest in their possible treatment. As Hollister (1981) has pointed out, the remaining uncertainty about etiology has not inhibited empirical approaches in this area any more than it ever has in other areas.

METABOLIC ENHANCERS   A variety of drugs were used on the mistaken assumption that arteriosclerotic narrowing was the primary pathology of dementia and that vasodilators might improve the ischemia. Some of those, most notably dihydroergotoxine (Hydergine), have been retained for their utility and are believed to have effects on cerebral metabolism. The most simplistic treatment, namely the administration of hyperbaric oxygen, has been proven ineffective in controlled studies (Thompson et al., 1976; Raskin et al., 1978). Similarly, no well-controlled studies have been done on anticoagulants, but Walsh and his colleagues have claimed their efficacy in open trials with heterogeneous patients (Walsh, 1968; 1969; Walsh and Walsh, 1978; Walsh et al., 1978).

(1) *Dihydroergotoxine.* Dihydroergotoxine (Hydergine) is the drug that is probably most frequently prescribed for cognitive impairment secondary to both cerebrovascular insufficiency and senile dementia. It may provide stimulation of nerve cell metabolism (Emmeneger and Meier-Ruge, 1968) and interference with norepinephrine uptake (Pacha and Salzman, 1970). Among the adequately controlled studies (Hicks and Funkenstein, 1980; Hughes et al., 1976; McDonald, 1979; Yesavage et al., 1979), consensus exists that some behavioral or psychological measures show practical and significant improvement. Higher doses produced the best results, and daily doses of 6.0 mg seem beneficial. Moreover, the longer the study the greater the improvement. The individual effects were small, and usually the depression scales showed the most improvement. Thus, the effects may be due to the drug's antidepressant quality. Shader and Goldsmith (1979) compared dihydroergotoxine and papaverine to placebo and found that both active drugs were superior to the placebo, but only after nine weeks of therapy. Although there is some modest improvement of general intelligence (Kugler et al., 1978; Dahl, 1972), it seems unlikely that the drug specifically enhances cognitive functioning. At best it may retard the underlying process of dementia.

(2) *Piracetam* (Ferris, 1981). This substance is a GABA derivative and is free from side effects. Weak effects on performance, cognitive, and global variables seem to be the general rule (Mindus et al., 1976), and some studies are negative (Dencker and Lindberg, 1977; Gustafson et al., 1978).

(3) *Centrophenoxine.* This substance reduces the accumulation of the age-related brain pigment lipofuscin (Nandy, 1978; 1981), and it seems to have positive effects, especially on new learning (Marcer and Hopkins, 1977). However, the issues of whether lipofuscin is harmful to cells and whether there is an increased amount in dementia are still controversial (Dowson, 1982; Mann and Sinclair, 1978).

(4) *Miscellaneous compounds.* Reisberg (1981) reviewed papaverine, nylidrin hydrochloride, vincamine, naftidrofuryl, and cyclandelate, which are all usually more effective than a placebo. Whether they have a role to play in the treatment of Alzheimer's disease remains to be proven. Even more unknown is whether they have any prophylactic value in milder cases.

PSYCHOSTIMULANTS Procaine hydrochloride (Gerovital-H$_3$) probably owes its unsubstantiated reputation as a panacea in old age (Jarvik and Milne, 1975; Ostfeld et al., 1977) to its possible mild antidepressant properties (Zung et al., 1974). However, Olsen et al. (1978) failed to confirm even this antidepressant action.

NEUROPEPTIDES   The opiate peptides and their antagonists may possibly interact with the hippocampus during consolidation of memory (Kastin et al., 1981). Naloxone enhances memory consolidation. Fragments of adrenocorticotrophic hormone (ACTH) and also thyrotropin-releasing hormone (TRH) may also have some effect on learning, either alone or synergically. Hollister (1981) suggests taking a skeptically optimistic view of these compounds at present.

CHOLINERGIC AGENTS   Davis et al. (1981) review the extant open and closed trials with cholinergic agents. The trials are not encouraging, even when combined with memory training (Brinkman et al., 1982). Christie et al. (1981) did demonstrate significantly improved picture recognition with both intravenous arecoline and physostigmine. Fisman et al. (1981) found no consistent direction of change in serum choline with lecithin as compared with the findings of Glen et al. (1981). They found no impairment of choline transport in CSF or erythrocytes.

One problem with these therapeutic approaches lies in the pathological heterogeneity of the demented sample, some having senile plaques and some presumptively having normal CAT activity (Zeisel et al., 1981). Although anticholinesterases seem to work, systemic effects and the difficulty of maintaining a sustained dose make them unlikely treatment agents.

TREATMENT WITH OTHER NEUROTRANSMITTERS   Treatment with L-dopa, tyrosine, and 5-hydroxytryptophan (5-HTP) have produced conflicting results (Gottfries, 1981).

Marchbanks (1980) suggests using the practical approach of a diet rich in meat, fish, and eggs to increase dietary lecithin and searching for a suitable inhibitor of cholineoxidase which breaks down choline in the liver.

Amidst this flood of approaches there is little solid ground.

General Drug Treatment

Important physiological changes in age affect pharmacokinetics. Decreases occur in cardiac output (30 to 40 percent), glomerular filtration rate, hepatic enzyme activity, and the concentration of albumin to globulin. Sugars, fats, and vitamins are less well absorbed by the GI tract and drug distribution is altered as fat replaces lean muscle mass (Hicks et al., 1980). The most important effects on pharmacokinetics are a prolongation of drug elimination half-life and a reduction in total drug clearance. Many drugs, including hypnotics, seem to be absorbed or seem to act more slowly.

For both Alzheimer's disease and multiinfarct dementia, antipsychotic drugs may be necessary at times for the acute disturbed states or even for the extreme restlessness and rambunctiousness seen in the aged. Thiothixene and haloperidol in very small divided doses of 1.0 or 2.0 mg are probably the safest and most effective ones to use. Both give rise to extrapyramidal symptoms for which anticholinergic agents should be used with caution, because they are apt to cause urinary retention, constipation, glaucoma, and confusion more readily in elderly people. Thioridazine is frequently given in doses of 25 mg three times a day, or up to 100 mg at bedtime. However, it may produce a fall in blood pressure and cardiac arrhythmias (Branchey et al., 1978). Long usage has shown it to be a very safe drug.

General Measures

In a somewhat negative editorial in the *British Medical Journal* (1979), the editor cautions that drug treatment is only a minor part of the management of dementia. Indeed, he adds that it may actually deflect the physician from the really important task of providing the family with sympathy, practical advice, and social support. To this list the author would add a wealth of both symptomatic treatment (Burnside, 1980; Charatan, 1980) and psychotherapy.

Psychotherapists have tended to avoid the older patient, especially the demented one. The therapist may not only need to be more active, problem oriented, and realistic, but also more empathic. The general principles of relationship therapy, namely, accepting the patient as someone of worth and allowing for gradual identification with the therapist's views and for modifying experiences within the therapy, work as well for the old as for the young.

Behavioral approaches have been well reviewed by Gotestam (1980). These may take the form of environmental stimulation, introducing such objects and activities as live plants, family pictures and other mementos, daily calendars and clocks, musical presentations, religious services, and bedside visiting (Loew and Silverstone, 1971). Studies have shown that socialization may be enhanced by the introduction of modest amounts of alcohol (Carroll, 1978; Black, 1969),* by milieu sessions (Quilitch, 1974), by token economy systems (Libb and Clements, 1969), and even by rearranging furniture (Sommer and Ross, 1958). For the unstable bladder, toileting regimes (Castelden and Duffin, 1981) work far better than naive token economies. Reality orientation greatly improves overall behavior (Gotestam and Melin, 1979). Alteration of the physical and psychological environment and reminiscent memories especially motor ones, seems to be the most effective approach.

Our enthusiasm to keep the family supportive should not blind us to the stress that caring for an elderly relative causes in many families (Greene et al., 1982). Britain has established respite facilities where such patients may be admitted for short periods, and these have proven helpful. Since comparisons between New York and London show that many more demented patients are managed in the community in Britain, we should be hopeful that such programs will be introduced more widely in this country.

VASCULAR DISORDERS

Repeated or Multiinfarct Dementia

The pathology and severity of this disorder appears to be related to the number of repeated infarcts of the brain rather than to the extent of cerebral arteriosclerosis. Usually when more than 50 cc of brain tissue are lost, the symptoms of general intellectual impairment and focal neurological signs appear (Hachinski et al., 1974). Often the patient is hypertensive, and there is a high correlation between the presence of hypertension and stroke. Birkett and Raskin (1982) argue

*Preceptor's note: As the author discusses later, alcohol can also cause difficulties, and in his chapter Pfeiffer discusses the various effects that alcohol may have on insomnia.

from autopsy material that brain infarcts occur in a close and causal relationship to cerebral arteriosclerosis.

CLINICAL FEATURES   The incidence in males is about double that in females. Distinctive clinical features include cerebrovascular lesions, markedly remittent or fluctuating course, the preservation of the personality with a large measure of insight until a relatively late stage, explosiveness or incontinence of emotional expression, and epileptiform attack. The illness usually begins earlier than senile dementia. The syndrome may be ushered in by a delirium and often clears within a few weeks. Only careful testing will show residual intellectual disability. Frequently underlying the acute episodes is a steady but sawtooth personality deterioration, with a gradual caricature of personality traits and general dementing signs and symptoms.

TREATMENT   Anticoagulants are usually not indicated and may actually increase morbidity (Hill et al., 1960). Where angiography reveals the presence of an arterial blockage, a thromboendarterectomy may help. This procedure, however, remains somewhat controversial despite reports of beneficial results (Paulson et al., 1966; Stein et al., 1962; Williams and McGee, 1964). As in Alzheimer's disease, antipsychotic drugs may be necessary.

CHRONIC DRUG AND ALCOHOL ABUSE

The Amnestic Syndrome

An amnestic syndrome in the aged may be due to cerebrovascular damage, with or without chronic alcoholism, and such a syndrome may predominate in the early stage of presenile or senile dementia. The amnestic syndrome, although by no means specific, is common to both chronic drug use and alcohol dependence. Its importance is that it may be reversible. The essential features are clinical and are dominated by the patient's inability to retain memory for more than a few minutes. There is an inability to consolidate information to permanent memory stores and a gradual loss of past memories. Intellect and personality are preserved. The syndrome occurs in a number of conditions, all of which affect the regions of the hippocampus-fornix-mammillary memory body system bilaterally (Marsden, 1978). It is more generally recognized in chronic alcoholism as Korsakoff's syndrome. Some claim that it may progress into a full-blown dementia, although this is controversial. Serious drinking problems are common in older patients (Hartford and Samorajski, 1982).

Sedative Drugs

The reduced sleep needs of the elderly must not be mistaken for insomnia. Commonsense measures, such as a warm bath, hot milk, or even a small dose of the customary alcoholic beverage at night (mindful of the dangers of alcoholism), are all helpful. Chloral hydrate, 250 mg to 500 mg, given an hour before bedtime, is a safe and effective drug and unlikely to cause habituation. Flurazepam has the least effect on suppression of REM sleep, but its major active metabolite, N_1-desalkyl-flurazepam, has a long plasma half-life, ranging from 47 to 100 hours (Greenblatt et al., 1975). Doses of 15 mg or less rather than 30 mg are helpful, and the drug is best used on an episodic basis. However, both flurazepam and diazepam are often prescribed regularly. While the therapeutic half-life is prolonged four-and-a-half times at age 80 compared with age 20, the mean intravenous dose to attain anesthesia is reduced to one third. Initial doses of 2.0 to 3.0 mg in the evening hours are appropriate, and most elderly patients will attain a satisfactory hypnotic effect with doses of less than 10 mg. Thus, if they are used as hypnotics, both diazepam and flurazepam should be used no more than one night in three, and daytime doses should be extremely small. Much of the action of single doses is quickly terminated by redistribution of body fat, but this is not true of oxazepam and lorazepam (Hollister, 1981).

ASSESSMENT TECHNIQUES

History and Examination

The more systematic and standard the history taking and examination, the more likely they are to be accurate and unbiased (Gurland, 1980; Gurland et al., 1980). The Comprehensive Assessment and Referral Evaluation (CARE) (Gurland et al., 1977) allows the clinician to distinguish functional psychiatric disorders, especially depression, from organic brain syndrome and to evaluate changes with treatment, self-care capacity, and fulfillment of health needs. Until this approach becomes more common, Arie (1973) offers some down-to-earth advice from Britain, where home visits are still the fashion. He suggests seeing the relative before seeing the patient, especially since the state of the household is a good indicator of self-care. Arie suggests asking the relative a number of questions about the patient. What can the patient do independently—toileting, marketing, cooking? Does he or she wander? Is the patient aggressive, incontinent, suspicious, destructive, or up at night? What community resources are involved?

Examination of the mental state has often paid no more than lip service to higher cortical functioning, but many guides exist in standard texts (Sloane, 1980). Memory should be evaluated early, especially new learning, and this evaluation can blend into history taking. Formal ways of testing memory include the Mental Status Questionnaire of Kahn et al. (1977) or the Short Portable Mental Status Questionnaire (SPMSQ) of Pfeiffer (1975). Haglund and Schuckit (1976) concluded that a combination of the SPMSQ and the Face-Hand Test (FHT) of Green and Bender (1952) was the most empirically useful test.

To the usual mental status examination should be added a complete medical, and especially neurological, examination and an evaluation of the state of consciousness, orientation, language, and motor functions (aphasias and apraxias). Hare (1978) has shown that aphasic and parietal signs indicate a poor prognosis better than memory disturbance and are easier to test. Here a number of questions should be addressed. Can the patient write, read, repeat, and comprehend speech? Can he or she name and use common objects? Is he or she able to follow simple and complex purposeful movements involving laterality? Does the patient have visual, spatial, and constructional ability, imitating patterns of matches or simple designs, such as a circle, a cross, and a three-dimensional cube? Can he or she use numbers and make change, involving carry-over? Can the patient dress and undress easily, or is there a dressing apraxia? Can he or she find the way easily around the home or hospital? All these are important guides to living alone and marketing.

Investigations

Arie (1973) feels that it is not necessary to do elaborate investigations in a patient with a long history of progressive deterioration. Most U.S. authors disagree (Fox et al., 1975). Wells advises a small but comprehensive battery including urinalysis, chest roentgenogram, complete blood count, serological test for syphilis, standard metabolic screening battery, serum thyroxin by column (CT4), Vitamin B_{12} and folate levels, and computerized axial tomogram (CT) scan of the head (Wells, 1978a). In practice, the use of heroic investigative measures probably tends to diminish with the patient's advancing age and the duration of illness.

CT scans are best used for excluding treatable causes of dementia, since ventricular enlargement seems to correlate more with age than with dementia (Ford and Winter, 1981). Cognitive correlations, however, have been made (Tsai and Tsuang, 1979). Hendrickson et al. (1979) found significantly longer latencies of auditory responses in demented patients than in controls and found intermediate latencies in depressed patients. Although these findings confirm the work of Goodin et al. (1978), the diagnostic potential between dementing and depressive illness is actually rather low. In fact, the dexamethasone suppression test (DST) may also be abnormal in nondepressed dements (Spar and Gerner, 1982)!*

More promising, perhaps, is the approach of Bondareff et al. (1981a), who showed that mean CT numbers or Hounsfield Units (HU) are significantly lower bilaterally in the medial temporal lobe, anterior frontal lobe, and head of the caudate in senile demented patients compared with age-matched controls.

Finally, Farkas and his colleagues (1982; Ferris et al., 1980) showed by positron emission tomographic (PET) scans that the rate of glucose metabolism was significantly lower in patients with senile dementia and was significantly correlated with the degree of impairment. This finding suggests considerable potential for both diagnosis and research.

Psychological testing, which is beyond the scope of this review (Miller, 1980; Schaie, 1980), usually does not help with the differentiation of depression from dementia or in diagnosing early dementia. Comprehensive and sophisticated techniques do aid in localization and may also diagnose incipient change.

THE FUTURE

Slow virus, the CJD story, remains intriguing despite the present stalemate. Much remains to be done in studies of neuronal receptors and enzymes, including lysosomal ones. More brain banks are needed (Glenner, 1982). Further animal models, such as the use of scrapie agent in mice and aluminum in rabbits, need to be developed and evaluated.

Better coordination of the social and health systems would help everybody, and so would recognition by public and private insurors that dementia is a treatable—and fundable—illness.

Wells (1978a) holds that the psychiatrist should be the specialist best trained to meld the organic and functional aspects of the patient's problem. The general psychiatrist should firmly grasp the nettle of his

*Preceptor's note: Friedel offers a detailed discussion of the DST and complementary tests in his chapter.

or her own professional responsibility. From psychotherapy to the treatment of dementia is but a hop, skip, and a jump. Try it.

Chapter 9

Affective Disorders in the Geriatric Patient
by Robert O. Friedel, M.D.

INTRODUCTION

Although considerable room for discussion, controversy, and new information remains, increasing clarity has developed about some aspects of affective disorders. At all stages of life affective disorders are among the most common psychiatric illnesses. They represent a heterogeneous group of disturbances with different etiologies, different symptom clusters, and different responsiveness to treatments (Post, 1976; Winokur et al., 1978). Regardless of the diagnostic criteria used, the frequency of depression in the age group above 60 appears to be significantly greater than in other age groups. The older population also has more medical illnesses, takes more medications, suffers more personal losses, and is probably more poorly nourished than the younger groups, and these factors confound the diagnosis and treatment of any disease, including affective disorders.

Because of the complexity and breadth of these and other important topics related to affective disorders in the geriatric patient, this chapter cannot cover comprehensively all of the relevant information that is now available. Rather, the author discusses that which appears most useful in current practice, which promises to become so in the near future, or which enhances an understanding of critical basic concepts.

CLASSIFICATION

Recent advances in classifying psychiatric disorders with operational definitions such as those contained in DSM-III seem to be improving diagnostic validity and reliability in the field of geriatric psychiatry (American Psychiatric Association, 1980). Nonetheless, it is often difficult with the elderly patient to separate nonpathological changes in mood, such as sadness or grief, from subtle forms of the pathological mood alterations included in the DSM-III criteria for Affective Disorders.

In contrast to DSM-II, DSM-III criteria do not include the presence or absence of precipitating psychosocial events as an important diagnostic discriminator. This is consistent with the current position that psychosocial events themselves may result in affective disturbances which in turn require biological interventions, psychosocial therapy, or no treatment at all. In other words, the presence of a significant loss in the life of an elderly patient with a mood disturbance does not especially help us to define a precise psychiatric diagnosis or treatment plan. To do this, we must rather rely on a thorough medical and psychiatric evaluation, a personal and family history, modern diagnostic criteria, and laboratory findings.

Our diagnostic task with the geriatric patient is particularly difficult because of the confounding factors which may mask or underlie the mood disturbance. Physical illnesses such as occult carcinomas may present as depression, and the elderly patient should therefore receive a very careful and complete medical evaluation with laboratory studies. On the other hand, elderly people are more prone to experience emotional discomfort as somatic pain (Horn, 1975), and the patient may actually present with one or more significant medical illnesses. In this case, a depression of moderate to severe intensity may be overlooked. Such an oversight is unfortunate. Most affective disturbances are highly treatable, and many are curable, which is not true for many of the medical or other psychiatric problems afflicting the aged. Dementia is noteworthy among these other psychiatric problems because depression is one of several causes of pseudodementia, a reversible group of disorders which present clinically as dementia, but which are typically responsive to treatment (Libow, 1977; Caine, 1981).

DSM-III Diagnostic Criteria

Of the six categories of Affective Disorders defined in DSM-III, three appear to be the most prevalent in the elderly patient and are discussed in this chapter—Major Depression, Bipolar Disorder, and Dysthymic Disorder. Atypical Depression is also common among the elderly, but the chapter focuses on the classical syndrome described by West and Dally (1959), not on the Atypical Depression that DSM-III describes. Since little has been written about the frequency, diagnosis, and treatment in the geriatric patient of the remaining two Affective Disorders, Cyclothymic Disorder and Atypical Bipolar Disorder, they are not discussed here.

The DSM-III diagnostic criteria for Major Depression are outlined in Table 1, and Table 2 displays the additional criteria for diagnosing

Table 1.   DSM-III Diagnostic Criteria for Major Depressive Episode

A.   Dysphoric mood or loss of interest or pleasure in all or almost all usual activities or pastimes . . .

B.   At least four of the following symptoms have been present nearly every day for a period of at least two weeks . . . :
(1)   poor appetite and/or significant weight loss or increased appetite or significant weight gain . . .
(2)   insomnia or hypersomnia
(3)   psychomotor agitation or retardation . . .
(4)   loss of interest or pleasure in usual activities, or decrease in sexual drive . . .
(5)   loss of energy; fatigue
(6)   feelings of worthlessness, self-reproach, or excessive or inappropriate guilt . . .
(7)   complaints or evidence of diminished ability to think or concentrate, such as slowed thinking, or indecisiveness . . .
(8)   recurrent thoughts of death, suicidal ideation, wishes to be dead, or suicide attempt

C.   Neither of the following dominate the clinical picture when an affective syndrome (i.e., criteria A and B above) is not present, that is, before it developed or after it has remitted:
(1)   preoccupation with a mood-incongruent delusion or hallucination . . .
(2)   bizarre behavior

D.   Not superimposed on either Schizophrenia, Schizophreniform Disorder, or a Paranoid Disorder

E.   Not due to any Organic Mental Disorder or Uncomplicated Bereavement

Source: American Psychiatric Association (1980).

Table 2. Additional DSM-III Diagnostic Criteria for Major Depressive Episode with Melancholia or with Psychotic Features

WITH MELANCHOLIA
Loss of pleasure in all or almost all activities, lack of reactivity to pleasurable stimuli . . . and at least three of the following:
(a)   distinct quality of depressed mood . . .
(b)   the depression is regularly worse in the morning
(c)   early morning awakening
(d)   marked psychomotor retardation or agitation
(e)   significant anorexia or weight loss
(f)   excessive or inappropriate guilt
WITH PSYCHOTIC FEATURES
There is apparently gross impairment of reality testing, as when there are delusions, hallucinations or depressive stupor.

Source: American Psychiatric Association (1980).

Major Depression with Melancholia or with Psychotic Features. Table 3 displays the criteria for Dysthymic Disorder. These diagnostic distinctions are important because of the explicit therapeutic implications which are discussed below.

For the sake of brevity, the discussion which follows refers to Major Depression with Melancholia, Bipolar Disorder, and Atypical Depression (described below) as *autonomous* affective disorders, and to Major Depression without Melancholia and Dysthymic Disorder as *non-*

Table 3. DSM-III Diagnostic Criteria for Dysthymic Disorder

A.   During the past two years . . . the individual has been bothered most or all of the time by symptoms characteristic of the depressive syndrome that are not of sufficient severity and duration to meet the criteria for major depressive episode.

B.   . . . periods of normal mood lasting a few days to a few weeks, but no more than a few months at a time.

C.   During the depressive periods there is either prominent depressed mood . . . or marked loss of interest or pleasure in . . . usual activities and pastimes.

D.   During the depressive periods at least three of the following symptoms are present:
   (1)   insomnia or hypersomnia
   (2)   low energy level or chronic tiredness
   (3)   feelings of inadequacy, loss of self-esteem, or self-depreciation
   (4)   decreased effectiveness or productivity at school, work, or home
   (5)   decreased attention, concentration, or ability to think clearly
   (6)   social withdrawal
   (7)   loss of interest in or enjoyment of pleasurable activities
   (8)   irritability or excessive anger (in children, expressed toward parents or caretakers)
   (9)   inability to respond with apparent pleasure to praise or rewards
   (10)   less active or talkative than usual, or feels slowed down or restless
   (11)   pessimistic attitude toward the future, brooding about past events, or feeling sorry for self
   (12)   tearfulness or crying
   (13)   recurrent thoughts of death or suicide

E.   There are no psychotic features, such as delusions, hallucinations, or incoherence.

Source: American Psychiatric Association (1980).

autonomous affective disorders. The distinction is principally one of treatment response. Regardless of etiology, the affective disturbances that are biologically driven or that do not respond to psychosocial interventions are considered autonomous (Nelson et al., 1981), while those that are responsive to psychosocial interventions and are not biologically driven are considered nonautonomous.

Laboratory Criteria

In addition to the clinical diagnostic criteria shown in Tables 1 through 3, several laboratory tests now appear to be useful in differentiating autonomous from nonautonomous affective disorders, supporting the contention that autonomous affective disorders are associated with significant CNS biological changes.

DEXAMETHASONE SUPPRESSION TEST (DST)   Developed by Bernard Carroll and his associates at the University of Michigan (Carroll et al., 1981), the DST is abnormal in approximately two thirds of the patients with symptoms of melancholia or bipolar depressive disorder. The patient takes 1.0 mg of dexamethasone at 11:30 P.M., and if an outpatient, returns to have a blood sample drawn at 4:00 P.M. the next afternoon. Inpatients have an additional sample taken at 11:00 P.M. that evening. A plasma cortisol level above 5.0 $\mu g/dl$ in either sample indicates an abnormal response to the usual suppressive effects of dexamethasone on plasma cortisol levels.

Excluding patients who are pregnant, patients who have Cushing's syndrome, anorexia nervosa, uncontrolled diabetes mellitus, a major physical illness, or temporal lobe epilepsy, and patients who are taking drugs inducing hepatic enzymes (see below), the test is 98 percent specific for Major Depression with Melancholia and for Bipolar Disorder, Depressed. As the DST is approximately 65 percent sensitive in patients who have two blood samples drawn and analyzed (50 percent for one sample), the test will only indicate the presence of these affective disorders, not their absence. The percentage of patients suffering from atypical depression who have an abnormal DST is unclear, but the author's clinical experience suggests that the number may be significant. The DST is not altered in patients receiving psychotropic or other medications, with the exception of diphenylhydantoin, barbiturates, meprobamate, and high doses of steroids or benzodiazepines. In elderly patients suspected of having autonomous depressions, including depressions associated with complicating behavioral or medical problems, the DST enhances the physician's certainty in making the correct diagnosis and in evaluating the usefulness of a trial on medications or ECT.

TRH/TSH RESPONSE TEST   The thyrotropin-releasing hormone/thyroid-stimulating hormone (TRH/TSH) response test, developed by Arthur Prange and his colleagues at the University of North Carolina (Loosen and Prange, 1982), is another neuroendocrine test which has been demonstrated to be abnormal in patients with autonomous depressions. This test is conducted on inpatients after an overnight fast with eight hours of bed rest. Protirelin (a synthetic TRH) is injected slowly at a dose of 500 μg at 9:30 A.M. after a baseline blood sample has been drawn. In the abbreviated form of the test recommended by Loosen and Prange, another blood sample is drawn thirty minutes later.

A stimulation of plasma TSH levels of 5.0 μU/ml or less is considered to be abnormal. Approximately 25 percent of patients with melancholia or bipolar depressive disorder will have a blunted TSH response as defined by this plasma TSH criterion. Using a less rigorous criterion, a TSH response of less than 7.0 μU/ml, Gold et al. (1981) have recently reported a blunted TSH response in 75 percent of unipolar depressed patients. An abnormal TSH response is nonspecific for autonomous depression. Patients with anorexia nervosa, patients in alcoholic withdrawal, patients with endocrine diseases or renal or hepatic failure, or patients taking estrogens, diphenylhydantoin, pimozide, or dopamine may all demonstrate a blunted TSH response.

The TRH/TSH response test is more complicated to perform than the DST. However, some patients with autonomous depressions will have a normal DST and prove to have an abnormal TSH response. The test is therefore especially useful in those elderly patients who have a clinical syndrome which suggests one of the autonomous depressions, who have a normal response to the DST, and for whom a confirmed diagnosis is critical in order to develop a rational and safe treatment plan.

EEG SLEEP STUDIES   Evaluated extensively by David Kupfer and his associates at the University of Pittsburgh (Kupfer et al., 1978), EEG sleep studies have also been shown to be helpful in diagnosis. In some autonomous depressions, shortened REM latency, increased REM activity, and increased REM density have been reported. Again, because EEG sleep studies complement the DST and the TRH/TSH response test, they are useful in confirming the diagnosis in those patients who are thought to have autonomous depressions, but who have a normal DST and TRH/TSH response.

DIAGNOSIS AND TREATMENT OF AUTONOMOUS AFFECTIVE DISORDERS

Major Depression with Melancholia and without Psychotic Features

Regardless of their age, patients suffering from Major Depression with Melancholia and without Psychotic Features respond significantly better to treatment with tricyclic antidepressants (TCAs) than to placebo (Bielski and Friedel, 1976). Among the clinical criteria for this subtype of depressive disorder, the treatment outcome literature indicates that the strongest clinical predictors of TCA response in depressed patients are psychomotor retardation and, to a lesser extent, early morning awakening and weight loss (Bielski and Friedel, 1976). Recently it has also been suggested that loss of interest and emotional withdrawal are important predictors of positive TCA response (Nelson et al., 1981). The presence of an abnormal DST, TRH/TSH response, or EEG sleep study, as noted above, confirms the diagnosis. As will be noted below, the presence of delusions appears to be a strong predictor of nonresponse to tricyclics (Friedel, 1983).

Certain guidelines for selecting and using TCAs with elderly patients are worth reviewing. Before initiating treatment, the physician should first conduct a thorough medical examination of the patient and perform routine blood and urine studies. In addition, an EKG should be done to determine the presence of prolonged intraventricular conduction, which, as noted below, presents a significant concern in the use of TCAs (Glassman and Bigger, 1981). The predisposition to orthostatic hypotension should be determined, because this appears to be one of the best predictors of severe, TCA-induced orthostatic hypotension (Glassman et al., 1979). This particular side effect occurs commonly in the elderly and has been reported to be associated with dizziness or falling in approximately 40 percent of elderly outpatients treated with TCAs (Blumenthal and Davie, 1980). Given the possible consequences of a fall in an elderly patient, this important side effect of TCA treatment must not be minimized. Finally, prior to TCA treatment, patients should be removed from all nonessential drugs, especially steroids, L-dopa, methyldopa (Aldomet), quanethadine, reserpine, propranolol, hydralazine, and cimetidine (Tagamet), which may cause depression themselves. Having done this, a TCA may be selected and treatment initiated.

Although some patients with melancholia clearly respond better to one TCA than to another, there is no reliable way to predict such responses at the present time. Experienced clinicians use a number of facts and clinical impressions about TCA responses to aid in their choice of a particular drug. First, it appears that TCAs have a tendency to cause either greater degrees of sedation (e.g., amitriptyline or doxepin) or lesser degrees (e.g., imipramine, desipramine, or nortriptyline). Therefore, patients who are not sleeping well and who are anxious or agitated may do better on one of the former drugs than the latter, which may increase "nervousness." Anticholinergic side effects of TCAs are more of a problem in the old than in the young patient because of the increased incidence of prostate disease, glaucoma, chronic constipation, and a greater susceptibility to CNS anticholinergic toxicity. Consequently, TCAs with less anticholinergic potencies, such as doxepin in the sedating group, and desipramine in the less sedating group, are preferred. As previously noted, TCA-induced orthostatic hypotension in the elderly must be kept at a minimum. Doxepin and nortriptyline appear to be less problematic in this respect than the other members of their respective classes. Finally, TCAs are known to have a quinidine-like action on the heart (Glassman and Bigger, 1981). Thus, the physician can use them in depressed patients who are also suffering from cardiac arrhythmias, even if they are being treated with quinidine. The dosage of the quinidine must of course be reduced appropriately. Since TCAs all significantly increase cardiac conduction time, heart block of any degree may be a contraindication to their use (Glassman and Bigger, 1981).

The initial dose of a TCA given to an elderly patient should be less than that given to a young patient. For example, 25 to 50 mg/day, usually given one to two hours before bedtime, is a reasonable starting dosage range. Daily doses are then increased by 25 to 50 mg, no more frequently than once a week, until symptoms begin to clear or side effects become problematic. It is not clear that pharmacodynamic responses to TCAs are altered in the aged patient with depression (Friedel, 1981). However, the pharmacokinetic processes of drug absorption, distribution, metabolism, and excretion are often, but not always, altered in the elderly patient (Friedel, 1978; Friedel, 1980). Because of this, monitoring TCA plasma levels in this patient group permits greater individualization of treatment, with improved response rate and decreased toxicity. To illustrate this point, a recent evaluation of elderly patients treated with doxepin achieved apparently therapeutic plasma levels of doxepin plus desmethyldoxepin in some patients on a daily dose of 100 mg, while others required as much as 300 mg to reach the same drug plasma level (Friedel, 1980). Table 4 lists the current best estimates of TCA therapeutic plasma levels derived from the research literature. It is important to recognize that most of these data were obtained from studies using nongeriatric patient populations (Friedel, in press) and that older patients might require somewhat lower or higher TCA plasma levels in order to achieve therapeutic responses. Nonetheless, the data can serve as general guidelines for the physician treating the elderly depressed patient.

Table 4.   Tricyclic Antidepressant Plasma Levels Associated with Maximal Response

Drug	Plasma Level (ng/ml)
Nortriptyline	50−150
Imipramine (plus desipramine)	> 200
Amitriptyline[1] (plus nortriptyline)	> 160 70−200
Doxepin[1] (plus desmethyldoxepin)	> 125
Desipramine[1]	40−160
Protriptyline[1]	165−240

[1]Data are insufficient to consider these values firm.
Source: adapted from Friedel (in press).

During the initial phases of TCA dosage adjustment, compliance can be enhanced, especially in outpatients, by alerting patients to the likely occurrence of certain side effects (drowsiness, dry mouth, and so forth) and to their usual transient nature. If side effects do not subside within three days after the start of treatment or after an increase of dosage, dosage reduction is often warranted. If improvement does not occur, changing to another TCA may be indicated. It is also helpful to tell patients that except for sleep disturbance their symptoms will probably not abate sooner than 10 to 14 days after treatment is initiated. Patients often need to be encouraged to stay on the medications during this period when side effects seem to be their primary reward for compliance. With TCA plasma levels the physician can detect the noncompliant patient. One should question the noncompliant patient gently and encourage him or her to take the medication every day as directed.

Patients who do not respond to a TCA of one class (e.g., doxepin or amitriptyline) despite the presence of therapeutic plasma levels for two weeks should be switched to a TCA of the other class (e.g., nortriptyline, desipramine, or imipramine) and not to a TCA of the same class. The above process of dosage adjustment should then be repeated. Patients who do not respond to thorough therapeutic trials on one TCA from each class require another form of somatic therapy, some of which are mentioned below. Before beginning another somatic therapy, however, the patient may be tried on a course of treatment with a new TCA recently approved by the FDA. Amoxapine (Asendin) is claimed to have an earlier onset of action than other TCAs currently used in this country and to have relatively minor anticholinergic and other side effects when given in the usual dosage range of 150 to 300 mg daily (Ayd, 1980). Since amoxapine also has the pharmocologic properties and side effects of neuroleptics, extrapyramidal symptoms, especially tardive dyskinesia, should be monitored carefully.

Although the literature on the subject contains no clear consensus, TCA dosages can probably be reduced safely in elderly depressed patients after about thirty days of improvement. A common technique is to reduce daily dosage by about 25 mg, no more often than once a week, until approximately half the therapeutic dosage is reached or symptoms recur. The maintenance dosage is then given for an additional three to four months, and then reduced again by the above schedule until the patient is off the medication. Approximately 15 percent of patients may require long-term maintenance on TCAs in order to control symptoms. At this time, there are no known deleterious effects of maintenance treatment on TCAs, and doxepin has been especially well researched (Ayd, 1978; 1979).

Major Depression with Melancholia and with Psychotic Features

The presence of psychotic features alters the response of melancholia to pharmacologic management (Bielski and Friedel, 1979; Friedel, 1983a). Delusions of worthlessness, guilt, somatic illness, visual and auditory hallucinations, and depressive stupor all predict that the response to TCAs will be no better than to placebo. The treatment of choice in such cases is to combine a neuroleptic with a TCA or to use ECT. When the former is determined to be the optimal clinical approach, low-dosage, nondepressing neuroleptics, such as thiothixene, trifluoperazine, or perphenazine, are recommended. It is especially important to monitor TCA plasma levels in patients treated concomitantly with neuroleptics. Research shows that neuroleptics increase plasma TCA levels, possibly by decreasing the rate of the metabolic pathways known to be reponsible for the conversion of TCAs to their metabolites (Nelson and Jatlow, 1980; Siris et al., 1982).

Bipolar Disorder

Bipolar disorders which develop earlier in life will often recur in advanced age. In addition, a small percentage of patients may develop a bipolar disorder for the first time after the age of 60.

BIPOLAR DISORDER, MANIC The diagnosis of mania in an elderly patient with a history of bipolar disorder usually does not present the physician with a significant diagnostic challenge. However, manic episodes may present atypically in the elderly (Langley, 1975) and may be mistaken for an agitated depression. Circumstantiality of speech, obsessive thought patterns, paranoid delusions, a mild organic mental syndrome with confusion, irritability, and anger may be the major symptoms on presentation, rather than the more typical symptoms of mania. Because of their decreased physiological capacities, elderly patients with mania are best treated promptly and vigorously, and in the hospital. It is important to remember that occult medical illnesses, as well as psychosocial stresses, may precipitate an apparent manic episode. These patients, like other elderly patients who present with affective disorders, require thorough medical and laboratory examinations upon admission.

Initially, a sedating neuroleptic that has minimal hypotensive and cardiac side effects, such as haloperidol, is indicated in patients with moderate to severe illness. Once the symptoms have decreased in severity with neuroleptic treatment, this medication can be gradually decreased while lithium carbonate is initiated and gradually increased. To initiate and use high doses of a neuroleptic and lithium concomitantly is not recommended because of the increased risks of neurotoxicity and cardiotoxicity in elderly patients. Furthermore, elderly patients appear to be more likely than younger patients to develop CNS toxicity due to lithium, even at therapeutic plasma levels (Foster et al., 1977). Careful evaluation of the patient's electrolyte status is also essential. Clearly, lithium must be used very carefully with elderly patients since this age group experiences therapeutic and toxic side effects at lower dosages and plasma levels than do younger groups (Foster et al., 1977). Because chronic lithium treatment is known to result occasionally in decreased thyroid and renal functions, these functions should be monitored carefully in all elderly patients treated with lithium (Klein et al., 1980). If elderly patients in a manic episode cannot be rapidly and safely treated with these pharmocological approaches, ECT is indicated (see below).

BIPOLAR DISORDER, DEPRESSED Bipolar depressive disorder in the elderly, as in the young, is most effectively treated with a combination of lithium carbonate and a TCA (Bielski and Friedel, 1979). The use of lithium with a TCA protects the patient against the development of a manic episode produced by the TCA. Since these medications appear to act synergistically, lower doses of both may be used. A starting dose of 300 mg of lithium twice a day and 25 to 50 mg of a TCA per day is often sufficient. Response to this treatment may be more rapid than in the case of melancholia, and the length of maintenance treatment with both medications may be substantially less, i.e., between two and four weeks. Between attacks, the use of maintenance lithium alone should be considered. As noted above, older patients are more sensitive to lithium CNS toxicity than younger patients, and any clouding of the sensorium of an elderly patient on lithium therefore warrants a lithium dosage reduction.

As was the case with major depressive disorder with melancholia, bipolar affective disorders presenting with psychotic features require the addition of a neuroleptic if pharmacologic management is to be employed. If using three medications presents a significant clinical problem, consideration should be given to the use of *unilateral* ECT, which causes significantly less memory loss than bilateral ECT (Squire, 1977; Fink, 1979). The efficacy of ECT in affective disorders with psychotic symptoms is approximately 85 percent, while that of medications is typically no better than 65 percent. Consequently, when medical illnesses contraindicate pharmacologic treatment or when pharmacologic management has been unsuccessful, elderly patients deserve a trial on this safe and effective treatment. Prior to the use of electroconvulsive therapy, an EEG, an EKG, and thoracic spine films are recommended (Weiner, 1979).

Classical Atypical Depression

In 1959, West and Dally described a syndrome in which usually well-adjusted patients become depressed after a precipitating stress. The depressive symptoms are typically mild to moderate in severity, vary from day to day, and are often masked by moderate to severe phobic anxiety, somatic complaints, and histrionic behaviors. Restless sleep and fatigue are also common during the illness. Vegetative symptoms, such as weight loss and early morning awakening, occur infrequently. In the early reports, monoamine oxidase (MAO) inhibitors appeared to be the treatment of choice for this disorder, a finding which has been supported by more recent work reviewed by Quitkin et al. (1979). These authors have cautioned that this syndrome, commonly referred to as atypical depression, be differentiated from the panic disorder syndrome, which is characterized by feelings of sudden and extreme fear and terror, accompanied by sympathetic nervous system discharge, and which can occur without the symptoms of atypical depression. In addition, the classical syndrome of atypical depression should not be confused with the DSM-III disorder of the same name.

MAO inhibitors, especially phenelzine, have recently been reported to be effective and safe in the treatment of depression in the elderly (Ashford and Ford, 1979; Robinson, 1981). That MAO inhibitors are effective with the elderly is not surprising considering the increased MAO activity observed in samples of human tissues, including brain and platelets (Robinson et al., 1971; 1977). In addition the increased MAO activity has been found to accompany a decline in norepinephrine levels in older subjects, while concentrations of serotonin do not appear to change with age (Robinson et al., 1977).

Robinson and his colleagues have recently reported a positive association between patients' age and a favorable response of their depressions to phenelzine treatment (Robinson, 1981). Contrary to conventional wisdom, these researchers have also found that phenelzine is well tolerated in the elderly patient and causes no greater incidence of side effects than in younger patients. Furthermore, they found that side effects occurred less frequently in patients over 50 treated with phenelzine than they did in a similar age group treated with amitriptyline. The most common side effects with phenelzine were sedation, dry mouth, and orthostatic dizziness, and they had a frequency between 48 and 54 percent.

In an open trial of 14 elderly patients with different subtypes of autonomous depressions, Ashford and Ford (1979) found that a majority of patients responded favorably to treatment with phenelzine or tranylcypromine. As in the Robinson study, elderly patients treated with MAO inhibitors seemed to experience fewer and less persistent side effects than those treated with TCAs. Ashford and Ford also found MAO inhibitors to be especially effective in treating depression related to dementia. This finding is consistent with the anecdotal reports that amphetamine is useful for demented patients because of its stimulatory action on noradrenergic and dopaminergic CNS activity.

Because Robinson's experience using phenelzine with the elderly appears more extensive than reported experiences using other MAO inhibitors with the elderly, the guidelines for the safe use of phenelzine with the elderly are probably sounder than for any of the other MAO inhibitors. Prior to treatment, patients should be thoroughly informed, both in writing and verbally, about the rigorous food, alcohol, and medication constraints during treatment (Gelenberg, 1982). The physician should also determine that a reliable family member can ensure compliance with these constraints and with the medication dosages.

Finally, the physician should be aware of the conditions that complicate treatment with MAO inhibitors, such as carcinoid syndrome, pheochromocytoma, Parkinson's disease, ischemic cardiac disease, and liver disease (Gelenberg, 1982).

Patients may be started on 15 mg of phenelzine twice a day. After at least five days of treatment, the dosage may be increased to 60 mg a day for the remainder of treatment. Obviously, if side effects become problematic, dosage should be adjusted accordingly. Doses of 45 to 60 mg per day of phenelzine should be employed for a minimum of four to six weeks in order to give the elderly depressed patient a thorough therapeutic trial. Robinson (1981) has reported a pattern of higher phenelzine plasma levels in patients over 50 years of age, a finding which suggests decreased biotransformation and metabolism of this drug by the elderly patient.*

Combined Use of Pharmacotherapy and Psychotherapy

The treatment of autonomous depressions in the geriatric patient is best accomplished by integrating the pharmacotherapeutic approaches noted above with the psychotherapeutic approaches discussed in the next section. The evidence increasingly indicates that pharmacotherapy and psychotherapy combined are more effective in the treatment of affective disorders than either treatment alone (Weissman, 1979; Weissman et al., 1981).

DIAGNOSIS AND TREATMENT OF NONAUTONOMOUS AFFECTIVE DISORDERS

The two nonautonomous affective disorders which probably occur most frequently in the geriatric patient are Major Depression without Melancholia (Table 1) and Dysthymic Disorder (Table 3). Autonomous affective disorders and other psychiatric and medical disorders should first be ruled out by thorough psychiatric, medical, and laboratory investigations. These conditions are best treated with medical interventions and do not respond to the exclusive use of psychosocial therapies.

Psychotherapy

The treatment of choice for nonautonomous affective disorders in the elderly patient is the same as that for the younger patient—psychotherapy. This statement seems gratuitous only if we fail to recognize that patients over the age of 65 are less likely to receive psychotherapy than younger patients, while they are much more likely to receive long-term institutionalization and the physical or custodial forms of treatment commonly associated with institutions. The prevalent attitude apparently holds that since the normal process of aging results in instability, decreased memory, dysphoria, and withdrawal, psychotherapeutic efforts are not warranted (Tuckman and Lorge, 1953). However, a careful analysis of treatment outcome data from controlled research studies indicates that some forms of psychotherapies are clearly effective with elderly patients (Götestam, 1980).

*Editor's note: In Part V Cole and Schatzberg discuss TCAs and MAO inhibitors in further detail, and Perel discusses TCA pharmacokinetics and plasma-level monitoring. In Part IV Dunner reviews the current knowledge concerning lithium treatment. Each chapter describes the particular issues involved in treating elderly patients.

Some general treatment principles are discussed here, although the specific indications and strategies for insight-oriented, supportive, group, and family therapies with elderly patients who have nonautonomous affective disorders cannot be reviewed comprehensively. Several recent and excellent reviews are available elsewhere (Götestam, 1980; Hartford, 1980; Blum and Tross, 1980).

In discussing those elements of geriatric psychotherapy which he believes are most critical to success, Comfort (1980) suggests that the decline of self-value in elderly depressed patients should be the central focus of psychotherapeutic intervention. Each patient's sources of self-value should be determined, sources which may include sexual desirability, strength, work performance, ability to get and retain possessions, artistic skill and reputation, or independence. An elderly patient's self-value is also related to how he or she perceives personal change. Elderly people rarely perceive and experience changes in themselves, but rather in the manner in which they are treated by others, and this results in feelings of bewilderment, anxiety, and resentment which they seldom express. Others generally expect old people to be dysphoric and tolerate somatization, but they are often relatively intolerant of unhappiness.

In Comfort's view, psychotherapy with older people most commonly begins with crisis intervention because it may often take a critical situation to bring elderly people to place themselves in the hands of psychiatrists. Elderly people distrust psychiatrists as a group and assume that psychiatrists will see them as being crazy because of their age. In addition, the generation of people who are now elderly were raised in a time when people believed that only the very crazy ever saw a psychiatrist.

Comfort considers respect to be the major force for social reintegration and for helping people deal with the problems of loss that accompany age. He contends that effective geriatric therapists must combine equality with respect and liking in order to differentiate themselves from a world which at some level the elderly experience as rejecting. Moreover, elderly people themselves expect the therapist to give them validation and love more than they expect permission and approval. Specific therapeutic measures should be focused around the self-value model, with attempts to search for new sources of self-value to replace the old and lost ones. Comfort believes that half of the therapist's work may need to be directed toward altering the attitudes of the staff or family, with the goal of enhancing the environmental support systems upon which the patient depends. Although old patients, as young, may require help to express dysphoric feelings of grief, anger, hostility, and disappointment, self-respect in the elderly may be indicated by only a modest expression of these affects.

Finally, Comfort points out that families with a geriatric patient often come into family therapy presenting with tension and ambivalence between the generations. Family therapy in such cases requires skill and empathy. The therapist must determine whether family therapy should be directed toward working through the normal frictions or whether radical solutions, such as a separation, are indicated.

Pfeiffer (1976) states that effective treatment of the geriatric patient requires a multidisciplinary approach because successful adaptation in the elderly depends on multiple factors, not just on psychological or personality issues. He and his colleagues have developed a schema of five areas of functioning to evaluate and address in geriatric patients: mental health, physical health, social health-social network, economic resources, and capacity for self-care or activities of daily living. The techniques of psychotherapy must be modified to accommodate the special limitations and needs of older people. Psychotherapy with older people requires several modifications: (1) greater activity on the part of the therapist; (2) symbolic giving within the therapeutic relationship; (3) specific or limited goals in therapy; (4) increased awareness of the differences in transference and countertransference phenomena; and (5) empathetic understanding of the particular problems of elderly patients.

Given the realistic assumption that many depressions in older people are the result of a loss of relationships, Pfeiffer emphasizes that the first step in therapy is to develop the therapeutic relationship. After initial improvement, when it is clear that the therapist cannot fill all of the patient's needs, the treatment will need to focus on the patient's disappointment. Finally, to help the patient establish new relationships and to enhance self-esteem, group therapy can be extremely valuable for elderly patients.

Chapter 10 # Late-Onset Schizophrenia and Paranoia in the Elderly
by Carl Eisdorfer, Ph.D., M.D. and Donna Cohen, Ph.D.

INTRODUCTION

Although geriatric psychiatry is often identified with the disorders of dementia and depression, the psychiatric disorders of older adults are by no means this narrowly confined. Not long ago, approximately half of all persons in state mental hospitals were over the age of 65, and a substantial number had the diagnosis of schizophrenia (Kramer, 1976; Redick, 1975). Schizophrenia, or more properly the Schizophrenic Disorders, involves a wide array of symptoms ranging from bizarre behaviors and ideation, including delusions and perceptual dysfunctions such as hallucinations, to flattened affect, autism, and a history of inability to relate interpersonally (Strauss and Carpenter, 1982). With time the apparent chronicity of the disorder leads to the presence of two groups of older patients, some who carry an active diagnosis and some who were previously diagnosed but who are currently in remission.

As a group many older, long-term schizophrenic individuals have received relatively poor care, and they often become the subjects of community concern. Many of these people gravitate to urban areas where they occupy single-room dwellings, have interpersonal contacts limited primarily to aftercare drug programs, and live out a relatively marginal existence. Another group of such individuals living in large cities have no housing and are therefore lost to the census, and they present a significant social challenge. Finally, many aged schizophrenics live in institutions, primarily nursing homes, state psychiatric hospitals, and Veterans Administration facilities, where they are often confused with another major population segment, those with the irreversible dementias of late life. The problems of older chronic schizophrenic patients are severe. They are likely to have untoward reactions to antipsychotic medication, and they tend to be socially isolated, with no support from the family or the community. Important as the issues and problems surrounding the older chronic schizophrenic patients may be, they are not the focus of this chapter. Rather, this review addresses problems germane to the onset de novo of paranoia and schizophrenia in the aged.*

Onset of schizophrenia in late life is relatively rare and is the subject of some controversy. Paranoid ideation, paranoid reactions, and suspiciousness, however, are quite frequently observed among elderly patients. The symptom cluster of the schizophrenic disorders often includes paranoia as a major, if not dominant feature. Perhaps because of this, there has been a long-standing confusion over the meaning of the presence of paranoia (suspiciousness), a delusional system, and hallucinations when other aspects of thinking and affective life are not deteriorated. The question is whether these symptoms signify a separate condition or are merely an early sign of a global schizophrenic disease process in which the other symptoms will develop with the passage of time. The differential diagnosis of paranoia as a symptom or a syndrome separate from schizophrenia is discussed by Bridge et al. (1978), Bridge and Wyatt (1980a; 1980b), Post (1966; 1980), and Manschreck (1979), among others.

By tradition schizophrenia is considered a disease entity, albeit with a long-standing history of periodic changes in subcategories of the disorder. Kraepelin's own work (1919) was based upon a separation of the entities and recognized that a substantial proportion of patients with paranoid illness would progress to be later diagnosed as schizophrenic (labeled paraphrenic by Kraepelin). Unfortunately, there were no recognizable prognostic signs to distinguish from among those patients who were initially identified as manifesting paranoia without schizophrenia those patients who would later become schizophrenic.

Roth (1955) observed that despite frequent failures to distinguish paranoid ideation from the organic dementias, about 10 percent of first-admission psychotic patients could be identified as nondemented and as late-onset schizophrenics and paraphrenics. While the use of the term *paraphrenic* is still controversial, there still seems to be agreement that about 10 percent of first-admission older patients appear to be psychotic, without primary affective disorder, and exhibiting significant paranoid ideation (Bridge and Wyatt, 1980a; 1980b).

The differentiation between paranoia and schizophrenia among the aged has recently been further complicated by DSM-III (American Psychiatric Association, 1980). One of the DSM-III differentiating features of schizophrenic illness is the onset of symptomatology before age 45. In order to accommodate similar personality changes in later life the category schizophreniform illness must be employed, but this class of disorders is rather infrequently addressed or followed in clinical research on the aged. DSM-III also describes schizophrenia as "not limited to illness with a deteriorating course," while proposing that "schizophrenia always involves deterioration from a previous level of functioning during some phase of the illness such as work, social relations and self-care" (American Psychiatric Association, 1980, 181). The diagnosis of the aging patient thus becomes even more confusing.

*Editor's note: For a comprehensive review of the concept of schizophrenia and the diagnosis and treatment of the schizophrenic disorders, see Psychiatry 1982 (Psychiatry Update: Volume I), Part II, pages 79 to 255.

The development of observable paranoia and suspiciousness is frequent enough in the elderly to suggest that paranoia, paraphrenia, and schizophreniform illness (but not schizophrenia?) may be important disorders in older persons, albeit not well studied. At this time the focus of controversy appears to have shifted from paranoia versus schizophrenia to paranoia versus schizophreniform illness. But clearly this shift has not helped to resolve the underlying question. The question remains, Is there a clinical entity in which paranoia is the initial dominant feature and in which broader cognitive and personality involvement do result in the deterioration of higher-order thinking, affective, and functional capacities, but which is unrelated to the dementias of organic etiology?

PREVALENCE

Paranoid states and reactions occur frequently in older persons (for reviews see Eisdorfer et al., 1981b; Berger and Zarit, 1980; Post, 1980). Although they are probably not as prevalent as depressive disorders, the nature of the paranoid delusions and hallucinations are more disturbing (Stotsky, 1967). Consequently, affected individuals are more likely to come to the attention of health professionals. To date most of the clinical research reports on paranoid illness in later life are based upon data collected in Western Europe (Ciompi, 1980; Bridge and Wyatt, 1980a; 1980b), and they are derived from hospital admission statistics. Kay and Roth (1961) and Kay (1972) report that about 4 percent of all schizophrenic illnesses in males and about 14 percent in females appear after age 65. Fish (1959) observed that 9.4 percent of all persons aged 60 and older admitted to inpatient care in four Edinburgh hospitals showed paranoid ideation, and one fourth to a third of late-onset paranoid states did not appear related to other diagnoses.

There have been no prevalence studies of later-life paranoia and schizophrenia in the United States (Bridge and Wyatt, 1980b). An early San Francisco survey by Lowenthal and her colleagues (1964) did report that 17 percent of a sample of psychiatrically impaired elderly exhibited some degree of "suspiciousness." Paranoia has been shown to occur as a feature of dementia (Eisdorfer et al., 1981b) and of depression in later life (Blazer, 1981), adding to the importance of the condition and complicating its epidemiology.

ETIOLOGY

The etiology of paranoid states and of schizophreniform illness in older persons is poorly understood. Some evidence indicates that family members of older persons with late-life onset of paranoid syndromes are at greater risk than the general population (Herbert and Jacobson, 1967; Post, 1966; Kay, 1972; Kay and Roth, 1963; Funding, 1961). However, that risk is lower than the risk observed for the relatives of family members who develop schizophrenia earlier in their adult life. These results are consistent with a polygenic hypothesis for schizophrenia, even in later life, and we are again faced with a paucity of family studies that limits our knowledge of these disorders among relatives.

The biologic basis of late-life paranoid and schizophrenic states has not been studied. Alterations in the adrenergic system may be related to paranoid symptomatology. Recent results suggest that brain norepinephrine is higher among paranoid compared with nonparanoid schizophrenics (Kendler and Davis, 1981). Increased sympathetic nervous system activity in healthy older adults has been related to poorer performance on learning tasks (a consequence of diminished responsivity) and potentially on other behaviors (Eisdorfer, 1972; Rowe and Troen, 1980). Heightened levels of serum catecholamines have been found in older men (Prinz et al., 1979; Wilkie et al., 1980), and the behavioral consequences of this biologic change bear further examination.

Social Isolation and Sensory Deficits

Among the more vigorously proposed causes of paranoia are communication defects, social isolation, and hearing loss (Kay and Roth, 1961; Berger and Zarit, 1978; Cooper et al., 1976). The role of hearing loss has been a special focus of research. Kay and Roth (1961) studied 99 patients who were 60 years and over and were suffering from "late paraphrenia." Females outnumbered males seven to one, and many were socially isolated. Half of the women were unmarried, and 40 percent of the sample lived alone. The rate of people living alone was twice the rate found for a comparison group with dementing disorders (16 percent living alone), and over three times the rate found for patients with affective illness (12 percent living alone). Three factors that seemed responsible for this isolation were impaired hearing, personality difficulties, and fewer surviving relations. The three factors may not be independent of one another. The social isolation of these patients may have resulted from their largely schizoid personality types, which in turn may have been related to communication problems secondary to hearing deficit. Social isolation and auditory impairment thus emerged as important etiologic factors in this study.

In a series of reports on the influence of hearing loss in paranoid ideation, Cooper and his colleagues described the influence of deafness in 132 patients who were over age 50 and were hospitalized with a diagnosis of paranoid or affective psychosis with no history of prior psychiatric illness (Cooper, 1976; Cooper et al., 1974; 1976; Cooper and Curry, 1976). The paranoid patients were lower in social class than those with affective disorders and more likely to be divorced, separated, or living alone. They also showed more "social deafness." In a subsequent study with an expanded group of 137 patients, 69 with paranoid disorders and 68 with affective disorders, 27 of the paranoid group and 18 of the affective disorders group were diagnosed as socially deaf (Cooper et al., 1976). The authors interpreted the data as giving limited support to the contention that there is a paranoid type of psychosis associated with deafness.

Not only was the incidence of hearing loss greater in the paranoid compared with the affective disorders group, but the quality of hearing loss differed (Cooper and Curry, 1976). Ninety percent of the hearing loss in the affective group was sensorineural (presbycusis), whereas 52 percent of the hearing loss in the paranoid group was conductive or mixed in nature. Conductive deafness has an earlier age of onset, a longer duration, and an arguably greater impact upon communication than presbycusis. Cooper and Curry therefore suggest that the etiologic significance of the conductive deafness in the paranoid group could be traced to the longer-standing and more severe hearing loss.[*]

Cooper and Porter (1976) examined the vision of the same sample of patients to see whether a relationship existed between the paranoid

[*]Preceptor's note: For further discussion of the physiological bases of various kinds of hearing and other perceptual losses, see the chapter by the Preceptor.

or affective disorders and a loss of sight. Visual acuity in the paranoid group was considerably worse than in the affective group, and members of the paranoid group had significantly more ocular pathology (cataracts) in their better eyes. Furthermore, a significant association was found between deafness and cataracts in the paranoid group, which could not be due to age since the paranoid group was younger. Cooper and Porter hypothesized that the relationship between loss of sight and hearing in the paranoid group may be an association with an underlying tendency to accelerated biologic aging. "The paranoid illnesses of the elderly are probably of multifactorial aetiology and . . . as well as adverse social factors, abnormal premorbid personality, deafness, and genetic influences, non-specific factors such as increased biological ageing may contribute to breakdown in old age" (Cooper and Porter, 1976, 113).

One of the authors (Eisdorfer, 1960) has reported that among aged men in the Duke longitudinal sample, the group with auditory impairment had developmentally lower levels of verbal communication and more poorly integrated personalities. The group with visual as well as auditory difficulty, however, did not perform any more poorly than those with auditory problems alone. Zimbardo and Andersen (1981) demonstrated that hearing deficits induced by posthypnotic suggestion led to paranoia and suggested a mechanism by which this might influence the older, hard-of-hearing patient.

Moore (1981) examined 340 older psychiatric patients to determine the relationship between sensory deficits and paranoia or affective disorders. He reviewed the records of all patients over age 60 admitted to the Bethlem Royal and Maudsley Hospitals from 1970 to 1972. Twenty percent of paranoid patients were deaf, and 7 percent were blind, compared with 6 percent of patients with affective disorders who were deaf and 5 percent who were blind. The deaf paranoid patients had fewer delusions of guilt, and the blind tended to have delusions of persecution, which Moore attributed to the blind patients' advanced age. Moore concluded that closer attention should be given to the relationships between age itself, auditory and visual deficit, and the distinction between paranoid illness and the affective disorders, which have a paranoid component in later life.

CLINICAL CHARACTERISTICS

The phenomenology of paranoia may range from suspiciousness to frank delusional states. At the outset, the clinician must examine the patient carefully to determine the scope, depth, and focus of the symptom complex and must also assess the impact of the disorder on the life of the patient. Is the problem limited to suspicion about theft or rearrangement of property? Or does the patient have delusions that he or she is the target of a widespread conspiracy involving major alterations in the environment affecting his or her property? Are the outside forces individuals who are involved in the person's life such as neighbors, nurses, or relatives? Or are they organizations such as the FBI, CIA, or foreign governments? Are supernatural beings involved, e.g., the devil or spirits? How malevolent are the actions against the patient? It is important to establish how the individual perceives the power of the forces of evil (or good) and the consequences of what is happening. The patient's beliefs can be mildly upsetting and socially irritating, or they may be so threatening that a major crisis develops. Are hallucinations present and, if so, what form do they take? A careful description of the paranoid ideation and its interpersonal and intrapersonal impact should be established and evaluated over time.

The clinician should also bear in mind that there are several potential models for understanding late-life paranoia. It may represent a subtype of schizophrenia, a separate disorder, or a complex behavioral entity. Given the clear need for a more solid body of knowledge, the authors propose that for now the paranoid states of later life be regarded as a number of phenomenologic entities ranging from adaptive suspiciousness to schizophreniform illness (Eisdorfer, 1980).

Suspiciousness

Suspiciousness is a vague concept which does not fit easily into psychiatric diagnostic classifications. The DSM-III classification of Paranoid Personality Disorder is not always applicable. It requires a pervasive and persistent pattern of suspiciousness and mistrust which is characteristic of an individual's long-term functioning. This form of paranoia is seen in later life as individuals with this personality disorder grow older. But as a rule these individuals avoid mental health professionals and do not exhibit behavioral dysfunctions severe enough to warrant social intervention.

A significant degree of suspiciousness may develop de novo in some individuals later in life. These persons become uneasy and concerned about the external forces or individuals controlling their life. Their concerns may be diffuse and generalized, or they may focus on a limited number of targets. Usually persons in the immediate environment emerge as malevolent, and they may include landlords, bosses, children, or spouses. The person may be someone who is close to the individual, like the grandchild who seems to be making noise purposefully to disturb the individual, or the son- or daughter-in-law who seems to want the individual to live elsewhere and seems to speak in hostile tones. A generalized feeling of having been deserted (by children, spouse, or even God) may emerge, and the individual may complain of abuse by the younger generation, by the government, or by other vaguely defined outside forces.

Any outsider or insider may play a negative role in the life of the conspicuously suspicious individual. In most instances, the symptoms are poorly formed and troublesome rather than disabling. However, the interpersonal consequences of suspicious behavior clearly put the individual at risk for social isolation. The symptoms themselves do not involve subjective perceptions of influence over the patient's body or mind. Furthermore, they are not accompanied by disturbed reality such as hallucinations, and they usually do not involve outside organizations in any systematic pattern of untoward behavior. Fortunately, the suspicious individual is often able to relate to someone for help. The complaints tend to be narrowly focused and seem reversible with appropriate treatment. Since there is no diagnostic category for this disturbance, clinical studies of suspiciousness do not exist and the etiology and prognosis are not understood.

THE ROLE OF LOSS   One hypothesis that may have heuristic value for investigation involves the role that loss plays in the development of suspiciousness and paranoid symptoms among older people (Eisdorfer, 1980). For many persons, later life involves traumatic changes with multiple psychosocial and physical losses. These losses are subtle and may not be readily identified as they occur. Loss of physical performance occurs gradually, and perceptual abilities, hearing in particular, may diminish over time. Both of these types of changes have been associated with an increase in paranoid symptomatology and with reduced attentional and mnemonic performance (Eisdorfer, 1960). The death of a spouse, decreases in interpersonal contacts, and loss of income and purchasing power all contribute to a heightening of anxiety at the same time that they reduce the individual's coping capacity. The possibility for isolation and paranoid ideation may thus escalate, particularly where the process of loss is subtle and not readily detected by the individual. What also characterizes many of these losses is that they are not under the individual's control and they actually do diminish his or her ability to deal with the environment.

Multiple losses in later life may require that an individual change how he or she perceives the world. In the absence of clear targets, and given certain predispositions in character structure, some individuals may resort to the mystical or regress to primitive interpretations of the world in a reasonable effort to reduce the ambiguity of the unknown (La Barre, 1972). Thus, an individual may well come to perceive that the problems result from the machinations of some outside person, group, or force and consequently have good reason to be on guard and suspicious of others.

While depression and depressive illness are the most frequent concomitants of loss, suspicion, particularly in the early stages, may be an alternative or coexisting reaction to unexplained, unconsciously perceived, or progressively subtle losses. In this context the loss of sensory acuity, especially auditory loss, has been associated with paranoia at many stages in the life span, including old age (Cooper et al., 1974). Perceived loss of control may be a particular factor in view of the data on the importance of this dimension (Eisdorfer et al., 1981a). Although supporting data are only suggestive, paranoid ideation frequently accompanies social hearing loss. The individual senses that the impaired communication is between him- or herself and others and projects the basis for the difficulty to others. Therefore, since hearing loss is much more frequent among the aged than among the young, suspiciousness verging on paranoia may indeed be anticipated with greater frequency among older persons. Less well-organized thinking and more immature perception and language have been empirically associated with hearing loss among older men who had no psychiatric diagnosis, and this is another basis for an older person's projection (Eisdorfer, 1960). Sparacino (1978) has argued that communication defects and reduced social contacts increase the probability of bizarre ideation, a possibility at any age.

Transient Paranoid Reaction

Post (1973) described a condition which he called paranoid hallucinosis. It is analogous to a transient paranoid reaction in which an individual exhibits severe paranoid thinking of a relatively focal nature. While such patients' distortions are limited and easily related to the immediate environment, they are typically persecutory in quality and quite disturbing both to patients and to those around them. The external focus is usually on someone close, such as a neighbor, a landlord, or a daughter-in-law. These reactions may be accompanied by hallucinations, which are often directly related to the focal delusion. Delusions of grandeur are not reported, and there is no evidence that patients feel possessed by spirits or extraterrestrial forces which make them do things against their will. A conspicuous feature of this form of paranoia is the individual's social isolation. Hearing or other communication impairments may also be observed. In many instances, the patient has recently moved or is separated from friends, relatives, and neighbors. To compound the problem, the nature of this paranoid syndrome typically exacerbates the interpersonal problems and thus further isolates the individual.

Environmental manipulation is often effective in treating the transient paranoid syndrome. Twenty-nine of Post's 93 patients (1966) improved markedly each time they were admitted to the hospital or stayed with friends. These 29 patients included patients judged to have either paranoid hallucinosis or a schizophreniform syndrome. Those patients whose symptoms were susceptible to environmental changes did not differ from the rest of the sample on any of the social or demographic variables measured. The objectives of the environmental changes are to reduce cognitive and social isolation. Attention to auditory loss may also be helpful, and a good relationship with someone who will make brief scheduled visits to the patient helps to maintain and monitor the patient's progress.

The paranoid symptoms may remit without any treatment beyond the social interventions, but where delirium or dementia exists, the possibility of some physical (metabolic) etiology should be explored and appropriate treatment pursued. Short-term psychopharmacologic treatment with antipsychotic medications in small doses may also be indicated (Langley, 1975; Branchley et al., 1978). Generally, however, pharmacotherapy is adjunctive, not alternative to psychosocial interventions.

Paraphrenia

Roth (1955) and Kay and Roth (1963) differentiate between paraphrenia and paranoid schizophrenia. They report that while delusional ideation and hallucinations are quite prominent in paraphrenia, the cognitive deficits, affective blunting, and bizarre personality attributes of schizophrenia (including impairment of volition) are not demonstrable. Nor does the deterioration typical of schizophrenia occur in paraphrenia. Nonetheless, the features which would clearly distinguish late-life paraphrenia from late-onset paranoid schizophrenia or schizophreniform illness remain to be identified. The European data suggest that the distinction may be more a difference of degree than a difference of quality and that paraphrenia should be included in the spectrum of schizophrenic or schizophreniform disorders. Clarifying the spectrum of illnesses involving a significant degree of late-onset paranoia with or without other schizophrenic ideation should be a goal of the next edition of the *Diagnostic and Statistical Manual of Mental Disorders*.

The natural history of paraphrenia (defined as a severe paranoid illness without deterioration of other cognitive or affective processes) remains to be elucidated. Kraepelin originally described the typical paraphrenic patient as *not* progressing to a more deteriorated state. However, it is not yet clear whether these older paraphrenic patients would or would not in the long run exhibit the entire range of disturbances typifying schizophrenia if they were to survive. At a three-year follow-up, Post found that the symptomatology of his 93 paranoid patients had remained constant (Post, 1966). Janzarik studied 50 late-onset schizophrenics observed prior to the availability of psychotropic drugs and reported that they tended to progress from one type of symptomatology to another (reported by Post, 1980).

Where schizophreniform illness is observed in the aged, it typically manifests with hallucinations and a more or less well-organized delusional system (Post, 1980). Delusions among older patients often appear rather banal compared with those of younger schizophrenic patients. Ideas of reference, grandiosity, and persecution may appear in more seriously impaired patients, and persons in relatively close proximity are often accused of interfering in patients' lives. The seriously impaired patient frequently does report a well-developed delusional system with auditory hallucinations. Affect is usually appropriate to the content of what is reported (Post, 1966), and orientation and memory are typically unimpaired. Post (1973) observed that patients with late-onset schizophrenia manifest some but not all of Schneider's (1957) first-rank symptoms, including thought intrusions, depersonalization, experiences of influence, and voices discussing them in the third person. Post also found that environmental manipulation alone does not influence the course of the disease.

MANAGEMENT AND TREATMENT

Effective treatment and management of severe paranoid symptoms in the aged depends on careful evaluation of the quality and intensity of the symptoms and prompt initiation of the chosen intervention. For any type of paranoid disturbance, at least five types of intervention should be considered: (1) identification of losses and/or substitution for them; (2) situational and environmental manipulations; (3) psychopharmacologic strategies; (4) observation and follow-up; and (5) psychotherapies. Due to space limitations in this brief chapter, the discussion which follows focuses only on the first three strategies.

Premorbid personality aside, the development of suspiciousness may be a function of physical and social losses and the context in which individuals find themselves. An important issue in care thus resides in attempts to deal with the perceived losses and to restore control and decision making to the individual. Helping the patient gain greater mastery over his or her life may be valuable (for review see Eisdorfer et al., 1981a). In institutional settings, more decision-making activity on the part of the residents often proves salutary. This may include opportunities to select and structure visiting hours, greater access to information, choices concerning activities, and other options that will facilitate the general restoration of dignity to the individual. The goal is to help the patient feel like a real person rather than an inmate, client, or patient. Counseling with other members of the family and staff concerning the fears and needs of the patient may also be helpful.

The restoration or prevention of loss is an extremely important treatment strategy. In the case of hearing loss, the use of appropriate appliances, in conjunction with individual counseling, may be crucial in helping the person (Eastwood et al., 1981). Counseling should address a number of issues, including the patient's attitudes and feelings about the appliance, the distorted quality of the amplified sounds, and the concerns and feelings attendant to the impaired hearing itself. Programs of exercise, physical fitness, alternative hobbies, and active participation in the community, either as a volunteer or through full- or part-time occupations, may be helpful though seemingly commonplace. The clinician may also need to address the potential impact of the patient's behavior on others in the immediate community and should explore how other professionals may be able to help to increase the patient's social interactions.

An older patient's impaired cognitive abilities may lead to difficulty locating objects and the consequent suspicion of theft or the belief that someone has intentionally moved them. The patient may benefit from specific assistance with organizing possessions, keeping personal objects such as eyeglasses in a consistent place, and having staff members and family recognize the nature of the problem. Memory enhancement techniques, perceptual aids, and a supportive learning environment should all be considered. Of course, it may be that individuals are inadvertently removing the patient's possessions or purposefully moving them for the sake of safety or good housekeeping, and this possibility should not be excluded. Tension between patients and staff or relatives can be reduced by helping the staff or relatives deal with the patient's accusations as psychopathology, loss, and anxiety rather than as attacks on their honesty. The secondary hostility and social isolation that staff or relatives mobilize in response to the patient's accusations exacerbate the patient's problem.

Major environmental changes typically bring on heightened anxiety or stress, particularly when the change is complicated by other trauma, and this may in turn be reflected in paranoid ideation, even in the young. Paranoid thinking is one aspect of the culture shock observed among previously intact foreign students who are reacting to environmental changes (Alexander et al., 1976; Chu et al., 1971). Supportive environmental manipulation has been reported to have a salutary effect even in instances of severe paranoid ideation (Post, 1966).

While treatment with antipsychotic medication is not indicated for the mildly suspicious, there is evidence that it is effective with the paraphrenic patient. Herbert and Jacobson (1967) and Post (1966) have reported some success in treating paraphrenic patients with phenothiazines. Although removing the paranoid symptoms may rarely lead to an improvement in social circumstances, Post maintains that all paraphrenic patients deserve a phenothiazine trial (Bridge, 1980a). Raskind et al. (1979) studied the effectiveness of oral antipsychotic medication in a group of paraphrenic outpatients compared with very low doses of the intramuscular depot medication, fluphenazine enanthate. They found far greater improvement and a high rate of success among the group receiving the depot antipsychotic medications and attributed this effect to differences in compliance. The patients in both groups also received social interventions to overcome their social isolation and to diminish the existing concerns of the immediate neighbors, many of whom were targets for the patients' suspicious accusations. Unfortunately, the study entailed open clinical observation without controls, which limits its generalizability, but it is worth replicating.

CONCLUSION

The diagnosis and treatment of the older patient with severe thought disturbance and paranoid ideation merit further careful clinical investigation. Clearly, our knowledge base is still diffuse and lacks sufficient clinical research studies. The confusing diagnostic nomenclature and the limited knowledge of valid prognostic signs are of little help to the clinician and the investigator. Genetic vulnerability, losses, social isolation, and sensory impairment all appear to play roles in the etiology of paranoia, but their specific influences are not clearly defined. To determine which models of etiology and classification are useful in understanding late-life paranoia and late-onset schizophrenia, further research is necessary. Is paranoia a subtype of schizophrenia? Is it a separate disorder? Or is paranoia broadly defined as a complex behavioral entity? These questions are important because so many patients suffer from this problem and because with proper understanding the possibilities for therapeutic success and prevention are enhanced.

Chapter 11 # Psychiatric Disorders Related to Physiological Changes in Aging
by Eric Pfeiffer, M.D.

INTRODUCTION

This chapter discusses a number of psychiatric disorders which result from the physiological changes that accompany old age or which present with somatic manifestations. The scope of the chapter is therefore broad, and a rather far-ranging array of topics is covered. The chapter begins by discussing acute and chronic anxiety states, transient situational disturbances, and adjustment reactions of late life. A variety of somatoform disorders are then reviewed, including hypochondriasis, somatic delusions, and pain syndromes associated with depression (depressive equivalents). Sleep disorders are the third major topic, and the final section reviews psychosexual changes.

ANXIETY REACTIONS

A few words on nomenclature are in order before launching into a discussion of the anxiety reactions seen in old age. By far the most frequent of these are adjustment reactions of late life, and in the author's experience these are essentially indistinguishable from acute anxiety reactions in old age, despite the fact that they receive quite separate treatment in DSM-III (American Psychiatric Association, 1980). The second most common of the anxiety reactions in old age are chronic anxiety states. Panic disorders rarely arise de novo in old age, but they may become more pronounced or disabling with advancing age.

Adjustment Reactions of Late Life

SYMPTOMS Adjustment reactions of late life are common, dramatic, disturbing, and highly treatable. Generally they are the consequence of a sudden and usually adverse change in an older person's life circumstances. Symptoms consist of all of the mental and physical manifestations of anxiety or panic: fear, confusion, bewilderment, helplessness, and even terror, along with rapid heart beat, shallow and rapid breath, sweating, widened palpebral fissure, tremulousness, and disturbed sleep that may involve nightmares. While much of psychiatry ascribes various psychiatric symptoms to anxiety that has been converted into this or that more complicated or more sophisticated response, what one sees in the adjustment disorders in late life is relatively naked, unmodified anxiety or raw panic.

PRECIPITATING CIRCUMSTANCES The potential precipitating circumstances are many and varied. Sudden losses, of a spouse, a close friend, or a trusted ally are common circumstances. Sudden news of having to move or being told that a friend or oneself will have to move to a nursing home or be admitted to the hospital can be precipitants. News of financial reverses is a frequent precipitating circumstance. A disappointing turn of events in a child's or a grandchild's life (divorce of a child, drug bust of a favorite grandchild) is also a possible precipitant.

TREATMENT APPROACHES With some modification to fit the special circumstances of older persons (Pfeiffer, 1971), treatment approaches are those generally used in crisis intervention. The therapist allows the patient to ventilate his or her full feelings about the event, gives correct empathic understanding, and rapidly explores alternative courses of action open to the patient, emphasizing the importance of exploring more than just one alternative. When these techniques are not sufficient to restore equilibrium, the short-term use of the minor tranquilizers, especially the benzodiazepines, both for daytime tranquilization and for nighttime sedation, are indicated. These drugs, however, must not be used as a permanent solution to the problem. Rather, substitute relationships, alternate housing, thorough familiarization with new housing, and so forth are the more enduring adaptations that the older person needs. Effectively treated, such episodes should be relatively fleeting perturbations. Left untreated, they can give rise to chronic anxiety states, depression, or various somatoform disorders with attendant long-term disability.

Chronic Anxiety States

SYMPTOMS The symptoms in chronic anxiety states are generally less severe but vastly more persistent. We usually do not consider the anxiety state chronic unless the symptoms have been present for more than three months. In addition to the psychological and physical symptoms described for adjustment reactions of late life, chronic insomnia, various somatic symptoms, and impaired social functioning are generally present.

PRECIPITATING CIRCUMSTANCES Precipitating circumstances either cannot be identified, or they may have occurred more than three months prior to the onset of the anxiety state. Generally, adverse life changes or factors undermining self-esteem are cited, but the relationship between these factors and the symptomatology is difficult to document. Patients usually present a history of always having been "nervous" or of previous episodes of acute or chronic anxiety.

TREATMENT APPROACHES Treatment approaches for chronic anxiety states are different from those used with acute anxiety states or adjustment reactions of late life. Both drug and nondrug approaches can be used. Benzodiazepines are the anxiolytic agents par excellence. However, the effective dosage should be kept to a minimum in order to avoid the hazards of habituation, addiction, and withdrawal, as well as daytime clouding of consciousness, unsteadiness of gait, falls, and fractures (Shader and Greenblatt, 1975). Nondrug approaches which have proven useful include assertiveness training, progressive muscular relaxation, transcendental meditation, and moderate amounts of regular exercise not contraindicated by coexisting medical disease.

Panic Disorders

Panic disorders are rare in old age. Sometimes they represent an exacerbation of a previous tendency to have panic attacks. More rarely, they make their first appearance in late life, usually as a consequence of a specific identifiable dramatic and traumatic event.

Panic reactions are, simply put, focused, acute, and massive anxiety reactions. Usually panic reactions are tied to a specific set of circumstances, such as riding in airplanes or crossing bridges, and the frightening circumstances are plausible but not probable. Clinical evidence suggests that older patients with panic reactions are also generally depressed. This view is strengthened by the fact that panic disorders in old age have been at least partially responsive to the use of tricyclic antidepressant drugs (Rifkin et al., 1981). More recently, it has been shown that panic reactions may also be responsive to some of the newer antidepressant drugs with marked antianxiety properties (Gelenberg, 1982). Understanding and treating the underlying depression in such patients is probably more important than trying to eradicate the phobic disorder, unless it is seriously limiting the patient's overall functioning. Again, it must be emphasized that the drugs mentioned are not free of side effects. Clinical judgment must determine the most suitable approach.

SOMATOFORM DISORDERS

Hypochondriasis

Hypochondriasis is the most common of the somatoform psychiatric disorders in late life. Hypochondriasis is a preoccupation with one's own body or with a portion of one's body that one believes to be either diseased or functioning improperly. For many years hypochondriasis was considered a syndrome rather than a distinct disease entity, but DSM-III has now established hypochondriasis as a separate entity. Hypochondriasis is far more common in older women than in older men, although the reasons for this are speculative.

Much of the early work on hypochondriasis in old age was carried out by Busse (1954; 1975; 1982). Hypochondriasis is characterized by (1) multiple physical complaints for which little or no organic basis can be found; (2) presentation of symptoms in a somewhat rehearsed but basically unconvincing manner; (3) rejection of any suggestion that the symptoms might be emotionally based; and (4) a history of having seen many physicians (Busse and Pfeiffer, 1977).

DYNAMICS To understand why some persons develop physical complaints as a way of solving their psychological problems, we must understand the "sick role" in our society. Our culture places great emphasis on personal independence, financial success, and social prestige. There is little tolerance for the nonachiever. When a person falls ill, however, a different set of rules applies. Talcott Parsons (1951) has outlined the sick role in our society as follows. The sick person is exempted from normal social responsibilities. It is assumed that the sick person became sick through no fault of his own and that he or she therefore has a right to be taken care of. It is further assumed that the person will desire to get well, will seek competent medical help, and will cooperate fully in the process of getting well. When a person becomes emotionally ill, society regards that person with much greater ambivalence than the person with a physical illness. While gross psychosis may be acceptable as an excuse for nonperformance, the lesser, so-called neurotic complaints are often seen as an unacceptable admission of personal failure.

Escape from personal failure into the sick role is available at all ages, but elderly people seem particularly disposed to this recourse. While the escape may appear successful for some time, if no organic illness exists, family members and associates ultimately recognize this and begin to change their attitudes toward the "sick" person. Recognition that the illness excuse is physically unjustified makes the other people feel exploited. As a result, the hypochondriac's problems increase.

Three psychological mechanisms play a major role in the dynamics of hypochondriasis: (1) a withdrawal of psychic interest from other persons or objects onto oneself and onto one's own body; (2) a shift of anxiety from a specific psychic area to a less threatening area of bodily concern; and (3) the use of physical symptoms as a means of self-punishment for unacceptable hostile impulses toward others. An awareness of these mechanisms facilitates designing an appropriate treatment program (Busse and Pfeiffer, 1977; Stone and Neale, 1981).

TREATMENT The treatment of hypochondriacal patients can be frustrating and time-consuming but will be less so if a few techniques of proven value are used as soon as the physician suspects that he or she is dealing with hypochondriasis. Timing is of the essence, since any delay in recognition can seriously impede effective treatment.

The most important element in the treatment of hypochondriasis is to tell the patient and any interested family members that *the patient is indeed sick and in need of care*. No specific diagnosis needs to be given to the patient, since the patient generally does not ask for one. When family members press for a specific diagnosis, a simple description of the patient's problems will usually suffice (e.g., "Your mother has a lot of problems with her stomach").

It is important to see hypochondriacal patients on a regular schedule. Such visits need be neither very frequent nor very long. But they must be scheduled. "As needed" visits will not work. For the hypochondriacal patient "as needed" is *now*.

The use of placebo medication has been found useful in hypochondriacal patients, but only if the prescribing physician understands and appreciates the very significant improvements in functioning which can result from placebos. For the hypochondriacal patient, receiving even a placebo medication documents that he or she *is sick* and *is* in fact *receiving care*. Under these circumstances, the hypochondriacal patient can permit himself or herself to feel better.

Hypochondriacal persons of course deserve a thorough but not esoteric physical and laboratory examination first to rule out other diagnoses and to serve as a baseline for future comparisons. Especially in older hypochondriacal patients, acute and chronic illnesses do develop and require additional medical attention. A record of initial physical and laboratory findings helps to distinguish "real" physical symptoms from simply increased hypochondriacal complaints. Interestingly, the patient will generally present the symptoms of "real" disease in a more "real" manner than the usually recited symptoms.

Once the hypochondriacal patient feels secure in the relationship with the doctor and is no longer worried about being found out, he or she may finally begin to bring up psychological problems for discussion. At this point the patient is willing to receive psychological help, in addition to the ongoing medical care for which he or she has continued in treatment.

Somatic Complaints in Nonmedical Settings

The somatoform disorders discussed above are found principally in patients who seek medical care repeatedly. A study of elderly people in the community, however, revealed that some 30 percent of the elderly population had high levels of bodily concern (Maddox, 1964), although most did not seek treatment. The term *high bodily concern* was used in the study to identify a level of concern regardless of the basis of this concern. The concern could be reality based, consistent with the presence of organic disease, or it could be psychogenic. Of the 30 percent with high bodily concern, one half had psychogenic concerns, and at least another one fourth had a physical basis for their concern but with some psychogenic overlay. As noted, most of these patients did not seek medical care. Instead they used their concern as a social crutch, a way of defending against anxiety and soliciting the sympathy, forgiveness, and help of others.

Depressive Equivalents

A depressive equivalent is generally considered part of the affective disorders. Depressive equivalents are included in this discussion, however, because of their presenting symptoms. The typical patient is middle-aged or older and complains of severe and persistent back pain, chest pain, neckache, or headache (Bradley, 1963; Gallemore and Wilson, 1969; Pfeiffer, 1971). No current organic basis for the pain can be found, although there may be a history of previous injury at the site of the pain. While the patient denies depressive feelings, somatic signs of depression may be present and can include anorexia, weight loss, and sleep disturbances. The patient often says that he or she would be just fine if only someone could remove the pain. The treatment approach for the patient with a depressive equivalent is basically the same as with severe affective disorders generally.*

Somatic Delusions

Pain which has no identifiable organic basis may be the manifestation of yet another psychiatric disorder, paranoid schizophrenia. In these cases, the pain constitutes a somatic delusion. It is typically located in the areas of the body endowed with symbolic importance, such as the genitals, the rectum, or the lower abdomen or back. Patients usually describe the pain very graphically, e.g., "It's like somebody is driving

*Preceptor's note: See the earlier chapter by Friedel for a discussion of treatment for affective disorders.

nails into my rectum." These patients are basically psychotic and must be treated as such. Surgical approaches are to be avoided at all costs, since such patients respond quite well to antipsychotic drugs and hospitalization.

SLEEP DISTURBANCES

Normal Sleep Patterns of the Elderly

Self-reports, observational data, and laboratory data, including 24-hour sleep studies, have begun to identify the normal sleep patterns of elderly people. While the diverse types of studies do not agree with one another on all points, there is a consensus, however, that the sleep patterns of elderly people differ from those of young people and of middle-aged adults. Both self-reported data (sleep diaries) (Tune, 1969a; 1969b) and laboratory studies (Feinberg et al., 1967) indicate that sleep in old age is associated with earlier onset, more frequent and longer nocturnal arousals, and daytime naps. A further distinction between the sleep patterns of elderly people and those of younger people relates to actual time spent asleep as opposed to time spent in bed. The observational study of Webb and Swinburne (1971) discovered that the average time spent in bed by elderly subjects was 12.1 hours per day in males and 11.7 hours in females, both considerably higher than in young adults.

Sleep-stage findings lend detailed confirmation to these global observations. Stage 1 sleep (light sleep) is much greater in the elderly than in younger subjects. Stage 2 sleep is generally difficult to assess in the elderly. Stage 3 and Stage 4 sleep (deep sleep) decline markedly among older people, sometimes to negligible levels (Feinberg, 1968; Kales et al., 1966; Williams et al., 1974). The absolute amount of REM sleep declines in the elderly, but the proportion of REM sleep time to total sleep time remains relatively unchanged (Williams et al., 1974).

The exact significance of these findings is by no means clear. Feinberg et al. (1967) found that patients with organic brain syndromes showed more pronounced changes in sleep than did older persons generally, but the changes were in the same direction. The finding invites speculation that changes in sleep patterns are related to neuronal depopulation both in elderly persons who are healthy and in elderly persons who have dementing disorders. But this relationship is still speculative. Of course, severe disruptions in sleep patterns, including continuous wakefulness, day-night reversals, and other grossly disrupted sleep patterns, are frequently seen in the advanced stages of dementia.

Insomnia

Many older patients complain about "insomnia." The term *insomnia* has different meanings to different individuals. For some, insomnia is the inability to fall asleep at a time when they would normally expect. For others, insomnia is a description of the altered sleep pattern that is normal for most older persons. For some, it simply means restless sleep. For still others, the complaint of insomnia is an expression of disappointment that the sleep they get does not leave them alert and refreshed on awakening. There is in fact little one-to-one correlation between complaints of insomnia in some patients and observed sleeplessness (where observations are made either by others or by EEG findings). The physician must therefore first clarify the exact nature of the insomnia before seeking to remedy it with medication or with advice for changed behavior prior to bedtime. Disrupted sleep patterns associated with depression (or mania), with anxiety reactions, and with advanced forms of dementia are discussed separately below.

The normal sleep pattern of the elderly does not require treatment, but the physician may need to explain that the pattern is normal. Older patients, their families, and institutional staff may be inclined to insist that the patient sleep "a good eight hours and not take any catnaps during the day." The author's advice is not to interfere with the normal sleep pattern of the elderly.

Other factors which may contribute to actual or perceived insomnia include unsatisfying or hostile social relationships prior to going to bed, boredom, use of caffeine, or the use of alcohol before bedtime. (In some patients alcohol may initially produce drowsiness and induce sleep, only to cause the patient to awaken and become alert a few hours later.) Behavioral changes can be prescribed to remedy some of these causes: resolution of social conflicts, development of more meaningful activities, avoidance of caffeine late in the day, or reduction or elimination of bedtime alcohol use. When physical exercise is not contraindicated by coexisting medical illnesses, moderate amounts during the early evening can also produce improved sleep. On the other hand, vigorous physical exertion just prior to going to bed may have the opposite effect.

The use of sleeping pills and their value, limitations, and serious risks have recently been reviewed by the Institute of Medicine (1979). The Institute concluded that only short-term use of nighttime hypnotics can be justified. Any long-term daily use of hypnotics is not only ineffective, but also brings substantial risks, including clouding of consciousness, impaired memory, and potential loss of equilibrium with the attendant danger of accidents and falls.

Sleep Disturbances Associated with Psychiatric Disorders

Sleep disturbance, especially early morning wakening, is regularly observed in serious depressive disorders and occurs in mania as well. The basic treatment of this symptom must be the treatment of the underlying affective disorder, as discussed in the earlier chapter by Friedel. Short-acting hypnotics, as well as sedation-producing antidepresssant drugs such as doxepin and maprotiline, taken at bedtime, have proven useful while the basic affective disorder is being brought under control.

Sleep disturbances are also a regular feature of the acute anxiety states, transient situational disturbances, and adjustment reactions of late life discussed earlier in this chapter. The specific sleep disturbances may include difficulty in falling asleep and difficulty in remaining asleep. The short-acting benzodiazepines of the hypnotic type are ideally suited for short-term use (one day to one week) in such situations.

A variety of sleep disturbances may be manifested in the later stages of dementia. Disturbances may include bedtime agitation, nightmares, restlessness, nighttime delusions, and occasionally complete disruption of the sleep-wakefulness cycle with 24-hour sleeplessness. Using one of the sedation-producing major tranquilizers in low doses at bedtime can be helpful. Benzodiazepines of the hypnotic type are well tolerated in some demented patients, but are definitely not tolerated in others, so that close monitoring is necesssary. When complete disruption of the sleep patterns occurs in a severely demented patient, it may be necessary to combine the above pharmacotherapeutic approaches and also provide one-to-one, 24-hour interaction with the patient, including the nonverbal techniques of holding, stroking, cuddling, and so forth. Such intensive treatment is warranted in view of the extremely disruptive effect of such sleep disturbances on the family or the institutional setting.

Sleep Apnea

Sleep apnea is neither a subjective symptom nor a complaint brought to the doctor by the patient. Rather, it is an observation that is optimally made in a sleep laboratory with multiple channels of somatographic analysis (Coleman et al., 1981). Sleep apnea is the repeated cessation of breathing during sleep, caused either centrally or by recurrent obstruction of the upper airway (Clark et al., 1979). It is substantially more common in elderly than in younger patients (Dement et al., 1982). Carskodan et al. (1980) have suggested that sleep apnea in the elderly is at least partially related to their changed sleep patterns. Their study further suggests that daytime sleepiness is correlated with the frequency of sleep apnea. The full meaning of the increased incidence and frequency of apneic episodes among older persons remains to be fully understood. While protriptyline has reportedly been used in the treatment of severe cases of sleep apnea (Clark et al., 1979), many unanswered questions militate against recommending this as a routine treatment. The drug is by no means risk free.

PSYCHOSEXUAL CHANGES*

Attitudes and Perceptions

In a society which has become increasingly open about sex for most of its members, a taboo regarding sexual expression for the elderly persists. Many physicians share in this attitude. With the lay public, they wrongly assume that sex plays no important role in the lives of older individuals. Prejudice, not scientific fact, underlies this assumption.

Elderly persons are interested in discussing this intimate area of their lives with professionals who are knowledgeable and who are themselves comfortable with the area. If this is already true of the present generation of older persons who were born around the turn of the century, it is likely to be even more true of future generations. Having grown up in a less restrictive era, future generations of elderly people will make even greater demands on health care professionals for information, education, treatment alternatives, and innovative living arrangements. They will increase their efforts to maintain their sexuality as an integral and valuable part of their lives. Tomorrow even more than today, health professionals will have to accept the fact that aging persons retain their rights to sexual expression and will need to understand the ways that they may be helped in this area.

Research Observations

During the past two decades, the author, his colleagues, and others have conducted a number of studies of sexuality in later life (Pfeiffer, 1979; Pfeiffer and Davis, 1972; Pfeiffer et al., 1968; 1969; 1972; Verwoerdt

*Editor's note: In Part I of *Psychiatry 1982* (*Psychiatry Update: Volume I*), Dr. Ira B. Pauly previewed this topic on pages 41–47.

et al., 1969a; 1969b; Masters and Johnson, 1966; 1970). An interesting and varied picture of sexual expression in old age emerges from these important studies.

Based on interviews with 254 persons in the age range of 60 to 94, including men and women in roughly equal proportion, the author and his colleagues found that the proportion of older men who continued to express an active interest in sex varied from 77 to 88 percent in the age group 60 to 65 and was between 50 and 72 percent in the age group 78 and over (Pfeiffer et al., 1968; 1969). Among women, the proportion who remained sexually interested ranged from 50 to 71 percent in the age group 60 to 65 and was between 19 and 33 percent in the age group 78 and over. Sexual interest had not disappeared from any age group.

Of the men aged 60 to 65 years, 67 to 71 percent reported continuing sexual intercourse, as did 21 to 39 percent of men aged 78 years or older. Among women aged 60 to 65, from 42 to 57 percent reported continuing sexual intercourse, and the percentage was between 7 and 39 percent among women aged 78 years of age and older. There was no age group in which sexual intercourse had disappeared.

FACTORS INFLUENCING CONTINUED SEXUAL EXPRESSION
From available data (Pfeiffer and Davis, 1972; Pfeiffer et al., 1972), the factors that contribute to continued sexual activity in later life appear to differ somewhat for men and women. Marital status is a significant distinguishing factor between the two sexes. For women, having a sexually capable and socially sanctioned sexual partner appears to be the most important factor. With men, marital status appears to be almost totally irrelevant to continued sexual activity. The persistent double standard about sexual activity for men and women is reflected in this finding, and so is the numerical imbalance between older unmarried men and older unmarried women. About 20 percent of older men are unmarried, compared with about 60 percent of older women. Among older unmarried women, the studies found that sexual intercourse was extremely rare. Even their levels of sexual interest were low, apparently because they had inhibited their sexual interest secondary to the unavailability of a socially acceptable partner. In contrast, levels of sexual interest among the older men tended to stay the same regardless of their marital status. As our society moves toward more equal standards for the sexes, these differences may narrow in future generations.

For the men, the most important factor underlying continued sexual activity in later years was the level of sexual interest and activity they had during their younger years. The men who had high sexual interest and extensive sexual activity in youth were far more likely to remain sexually active in later years. This was also true for women, though not as much as for men. As with so many other activities and capabilities in old age, sexual expression appears to be a matter of "use it or lose it." Of roughly equal significance to men and women were factors such as general health status and, to a lesser degree, adequate income.

De Nicola and Peruzza (1974) conducted a study in Italy and had findings similar to these. They found that among subjects aged 62 to 81 years, 80 percent of the men and 53 percent of the women were still active sexually, with a maximum frequency of intercourse of five times a week and a minimum frequency of once a month. A few persons reported increased subjective satisfaction after age 60, but most evaluated their experiences as giving them about as much satisfaction as their earlier experiences.

PHYSIOLOGICAL CHANGES Masters and Johnson (1966) have documented the changes in sexual physiology that normally occur with older age. A thorough knowledge of these changes is essential to understanding sexual behavior in older men and women. Without such knowledge, people can misinterpret the normal changes and come to the unwarranted conclusion that "it is all over." Such misinterpretations can prematurely and sometimes irreversibly terminate a profoundly gratifying human activity. Changes in sexual physiology occur with age in both men and women. Correctly interpreted and understood, they can actually enhance rather than decrease sexual satisfaction. Partners need to shift their orientation from performance to giving and receiving pleasure.

Aging men are generally slower to achieve an erection. Psychological stimulation alone may be insufficient, and older men may require physical stimulation of the penis in order to achieve full erection. Once achieved, an older man's erection may be maintained for extended periods of time without ejaculation, thus permitting more extended periods of sexual intercourse.

Masters and Johnson close their chapter on "The Aging Female" with the ringing conclusion that for women's sexuality "there is no time limit drawn by the advancing years" (Masters and Johnson, 1966, 247). Their findings reveal that the physiological changes occurring in older women need not affect continued sexual expression. Alas, the social changes do affect older women's sexual expression. The increasing unavailability of socially acceptable sexual partners poses a very real limitation. One major physiological change occurs as a result of menopause and the consequent decrease in estrogen production. A thinning of the vaginal mucosa may result in discomfort during intercourse. In many instances, the use of lubricants is a sufficient corrective measure. Due to the frequency of uterine carcinoma in women who have had hormone therapy, routine hormone replacement therapy cannot be recommended. When sexual functioning is severely impaired, however, clinical risks and benefits must be weighed against each other. If replacement therapy is chosen, it should be administered on a cyclical, not a continuous basis. Frequent examinations, including cytological examinations, are required.

Clinical Observations

The important role that sex continues to play in the lives of many older patients can be a source of profound gratification but is sometimes a source of extreme frustration. Before proceeding to discuss their sexual concerns, elderly patients will generally first test the clinician about his or her comfort, acceptance, and knowledgeability in dealing with sexual matters.

The clinician must be prepared to offer a wide range of responses, including empathic listening, active clarification, sex counseling, specific treatment recommendations, or sex education. Although older persons are often quite comfortable in discussing sexual matters, many do not have thorough knowledge in this area. Courses in sex education were not available to them, and they often have a thirst for sexual information.

NEED FOR PRIVACY As a manifestation of our society's disapproval of continued sexual expression by older persons, their right to privacy is often restricted. This is true both in private residences where they live with their grown children and in institutions. Family members, especially adult children, not infrequently regard the older person's sexual or affectionate relationships as objectionable or inappropriate. Health professionals can and ought to insist on the rights of the elderly to privacy, including privacy for sexual expression.

Implications for Clinical Practice

Certain illnesses and medical treatments are likely to affect sexual behavior in later life. The practicing clinician should therefore keep in mind several principles and assumptions that underlie an effective approach to the sexual needs of an elderly person in treatment. First, it is assumed that it is desirable for older persons to maintain an active sex life for as long as possible. Second, the clinician's role is to serve as an objective, sympathetic, accepting, and informed sexual counselor toward achieving this goal. Third, the clinician must not impose his or her own sexual standards on the patient and should suggest modifications rather than radical departures from the patient's own sexual patterns and value system. Finally, although the clinician must deal explicitly with sexual matters, he or she must deal with them in the context of the patient's overall health picture and overall affectionate relationships (Pfeiffer, 1979).

An inquiry about the patient's sex life should be part of any general examination, medical or psychiatric. The possible effects of illness or treatments on the patient's sexual behavior should be discussed. Many physical and psychological illnesses have temporary effects on sexual behavior. Depression, myocardial infarction, long-term hospitalization, or absence from the marital partner for any reason can all have temporary effects. All too often a permanent cessation of sexual activity results, since partners may assume quite incorrectly that "it's all over." These negative assumptions become self-fulfilling prophecies and lead to a permanent psychogenic stoppage of an enjoyable sex life. The clinician needs to counsel the patient and spouse that sex activities can and should be resumed after illness or separation. The longer an older patient has abstained from sexual activity, the less likely he or she is to return to regular sexual activity. For these reasons, clinicians should facilitate maintenance of regular sexual expression where it exists and when the medical condition permits.

Many medications, singly or in combination, have a tendency to suppress sexual drive. Sedatives, narcotics, antianxiety agents, antidepressants, major tranquilizers, and antihypertensive and antispasmodic drugs all may have this effect (Glover, 1977). If side effects do appear to be affecting the patient's sex life, the clinician must weigh the potential risks and benefits of the medications. A regular drug review with adjustment of the medication to the lowest effective dosage is clearly indicated. The issues involved in drug administration with elderly patients are discussed elsewhere in greater detail (Davis, 1973; Eisdorfer and Fann, 1973; Fann and Maddox, 1974).

Differential Diagnosis of Sexual Decline

Women rarely seek help in regard to their own declining sexual interest or activity. If a woman seeks help at all, she is more likely to discuss her husband's declining interest or activity or to bring her husband with her, again complaining of his "impotence." The word *impotence* is itself a problem. Applied to an aging male with somewhat diminished sexual vigor, the label itself can worsen the situation, lowering his self-esteem and contributing further to his sexual decline. Thus, reports of impotence in an aging man must be examined in light of the Masters and Johnson (1966) data already cited and in light of earlier data reported by Kinsey et al. (1948). Kinsey et al. made it clear that the total number of orgasmic episodes declines steadily with age after reaching a peak between 16 to 20 years of age. Both husband and wife should be reassured that some decline in frequency of sexual activity is normal and expected.

When the woman has greater needs than the man is able to satisfy through vaginal sexual intercourse, the couple can be introduced to a broader range of sexual activities and encouraged to engage in them. Oral or manual sexual stimulation depends less on complex physiological mechanisms than penile erection. The physician can counsel the couple to shift to a pleasure-giving, pleasure-receiving orientation. This orientation can involve a combination of fondling and cuddling and manual, oral, and penile sexual stimulation. With such a shift, many husbands and wives report greater satisfaction from their sex lives.

PSYCHOGENIC VERSUS ORGANICALLY BASED SEXUAL DECLINE Sexual decline in aging men may be precipitated by such psychogenic factors as excessive use of alcohol, preoccupation with major work-related problems, boredom or monotony in the marital relationship, and anger within the couple stemming from sexual or other areas of disagreement. Many men are quite aware of the psychogenic circumstances which lead to lessened sexual drive and activity. Other men lack the capacity for introspection and blame their decline on old age or illness, real or imagined. When possible, the wife should be included in the history-taking process, since her attitudes and observations can contribute to understanding the problem. Her early inclusion can also contribute to the restoration of sexual drive and activity. Involvement of the sexual partner from evaluation through treatment markedly improves the chances of a favorable result.

Psychogenic sexual decline must be differentiated from organically based decline. Clues which favor the diagnosis of psychogenic decline are intermittent ability to have erections, persistence of nocturnal or early morning erections with an inability to achieve erections when attempting sexual intercourse, or the ability to have erections with a mistress but not the wife (Karacan et al., 1978).

A complete absence of erections under all circumstances strongly favors an organic basis. Diabetes, severe atherosclerosis in the pelvic vessels, and extensive pelvic surgery are among the most common causes of organic erectile malfunction. In such instances, surgical techniques may be considered, such as the penile prostheses described by Gee (1974) and by Scott et al. (1973). The patient, of course, should strongly wish such a procedure and be reasonably psychologically stable.

References for the Introduction

American Psychiatric Association: Operations Manual of the American Psychiatric Association. Washington, D.C., American Psychiatric Association, 1981.

Busse E.W.: Prejudice and gerontology.The Gerontologist. 8:129–130, 1968.

Busse E.W.: Are the elderly a minority group? in Behavior and Adaptation in Late Life, 2nd ed. Edited by Busse E.W., Pfeiffer E. Boston, Little, Brown & Co., 1977.

Busse E.W.: Old age, in The Course of Life: Psychoanalytic Contributions Toward Understanding Personality Development, vol. 3: Adulthood and the Aging Process. Edited by Greenspan S.I., Pollock G.H. Bethesda, MD., National Institute of Mental Health, 1981.

Butler R.N.: Why Survive? Being Old in America. New York, Harper & Row, 1975.

Comfort A.: On gerontophobia. Med. Opinion Rev. Sept.: 30–37, 1967

Erikson E.H.: Gandhi's Truth on the Origins of Militant Nonviolence. New York, W.W. Norton, 1969.

Goldfarb A.I.: One aspect of the psychodynamics of the therapeutic situation with the aged patients. Psychoanal. Rev. 42:180, 1955.

Goldfarb A.I.: Minor maladjustments in the aged, in American Handbook of Psychiatry. Edited by Arieti S. NewYork, Basic Books, 1959.

Gruman G.W.: A History of Ideas about the Prolongation of Life: The Evolution of Prolongevity Hypotheses to 1800. Philadelphia, American Philosophical Society, 1966.

Kerenyi C.: The Gods of the Greeks. London, Thames & Hudson, 1974.

Weinberg J.: Psychopathology, in Modern Perspectives in the Psychiatry of Old Age. Edited by Howells J.G. New York, Brunner/Mazel, 1975.

References for Chapter 6

The Epidemiology of Psychiatric Disorders in the Elderly Population

American Psychiatric Association: Diagnostic and Statistical Manual of Mental Disorders, 3rd ed. Washington, D.C., American Psychiatric Association, 1980.

Balter M.D., Bauer M.L.: Patterns of prescribing and use of hypnotic drugs in the U.S., in Sleep Disturbance and Hypnotic Drug Dependence. Edited by Clift A.D. Amsterdam, Excerpta Medica, 1975.

Barker D.J.P., Rose G.: Epidemiology in Medical Practice. London, Churchill Livingstone, 1979.

Blazer D.G.: The diagnosis of depression in the elderly. J. Am. Geriatr. Soc. 28:52–58, 1980a.

Blazer D.G.: The epidemiology of mental illness in late life, in Handbook of Geriatric Psychiatry. Edited by Busse E.W., Blazer D.G. New York, Van Nostrand, 1980b.

Blazer D.G.: Life events, mental health functioning and the use of health care services by the elderly. Am. J. Public Health 70:1174–1179, 1980c.

Blazer, D.G., Houpt J.L.: Perception of poor health in the healthy older adult. J. Am. Geriatr. Soc. 27:330–334, 1979.

Blazer D.G., Maddox G.: Using epidemiologic survey data to plan geriatric mental health services. Hosp. Community Psychiatry 33:42–45, 1982.

Blazer D.G., Williams C.D.: The epidemiology of dysphoria and depression in an elderly population. Am. J. Psychiatry 137:439–444, 1980.

Brown G.W., Harris T.: Social Origins of Depression: A Study of Psychiatric Disorder in Women. London, Tavistock Publications, 1978.

Bureau of the Census: 1980 Census of the Population—Age, Sex, Race and Spanish Origin of the Population by Regions, Divisions and States, 1980. Supplementary Report, U.S. Department of Commerce, 1981.

Dement W.C., Laughton, E.M., Carskadon M.A.: "White paper" on sleep in aging. J. Am. Geriatr. Soc. 30:25–50, 1982.

Eaton W.E., Regier D.A., Locke B.Z., et al.: The NIMH epidemiologic catchment area program, in What is a Case? Edited by Wing J.K., Beddington, P., Robins L.N. London, Grant McIntyre, 1981.

Goodwin D.W., Guze S.B.: Psychiatric Diagnosis, 2nd ed. New York, Oxford University Press, 1979.

Hollingshead A.B., Redlich F.C.: Social Class and Mental Illness. New York, John Wiley & Sons, 1958.

Kay D.W., Beamish P., Roth M.: Old age mental disorders in Newcastle-upon-Tyne: a study of prevalence. Br. J. Psychiatry 110:146–158, 668–682, 1964.

Langer T.S., Michael S.T.: Life Stress and Mental Disorder. London, The Free Press of Glencoe, 1963.

Leighton D.C., Harding J.S., Macklin D.B., et al.: The Character of Danger. New York, Basic Books, 1963.

Lowenthal M.F., Berkman P.L.: Aging and Mental Disorder in San Francisco. San Francisco, Jossey-Bass, 1967.

MacMahon B., Pugh T.F.: Epidemiology: Principles and Methods. Boston, Little, Brown & Co., 1970.

Manton K.G.: Changing concepts of morbidity and mortality in the elderly population. Milbank Mem. Fund. Q. (in press).

McGhie A., Russell S.: The subjective assessment of normal sleep patterns. J. Ment. Science 108:642, 1962.

Mellinger G.D., Balter M.D., Perry H.S., et al.: An overview of psychotherapeutic drug use in the U.S., in Drug Use: Epidemiology and Sociological Approaches. Edited by Josephson E., Carroll E.E. New York, Hemisphere Publication Co., 1971.

Miles A.: The Mentally Ill in Contemporary Society. Oxford, Martin Robertson, 1981.

Morris J.N.: Uses of Epidemiology, 3rd ed. London, Churchill Livingstone, 1975.

National Nursing Home Survey: 1977 Summary for the United States. Rockville, MD., DHEW Publication Number (PHS) 79–1794, 1979.

Nielson J.: Geronto-psychiatric period—prevalence investigation in a geographically limited population. Acta Psychiatr. Scand. 38:307–330, 1963.

Ray W.A., Federspiel C.F., Schaffner W.A.: A study of antipsychotic drug use in nursing homes: epidemiological evidence suggesting misuse. Am. J. Public Health 70:485–491, 1980.

Redick R.W., Kramer M., Taube C.A.: Epidemiology of mental illness and utilization of psychiatric facilities among older persons, in Mental Illness in Later Life. Edited by Busse E.W., Pfeiffer E. Washington, D.C., American Psychiatric Association, 1973.

Regier D.A., Taube C.A.: The delivery of mental health services, in Advances and New Directions, American

Handbook of Psychiatry, 2nd ed, vol. VII. Edited by Arieti S., Brodie H.K.H. New York, Basic Books, 1981.

Robins L.N., Helzer J.E., Croughan J.L., et al.: The NIMH diagnostic interview schedule: its history, characteristics and validity, in What is a Case? Edited by Wing J.K., Beddington P., Robins L.N. London, Grant McIntyre, 1981.

Schwab J.J., Schwab M.E.: Sociocultural Roots of Mental Illness: An Epidemiologic Survey. New York, Plenum Medical Book Co., 1978.

Sheldon J.H.: The Social Medicine of Old Age: Report of an Inquiry in Wolfe Hampton. London, Oxford University Press, 1948.

Shephard M., Cooper B., Brown A.C.: Psychiatric Illness in General Practice. London, Oxford University Press, 1966.

Sourcebook on Aging, 1st ed. Chicago, Marquis Academic Media, 1977.

Srole L., Fischer A.K.: Perspective: the mid-town Manhattan longitudinal study vs. "the mental health paradise lost" doctrine. Arch. Gen. Psychiatry 37:209–221, 1980.

Tsuang M.T., Wilson R.F., Fleming J.A.: Premature deaths in schizophrenia and affective disorders. Arch. Gen. Psychiatry 37:979–983, 1980.

Weissman M.M., Klerman G.L.: Sex differences and epidemiology of depression. Arch. Gen. Psychiatry 34:98–111, 1977.

Weissman M.M., Myers J.K.: Affective disorders in a U.S. urban community. Arch. Gen. Psychiatry 35:1304–1311, 1978.

Wells C.E.: Pseudodementia. Am. J. Psychiatry 136:895–900, 1979.

References for Chapter 7

Biologic and Psychosocial Bases of Behavioral Changes in Aging

Anderson B., Palmore E.: Longitudinal evaluation of ocular function, in Normal Aging II: Reports from the Duke Longitudinal Studies. Edited by Palmore E. Durham, Duke University Press, 1974.

Barchas J.: Behavioral neurochemistry, neuroregulators, and behavioral states. Science 200:963–968, 1978.

Brodie H.K.H.: Neuroanatomy and neuropathology, in Handbook of Geriatric Psychiatry. Edited by Busse E.W., Blazer D.G. New York, Van Nostrand Reinhold Co., 1980.

Brodie H.K.H.: Neuron loss, in Biological Mechanisms in Aging (NIA Conference Proceedings). Edited by Schimke R.T. Bethesda, MD., 1981.

Busse E.W.: Eating in late life: physiological and psychological factors. Am. Pharmacy NS20:36–40, 1980.

Busse, E.W., Wang H.S.: The electroencephalographic changes in late life: a longitudinal study. J. Clin. Exp. Geront. 1:145–158, 1979.

Cumming E., Henry W.: Growing Old. New York, Basic Books, 1961.

Fridovich I.: The two faces of oxygen: benign and malignant. Duke University Letters 1–4, November 1979.

Hart R.W.: Pathology of DNA, in Biological Mechanisms in Aging (NIA Conference Proceedings, June 1980). Edited by Schimke R.T. Bethesda, MD., 1981.

Havighurst R.: Successful aging, in Processes of Aging. Edited by Williams R., Tibbitts C., Donahue W. New York, Atherton Press, 1963.

Hayflick L., Moorhead P.S.: The serial cultivation of human diploid cells. Exp. Cell. Res. 25:585–621, 1961.

Heston L.L., Mastri A.R.: The genetics of Alzheimer's disease. Arch. Gen. Psychiatry 35:976–981, 1977.

Jarvik L.F.: The aging central nervous system: clinical aspects, in Aging: Clinical, Morphologic, and Neurochemical Aspects in the Central Nervous System. Edited by Brodie H.K.H., Harman D., Ordy J.M. New York, Raven Press, 1975.

Marx J.L.: Hormones and their effects in the aging body. Science 206:805–806, 1979.

Meier-Ruge W., Enz A., Gugax P., et al.: Experimental pathology in basic research of the aging brain, in Aging, Vol. 2: Genesis and Treatment of Psychologic Disorders in the Elderly. Edited by Gershon E.S., Raskin A. New York, Raven Press, 1975.

Nies A.: Changes in monoamine oxidase with aging, in Psychopharmacology and Aging. Edited by Eisdorfer C., Fann, W.E. New York, Plenum Press, 1973.

Palmore E.: Social Patterns in Normal Aging—Findings from the Duke Longitudinal Study. Durham, Duke University Press, 1982.

Reinberg A.: Chronopharmacology in man, in Chronobiological Aspects of Endocrinology. Edited by Aschoff J., Cersa F., Halberg G. Stuttgart and New York, F. K. Schattauer Verlag, 1974.

Rogers D.E., Blendon R.J., Moloney T.J.: Providing medical care for the elderly and the poor: a serious problem for the downsizing 1980's, in The Proceedings of the 7th Private Sector Conference. Durham, Duke University Medical Center, March 1982.

Samorajski T., Hartford J.: Brain physiology of aging, in Handbook of Geriatric Psychiatry. Edited by Busse E.W., Blazer, D.G. New York, Van Nostrand Reinhold Co., 1980.

Sandoz Pharmaceuticals: Loss of vision. Sensory Loss in the Elderly: An Overview, 7–11, 1980a.

Sandoz Pharmaceuticals: Loss of hearing. Sensory Loss in the Elderly: An Overview, 13–16, 1980b.

Scheibel M.E., Scheibel A.G.: Structural changes in the aging brain, in Aging: Clinical, Morphologic, and Neurochemical Aspects in the Central Nervous System. Edited by Brodie H.K.H., Harman D., Ordy J.M. New York, Raven Press, 1975.

Schiffman S.: Changes in taste and smell with age: psychophysical aspects, in Sensory Systems and Communication in the Elderly, Aging, vol 10. Edited by Ordy J.M., Brizzee K.R. New York, Raven Press, 1979.

Snyder S.H.: Brain peptides as neurotransmitters. Science 209:976–983, 1980.

Suskind G.W.: Immunological aspects of aging: an overview, in Biological Mechanisms in Aging (NIA Conference Proceedings). Edited by Schimke R.T. Bethesda, MD., 1981.

Wisniewski H.M., Terry R.D.: Neuropathology of the aging brain, in Neurobiology of Aging. Edited by Terry R.D. New York, Raven Press, 1976.

References for Chapter 8

Organic Mental Disorders

Alfrey A.C., LeGendre G.R., Kaehny W.D.: The dialysis encephalopathy syndrome. New Eng. J. Med. 294:184–188, 1976.

American Psychiatric Association: Diagnostic and Statistical Manual of Mental Disorders, 3rd ed. Washington, D.C., American Psychiatric Association, 1980.

Arie T.: Dementia in the elderly: diagnosis and assessment. Br. Med. J. 4:540–543, 1973.

Baringer J.R., Gajdusek D.C., Gibbs C.J., et al.: Transmissible dementias: current problems in tissue handling. Neurology 30:302–303, 1980.

Barnes R.F., Raskind M.A.: DSM-III criteria and the clinical diagnosis of dementia: a nursing home study. J. Gerontol. 36:20–27, 1981.

Birkett D.P., Raskin A.: Arteriosclerosis, infarcts, and dementia. J. Am. Geriatr. Soc. 30:261–266, 1982.

Birren J.E., Sloane R.B., (eds.): Handbook of Mental Health and Aging. Englewood Cliffs, N.J., Prentice-Hall, 1980.

Black A.L.: Altering behavior of geriatric patients with beer. Northwest Medicine 68:453–456, 1969.

Bondareff W., Baldy R., Levy R.: Quantitative computed tomography in senile dementia. Arch. Gen. Psychiatry 38:1365–1368, 1981a.

Bondareff W., Mountjoy C.O., Roth M.: Selective loss of neurons of origin of adrenergic projection to cerebral cortex (nucleus locus coeruleus) in senile dementia (letter). Lancet 1:783–784, 1981b.

Bondareff W., Mountjoy C.O., Roth M.: Loss of neurons of origin of the adrenergic projection to cerebral cortex (nucleus locus coeruleus) in senile dementia. Neurology (Ny) 32:164–168, 1982.

Bowen D.M., Davison A.N.: Biochemical changes in the cholinergic system of the aging brain in senile dementia. Psychol. Med. 10:315–319, 1980.

Bowen D.M., Goodhardt M.J., Strong A.J., et al.: Biochemical indices of brain structure, function and "hypoxia" in cortex from baboons with middle cerebral artery occlusion. Brain Res. 117:503–507, 1976a.

Bowen D.M., Smith C.B., White P., et al.: Neurotransmitter-related enzymes and indices of hypoxia in senile dementia and other abiotrophies. Brain 99:459–496, 1976b.

Bowen D.M., White P., Spillane J.A., et al.: Accelerated ageing or selective neuronal loss as an important cause of dementia? Lancet 1:11–14, 1979.

Branchley M.H., Lee J.H., Amin. R., et al.: High and low potency neuroleptics in elderly psychiatric patients. JAMA 239:1860–1862, 1978.

Brinkman S.D., Smith R.C., Meyer J.S., et al.: Lecithin and memory training in suspected Alzheimer's disease. J. Gerontol. 37:104–109, 1982.

British Medical Journal: Vasodilators in senile dementia (editorial). 2:511–512, 1979.

Burnet F.M.: A possible role of zinc in the pathology of dementia. Lancet 1:186–187, 1981.

Burnside I.M.: Symptomatic behaviors in the elderly, in Handbook of Mental Health and Aging. Edited by Birren J.E., Sloane R.B. Englewood Cliffs, N.J., Prentice-Hall, 1980.

Carroll P.J.: The social hour for geropsychiatric patients. J. Am. Geriatr. Soc. 26:32–35, 1978.

Castleden C.M., Duffin H.M.: Guidelines for controlling urinary incontinence without drugs or catheters. Age and Ageing 10:186–190, 1981.

Charatan F.B.: Therapeutic supports for the patient with OBS. Geriatrics 35:100–102, 1980.

Christie A.B.: Changing patterns of mental illness in the elderly. Br. J. Psychiatry 140:154–159, 1982.

Christie J.E., Shering A., Gerguson J., et al.: Physostigmine and arecoline: effects of intravenous infusions in Alzheimer presenile dementia. Br. J. Psychiatry 138:46–50, 1981.

Coblentz J.M., Mattis S., Zingesser L.H., et al.: Presenile dementia. Clinical aspects and evaluation of cerebrospinal fluid dynamics. Arch. Neurol. 29:299–308, 1973.

Constantinidis J.: Zinc metabolism in presenile dementias, in Alzheimer's Disease: Early Recognition of Potentially Reversible Deficits. Edited by Glen A.I.M., Whalley L.J. Edinburgh, Churchill Livingstone, 1979.

Constantinidis J., Tissot R.: Role of glutamate and zinc in the hippocampal lesions of Pick's disease, in Glutamate as a Neurotransmitter. Edited by Di Chiara G., Gessa G.L. New York, Raven Press, 1981.

Crapper D.R., De Boni U.: Brain aging and Alzheimer's disease. Can. Psychiatric Assoc. J. 23:229–233, 1978.

Crapper D.R., Krishnan S.S., Quittkat S.: Aluminum, neurofibrillary degeneration and Alzheimer's disease. Brain 99:67–80, 1976.

Crapper D.R., Quittkat S., De Boni U.: Altered chromatin confirmation in Alzheimer's disease. Brain 102:483–495, 1979.

Dahl G.: WIP-Reduzierter Wechsler-Intelligenz Test. Meisenheim, 1972.

Davies P., Maloney A.J.F.: Selective loss of central cholinergic neurons in Alzheimer's disease. Lancet 2:1403, 1976.

Davis K.L., Mohs R.C., Davis B.M., et al.: Cholinomimetic agents and human memory: clinical studies in Alzheimer's disease and scopolamine dementia, in Strategies for the Development of an Effective Treatment for Senile Dementia. Edited by Crook T., Gershon E.S. New Canaan, CT., Mark Powley Associates, 1981.

Dencker S.J., Lindberg D.: A controlled double-blind study of piracetam in the treatment of senile dementia. Nord Psykiatr Tidskreft 31:48–52, 1977.

Dowson J.H.: Neuronal lipofuscin accumulation in ageing and Alzheimer dementia: a pathogenic mechanism? Br. J. Psychiatry 140:142–148, 1982.

Duckworth G.S., Ross H.: Diagnostic differences in psychogeriatric patients in Toronto, New York and London, England. Can. Med. Assoc. J. 112:847–851, 1975.

Dunea G., Mahurkar S.D., Mamdani B., et al.: Role of aluminum in dialysis dementia. Ann. Int. Med. 88:502–504, 1978.

Emmeneger H., Meier-Ruge W.: Actions of hydergine on the brain. Pharmacology 1:65–78, 1968.

Engel G.L., Romano J.: Studies of delirium. II. Reversibility of the encephalogram with experimental procedures. Arch. Neurology Psychiatry 51:378–392, 1944.

Engel G.L., Romano J.: Delirium: a syndrome of cerebral insufficiency. J. Chronic. Dis. 9:260–277, 1959.

Farkas T., Ferris S.H., Wolf A.P., et al.: F-2-Deoxy-2-fluoro-D-glucose as a tracer in the positron emission tomographic study of senile dementia. Am. J. Psychiatry 139:352–353, 1982.

Farmer P.M., Peck A., Terry R.D.: Correlations among neuritic plaques, neurofibrillary tangles and the severity of senile dementia (abstract). J. Neuropathol. Exp. Neurol. 35:367, 1976.

Ferris S.H.: Empirical studies in senile dementia with central nervous system stimulants and metabolic enhancers, in Strategies for the Development of an Effective Treatment for Senile Dementia. Edited by Crook T., Gershon E.S. New Canaan, CT., Mark Powley Associates, 1981.

Ferris S.H., De Leon M.J., Wolf A.P., et al.: Positron emission tomography in the study of aging and senile dementia. Neurobiol. Aging 1:127–131, 1980.

Fisman M., Mersky H., Helmes E., et al.: Double-blind study of lecithin in patients with Alzheimer's disease. Can. J. Psychiatry 26:426–428, 1981.

Folstein M.F., McHugh P.R.: Dementia syndrome of depression, in Alzheimer's Disease: Senile Dementia and

Related Disorders. Edited by Katzman R., Terry R.D., Bick K.L. New York, Raven Press, 1978.

Ford C.V., Winter J.: Computerized axial tomograms in dementia in elderly patients. J. Gerontology 36:164–169, 1981.

Fox J.H., Topel J.L., Huckman M.S.: Dementia in the elderly—a search for treatable illnesses. J. Gerontol. 330:557–564, 1975.

Freemon F.R.: Evaluation of patients with progressive intellectual deterioration. Arch. Neurol. 33:658–659, 1976.

Glen A.I.M., Yates C.M., Simpson J., et al.: Choline uptake in patients with Alzheimer pre-senile dementia. Psychol. Med. 11:469–476, 1981.

Glenner G.G.: Alzheimer's disease (senile dementia): a research update and critique with recommendations. J. Am. Geriatr. Soc. 30:59–62, 1982.

Good M.I.: Pseudodementia and physical findings masking significant psychopathology. Am. J. Psychiatry 138:811–814, 1981.

Goodin D.S., Squires K.C., Starr A.: Long latency event-related components of the auditory evoked potential in dementia. Brain 101:635–648, 1978.

Götestam K.G.: Behavioral and dynamic psychotherapy with the elderly, in Handbook of Mental Health and Aging. Edited by Birren J.E., Sloane R.B. Englewood Cliffs, N.J., Prentice-Hall, 1980.

Götestam K.G., Melin L.: Improving well-being for patients with senile dementia by minor changes in the ward environment, in Society, Stress and Disease: Aging and Old Age. Edited by Levi L. London, Oxford University Press, 1979.

Gottfries C.G.: Etiological and treatment considerations in SDAT, in Strategies for the Development of an Effective Treatment for Senile Dementia. Edited by Crook T., Gershon E.S. New Canaan, CT., Mark Powley Associates, 1981.

Goudsmit J., Morrow C.H., Asher D.M., et al.: Evidence for and against the transmissibility of Alzheimer disease. Neurology 30:945–950, 1980.

Green M.A., Bender M.B.: The face-hand test as a diagnostic sign of organic mental syndrome. Neurology 2:46–58, 1952.

Greenblatt D., Allen M.D., Shader R.: Fluorazepam hydrochloride. Clinic. Pharmacol. Ther. 17:1–14, 1975.

Greene J.G., Smith R., Gardiner M., et al.: Measuring behavioral disturbance of elderly demented patients in the community and its effect on relatives: a factor analytic study. Age and Ageing 11:121–126, 1982.

Gurland B.J.: The assessment of the mental health status of older adults, in Handbook of Mental Health and Aging. Edited by Birren J.E., Sloane R.B. Englewood Cliffs, N.J., Prentice-Hall, 1980.

Gurland B.J., Dean L., Cross P., et al.: The epidemiology of dementia and depression in the elderly: the use of multiple indicators of these conditions, in Psychopathology in the Aged. Edited by Cole J.O., Barrett J.E. New York, Raven Press, 1980.

Gurland B.J., Kuriansky J., Sharpe L., et al.: The Comprehensive Assessment and Referral Evaluation (CARE)—rationale, development and reliability. Int'l J. Aging and Human Development 8:9–42, 1977.

Gustafson L., Risberg J., Johanson M., et al.: Effects of piracetam on regional cerebral blood flow and mental functions in patients with organic dementia. Psychopharmacol. 56:115–117, 1978.

Habot B., Lobow L.: The interrelationship of mental and physical status and its assessment in the older adult: mind-body interaction, in Handbook of Mental Health

and Aging. Edited by Birren J.E., Sloane R.B. Englewood Cliffs, N.J., Prentice-Hall, 1980.

Hachinski V.C., Lassen N.A., Marshall J.: Multi-infarct dementia: a cause of mental deterioration in the elderly. Lancet 2:207–210, 1974.

Haglund R.M., Schuckit M.A.: A clinical comparison of tests of organicity in elderly patients. J. Gerontol. 31:654–659, 1976.

Hare M.: Clinical checklist for diagnosis of dementia. Br. Med. J. 2:266–267, 1978.

Harris R.: The relationship between organic brain disease and physical status, in Aging and the Brain. Edited by Gaitz C.M. New York/London, Plenum Press, 1972.

Harrison M.J.G., Marsden C.D.: Progressive intellectual deterioration (letter to editor). Arch. Neurol. 34:199, 1977.

Hartford J.T., Samorajski T.: Alcoholism in the geriatric population. J. Am. Geriatr. Soc. 30:18–24, 1982.

Hendrickson E., Levy R., Post F.: Averaged evoked responses in relation to cognitive and affective state of elderly psychiatric patients. Br. J. Psychiatry 134:494–501, 1979.

Henschke P.J., Bell D.A., Cape R.D.T.: Alzheimer's disease and HLA. Tissue Antigens 12:132–135, 1978.

Heston L.L., Mastri A.R.: The genetics of Alzheimer's disease: associations with hematological malignancy and Down's syndrome. Arch. Gen. Psychiatry 34:976–981, 1977.

Hicks R., Funkenstein H.H., Dysken M.W., et al.: Geriatric psychopharmacology, in Handbook of Mental Health and Aging. Edited by Birren J.E., Sloane R.B. Englewood Cliffs, N.J., Prentice-Hall, 1980.

Hill A.B., Marshall J., Shaw D.A.: A controlled clinical trial of long-term anticoagulant therapy in cerebrovascular disease. Quart. J. Med. 29:597–609, 1960.

Hollister L.F.: An overview of strategies for the development of an effective treatment for senile dementia, in Strategies for the Development of an Effective Treatment for Senile Dementia. Edited by Crook T., Gershon E.S. New Canaan, CT., Mark Powley Associates, 1981.

Hughes J.R., Williams J.G., Currier R.D.: An ergot alkaloid preparation (Hydergine) in the treatment of dementia: critical review of the literature. J. Am. Geriatr. Soc. 24:490–497, 1976.

Jarvik L.F., Milne J.F.: Gerovital-H$_x$: a review of the literature, in Aging, vol. 2. Genesis and Treatment of Psychologic Disorders in the Elderly. Edited by Gershon E.S., Raskin A. New York, Raven Press, 1975.

Kahn R.L., Goldfarb A.I., Pollack M., et al.: Brief objective measures for the determination of mental status in the aged. Am. J. Psychiatry 117:326–328, 1977.

Kahn R.L., Zarit S.H., Hilbert N.M., et al.: Memory complaint and impairment in the aged. The effect of depression and altered brain function. Arch. Gen. Psychiatry 32:1569, 1975.

Kastin A.J., Olson G.A., Sandman C.A., et al.: Possible role of peptides in senile dementia, in Strategies for the Development of an Effective Treatment for Senile Dementia. Edited by Crook T., Gershon E.S. New Canaan, CT., Mark Powley Associates, 1981.

Katzman R.: The prevalence and malignancy of Alzheimer disease. Arch. Neurol. 33:217–218, 1976.

Katzman R., Karasu T.B.: Differential diagnosis in dementia, in Neurological and Sensory Disorders in the Elderly. Edited by Fields W.S. New York, Stratton Intercontinental, 1975.

Kay D.W.K., Beamish P., Roth M.: Old age mental disorders in Newcastle-upon-Tyne, Part I: a study of prevalence. Br. J. Psychiatry 110:146–158, 1964.

Kay D.W.K., Bergmann K.: Epidemiology of mental disorders among the aged in the community, in Handbook of Mental Health and Aging. Edited by Birren J.E., Sloane R.B. Englewood Cliffs, N.J., Prentice-Hall, 1980.

Kay D.W.K., Roth M.: Physical accompaniments of mental disorders in old age. Lancet 2:740, 1955.

Kiloh L.G.: Pseudo-dementia. Acta Psychiat. Scand. 37:336, 1961.

Kral V.A.: Benign senescent forgetfulness, in Aging, vol. 7, Alzheimer's Disease: Senile Dementia and Related Disorders. Edited by Katzman R., Terry R.D., Bick K.L. New York, Raven Press, 1978.

Kubanis P., Zornetzer S.F.: Age-related behavioral and neurobiological changes: a review with an emphasis on memory. Behav. Neurol. Biology 31:115–172, 1981.

Kugler J., Oswald W.D., Hersfeld U.: Langzeittherapie altersbedingter Insuffizienzerscheinungen des Gehirns. Deutsch. Med. Wochenschr. 103:456–462, 1978.

Kurucz J., Charbonneau R., Kurucz A., et al.: Quantitative clinicopathologic study of senile dementia. J. Am. Geriatr. Soc. 29:158–163, 1981.

Larsson T., Sjogren T., Jacobson G.: Senile dementia. Acta Psychiat. Scand. 39:(suppl. 167) 3–259, 1963.

Libb J.W., Clements C.B.: Token reinforcement in an exercise program for hospitalized geriatric patients. Percept. Motor Skills 28:957–958, 1969.

Libow L.S.: Pseudosenility: acute and reversible organic brain syndrome. J. Am. Geriatr. Soc. 21:112–120, 1973.

Lipowski Z.J.: Delirium updated. Compr. Psychiatry 31: 190–196, 1980.

Liston E.J., Jr.: Occult presenile dementia. J. Nerv. Ment. Dis. 164:263–267, 1977.

Loew C.A., Silverstone B.M.: A program of intensified stimulation and response facilitation for the senile aged. Gerontologist 11:341–347, 1971.

Mann D.M.A., Sinclair K.G.A.: The quantitative assessment of lipofuscin pigment cytoplasmic DNA and nucleolar volume in senile dementia. Neuropath. Neurobiol. 4:129–135, 1978.

Mann D.M.A., Yates P.O.: Dementia and cerebral noradrenergic innervation. Br. Med. J. 282:474–475, 1981.

Marcer D., Hopkins S.M.: The differential effects of meclofenoxate on memory loss in the elderly. Age and Ageing 6:123–131, 1977.

Marchbanks R.M.: Choline, acetylcholine and dementia (editorial). Psychol. Med. 10:1–3, 1980.

Marsden C.D.: The diagnosis of dementia, in Studies in Geriatric Psychiatry. Edited by Isaacs A.D., Post F. Chichester, N.Y., John Wiley & Sons, 1978.

Marsden C.D., Harrison M.J.G.: Outcome of investigation of patients with presenile dementia. Br. Med. J. 2:249–252, 1972.

Mayer V., Orolin D., Mitrova E., et al.: Transmissible virus dementia. I. An unusual space and time clustering of Creutzfeldt-Jakob disease and of other organic presenile dementia cases. Acta Virol. 22:146–153, 1978.

McAllister T.W., Price T.R.P.: Depressive pseudodementia. Am. J. Psychiatry 139:626–629, 1982.

McDermott J.R., Smith A.I., Iqbal K., et al.: Aluminum and Alzheimer's disease. Lancet 2:710–711, 1977.

McDermott J.R., Smith A.I., Iqbal K., et al.: Brain aluminum in aging and Alzheimer's disease. Neurol. 29:809–814, 1979.

McDonald R.J.: Hydergine: a review of 26 clinical studies. Pharmakopsychiatrie 12:407–422, 1979.

McLaughlin A.I.G., Kazantis G., King E., et al.: Pulmonary fibrosis and encephalopathy associated with the inhalation of aluminum dust. Br. J. Indus. Med. 9: 253–263, 1962.

Miller E.: Cognitive assessment of the older adult, in Handbook of Mental Health and Aging. Edited by Birren J.E., Sloane R.B. Englewood Cliffs, N.J., Prentice-Hall, 1980.

Miller A.E., Neighbour P.A., Katzman R., et al.: Immunological studies in senile dementia of the Alzheimer type: evidence for enhanced suppressor cell activity. Ann. Neurol. 10:506–510, 1981.

Mindus P., Cronholm B., Levander S.E.: Piracetam-induced improvement of mental performance: a controlled study on normally aging individuals. Acta Psychiatr. Scand. 54:150–160, 1976.

Mortimer J.A.: Epidemiologic aspects of Alzheimer's disease, in Advances in Neurogerontology, vol. 1, The Aging Nervous System. Edited by Maletta G.J., Pirozzolo F.J. New York, Praeger Publications, 1980.

Nandy K.: Centrophenoxine: effects on aging mammalian brain. J. Am. Geriatr. Soc. 27:74–81, 1978.

Nandy K.: Lipofuscin pigment and immunological factors in the pathogenesis and treatment of senile dementia, in Strategies for the Development of an Effective Treatment for Senile Dementia. Edited by Crook T., Gershon E.S. New Canaan, CT., Mark Powley Associates, 1981.

Nott P.N., Fleminger J.J.: Presenile dementia: the difficulties of early diagnosis. Acta Psychiatr. Scand. 51: 210–217, 1975.

Olsen E.J., Bank L., Jarvik L.F.: Gerovital-H_3: A clinical trial as an antidepressant. J. Gerontol. 33:514–520, 1978.

Op Den Velde W., Stam F.C.: Haptoglobin types in Alzheimer's disease and senile dementia. Br. J. Psychiatry 122:331–336, 1973.

Ostfeld A., Smith C.M., Stotsky B.A.: The systemic use of procaine in the treatment of the elderly: a review. J. Am. Geriatr. Soc. 25:1–19, 1977.

Pacha W., Salzman R.: Inhibition of the re-uptake of neuronally-liberated noradrenaline and receptor blocking action of some ergot alkaloids. Br. J. Pharmacol. 38: 439–440, 1970.

Paulson G.W., Kapp J., Cook W.: Dementia associated with bilateral carotid artery disease. Geriatrics 21: 159–166, 1966.

Perry E.K., Perry R.H., Blessed G., et al.: Necropsy evidence of central cholinergic deficits in senile dementia. Lancet 1:189, 1977.

Perry E.K., Tomlinson B.E., Blessed G., et al.: Correlation of cholinergic abnormalities with senile plaques and mental test scores in senile dementia. Br. Med. J. 2: 1457–1459, 1978.

Perry E.K., Tomlinson B.E., Blessed G., et al.: Noradrenergic and cholinergic systems in senile dementia of Alzheimer type (letter). Lancet 2:149, 1981.

Pfeiffer E.: A short portable mental status questionnaire for the assessment of organic brain deficit in elderly patients. J. Am. Geriatr. Soc. 23:433–441, 1975.

Posner J.B.: Delirium and exogenous metabolic brain disease, in Textbook of Medicine, ed. 14. Edited by Beeson P.B., McDermott W. Philadelphia, W.B. Saunders Co., 1975.

Post F.: The Clinical Psychiatry of Late Life, Oxford, Pergamon Press, 1965.

Pro J.D., Wells C.E.: The use of the electroencephalogram in the diagnosis of delirium. Dis. Nerv. Syst. 38: 804–808, 1977.

Quilitch H.R.: Purposeful activity increased in a geriatric ward through programmed recreation. J. Am. Geriatr. Soc. 22:226–229, 1974.

Robins, P.V., Folstein M.F.: Delirium and dementia: diagnostic criteria and fatality rates. Br. J. Psychiatry 140: 149–153, 1982.

Raskin A.S., Gershon E.S., Crook T.: The effects of hyperbaric and normobaric oxygen on cognitive impairment in the elderly. Arch. Gen. Psychiatry 35:50–58, 1978.

Reifler B., Larson E., Hanley R.: Coexistence of cognitive impairment in depression in geriatric outpatients. Am. J. Psychiatry 139:623–626, 1982.

Reisberg B.: Empirical studies in senile dementia with metabolic enhancers and agents that alter blood flow and oxygen utilization, in Strategies for the Development of an Effective Treatment for Senile Dementia. Edited by Crook T., Gershon E.S. New Canaan, CT., Mark Powley Associates, 1981.

Reisine T.D., Bird E.D., Spokes E., et al.: Pre- and postsynaptic neurochemical alterations in Alzheimer's disease. Trans. Am. Soc. Neurochem. 9:203, 1978.

Ron M.A., Toone B.K., Garralda M.E., et al.: Diagnostic accuracy in presenile dementia. Br. J. Psychiatry 134: 161–168, 1979.

Rossor, M.N., Rehfeld J.F., Emson P.C., et al.: Normal cortical concentration of cholecystokinin-like immunoreactivity with reduced choline acetyltransferase activity in senile dementia of Alzheimer type. Life Sciences 29:405–410, 1981.

Roth M.: The psychiatric disorders of later life. Psych. Ann. 69:57–98, 1976.

Roth M., Kay D.W.K.: Affective disorders arising in the senium. II. Physical disability as an aetiological factor. J. Ment. Sci. 102:141–150, 1956.

Roth M., Morrissey J.D.: Problems in the diagnosis and classification of mental disorder in old age. J. Ment. Sci. 98:66, 1952.

Salk D.: Can we learn about aging from a study of Werner's syndrome? J. Am. Geriatr. Soc. 30:334–339, 1982.

Schaie K.W.: Intelligence and problem solving, in Handbook of Mental Health and Aging. Edited by Birren J.E., Sloane R.B. Englewood Cliffs, N.J., Prentice-Hall, 1980.

Schneck M.K., Reisberg B., Ferris S.H.: An overview of current concepts of Alzheimer's disease. Am. J. Psychiatry 139:165–173, 1982.

Seltzer B., Sherwin I.: "Organic brain syndromes:" an empirical study and critical review. Am. J. Psychiatry 135:13–21, 1978.

Shader R.I., Goldsmith G.N.: Dihydrogerated ergot alkaloids and papaverine: a status report on their effects in senile mental deterioration, in Progress in Psychiatric Drug Treatment. Edited by Klein D.F., Gittelman-Klein R. New York, Brunner/Mazel, 1979.

Shore D., Millson M., Holtz J.L., et al.: Serum aluminum in primary degenerative dementia. Biol. Psychiatry 15: 971–977, 1980.

Slater E., Roth M.: Clinical Psychiatry, 3rd ed. Baltimore, Williams & Wilkins, 1977.

Sloane R.B.: Organic brain syndrome, in Handbook of Mental Health and Aging. Edited by Birren J.E., Sloane R.B. Englewood Cliffs, N.J., Prentice-Hall, 1980.

Smith J.S., Kiloh L.G., Ratnavale G.S.: The investigation of dementia. The results of 100 consecutive admissions. Med. J. Australia 2:403–405, 1976.

Snowden P.R., Woodrow J.C., Copeland J.R.M.: HLA antigens in senile dementia and multiple infarct dementia. Age and Ageing 10:259–263, 1981.

Snowdon J.: When is dementia presenile? Br. Med. J. 2:465, 1972.

Soininen H., Halonen T., Riekkinen P.J.: Acetylcholinesterase activity in cerebrospinal fluid in patients with senile dementia of Alzheimer type. Acta Neurol. Scand. 64:217–224, 1981.

Sommer R., Ross H.: Social interaction on a geriatric ward. Inter. J. Social Psychiatry 4:128–133, 1958.

Spar J.E., Gerner R.: Does the dexamethasone suppression test distinguish dementia from depression? Am. J. Psychiatry 139:238–240, 1982.

Stein B.M., McCormick W.F., Rodriguez J.N., et al.: Postmortem angiography of cerebral vascular system. Arch. Neurol. (Chic.) 7:545–569, 1962.

Terry R.D.: Dementia: a brief and selective review. Arch. Neurol. 33:1–4, 1976.

Terry R.D., Davies P.: Dementia of the Alzheimer type. Ann. Rev. Neurosci. 3:77–95, 1980.

Thompson L.W., Glenn C.D., Obrist W.D., et al.: Effects of hyperbaric oxygen on behavioral and physiological measures in elderly demented patients. J. Gerontol. 31:23–28, 1976.

Tomlinson B.E., Blessed G., Roth M.: Observations on the brains of demented old people. J. Neurol. Sci. 11: 205–242, 1970.

Tomlinson B.E., Irving D., Blessed G.: Cell loss in the locus coeruleus in senile dementia of Alzheimer type. J. Neurol. Sci. 49:419–428, 1981.

Traub R.D., Gajdusek D.C., Gibbs C.J., Jr.: Transmissible virus dementias: the relation of transmissible spongiform encephalopathy to Creutzfeldt-Jakob disease, in Aging and Dementia. Edited by Smith L., Kinsbourne M. New York, Spectrum, 1977.

Tsai L., Tsuang M.T.: The mini-mental state test and computerized tomography. Am. J. Psychiatry 136:4A: 436–438, 1979.

Victoratos G.C., Lenman J.A.R., Herzberg L.: Neurological investigation of dementia. Br. J. Psychiatry 130: 131–133, 1977.

Walford R.L., Hodge S.E.: HLA distribution in Alzheimer's disease, in Histocompatibility Testing. Edited by Peresaki P.I. Los Angeles, UCLA Tissue Typing Lab, 1980.

Walsh A.C.: Senile dementia: a report on the anticoagulant treatment of thirteen patients. Pennsylvania Med. 71:65–72, 1968.

Walsh A.C.: Prevention of senile and presenile dementia by bibishydroxycoumarin (Dicumarol) therapy. J. Am. Geriatr. Soc. 17:477–487, 1969.

Walsh A.C., Walsh B.H., Melaney C.: Senile-presenile dementia: follow-up data on an effective psychotherapy-anticoagulant regimen. J. Am. Geriatr. Soc. 26:467–470, 1978.

Ward B.E., Cook R.H., Robinson A., et al.: Increased aneuploidy in Alzheimer disease. Am. J. Med. Genet. 3:137–144, 1979.

Weingartner H., Cohen R.M., Murphy D.L., et al.: Cognitive processes in depression. Arch. Gen. Psychiatry 38:42–47, 1981.

Wells C.E. (ed.): Dementia, 2nd ed. Philadelphia, F.A. Davis Co., 1977.

Wells C.E.: Chronic brain disease: An overview. Am. J. Psychiatry 135(1):1–12, 1978a.

Wells C.E.: Role of stroke in dementia. Stroke 9:1–3, 1978b.

Wells C.E.: Diagnosis of dementia. Psychosomatics 20:517–522, 1979a.

Wells C.E.: Pseudodementia. Am. J. Psychiatry 136:895–900, 1979b.

Wells C.E.: Refinements in the diagnosis of dementia. Am. J. Psychiatry 139:621–622, 1982.

Whalley L.J., Urbaniak S.J., Darg C., et al.: Histocompatibility antigens and antibodies to viral and other antigens in Alzheimer's presenile dementia. Acta Psychiat. Scand. 61:1–7, 1980.

White B.J., Crandall C., Goudsmit J., et al.: Cytogenetic studies of familial and sporadic Alzheimer disease. Am. J. Med. Genet. 10:77–89, 1981.

White P., Goodhardt M.J., Keet J.P., et al.: Neocortical cholinergic neurons in elderly people. Lancet 1:668–670, 1977.

Wilcox C.B., Caspary E.A., Behan P.O.: Histocompatibility antigens associated with Alzheimer's disease. European Neurol. 19(4): 262–265, 1980.

Williams M., McGee T.E.: Psychological study of carotid occlusion and endarterectomy. Arch. Neurol. 10:292–297, 1964.

Yates C.M.: Aluminum and Alzheimer's disease, in Alzheimer's Disease: Early Recognition of Potentially Reversible Deficits. Edited by Glen. A.I.M., Whalley L.J. Edinburgh, Churchill Livingstone, 1979.

Yesavage J.A., Tinklenberg J.R., Hollister L.E., et al.: Vasodilators in senile dementia: a review of the literature. Arch. Gen. Psychiatry 36:220–223, 1979.

Zeisel S., Reinstein D., Corkin S., et al.: Cholinergic neurons and memory. Nature 293:187–188, 1981.

Zung W.W.K., Gianturco D., Pfeiffer E., et al.: Pharmacology of depression in the aged: evaluation of Gerovital-H_3 as an antidepressant drug. Psychosomatics 15:127–131, 1974.

References for Chapter 9

Affective Disorders in the Geriatric Patient

American Psychiatric Association: Diagnostic and Statistical Manual of Mental Disorders, 3rd ed. Washington, D.C., American Psychiatric Association, 1980.

Ashford W., Ford C.V.: Use of MAO inhibitors in elderly patients. Am. J. Psychiatry 136:1466–1467, 1979.

Ayd F.J.: Guidelines for treating cardiac patients with tricyclic and tetracyclic antidepressants. Int. Drug Ther. Newsletter 13:9–12, 1978.

Ayd F.J.: Continuation and maintenance doxepin (Sinequan) therapy: ten years' experience. Int. Drug Ther. Newsletter 14:9–16, 1979.

Ayd F.J.: Amoxapine: a new tricyclic antidepressant. Int. Drug Ther. Newsletter 15:33–38, 1980.

Bielski R.J., Friedel R.O.: Prediction of tricyclic antidepressant response: a critical review. Arch. Gen. Psychiatry 33:1479–1489, 1976.

Bielski R. J., Friedel R.O.: Depressive subtypes defined by response to pharmacotherapy, in Affective Disorders. Guest editor Akiskal H.S. Psychiatr. Clin. North Am. vol. II, No. 3, December 1979.

Blum J.E., Tross S.: Psychodynamic treatment of the elderly: a review of issues in theory and practice, in Annual Review of Gerontology and Geriatrics, vol. 1. Edited by Eisdorfer C. New York, Springer Publishing Co., 1980.

Blumenthal M.D., Davie J.W.: Dizziness and falling in elderly psychiatric outpatients. Am. J. Psychiatry 137:203–206, 1980.

Caine E.D.: Pseudodementia: current concepts and future directions. Arch. Gen. Psychiatry 38:1359–1364, 1981.

Carroll B.J., Feinberg M., Greden J.F., et al.: A specific laboratory test for the diagnosis of melancholia. Arch. Gen. Psychiatry 38:15–22, 1981.

Comfort A.: Geriatric psychotherapy, in Practice of Geriatric Psychiatry. New York, Elsevier-North Holland, 1980.

Fink M.: Convulsive Therapy: Theory and Practice. New York, Raven Press, 1979.

Foster J.R., Gershell W.J., Goldfarb A.I.: Lithium treatment in the elderly. I. Clinical usage. J. Gerontol. 32:299–392, 1977.

Friedel R.O.: Pharmacokinetics in the geropsychiatric patient, in Psychopharmacology: A Generation of Progress. Edited by Lipton M.A., DiMascio A., Killam K.F. New York, Raven Press, 1978.

Friedel R.O.: The pharmacotherapy of depression in the elderly: Pharmacokinetic considerations, in Psychopathology in the Aged. Edited by Cole J.O., Barrett J.E. New York, Raven Press, 1980.

Friedel R.O.: Effects of age on the pharmacology of tricyclic antidepressants, in Age and the Pharmacology of Psychoactive Drugs. Edited by Raskin A., Robinson D.S., Levine J. New York, Elsevier-North Holland, 1981.

Friedel R.O.: Clinical predictors of treatment response: an update, in Affective Disorders. Edited by Davis J., Maas J. Washington, American Psychiatric Press, Inc., 1983.

Friedel R.O.: The relationship of therapeutic response and antidepressant plasma levels: an update. J. Clin. Psychiatry, in press.

Gelenberg A.J. (ed.): MAO inhibitors in sickness and health, in Biological Therapies in Psychiatry, Massachusetts General Hospital Newsletter, vol. 5, no 7. Littleton, John Wright-PSG, Inc., 1982.

Glassman A.H., Bigger J.T.: Cardiovascular effects of therapeutic doses of tricyclic antidepressants: a review. Arch. Gen. Psychiatry 38:815–820, 1981.

Glassman A.H., Giardine E.U., Perel J.M., et al.: Clinical characteristics of imipramine-induced orthostatic hypotension. Lancet 1:468–472, 1979.

Gold M.S., Pottash A.L.C., Extein I: The TRH test in the diagnosis of major and minor depression. Psychoneuroendocrinology 6:159–169, 1981.

Götestam K.G.: Behavioral and dynamic psychotherapy with the elderly, in Handbook of Mental Health and Aging. Edited by Birren J.E., Sloane R.B. Englewood Cliffs, N.J., Prentice-Hall, Inc., 1980.

Hartford M.E.: The use of group methods for work with the aged, in Handbook of Mental Health and Aging. Edited by Birren J.E., Sloane R.B. Englewood Cliffs, N.J., Prentice-Hall, 1980.

Horn J.L.: Psychometric studies of aging and intelligence, in Aging: Genesis and Treatment of Psychologic Disorders in the Elderly. Edited by Gershon E.S., Raskin A. New York, Raven Press, 1975.

Klein D.F., Gittelman R., Quitkin E., et al.: Diagnosis and Drug Treatment of Psychiatric Disorders: Adults and Children, 2nd ed. Baltimore, Williams & Wilkins, 1980.

Kupfer D.J., Foster F.G., Coble P., et al.: The application of EEG sleep for the differential diagnosis of affective disorders. Am. J. Psychiatry 135:69–74, 1978.

Langley G.E.: Functional psychoses, in Modern Perspectives in the Psychiatry of Old Age. Edited by Howells J.G. New York, Brunner/Mazel, 1975.

Libow L.S.: Senile dementia and "pseudosenility": clinical diagnosis, in Cognitive and Emotional Disturbance in the Elderly: Clinical Issues. Edited by Eisdorfer C., Friedel R.O. Chicago, Year Book Medical Publications, 1977.

Loosen P.T., Prange A.J.: Serum thyrotropin response to thyrotropin-releasing hormone in psychiatric patients: a review. Am. J. Psychiatry 139:405–416, 1982.

Nelson J.C., Charney D.S., Quinlan D.M.: Evaluation of the DSM-III criteria for melancholia. Arch. Gen. Psychiatry 38:555–559, 1981.

Nelson J.C., Jatlow P.I.: Neuroleptic effect on desipramine steady-state plasma concentrations. Am. J. Psychiatry 137:1232–1234, 1980.

Pfeiffer E.: Psychotherapy with elderly patients, in Geriatric Psychiatry. Edited by Bellak L., Karasu T.B. New York, Grune & Stratton, 1976.

Post F.: Diagnosis of depression in geriatric patients and treatment modalities appropriate for the population, in Depression: Behavioral, Biochemical, Diagnostic and Treatment Concepts. Edited by Gallant D.M., Simpson C.M. New York, Spectrum Publications, 1976.

Quitkin F., Rifkin A., Klein D.F.: Monoamine oxidase inhibitors. Arch. Gen. Psychiatry 36:749–764, 1979.

Robinson D.S.: Monoamine oxidase inhibitors and the elderly, in Age and the Pharmacology of Psychoactive Drugs. Edited by Raskin A., Robinson D.S., Levine J. New York, Elsevier-North Holland, 1981.

Robinson D.S., Davis J.M., Nies A., et al.: Relation of sex and aging to monoamine oxidase activity of human brain, plasma and platelets. Arch. Gen. Psychiatry 24:536–539, 1971.

Robinson D.S., Sourkes T.L., Nies A., et al.: Monoamine metabolism in human brain. Arch. Gen. Psychiatry 34:89–92, 1977.

Siris S.G., Cooper T.B., Rifkin A.E.: Plasma imipramine concentrations in patients receiving concomitant fluphenazine decanoate. Am. J. Psychiatry 139:104–106, 1982.

Squire L.R.: ECT and memory loss. Am. J. Psychiatry 134:997–1001, 1977.

Tuckman J., Lorge I.: Attitudes toward old people. J. Soc. Psychol. 37:249–260, 1953.

Weissman M.M.: The psychological treatment of depression: evidence for the efficacy of psychotherapy alone in comparison with, and in combination with pharmacotherapy. Arch. Gen. Psychiatry 36:1261–1296, 1979.

Weissman M.M., Klerman G.L., Prusoff B.A., et al.: Depressed outpatients. Arch. Gen. Psychiatry 38:51–55, 1981.

West E.D., Dally P.J.: Effects of iproniazid in depressive syndromes. Br. Med. J. 1:1491–1494, 1959.

Winokur G., Behar D., Vanvalkenburg C., et al.: Is a familial definition of depression both feasible and valid? J. Nerv. Ment. Dis. 1966:764–768, 1978.

References for Chapter 10

Late-Onset Schizophrenia and Paranoia in the Elderly

Alexander A.A., Workneh F., Klein M.H., et al.: Psychotherapy and the foreign student, in Cross-Cultural Counseling. Edited by Pederson P., Wintrob R. Honolulu, Cultural Learning Institute, University of Hawaii, 1976.

American Psychiatric Association: Diagnostic and Statistical Manual of Mental Disorders, 3rd ed. Washington, D.C., American Psychiatric Association, 1980.

Berger K.S., Zarit S.N.: Late-life paranoid states: assessment and treatment. Am. J. Orthopsychiatry 48:528–537, 1978.

Blazer D.G.: Depression in Late Life. St. Louis, C.V. Mosby Co., 1981.

Branchley M.H., Lee J.H., Amin R., et al.: High- and low-potency neuroleptics in elderly psychiatric patients. JAMA 239:1860–1862, 1978.

Bridge T.P., Cannon H.E., Wyatt R.J.: Burned-out schizophrenia: evidence for age effects on schizophrenic symptomatology. J. Gerontol. 33:835–839, 1978.

Bridge T.P., Wyatt, R.J.: Paraphrenia: paranoid states in late life, I. European research. J. Am. Geriatr. Soc. 28:193–200, 1980a.

Bridge T.P., Wyatt, R.J.: Paraphrenia: paranoid states in late life, II. American research. J. Am. Geriatr. Soc. 28:201–205, 1980b.

Chu H.M., Yeh E.K., Klein M.H., et al.: A study of Chinese students' adjustment in the U.S.A. Acta Psychologica Taiwanica 13:206–218, 1971.

Ciompi L.: The natural history of schizophrenia in the long term. Br. J. Psychiatry 136:413–420, 1980.

Cooper A.F.: Deafness and psychiatric illness. Br. J. Psychiatry 129:216–226, 1976.

Cooper A.F., Curry A.R.: The pathology of deafness in the paranoid and affective psychoses of later life. J. Psychosomatic Res. 20:97–105, 1976.

Cooper A.F., Curry A.R., Kay D.W.K., et al.: Hearing loss in paranoid and affective psychoses of the elderly. Lancet ii:851–854, 1974.

Cooper A.F., Garside R.F., Kay D.W.K.: A comparison of deaf and non-deaf patients with paranoid and affective psychoses. Br. J. Psychiatry 129:532–538, 1976.

Cooper A.F., Porter R: Visual acuity and ocular pathology in the paranoid and affective psychoses in later life. J. Psychosomatic Res. 20:107–114, 1976.

Eastwood R., Corbin S., Reed M.: Hearing impairment and paraphrenia. J. Otolaryngol 10:306–308, 1981.

Eisdorfer C.: Rorschach rigidity and sensory decrement in a senescent population. J. Gerontol. 15:188–202, 1960.

Eisdorfer C.: Mental health in later life, in Handbook of Community Mental Health. Edited by Golann S., Eisdorfer C. New York, Appleton-Century-Crofts, 1972.

Eisdorfer C.: Paranoia and schizophrenic disorders in later life, in Handbook of Geriatric Psychiatry. Edited by Busse E., Blazer D. New York, Van Nostrand Reinhold, 1980.

Eisdorfer C., Cohen D., Preston C.: Psychological and behavioral therapies with the cognitively impaired aged, in Clinical Aspects of Alzheimer's Disease. Edited by Miller N., Cohen G. New York, Raven Press, 1981a.

Eisdorfer C., Cohen D., Veith R.: The Psychopathology of Aging. Kalamazoo, MI, Scope, 1981b.

Fish F.J.: Senile paranoid states. Gerontologica Clinica. I. 1959.

Funding T.: Genetics of paranoid psychoses of later life. Acta Psychiatr. Scand. 37:267, 1961.

Herbert M.E., Jacobson S.: Late paraphrenia. Br. J. Psychiatry 113:461–469, 1967.

Kay D.W.K.: Schizophrenia and schizophrenia-like states in the elderly. Br. J. Hosp. Med. 8:369–373, 1972.

Kay D.W.K., Roth M: Environmental and hereditary factors in schizophrenia of old age. J. Ment. Med. 107:649–686, 1961.

Kay D.W.K., Roth M.: Schizophrenias of old age, in Process of Aging: I. Edited by Williams R.H., Tibbits C., Donahue W. New York, Atherton Press, 1963.

Kendler K.S., Davis K.L.: The genetics and biochemistry of paranoid schizophrenia and other paranoid psychoses. Schizophr. Bull. 7:689–709, 1981.

Kraepelin E.: Dementia Praecox and Paraphrenia, reprint of 1919 ed. New York, Krieger, 1971.

Kramer M.: Population changes and schizophrenia, 1970–1985. Second Rochester International Conference on Schizophrenia. Rochester, N.Y., 1976.

La Barre W.: The Ghost Dance: Origins of Religion. New York, Doubleday (Delta), 1972.

Langley G.E.: Functional psychoses, in Modern Perspectives in the Psychiatry of Old Age. Edited by Howells J.G. New York, Brunner/Mazel, 1975.

Lowenthal M.F.: Lives in Distress: The Paths of the Elderly to the Psychiatric Ward. New York, Basic Books, 1964.

Manschreck T.C.: The assessment of paranoid features. Compr. Psychiatry 20:370–377, 1979.

Moore N.C.: Is paranoid illness associated with sensory defects in the elderly? J. Psychosomatic Res. 25:69–74, 1981.

Post F.: Persistent Persecutory State of the Elderly. Oxford, Pergamon Press, 1966.

Post F.: Psychiatric disorders, in Textbook of Geriatric Medicine and Gerontology. Edited by Brockleyhurst J.C. Edinburgh and London, Churchill Livingstone, 1973.

Post F.: Paranoid, schizophrenia-like, and schizophrenic states in the aged, in Handbook of Mental Health and Aging. Edited by Birren J.E., Sloane R.B. Englewood Cliffs, N.J., Prentice-Hall, 1980.

Prinz P., Halter J., Benedetti J., et al.: Circadian variation in plasma catecholamine in young and old men: relation to eye movement and slow wave sleep. J. Clin. Endocr. Metab. 49:300–304, 1979.

Raskind M., Alvarez C., Herlin S.: Fluphenazine enanthate in the out-patient treatment of late paraphrenia. J. Am. Geriatr. Soc. 27:451–463, 1979.

Redick R: Changes in the age, sex and diagnostic composition of additions to state and county mental hospitals, United States 1969–1973 (Statistical Note 117). Survey and Reports Section, Biometrics Branch, National Institute of Mental Health, 1975.

Roth M: The natural history of mental disorders in old age. J. Ment. Science 101:281–301, 1955.

Rowe J.W., Troen B.R.: Sympathetic nervous system and aging in man. Endocrine Rev. 1:167–179, 1980.

Schneider K.: Primare und sekundare symptome bei schizophrenie. Fortschrft. Neurol. Psychiat. 25:487, 1957.

Sparacino J.: An attributional approach to psychotherapy with the aged. J. Am. Geriatr. Soc. 26:9–130, 1978.

Stotsky B.: Nursing home or mental hospital: which is better for the geriatric mental patient? J. Genetic. Psychol. 3:1130–1137, 1967.

Strauss J.S., Carpenter W.T.: Schizophrenia. New York, Plenum Press, 1982.

Wilkie F., Halter J., Eisdorfer C., et al.: Effects of age on metabolism and metabolic effects of epinephrine in man, Part II. Gerontologist 20:1980.

Zimbardo P.G., Andersen S.M.: Induced hearing deficit generates experimental paranoia. Science 212:1529–1531, 1981.

References for Chapter 11

Psychiatric Disorders Related to Physiological Changes in Aging

American Psychiatric Association: Diagnostic and Statistical Manual of Mental Disorders. Washington, D.C., American Psychiatric Association, 1980.

Bradley J.: Severe localized pain associated with the depressive syndrome. Br. J. Psychiatry 109:741–745, 1963.

Busse E.W.: The treatment of hypochondriasis. Tri-State Med. J. 2:7, 1954.

Busse E.W.: Hypochondriasis in the elderly: a reaction to social stress. Paper presented at the Tenth International Congress of Gerontology, Jerusalem, Israel, July 1975.

Busse E.W.: Hypochondriasis in the elderly. Am. Fam. Physician 25:199–202, 1982.

Busse E.W., Pfeiffer E.: Functional psychiatric disorders in old age, in Behavior and Adaptation in Late Life, 2nd ed, Edited by Busse E. W., Pfeiffer E. Boston, Little, Brown & Co., 1977.

Carskadon M., van den Hoed J., Dement W.: Sleep and daytime sleepiness in the elderly. J. Geriatr. Psychiatry 13:135–151, 1980.

Clark R., Schmidt H., Schael S., et al.: Sleep apnea: treatment with protriptyline. Neurology 29:1287–1289, 1979.

Coleman R., Miles L., Guilleminault C., et al.: Sleep-wake disorders in the elderly: polysomnographic analysis. J. Am. Geriatr. Soc. 29:289–296, 1981.

Davis R.H.: Drugs and the Elderly. Los Angeles, University of Southern California, 1973.

Dement W., Miles L., Carskadon M.: "White Paper" on sleep and aging. J. Am. Geriatr. Soc. 30:25–50, 1982.

De Nicola P., Peruzza M.: Sex in the aged. J. Am. Geriatr. Soc. 22:380–382, 1974.

Eisdorfer C., Fann W.E.: Psychopharmacology and Aging. New York, Plenum Press, 1973.

Fann W.E., Maddox G.L.: Drug Issues in Geropsychiatry. Baltimore, Williams & Wilkins Co., 1974.

Feinberg I.: The ontogenesis of human sleep and the relationship of sleep variables to intellectual function in the aged. Compr. Psychiatry 9:138–147, 1968.

Feinberg I., Koresko R., Heller N.: EEG sleep patterns as a function of normal and pathological aging in man. J. Psychiatr. Res. 1:107–144, 1967.

Gallemore J., Wilson W.: The complaint of pain in the clinical setting of affective disorders. Southern Med. J. 62:551–555, 1969.

Gee W.F.: The impotent patient: surgical treatment with penile prosthesis and psychiatric evaluation. J. Urol. 111:41–43, 1974.

Gelenberg A.: Treating panic attacks. Massachusetts General Hospital Newsletter 5:1–2, 1982.

Glover B.H.: Sex counseling of the elderly. Hosp. Pract. 12:101–113, 1977.

Guilleminault C., Tilkian A., Dement W.: The sleep apnea syndrome. Annu. Rev. Med. 27:465, 1976.

Institute of Medicine: Sleeping Pills, Insomnia and Medical Practice. Washington D.C., National Academy of Science, 1979.

Kales A., Kales J., Jacobson A., et al.: All night EEG studies: children and elderly. Electroencephalo. Clin. Neurophysiol. 21:415, 1966.

Kales J.: Aging and sleep, in the Physiology and Pathology of Human Aging. Edited by Goldman R., Rockstein M. New York, Academic Press, 1975.

Karacan I., Salis P.J., Ware J.C., et al.: Nocturnal penile tumescence and diagnosis in diabetic impotence. Am. J. Psychiatry 135:191–197, 1978.

Kinsey A.C., Pomeroy W.P., Martin C.E.: Sexual Behavior in the Human Male. Philadelphia, W.B. Saunders, 1948.

Maddox G.L.: Self-assessment of health status. A longitudinal study of selected elderly subjects. J. Chronic. Dis. 17:449, 1964.

Masters W.H., Johnson V.E.: Human Sexual Response. Boston, Little, Brown & Co., 1966.

Masters W.H., Johnson V.E.: Human Sexual Inadequacy. Boston, Little, Brown & Co., 1970.

Parsons T.: The Social System. Glencoe IL, Free Press, 1951.

Pfeiffer E.: Psychotherapy with elderly patients. Postgrad. Med. 50:254, 1971.

Pfeiffer E.: Treating the patient with confirmed functional pain. Hosp. Phys. 6:68–92, 1971.

Pfeiffer E.: Sexuality and the aging patient, in Human Sexuality: A Health Practitioner's Text, 2nd ed. Edited by Green R. Baltimore, Williams & Wilkins, 1979.

Pfeiffer E., Verwoerdt A., Wang H.S.: Sexual behavior in aged men and women: observations on 254 community volunteers. Arch. Gen. Psychiatry 19:641–646, 1968.

Pfeiffer E., Verwoerdt A., Wang H.S.: The natural history of sexual behavior in a biologically advantaged group of aged individuals. J. Gerontol. 24:193–198, 1969.

Pfeiffer E., Davis G.C.: Determinants of sexual behavior in middle and old age. J. Am. Geriat. Soc. 20:151–158, 1972.

Pfeiffer E., Verwoerdt A., Davis G.C.: Sexual behavior in middle life. Am. J. Psychiatry 128:1262–1267, 1972.

Rifkin A., Klein D., Dillon D., et al.: Blockage by imipramine or desipramine of panic induced by sodium lactate. Am. J. Psychiatry 138:676–677, 1981.

Scott F.B., Bradley W.E., Timm G.W.: Management of erectile impotence. Use of implantable inflatable prosthesis. Urology 2:80–82, 1973.

Shader R., Greenblatt D.: The psychopharmacological treatment of anxiety states, in Manual of Psychiatric Therapeutics. Edited by Shader R. Boston, Little, Brown & Co., 1975.

Stone A., Neale J.: Hypochondriasis and tendency to adopt the sick role as moderators and somatic symptomatology. Br. J. Med. Psychol. 54:75–81, 1981.

Tune G.: The influence of age and temperament on the adult human sleep-wakefulness pattern. Br. J. Psychol. 60:431–441, 1969a.

Tune G.: Sleep and wakefulness in 509 normal adults. Br. J. Med. Psychol. 42:75–80, 1969b.

Verwoerdt A., Pfeiffer E., Wang H.S.: Sexual behavior in senescence. Changes in sexual activity and interest in aging men and women. J. Geriat. Psychiatry 2:163–180, 1969a.

Verwoerdt A., Pfeiffer E., Wang H.S.: Sexual behavior in senescence. Patterns of sexual activity and interest. Geriatrics 24:137–154, 1969b.

Webb W., Swinburne H.: An observational study of sleep in the aged. Percept. Mot. Skills 32:895–898, 1971.

Williams R., Karacan I., Hursch J.: EEG of Human Sleep: Clinical Applications. New York, John Wiley & Sons, 1974.

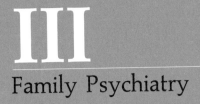

III

Family Psychiatry

Family Psychiatry

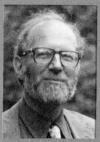

Henry Grunebaum, M.D., Preceptor

Clinical Professor of Psychiatry
Harvard Medical School and
Director, Group and Family
  Psychotherapy Training
The Cambridge Hospital

Authors for Part III

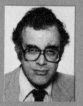

David Reiss, M.D.
Professor and Director
Center for Family Research
George Washington University
  Medical Center

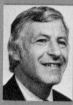

Ira D. Glick, M.D.
Professor of Psychiatry
Cornell University Medical College
Associate Medical Director
  for Inpatient Services
Payne Whitney Clinic
The New York Hospital-
  Cornell Medical Center

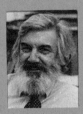

Donald A. Bloch, M.D.

Ackerman Institute for
  Family Therapy
New York

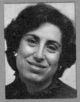

Ellen Berman, M.D.

Associate Professor of Psychiatry
University of Pennsylvania
Director of Training
Marriage Council of Philadelphia

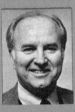

Charles A. Malone, M.D.

Professor and Director
Division of Child Psychiatry
Case Western Reserve University
  School of Medicine and
University Hospitals of Cleveland

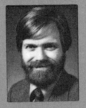

William R. McFarlane, M.D.

Associate Director
Fellowship in Public Psychiatry
Department of Psychiatry
College of Physicians
  and Surgeons
Columbia University and New York State
  Psychiatric Institute

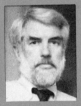

C. Christian Beels, M.D., M.S.

Director
Fellowship in Public Psychiatry
Department of Psychiatry
College of Physicians
  and Surgeons
Columbia University and New York State
  Psychiatric Institute

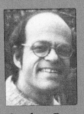

Stephen Rosenheck, M.S.W.

Training Coordinator
Fellowship in Public Psychiatry
Department of Psychiatry
College of Physicians
  and Surgeons
Columbia University and New York State
  Psychiatric Institute

III

Family
Psychiatry

Introduction
by Henry Grunebaum, M.D.

Family psychiatry—is there any other kind? All human beings live in relation to their families, sometimes on good terms and sometimes not. And how we get along with our families influences the texture and quality of our lives. Curiously, however, psychiatrists for many years acted as though they believed that patients were either so little influenced or so destructively affected by their families that patients should be helped in isolation from the very families that brought them to the hospital in the first place and later paid the bills. Freud himself and psychoanalysts in general regarded the patient's family more as an interference to be avoided than as an opportunity to be investigated or intervened with, despite the fact that the first child treated psycho-analytically was helped by his father.

Perhaps this traditional view of the family explains why the ideal psychotherapy case has been thought to be the intelligent young adult who is single, who lives independently, and who has independent means. Gradually, we have come to realize that this state is unusual. Even young adults visit home, take money from parents, and are much influenced by them. The immediate impact of families is clearly even greater for children, adolescents, and married couples and for those who are unable to separate by virtue of psychosis. More recently, we have learned that certain psychosomatic conditions, such as anorexia nervosa, are better treated in a family context. We have also seen that many physically ill patients, such as those with myocardial infarctions and mastectomies, will make much better posthospitalization adjustments if the impacts of the illness on their relationships are taken into account and dealt with before the discharge.

The family of the psychiatric patient has always been with us, although unnoticed or avoided. However, it is a recent and revolutionary development to view the family itself as the psychiatric patient, even when the family may come to attention due to the symptoms of a single member. Only recently have we come to see that the difficulties in functioning or the symptoms themselves can arise because of malfunctioning in relationships in a system and that the family can be the locus of investigations and intervention. These developments represent a dual vision of etiology and treatment: the family *of* the patient and the family *as* the patient. The counterpoint and dialectic between these elements is a major theme of this Part.

Recent advances in clinical work with families and theories of family structure, dynamics, and therapy had their beginnings after World War II. The soil in this country was relatively fertile for these advances because of a long and honorable tradition of interest in families. Social workers in particular, such as Jane Addams, were deeply involved with families in settlement houses in the late 1800s. In 1910 Mary Richmond, for instance, began "to take notes, gather illustrations, and even draft a few chapters for a book on Social Work in Families" (Richmond, 1917, 5). And in her book, *Social Diagnosis*, Richmond states that one finds "that the good results of individual treatment crumble away, often because the case worker has been ignorant of his client's family history" (Richmond, 1917, 134). She then discusses the importance of seeing at the very beginning "several members of the family assembled in their own home environment, acting and reacting upon one another" (Richmond, 1917, 137).

Adolf Meyer, a major influence on American psychiatry, was also interested in the family of the patient. Meyer's wife, Mary Potter Brook, was one of the first people to visit the families of psychiatric patients. Another major influence was Harry Stack Sullivan. Calling his theory "the interpersonal theory of psychiatry," Sullivan believed that the phenomena of personality are conditional on a personal situation which invariably includes at least one other person who may or may not be immediately real or present. In Sullivan's view, personalities are entities which are inferred for the purpose of explaining interpersonal phenomena (Sullivan, 1953).

While little read or known today, the pioneering work of the early social workers and the influences of Meyer and Sullivan are still important. The main thrust of family therapy and theory, however, began in the 1950s. Nathan Ackerman, Gregory Bateson, John Bell, Ivan Boszormenyi-Nagy, Murray Bowen, Jay Haley, Don Jackson, and Theodore Lidz, together with John Spiegel, John Weakland, Carl Whitaker, and Lyman Wynne, are among those who began the serious exploration of conjoint family evaluation and therapy. Many of these pioneers are still active and productive in the field which they helped to open up, and the issues they confronted are still with us.

Despite the emphasis on clinical practice among these contributors, the primary contribution of family psychiatry today may be theoretical rather than therapeutic. A family forces the therapist to look beyond the individual patient to the field of forces, the context within which he or she lives, and beyond that to the community and society. Both the individual paradigm, which emphasizes development, dynamics, and deviations, and the systemic paradigm, which emphasizes relationships, their evolution, patterning, and potentialities, are relevant. Both offer to their proponents a meaningful basis for intervention, and thus the conviction necessary to act decisively. At the moment, in the absence of conclusive data, this may be their main significance. And these two paradigms and the dual vision they suggest may eventually be supplanted by a theory which encompasses both. Such a theory might emphasize the importance to the patient, the family, and the therapist of feeling that one's actions are contextually meaningful and that these actions have an effect on one's own life and, of equal importance, on the lives of others.

Among the critical questions that will be discussed in this Part are:

(1)   Are the symptoms of an individual the product of the workings of family dynamics, or does the family respond to the pathology arising within an individual, or both?

(2)   How should one enter, observe, and influence a family?

(3)   How active should the therapist be and in what ways, as a questioner, for example, or as one who assigns tasks?

(4)   To what extent is it important that the therapy occur in the here and now of the family session, and how should the past, the then and there, be dealt with?

(5) Is it important for the therapist to be involved empathically with the family, or should the therapist rather operate from the more distant position of authority?

(6) Are the primary forces which the therapist can mobilize to foster change the forces of affection, of power redistribution, or of the claims of intrafamilial fairness and justice?

Raising these questions is not meant to suggest that the chapters in this Part answer them. At the present time, there are no outcome data to indicate which family theories lead to the most effective therapy. On the other hand, as reviewed by Gurman and Kniskern (1981), studies do indicate clearly that the outcome of family therapy is in certain instances superior to the outcome of other forms of therapy. In particular, couples therapy is superior to individual therapy for couples with marital difficulties. Couples therapy leads to more positive outcomes and fewer negative outcomes than individual therapy for marital problems. Family therapy appears to lead to superior results for many behavior problems of children and adolescents and for certain psychosomatic illnesses, such as anorexia nervosa. In addition, psychoeducational approaches for the families of patients with schizophrenia appear from preliminary results to lower relapses and rehospitalization rates. As favorable outcome data accumulate on the therapeutic effectiveness of family and couples therapy, it seems appropriate to ask individual psychotherapists to consider with greater care the effects of individual treatment on the significant others of the patient. To end this part of the introduction where it began, we do not live in isolation, but rather in a human context.

What follows is an attempt at a basic course in the evaluation of couples and families and in the design of effective interventions with them. As such, some of the material may seem elementary to therapists who are familiar with family psychiatry. Since work with couples and families is a fairly new area, however, the Preceptor assumed that such an introduction would be useful at this time, and he prepared an annotated bibliography to accompany the Part. The annotated bibliography follows the references for this introduction after the last chapter in the Part.

In the first chapter, Dr. David Reiss compares traditional views of the doctor's role and the patient's problems with the new perspectives offered by family theory and therapy, and he reviews the research on family systems. Reiss also has prepared a brief annotated bibliography. The Preceptor and Dr. Ira Glick next present some of the basics of family treatment—the various approaches to family evaluation and treatment and a series of guidelines for family evaluation, differential therapeutics, and family interventions.

The remaining chapters deal with a variety of specific family therapy applications which will be of interest to a range of practitioners. In his chapter, Dr. Donald A. Bloch discusses the implications of family theory and therapy for the treatment of individuals, with a particular focus on the benefits of a family systems approach to life-cycle issues, illnesses, and crises. Dr. Ellen Berman then reviews approaches to the treatment of couples, covering a number of theoretical models and offering some guidelines for treating couples. Focusing on the treatment of children, Dr. Charles A. Malone discusses a number of diagnostic and therapeutic advantages of the family system orientation to childhood disorder. Dr.

William R. McFarlane, Dr. C. Christian Beels, and Mr. Stephen Rosen-heck describe the promising new developments which family systems perspectives and family treatment have generated in the treatment of schizophrenic patients and the developing knowledge of family treatments for persons with bipolar and unipolar disorders. McFarlane and his colleagues have also prepared two useful appendices.

Because it would be impossible to cover all theories relevant to the essential clinical areas, the Preceptor asked each author to deal in greater detail with certain theories and interventions and leave others to be covered in another chapter, rather than to have each author cover all applicable theories in less depth. Thus, structural theories and interventions are discussed by Malone, historical and contractual issues by Berman, and systems theory and the family life cycle by Bloch. The applicability of these theories is not confined to the population discussed in the chapter where they are described. Further, the psychoeducational efforts discussed by McFarlane and his colleagues are not confined to psychotic populations, but are useful for many couples and families who may not know necessary information about such things as sexual functioning or age-appropriate behavior of children. Finally, the chapter by Glick and the Preceptor is intended as an overview of evaluation and technique and, thus, as a primer to be read before the chapters which follow it.

Chapter 12

Family Studies:
Reframing the Illness,
the Patient, and the Doctor
by David Reiss, M.D.

INTRODUCTION

Psychiatry is returning to medicine. This is an unassailable fact in the history of our profession. It is reflected in the narrowing of our concerns from broad social problems to specific and circumscribed mental illnesses. It shows itself in the increasing specificity of our assessment of psychopathology and in the official manuals to guide and shape the diagnostic process. It is manifest in the increasing comfort of our profession in general hospitals and the extraordinary prevalence of psychopharmacology as a major treatment strategy. Indeed, the term *psychiatric medicine* is perfectly apt in describing the current thinking and practice in our profession. This term implies more than a mode of practice. It emphasizes a form of thinking: objectivity, precise categorization, instrumentation, and experimental design are the preferred means of accumulating knowledge.

For many, this has come to mean that the new psychiatric medicine is to be rooted in our expanding knowledge of the central nervous system, indeed someday to become another branch of an overarching neuroscience. Where do family studies—the formal, quantitative investigations of family process and the careful clinical descriptions of family life and family therapy—fit into this new configuration? Do these studies provide an alternative "truth," a second culture fated to stand in dialectic opposition to the expanding neuroscientific visions of psychiatric medicine? Or are they taking an integrated place within a newly developing whole? With some diffidence, the author maintains the latter, in an argument that mixes affirmation with hope.

The main thesis is this: as psychiatrists rejoin their fellow physicians, they encounter a dualism that has been present in medicine for centuries. On the one hand, man is regarded as a machine, and illness is seen as a consequence of a mechanical breakdown in one or more parts (Osherson and Amarasingham, 1981). On the other hand, man is also a member of one or more human communities, and his illness is a social fact (Scott, 1969). For the physician, the practice of medicine has always been a struggle to reconcile the detached objectivity which views the human patient as a machine and the intimate engagement necessary to learn about the patient as a person engaged in relationships (Lief and Fox, 1963; Zabarenko and Zabarenko, 1978). In this second domain, the understanding of human relationships, the physician has traditionally turned for guidance to religion, humanism, or personal intuition. Family studies, the author argues, provide a firmer base for that guidance. They constitute a coherent set of ideas and clinical observations and a growing corpus of fine empirical studies.

The chapter briefly reviews two areas to illustrate the current status of the field of family studies and its interface with psychiatric medicine. First, the chapter reports some recent findings on the roles of family process in the pathogenesis of major mental illness. Since this area of inquiry is still a modest scientific enterprise, the chapter focuses on perspectives currently being explored rather than on conclusions already established. In particular, this first section demonstrates how scientific inquiry is shifting its focus to the role of mental illness in maintaining the integrity of families and shows how data coming from such inquiries sheds new light on the pathogenesis of mental illness. Indeed, these studies and the clinical observations on which they are based provide the physician with a new conception of mental illness itself. To borrow a term from family therapy, family studies "reframe" the concept of mental illness.

Arising from the family studies and this new concept of mental illness is a new concept of the physician. This concept is the second area that the chapter reviews. Rather than focusing on the highly specialized and technical knowledge the physician must master before he attempts to heal a patient, the new concept of the physician focuses on the healing process itself. At the center of this new idea is a different conception of the physician's power, authority, and efficacy as a healer. Here the physician's power is granted by the patient and the family rather than by the august and priestly processes of the profession. Either directly or indirectly, the physician must gain temporary membership in the patient's family and then exploit the position as an insider to effect and provide healing. Thus, the physician draws strength from the patient and family, not the reverse. To be sure, other humanistic traditions in medicine have encouraged the physician to enter the experiential and social world of the patient in order to enhance empathy and to grasp the meaning of the patient's illness. Family studies encourage a more radical view: a physician's healing powers depend not only on entering the patient's social world, but also on the ability to gain authority from that world, an authority which is the patient's to give and to retrieve. As the chapter demonstrates, family studies have encouraged a reframing of illness and of the doctor, too.

REFRAMING THE ILLNESS

Since the middle 1960s, well-trained researchers have explored the role of family process in the etiology and pathogenesis of major mental illness. In this period, there has been a small but steady stream of well-designed studies which can be divided very roughly into two groups. The first group incorporates a great majority and reflects a fundamentally mechanistic conception of medical disorder. In the view of those who are conducting these studies, mental disorder is considered to be a significant deficiency in interpersonal, cognitive, or affective function, and the studies, like comparable studies in the neurosciences, search for the causes of these deficits. For the most part, the studies examine processes for their potentially toxic effects, and they follow two lines of inquiry. Are family processes toxic in the sense of distorting normal development and producing serious psychopathology? Or are they toxic in the sense that they retard recovery from psychopathology whatever its etiology? Several of the studies in the first group have been extremely well designed. They have produced striking results and, in turn, have had profound effects on clinical practice.

More recently, a second group of scientific studies has emerged. Investigators in this group have attempted to understand the pathogenesis of major mental illness from a different perspective. In a fundamental reframing of the problem of pathogenesis, they have investigated how pathology supports the integrity and continuity of family life. The investigators do not regard psychopathology simply as a deficit that drags its sufferer and the family into profound misery. They take the revised and paradoxical view that psychopathology is a potential source of strength. In this systems-level conception, psychopathology is viewed as a source of power and protection for the patient in the social world and a medium of communication, integration, and continuity for the family.

Psychopathology as Deficit: The Family as a Toxin

The first approach to investigating the family's role in the development of psychopathology has explored it from the standpoint of a number of mental disorders. During the last two decades the schizophrenic syndrome has been the most frequently explored. Some excellent reviews of these studies include those of Jacob (1975), Reiss (1976), Goldstein and Rodnick (1975), and Liem (1980). Other areas now receiving concentrated attention are substance abuse (Stanton, 1979), alcoholism (Steinglass and Robertson, in press), childhood psychosomatic disorders (Minuchin et al., 1978), and childhood conduct disorders (Patterson, 1979).[1]

A series of closely linked investigations illustrates the potential utility of this approach to family processes. Following some initial investigations by Brown, Birley, and Wing (1972), Vaughn and Leff (1976) reported some striking observations.[*] These British investigators had

---

[1]Many of these reviewers, particularly Stanton, Steinglass and Roberts, the Minuchin group, and Patterson, do not themselves subscribe to the deficit-toxin approach. Nonetheless, with the exception of Patterson, the reviews do cite and describe the gamut of work in this area. Patterson describes his own approach to behavioral analysis of coercive family systems and conduct disturbances in children.

[*]Editor's note: This group of studies is reviewed in detail by Dr. Robert Paul Liberman in Part II of Psychiatry 1982 (Psychiatry Update: Volume I), pages 103–106.

wondered whether some particularly malignant forms of emotional expression and interpersonal style in family members of schizophrenic or depressed patients might make patients more vulnerable to relapse. They conducted standardized interviews with relatives concerning various aspects of the identified patient. Then they measured the number of critical comments the relatives made about the patient, the amount of overhostility, and the amount of emotional overinvolvement, and termed this type of behavior expressed emotion. Based on these measures, the investigators separated a sample of 128 schizophrenic patients into one group with relatives who were high on expressed emotion and another group with relatives who were low on expressed emotion.

Three of their findings are particularly striking. First, the high-expressed-emotion group showed a much higher relapse rate than the low-expressed-emotion group. Second, this difference was particularly significant and dramatic for those patients not treated with antipsychotic medication. Third, patients in the high-expressed-emotion group who were "exposed" to their families less than 35 hours a week did far better than those who were exposed for more than 35 hours a week. This last finding and the way it was reported reveal the underlying assumptions of their approach. The recovered schizophrenic patient is viewed as if he or she were being exposed to various dosages of radiation, bacteria, or chemical waste.

Because these findings were so clear and because they were replicated, they galvanized a whole series of subsequent investigations. In one subsequent investigation, Michael Goldstein and his colleagues (Doane et al., 1981) followed a sample of 65 adolescents and their families. The families were admitted to the study years ago after they sought treatment for their adolescent children. At the time, none of the adolescents were psychotic or even borderline. Nonetheless, the investigators regarded them as being at risk for developing schizophrenia, and after the Vaughn and Leff studies appeared, they wondered if they could predict the schizophrenic outcome based on the nature of the family interaction process. After the families were admitted, the Goldstein group had completed videotapes of parents interacting with their troubled adolescents. Then, after the Vaughn and Leff studies, they designed a scale for measuring the levels of parental support, criticism, guilt induction, and intrusiveness in the family interaction patterns. These features seemed to duplicate the kind of emotional expression that Vaughn and Leff found had such a devastating effect on already established schizophrenia.

Coders who were blind to the subsequent clinical course of the adolescents carefully measured the style of the parents' emotional expression in the videotaped interactions. The parents who were high on support but low on criticism, guilt induction, and intrusiveness were categorized as "benign." Those with an opposite pattern were characterized as "poor." A third, in-between category was called "intermediate." As Table 1 shows, critical and intrusive parent behaviors at the time of admission predict the development of schizophrenia and schizophrenia-like disorders five years later.

Both the Vaughn and Leff and the Goldstein group studies have spurred a great deal of interest in therapeutic methods to reduce parental intrusion and overinvolvement. Early experience has been encouraging, as McFarlane, Beels, and Rosenheck discuss in their chapter.

Table 1. Parental Affective Style and Five-Year Outcome in 65
Troubled Adolescents*

Parental Affective Style		Disorders in Adolescents		
	Normal/ Neurotic	Drug Abuse/ Antisocial Personality	or	Schizoid; Probable Borderline	Definite Borderline; Schizophrenia
Benign	23	2		0
Intermediate	5	4		1
Poor	7	4		6

Note: $X^2 = 17.9$; $p < 0.005$
*Adapted from Doane et al. (1981).

Psychopathology as Asset: Its Role in Family Maintenance

The second view of family process emphasizes the adaptive aspects of psychopathology. This view is, quite emphatically, not simply the reverse of the view that psychopathology is a deficit: the concept of psychopathology is transformed. Symptoms are seen as being fully integrated into enduring, subtle, and complex patterns of family interaction. Examined closely, symptoms appear to be critical links in ongoing family life. Over time, they function to maintain family stability and integrity, however troubled. Symptoms are regarded as part of the central regulators of family life, not as indicators of defective mechanical operations of the individual.*

Whatever differences exist among family therapists, most agree on this central conception of psychopathology. But despite over two decades of family therapy practice, little scientific evidence exists to support the conception. The simple reason is that methods to explore this systems-level concept of psychopathology are still in a rudimentary stage. Several investigators, however, have recently contributed to the conceptualization and the methodology some well-designed research studies in this area. Two examples are the work of Straker and Jacobson (1979) and Wolin et al. (1980).

SYMPTOMS AND FAMILY INTERACTION PATTERNS   Straker and Jacobson (1979) have examined one key aspect of the systems-level conception of psychopathology in their study of encopresis. The systems-level conception as a whole views symptoms as components of regularly recurring cycles of family interaction patterns and also holds that their critical location in these chains gives the symptoms a central role in regulating family process. Straker and Jacobson examined the first aspect of this hypothesis. They explored whether the encopresis in a child was part of a regularly recurring cycle of family interaction patterns.

Their subjects were five families. Each was in family therapy for a period of twenty weeks. During the weeks between sessions the parents were asked to record the frequency of encopresis. Straker and Jacobson coded family process during the family therapy sessions in a number of

*Preceptor's note: At the same time that symptoms are seen as part of a system, they are also understood as having a particular meaning to the individual who has them, as well as to others.

ways. In particular, they focused on the frequency with which the parents thwarted any signs of self-assertion or aggression in the child, since previous clinical observations had suggested that encopresis is associated with parent-child struggles for autonomy. Coders, blind to the frequency of encopresis, noted all instances where the child took any verbal initiative: asking a question, expressing an idea, or revealing a feeling. Whenever the child's initiative was blunted, reprimanded, or ignored, the coder scored the family for a "thwarted assertion." Each family therapy session thus received a score reflecting levels of blocked autonomy in the child, and this score could, in turn, be correlated with the frequency of encopresis both before and after the session (Table 2 shows the results). While the correlations themselves were higher for the week following the session, they were also significant for the preceding week.

Table 2. The Relationship Between Encopresis and Thwarted Assertion*

Encopresis Measure	Corrected Correlation with Thwarted Assertion in Session[1]	$p <$
Week before Session	.25	.01
Week after Session	.45	.01

[1]N = 100 observations from five families corrected for variance due to families.
*Adapted from Straker and Jacobson (1979).

These data do suggest a cycle. The child is encopretic. This then leads the parents to thwart the child's milder and more socially acceptable forms of self-assertion. The parents' behavior leads, in turn, to an even higher frequency of encopresis. Beyond demonstrating the first (cyclical) aspect of the systems-level conception, these data also suggest the plausibility of the second. For these families, encopresis has become a central regulator of autonomy and control. It permits the child to struggle against the parents and the parents to exercise control over the child. This use of encopresis, however, may mean that the parents and the child never fully resolve struggles. The child's mastery and self-control is never clearly established; the parents' control is never relinquished. The family itself remains locked at an anal stage of struggle without having to experience the changes and losses that moving on to the next stage would entail.

SYMPTOMS IN FAMILY PATTERNS ACROSS GENERATIONS
Wolin et al. (1980) took another approach to examining psychopathology as a systems-level asset. Where Straker and Jacobson studied the effect of pathology in maintaining family patterns over a period of weeks, Wolin et al. were interested in how psychopathology can maintain family patterns across two generations.

These investigators centered their attention on what they call family identity. By this they mean the family's experience of itself as a group: its sense of openness to the outside world or its sense of distance and withdrawal from the outside world; its sense of tradition and continuity with the past; and its sense of internal cohesion or distance. Wolin et al. have argued that a family's identity is most clearly expressed and most effectively maintained by its rituals. Rituals are highly patterned sequences with great symbolic meaning for the family. The family practices them regularly, and they are a source of great family pride. The clearest example is the family's conduct at dinner time. Some families typically include all members at the table; others never do. Some families include religious or ethnic practices at mealtime; others exclude them. Members of some families are careful to plan their entire days in order to have dinner together at a set time each night; other families eat together once a week or even less. These variations, hypothesize Wolin et al., express differences in the family's underlying identity.

Wolin et al. focused their research on family identity and alcohol rituals in relation to alcoholism. Many families contain a member who is an alcoholic or an alcohol abuser. But families differ strikingly as to whether or not the alcoholic's drinking behavior is included in critical rituals such as dinner time. Some families expend great efforts to make sure no drinking occurs during critical rituals. Others allow the drinking to become a central part of the family ritual life. The latter group should be at greatest risk of transmitting alcoholism to subsequent generations. The alcoholism has, in effect, been admitted to the internal family structure; it has become a central part of the family's identity. Thus, children who come from such a family and who seek to maintain continuity with their family of origin must include drinking behavior in the structures of their own developing families. They could do so either by becoming alcoholics themselves or by marrying alcoholics. In this sense Wolin et al. do not consider drinking to be a deficit in one individual. Rather, drinking is a behavior which provides the couple with a sense of membership in, and continuity with, a particular family of origin. To put the matter another way, drinking gives both spouses a sense of continuity across time, a central function in both normal and pathologic families. Table 3 shows the results from their first study in this area (Wolin et al., 1980). In a retrospective study of 25 families, those who had excluded alcohol from key rituals were much less likely to have children who either had alcoholism themselves or who married alcoholics.

Table 3. Intrusion of Alcoholism into Family Rituals and Transmission from Parents to Children*

	Status of Offspring		
Alcohol in Rituals of Family of Origin[1]	No Transmission	Partial Transmission (≥ 1 Problem Drinker)	Full Transmission (≥ 1 Alcoholic)
None	4	2	1
Partial Intrusion	2	2	6
Full Intrusion	0	3	5

[1]N = 25 families
*Adapted from Wolin et al. (1980).

REFRAMING THE DOCTOR

The Doctor as Anthropologist

The doctor's job has always been diagnosis and treatment, and this holds true when the doctor becomes a family therapist. The examples just given illustrate that the family diagnostician must assess two complex areas in the effort to understand the relationship between psychopathology and family process. First, he or she must understand how the psychopathology fits into ongoing interaction patterns or cycles in the here and now. Toward this end, the doctor must locate precisely where symptoms appear in interaction sequences. The goal here is to understand how the symptoms connect various behaviors and feelings in a sequence, how they function as indirect forms of communication, and how they serve as fundamental regulators of relationships.

Second, the family diagnostician must delineate fundamental underlying structures in family life, including the family's belief about itself and its conceptions about the social world in which it lives. He or she must also learn about other critical structures, the family's hierarchy of power and influence and the openness of its boundaries to outsiders. Often the diagnostician must explore how these structures have developed over time and how vulnerable to change they are in the present. Family therapists vary as to whether they emphasize identifying the surface interaction patterns or the underlying structures and as to whether they concentrate on the present or on the past. But whatever the particular emphasis, the family therapist faces a formidable task. The therapist may be able to call on objective testing procedures and structured interviews for some of the work (one such procedure is described below). Most family therapists, however, believe they must immerse themselves directly in the life of the family. This immersion is required not only for adequate assessment, but also for the more important task of producing therapeutic change.

Considering this immersion, Salvador Minuchin likened family therapists to anthropologists. Both must join a foreign culture in order to learn about it. Minuchin describes "joining" the family by openly supporting its existing alignments among members, by fitting into its patterns, by grasping and accepting its values, and by behaving according to its standards (Minuchin et al., 1978). Thus, a therapist seeking to join a family will respect a particular alliance within it, will use language and examples the family can readily understand, and will pace interactions with the family to match its fast or slow rhythms. It is in this sense that the family therapist joins an indigenous, well-bounded culture.

Research has only recently begun to document the power of this indigenous family culture to regulate internally the norms and styles of interaction among members. Perhaps even more important are the recent insights about how this culture regulates the transactions between the family and its external social world, a world which includes treatment agencies and therapists.

THE INVESTIGATION OF INDIGENOUS FAMILY CULTURE

In their laboratory, the author and his colleagues have developed several precise methods for measuring some aspects of this indigenous family culture. One such procedure is illustrated in Figures 1 and 2. Family threesomes are asked to sit in booths (Figure 1). Each member is given a deck of cards (Figure 2). The family members can talk with one another over the telephone-like audio system. The family is asked to sort the cards into as many piles as they wish—up to seven. They are not told whether they have to work together as a group or as individuals. Nor do they receive any hints about how they should sort the cards.

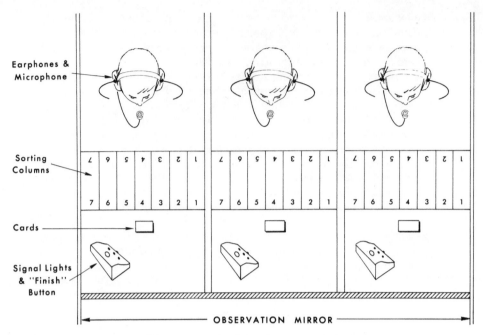

Figure 1. Bird's-eye view of the apparatus for the card-sorting procedure which assesses the indigenous family culture

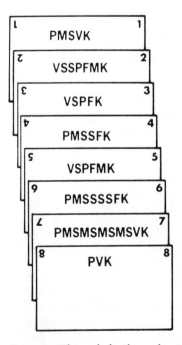

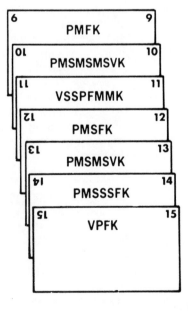

Figure 2. The cards for the card-sorting procedure

The author's studies have shown that a family's approach to this task is a clear index of its convictions about what the research staff is really up to (Reiss, 1981). For example, some families see the researchers as malevolent and out to trick them. As a consequence, their problem-solving efforts are hurried and superficial, permitting them a rapid, though decorous exit from the hostile scene. Other families trust the researchers. Feeling that the research staff have a genuine interest in how they as a group solve problems, they linger over the details of the task, collaboratively developing elegant solutions. Through a series of such studies, the author and his colleagues have shown that these beliefs about the laboratory reflect the family's enduring convictions about ambiguous social settings (Reiss, 1981). The laboratory procedure can thus be used to predict a family's conceptions and convictions about treatment agencies and therapists.

Two dimensions of family performance are of particular interest in this regard. The first is called coordination. Coordination is measured by the amount of agreement and cooperation families evidence as they work at the laboratory puzzles. Several studies suggest that this performance reflects the family's conception of how it is treated by the outside world. A high-coordination family feels that the world treats it as a unitary group; thus, what any one member does reflects on the entire group. A low-coordination family feels that the world treats its members as individuals. Such a family often believes the laboratory tasks are intelligence tests designed to see which member is the smartest. A second dimension is called configuration. Configuration is measured by quantitative estimates of how much information on the cards the family uses in its solution; high-configuration families recognize subtle patterns and sort the cards accordingly. Interestingly, this performance is unrelated to intelligence, education, occupation, or social class. Rather, many of the author's studies suggest, it reflects the family's trust that they have been given a soluble puzzle and their optimism that they can, with diligent work, master it.

These methods are useful for predicting how families will perceive and react to therapists and treatment programs. For example, in a study of families with an adolescent who had been hospitalized for severely disturbed behavior, high-coordination families attended therapy sessions more regularly, were better liked by other families, and participated more actively in therapeutic activities. In terms of their subjective experience in the treatment program, they felt more involved, experienced much less danger and unpredictability in the ward community, and had more typical and less idiosyncratic views of the psychiatric unit. Within the group of high-coordination families, an important difference emerged between those which were high and those which were low on the configuration dimensions. High-configuration families opened themselves up to a variety of relationships. In a ward setting these families seemed available and accessible to change through the many relationships they made with staff and other families. In contrast, low-configuration families withdrew from relationships with others. Their family boundaries were rigid, and they were less open to change.

These findings suggest an important link between therapy and the family's beliefs or indigenous culture. High-coordination families regard themselves as an integrated group. They embrace the concept of the family as a system. The behavior of one member, they are convinced, is intimately tied to the fate of the others. On their own terms, they already believe in a major tenet of the surrounding therapeutic culture. Thus, the ward's requirement that the whole family participate in treatment makes good sense to them, and they really become engaged. Within this group of high-coordination families, a special advantage accrues to high-configuration families, for their indigenous culture emphasizes a belief in the order, safety, and predictability of the social world. These families take chances. They open themselves to new relationships and new perspectives and are mostly ready for significant therapeutic change. The low-configuration family has a different indigenous culture which stresses the unpredictability and the possible danger of the social world. In their world view, the family is the best source of protection, and consequently they resist new relationships. Though engaged in the program, they resist therapeutic change.

THE DOCTOR AND THE FAMILY CULTURE Although these studies clearly demonstrate the power of the family's indigenous culture and suggest the utility of objective testing procedures, it will be a long time, if ever, before elaborate instrumentation can replace the immersion of the therapist into the family. Indeed, the results of formal testing must be constantly cross-checked by such immersion. But the therapist does not become immersed in the indigenous culture for the sole purpose of assessing the patterns and structures of family life. Successful therapeutic intervention, according to many experienced family therapists, also depends on such immersion. Indeed, the family therapist is in a paradoxical position. Although the family first comes to him or her for help, in order to become effective, the therapist becomes dependent on the authority and power he or she can derive from the family. This authority and power depend at the least on an early step of limited immersion. Since there are major differences among family therapists and their techniques, it is useful to clarify briefly in what sense immersion is so broadly, if not universally, important.

As Grunebaum and Glick discuss in their chapter, family therapy interventions may be divided into the three broad classes of understanding, transformation, and identification. Understanding, transformation, and identification cannot be successful without the active accession and participation of the family itself. In order to use understanding, the family must perceive the therapist as an authority about their family in particular. The therapist must convince them that it is possible for him or her to know something they do not, about them in particular. Suspicious families who feel threatened, such as the low-configuration families, will not readily see a therapist as authoritative about them. More likely, the therapist will be viewed as a potentially harmful intruder. The therapist must join the family emotionally and must convince them that he or she is on their side and can directly grasp their concerns.

Likewise, effective use of transformation or the manipulative strategies depends on the therapist's power or leadership, but it is leadership or power in a particular family. Leadership cannot effectively be imposed on the family through coercion but must be established with the family's willing consent. In effect, the therapist must rise from within the ranks. For example, in some highly coordinated families, members' autonomy may be smothered by overinvolvement and enmeshment with others. Here the therapist derives power from becoming partially involved with the family but keeping a strategic distance from these entanglements. The reverse is true for some poorly coordinated families where members are in painful isolation from each other. There power can be derived by making short-term strategic alliances with individuals or by serving as a go-between (Zuk, 1966).

The Doctor without a Profession

As a family therapist, the physician becomes preoccupied with the indigenous culture of the family that he or she treats. In an important experiential sense, the therapist must for extended periods abandon the culture of the profession for the culture of the family. This is not to say that a strong professional identification is not useful for the physician as family therapist or that technical or professional knowledge about family dynamics and therapeutic techniques is a less valuable tool. It does mean that the physician's authority and power to use that knowledge and those techniques come from the family and the physician's temporary membership in the family. This power cannot come from the culture of the profession.

The training of family therapists facilitates this shift from professional to family culture. Family therapy training programs are rarely restricted to a single discipline or even to doctoral-level disciplines. Indeed, all mental health disciplines have contributed leading family therapists, and some leading family therapists have had no formal training in mental health disciplines at all. This de-emphasis on membership in the disciplines is accentuated by family therapy's typical mode of clinical supervision. In sharp contrast to the supervisory style in the other psychotherapies, let alone the pharmacotherapies, family therapy supervision is immediate and alive. The supervisor directly observes the trainee through a one-way screen. Often the family knows that the therapist is being supervised, and in many training centers the supervisor directly phones instructions to the therapist-trainee in the course of a therapeutic hour.

Supervision, then, is not an occult procedure carried on in professional privacy without the knowledge of the family. In other therapeutic modes, the customarily private supervisory sessions facilitate an intense identification of the trainee not only with the supervisor, but also with the theories and techniques of the profession. Private supervision, while often successful in increasing the trainee's sensitivity to the patient, is also a professional ritual by which the trainee is ushered into the culture of the discipline. The live and interventionist supervision in family therapy training has an important difference. The published report of the experience of Gershenson and Cohen (1978) conveys the essence of the feeling. As supervisees, they felt themselves pinioned between the supervisor and the family. In effect, live supervision pushed them out of the profession and into the family.

FAMILY STUDIES AND THE PSYCHIATRIC PHYSICIAN

The chapter concludes with some further elaboration on its beginning topic, the practice of medicine and its traditional dualism. As previously argued, the competent physician has, for centuries, integrated two roles. As a detached professional, the physician has surveyed patients and their illnesses from a distance. From his vantage point, the physician's view has been mechanistic: the patient is a machine gone awry, and the treatment attempts a specific repair. In contrast, in the other role, the physician has abandoned professional distance and entered the world of the patient to grasp the social meaning of the illness and its cure. From this vantage point, the physician has tried to grasp how the patient's relationships with others may have brought on the illness and defined and influenced its cure. To conceive of these two roles as reflecting a distinction between the scientific and humanistic traditions in medicine is to misread the history of medicine. Indeed, mechanistic perspectives in medicine were, for a millenium, built on nonscientific fantasies such as the wandering uterus and the four humors. These fantasies persist today in the form of mechanistic excesses such as the high incidence of elective hysterectomies, the extravagant use of antibiotics, and the overzealous worship of the CT scan (particularly in children where its safety has been seriously questioned). On the other hand, solid scientific evidence is now accumulating to help the physician enter the world of the patient. These include elegant studies of the doctor-patient relationship (Hauser, 1981; Duff and Hollingshead, 1968), brilliant investigations of the social definition of illness (Scott, 1969; Mishler, 1981), and most conspicuous, in line with the chapter's fundamental point, studies of the interaction of illness and the family (Lewis, 1980).

In this light, the rise of science as the arbiter of medical practice may be unrelated to either the mechanistic view of the distant physician or the empathic view of the healer engaged in the world of the patient. Science in medicine is at once a new system of values and a new set of concepts and rules about gathering data and making inferences. As psychiatry returns to medicine, its own scientific traditions, which are long and honorable, can only be enhanced. Most notable and compelling among the scientific activities in psychiatry are the descriptive studies in the Kraepelinian tradition and in the neurosciences and psychopharmacology. This work is bound to bolster the physician's effectiveness in the first role: observing with detachment the failure of mechanisms in the patient.

Family studies offer a secure and vital source of scientific knowledge to improve the physician's effectiveness in the second role: entering the patient's world. Working with the family, the physician enters the world of the patient more completely than in any other form of therapeutics. To be sure, the physician retains some modest control. Families come to the physician's office at times that he or she specifies. They sit on furniture that the physician arranges next to a window which is open or closed at his or her discretion. But once the encounter begins, the relationships within the family, relationships which are formed and solidified long before the family first meets the therapist, subsume the therapist. In this respect, family therapy is different from all other psychotherapies. In group therapy and in psychoanalysis, for example, the therapeutically critical relationships start at the time of the first therapeutic encounter, not before. While these relationships do assume a life of their own in the other therapies, a life into which the physician enters, the relationships are contained or enclosed within a relational envelope the physician provides. In family therapy, the family itself is the envelope.

The family researcher and the family therapist thus begin from a different perspective, a perspective of potentially great importance to the working physician. But beginnings and perspectives are not enough, particularly for contemporary psychiatry. Contemporary psychiatry both recognizes the physician's dual role and also honors science. Clinically relevant family research is a modest enterprise, far too modest in the author's view. Although a small number of well-designed studies of the outcome of family therapy have had positive results (Gurman and Kniskern, 1978), and although some good, scientific results do illuminate the role of the family in normal and pathological behavior, the research enterprise must be nourished. The promising and novel ideas of family clinicians, for example, must be tested with rigorous, scientific methods, or the family field will become just another humanism lending moral, but not scientific support to the physician seeking entry into the patient's world. At this stage in the development of psychiatry, we need more than that.

Chapter *13*

The Basics of Family Treatment
by Henry Grunebaum, M.D. and Ira D. Glick, M.D.

In this chapter, the authors attempt the formidable task of presenting a primer of family therapy. Most family therapy texts delineate a particular theory of family function and dysfunction and develop a therapy based on that theory. A few texts describe many different theories and techniques and leave the reader to choose which are appropriate and when. In part for heuristic reasons, the authors take a different approach. They describe major techniques of family therapy and then suggest a rationale for deciding which to use and in what order. In general, the scheme of the chapter stems from the twofold task of the therapist. The first task is to deal with troubling behavior or dysfunctional interaction. The second task is to help family members improve communication and understand each other and themselves better so as to foster mutual support for common and individual goals and an improved emotional atmosphere in the family.

The thrust of the chapter is practical rather than theoretical, although the authors do believe that the major importance and impact of family therapy is theoretical. Family therapy embodies a nonlinear, systemic conceptual model of life in which meaning, power, love, and fairness are pivotal. Nonetheless, the chapter focuses on the practice of family treatment, in accord with the views of about half of all family therapists, because such a focus may be of greater value to most readers than a purely theoretical treatment.

BACKGROUND

Family therapy can be defined as a professionally organized attempt to produce beneficial changes in a disturbed marital or family unit by primarily nonpharmacological methods. It aims to establish more satisfying ways of living for the entire family, not just for a single family member. Family therapy is distinguished from other psychotherapies by its conceptual focus on the family system. In this conception beneficial alterations in the larger unit have positive consequences for the individual members as well as for the family system. The major emphasis is on understanding individual behavior patterns as differentiated parts of the complicated family matrix itself. The focus is on relationships rather than individuals, on patterns rather than forces, and on coherence rather than cause.

Generally speaking, family therapy is initiated after an individual family member has been identified as being in need of psychiatric assistance. Depending on what sort of label this individual carries, the person and the family may be seen in one of several types of helping facilities: psychiatric, correctional, or medical. Occasionally, however, a marital or family unit will present itself as being in trouble and will not single out an individual member. A married couple may realize that their marriage is in trouble and that it seems to be their interaction, rather than (or more than) anything about either one of them individually that is creating problems.

Families as Systems

Models for assessing and treating families are currently proliferating. Each model makes different assumptions, focuses on different data, and allows for different interventions. The theory most commonly used by family therapists is the "family systems theory."* From this standpoint, understanding families is based in part upon the notion that the capabilities of the system are greater than the sum of the capabilities of all its parts. A single person in a family must be studied in relation to all the other members of the family in which he or she interacts. And the family system is maintained coherently, often in a steady state, sometimes acting with creative novelty, but always evolving. The family systems theory of family evolution and change as life events occur (such as when a child goes away to college) is different from the physiological systems concept of a stable homeostasis. In the case of families, it could be said that the critical issue is which homeostasis to evolve toward.

The systems theory has a wide range of applications to diagnosis, therapy, and prevention in family psychiatry. In therapy, for example, alternate insights are obtained from viewing a family not simply as a set of individual persons, but as a system made up of interacting human beings. The therapist looks at the persons in a family as individual living systems, while viewing the family they constitute as a system of comparable subsystems. The task is to determine to what extent pathology lies in the family as a whole, in one or more individual members, in the suprasystem (the outer environment with which the entire family system interacts), or in a combination of these, and then to plan appropriate treatment interventions.

Perspectives and Approaches

Among the many theorists and theories in the field of family therapy, most start with a systems theory. They then diverge and begin to gather information about the family from three different perspectives: historical, interactional, and existential (Grunebaum and Chasin, 1980; in press). Treatment proceeds from each of three approaches: understanding, transformation, and identification. More advanced techniques such as strategic and paradoxical approaches are also important, but are not appropriate in this discussion of basic techniques. Evaluation thus entails three lines of inquiry. Historical inquiry asks the question, How

*Preceptor's note: Family systems are discussed in greater detail by Bloch in his chapter.

did this situation come about? Interactional inquiry focuses on the problem, asking, What behavioral sequences can be observed in the family now? Existential inquiry wonders, What does it feel like to be this member of the family? The therapist can then choose the appropriate approaches. He or she can (1) increase the family's knowledge and understanding of themselves or their situation; (2) alter family interactions (either dyadic or systemic) by making transforming moves such as assigning tasks; and (3) foster new identifications (for instance, with parents who may have changed but are still seen in the old ways, and also with the therapist). While therapists often tend to use historical data to develop understanding and insights and interactional data to transform or change behaviors, for instance by assigning tasks, these links between perspectives and approaches are not necessary. In fact, unlinking the perspectives from the approaches permits the therapist greater flexibility.

It is important to realize that families may respond to the therapist's interventions in ways that differ from the intended response. A comment offered as an insight to increase the family's understanding can be taken as a directive. For instance, a therapist was asked by parents why he thought they needed family therapy, and he told them, "The children are in charge of the family." The parents took this observation as though it were the command, "Take charge of your family," and they did so forthwith. What therapists teach and say that they are attempting to do may in fact be quite different from what careful reading and observation suggest. Thus, Minuchin (1974), who emphasizes transformational approaches, does a vast amount of teaching with the family and interacts with them in a warm and involving way. And Boszormenyi-Nagy not only explores with great skill the ethical balances and imbalances in families, but obviously cares deeply that families achieve a sense of justice and trust (Boszormenyi-Nagy and Krasner, 1980). What influences the family is how the family uses what the therapist does.

DECISION GUIDELINES

The authors believe that the final recommendation of a particular kind of family treatment results from a sequence of four clinical decisions. The discussion here reviews the first two of the four steps in the sequence. The second two steps are beyond the scope of a chapter on the basics of family treatment (but see Clarkin et al., 1981).

The process of choosing a particular family treatment is like a decision tree that a clinician might have in mind as he or she evaluates a patient. The first step addresses the question, *Is family evaluation indicated?* Presumably family treatment would never be recommended except after a family evaluation. The second step addresses the question of differential therapeutics. *Is the optimal treatment family therapy or a common alternative such as individual or hospital treatment?* The third step addresses the question of treatment format, in the event that family therapy is indicated. *How should the treatment format be specified in terms of intensity* (crisis versus noncrisis treatment), *duration* (brief versus open-ended), *focus* (sex versus marital), *subsystems involved* (marital versus family), *or as part of a sequence of various treatment modalities?* The fourth step addresses the question of methodology. *Is a particular methodology such as the systems or dynamic method of family intervention most indicated?*

Indications for Family or Marital Evaluation

Family evaluation is defined as one or more family interviews conducted to assess the structure and process of family interaction, to determine how the family influences and is influenced by the behavior and symptoms of its individual members, and to gather the data necessary to decide whether family treatment is possible and indicated. While the following material delineates the *indications* for family evaluation, many experts today would agree that a family evaluation is a necessary part of every evaluation of children, adolescents, and married people, *unless there are contraindications.* The following lists the indications for conducting a family evaluation.

(1) *Strong indications.* In certain cases, family or marital evaluation is almost essential in understanding the presenting situation and recommending appropriate treatment. For example:

a child or adolescent is the presenting patient;

the presenting problem is sexual difficulty or dissatisfaction;

the presenting issue is a family or marital problem serious enough to jeopardize the relationship, job stability, health, or parenting ability of a couple (child neglect or abuse, disruptive extramarital affairs, spouse battering, preoccupation with problems at work);

there has been a recent clear stress and emotional disruption to the family caused by family crisis (illness, injury, job loss, death) or a family milestone (graduation, marriage, birth) (Langsley et al., 1968); and/or

the family or marital pair defines the problem as a family issue, and there is motivation for family evaluation.

(2) *Usual indications: hospitalization considered.* Whenever psychiatric hospitalization is being considered, a family evaluation is usually indicated for one or more of the following reasons:

history gathering;

clarification of how the family interaction is influenced by and has influenced the course of illness; and/or

negotiating the treatment plan with the whole family (Is hospitalization necessary, or can the family manage with outpatient help? If hospitalization is necessary, what part will the family play?).

(3) *Other common indications.* The following are less powerful, but nonetheless common and important indications for family evaluation:

more than one family member is simultaneously in psychiatric treatment;

improvement in the individual patient is correlated with symptom formation in another family member or deterioration in the relationship between the member and the patient;

individual or group treatment is failing or has failed (Glick and Kessler, 1980; Greenberg et al., 1964) and:

  (a) the patient is much involved with family problems; or
  (b) the patient has difficulty dealing with family issues unless they are demonstrated directly in the room; or
  (c) the transference to the therapist is too intense or actualized and can be brought back to realistic proportions by including family members; or
  (d) family cooperation seems necessary to allow the individual to change; and/or

although the patient presents with symptoms that are not immediately related to family issues, the therapist decides during the individual evaluation that the primary or secondary gain of the symptoms is an important expression of family systems pathology (e.g., a wife's worsening agoraphobia when her husband works overtime) (Ackerman, 1966; Greenberg et al., 1964; Langsley et al., 1968; Satir, 1967).

Differential Therapeutics

The model of differential therapeutics presented here specifies those factors discovered in individual and family evaluation that are most crucial in guiding the clinician's choice between family treatment and individual treatment. When clinicians recommend a specific treatment modality, they consciously or intuitively match patients' needs with their own experience or fantasies about various treatments. The following guidelines are intended to broaden this perspective with a summary of general clinical opinion and currently available research data. As the results of accumulating outcome research indicate the specific characteristics of patients who succeed or fail in each treatment modality, the process of choosing a therapy will become increasingly precise.

THE CHOICE OF FAMILY OR MARITAL THERAPY VERSUS INDIVIDUAL THERAPY   A basic theoretical premise of family and marital therapy is that individual symptoms can be viewed as interpersonal in etiology or current maintenance or both and can be changed by altering the family system. Perhaps one of the most fundamental and common therapy decisions is whether to direct the treatment to the family or to focus on the symptomatic individual. Surprisingly, a survey of family therapists (Group for the Advancement of Psychiatry, 1970) showed that 83 percent were interested in the decision about how to combine individual and family therapies.

The authors' criteria (see Table 1) depend more on the characteristics of the family and how the members function than on the particular diagnosis or problem area presented by the identified patient(s). The choice of family therapy, as in most psychiatric treatment, is not determined in any simple or reliable way by patients' problems or diagnoses. The problem itself is a final common pathway for multiple causes and influences which may or may not include a preponderance of contributing factors from the family. Moreover, describing a problem in detail tells one less about how to change it than a functional analysis of the problem. The functional analysis shows how much the family in a particular case is maintaining or exacerbating the problem. For these reasons, the indications are not organized around particular diagnoses.

In some areas, limited research has shown that family therapy may be useful for specific symptom constellations. These areas include severe family pathology (Fleck, 1976); schizophrenia (Beels, 1975; Goldstein et al., 1978), marital therapy when one spouse is manic-depressive (Greene et al., 1975); alcoholism (Steinglass, 1976); adolescents with anorexia (Minuchin et al., 1978); parents of feminine boys (Newman, 1976); divorce (Kaplan, 1977); asthma (Liebman et al., 1974); gambling (Boyd and Bolen, 1970); and the deaf (Shapiro and Harris, 1976). In almost none of the existing studies is there a direct comparison between the benefits of marital or family therapy and those of other modalities. Thus, a discussion of differential therapeutics in these specific areas has limitations.

Table 1.   Criteria for Family or Marital and Individual Therapy

Family or Marital Therapy	*Individual Therapy*
INDICATIONS	

Family or Marital Therapy	Individual Therapy
Marital problems are presented as such, without either spouse or any family member designated as the identified patient; couple is committed to work on the marital problem; symptoms are predominantly within the marital relationship (Ackerman, 1966; Group for the Advancement of Psychiatry, 1970; Gurman, 1975; 1978; Gurman and Kniskern, 1978b; Hurvitz, 1967).	The presenting problem of the individual does not have a significant etiology in or effect upon the family system. The patient's symptom or character is based on firmly structured intrapsychic conflict that causes repetitive life patterns more or less transcending the particulars of the current family interaction.
Marital problems that are acute and ego-alien are an indication for conjoint treatment, while for marital problems which are chronic and ego-syntonic, couples group is indicated (Grunebaum et al., 1971).	Defensive misuse of family therapy to deny individual responsibility for major personality or character illness (Schomer, 1978).
Family presents with current structured difficulties in intrafamilial relationships, with each person contributing collusively or openly to the reciprocal interaction problems (Ackerman, 1966; Group for the Advancement of Psychiatry, 1970; Schomer, 1978; Wynne, 1965).	Massive but minimally relevant or unworkable parental pathology that indicates symptomatic child or adolescent should be treated alone (Schomer, 1978).
Family has fixed and severe deficits in perception and communication: (a) projective identification so that each member blames the other for all problems (Wynne, 1965); (b) family using paranoid/schizoid functioning, boundaries vague and fluctuating, parts of self readily projected onto other family members, trading of ego functions (Skynner, 1976); (c) a relentless fixity of distance maintained by pseudomutual and pseudo-hostile mechanisms (Wynne, 1965); (d) collective cognitive chaos and erratic distancing (Wynne, 1965); (e) amorphous, vague, undirected forms of communication that are pervasive (Wynne, 1965).	Individuation of one or more family members requires that they have their own separate treatment. Family treatment has stalemated or failed and has resolved what crises it can, and one or more individual members require additional individual treatment. There is a need for another modality of treatment prior to family therapy, e.g., detoxification, medication, and/or individual sessions, to establish trust.
Adolescent acting-out behavior, e.g., promiscuity, drug abuse, delinquency, perversion, vandalism, violent behavior (Ackerman, 1966; Alexander and Parsons, 1973; Anthony, 1978; Beck, 1975).	
The presence of sexual dysfunction (Sager, 1974).	
Reduction of secondary gain in one or more family members is a major goal (Ackerman, 1966).	
More than one person needs treatment, and resources are available for only one treatment.	

Table 1 *(continued)*

Family or Marital Therapy	*Individual Therapy*

ENABLING FACTORS

Motivation is strongest to be seen as a couple or family, or an individual patient will accept no other format.	Motivation is strong to be seen alone, e.g., adolescents who state emphatically that they have personal problems for which they want individual help (Offer and Vanderstoep, 1975).
No family member has psychopathology of such proportions that family therapy would be prevented, e.g., extreme agitation, mania, paranoia, severe distrust, dangerous hostility, or acute schizophrenia (Ackerman, 1966; Group for the Advancement of Psychiatry, 1970; Offer and Vanderstoep, 1975; Wynne, 1965).	
Parents are honest and open about family conflicts (Ackerman, 1966).	
Crucial members of a defined functional social system are available for family treatment.	

The major area with a growing body of research and consistent results is the treatment of marital difficulties. For a number of years, the prevalent clinical opinion has been that marital therapy is the treatment of choice for marital difficulties (Ackerman, 1966; Group for the Advancement of Psychiatry, 1970). Hurvitz (1967) has written of the dangers of doing individual therapy with only one spouse in such a situation. In a recent review of marital therapy research results, Gurman and Kniskern (1978b) summarize data that indicate that conjoint marital therapy is superior to conjoint-plus-individual therapy, concurrent individual therapy, or individual therapy for one partner. Another criterion for differential therapeutics is the comparative deterioration effect of each treatment modality. This approaches the question of treatment choice from the negative side, what treatment does the most harm. Gurman and Kniskern (1978a) report that for marital problems the rate of deterioration for conjoint, group, and concurrent-collaborative marital therapies is half that of individual therapy.

The authors' statement that marital treatment for marital difficulties is the major area where a marital or family intervention is the firmly established treatment of choice is probably conservative. Gurman and Kniskern (1978b) conclude their extensive review by saying that family treatment is the treatment of choice for marital difficulties, for decreasing hospitalization rates for some chronic and acute inpatients, for anorexia, for many childhood behavior problems, for juvenile delinquency, and for sexual dysfunction.

Other intimate interpersonal systems, less formally organized and sanctioned than marriages and families, may also lend themselves successfully to conjoint interventions. Partners who are involved significantly with each other, whether or not they are married or living together, whether they are heterosexual or homosexual, have also been effectively treated in conjoint modalities. Here the goal is to help the partners explore relevant issues and, if marriage is contemplated, the doubts and anticipations they may have (Gross, 1977).

Two particular differential decisions between individual and family therapy are controversial and frequent enough to warrant special discussion. The first pertains to treating children. Two disciplines with radically different therapeutic perspectives on the treatment of children are simultaneously flourishing, the family therapy discipline and the child psychotherapy and psychoanalysis discipline. From the point of view of most family therapists, the presenting symptoms in children usually represent dysfunction in the parental and family system. Troubled children thus present an especially strong indication for family therapy, particularly since the children are developmentally vulnerable and changes in the family will profoundly affect their maturation. Child analysts and therapists often take the contrary view that the psychopathology of even very young children results from established intrapsychic structure and conflict, that this is not easily altered by changing the family, and that individual treatment is indicated. Child analysis or therapy would be especially indicated if the child is expressive verbally or in play and can sustain a one-to-one relationship. Anthony (1978) has contributed a helpful discussion of the history of this controversy, as has Malone in this Part.

A second difference of opinion relates to the treatment of adolescents involved in symbiotic, mutually destructive parent-child relationships. Some therapists view this as an indication for family treatment, believing that family treatment can facilitate the weaning of the teenager (Haley, 1980). Other therapists believe that furthering separation and individuation in family treatment is difficult, since family treatment brings all members together and may therefore involve them even more in each other's lives. These therapists would instead recommend that the adolescents receive individual or group treatment to demonstrate concretely their individuation and to promote their growth outside the family. The parents might be seen together to solidify their attachment to each other and their ability to tolerate the loss of their child. Consensus seems to be growing that family therapy is most indicated when the symptomatic adolescent is exhibiting acting-out behavior. Furthermore, some adolescents are unequipped to deal with symbolic psychological processes or to benefit from the insight-oriented individual modes of treatment. Such people may, however, be quite amenable to an action oriented family modality which seems more understandable and practical. Finally, some adolescents refuse to participate in individual sessions, fearing that they will be stigmatized as suffering from some type of mental disorder, or that they will be made to feel guilty personally and individually for what has happened in the family. These people may often be more readily involved if they are included as part of an entire family and if common areas of family concern are addressed.

Before concluding this discussion of indications, two final sets of circumstances are worth noting, families which are breaking up and families in which a member has a severe illness. If the family is irrevocably committed to dissolution, such as when the actual divorce process is going on, family or couples therapy can help to permit the breakup to occur in the most positive manner possible and with the fewest raw edges of unresolved feelings. Divorce therapy can often lead to a less painful experience for each family member (Toomin, 1972). Of course, if the family members do not care about one another, they will usually fail in any form of family therapy. Inexperienced therapists, however, may be overly pessimistic (or overly optimistic) about the changes that can be brought about in families. Marital couples or families may begin therapy by talking about breaking up and appear more chaotic in the early sessions than they will later. Many families start treatment by emphasizing their worst aspects. During a first interview, the therapist may feel that the situation is more hopeless than it is. Once the therapist knows the family better, he or she can usually see positive aspects that the family may have overlooked. The fact that the family members come for treatment should in itself be taken as an indication that they are potentially seeking help for their difficulties. If the marital partners were determined to break up or divorce, and if this were not a conflicted or difficult issue for them, they would see a divorce lawyer rather than seek family therapy.

Although no amount of family therapy can change the course of an organic disease such as a tumor, the family may be helped to live more comfortably with the secondary consequences of the illness. What might be changed are the reactions of the patient and family to the symptoms and dysfunctions.

THE PROCESS OF FAMILY EVALUATION

In this section, and in the next section on therapy, the authors offer a basic approach rather than a comprehensive scheme (for a more comprehensive scheme, see Glick and Kessler, 1980).

(1) *Bring all relevant members of the family unit together.* Observing a couple, a family unit, or several generations of a family together offers the opportunity to gather new data, data which are different from what one can gather from an individual with his or her necessarily limited perspective. It offers the opportunity to observe interaction, to hear the points of view of different participants, and to assess the emotional climate of the family and the feelings, thoughts, and behaviors of each person. As Wynne says, "in comparison with psychoanalytic psychotherapy, in family therapy its focus is more on *unnoticed* but *observable*, rather than on *unnoticed* but *inferable* [phenomena]" (Wynne, 1965, 291). For no other reason than the fact that the perspectives of individuals are so much influenced by their feelings and views, conjoint interviews with the significant others in the patient's life are invaluable. In addition, bringing the family together permits the therapist to influence directly the family's patterns of relating and interacting.

Sometimes who should attend is obvious, such as the wife of a depressed middle-aged man or the parents and siblings of a troubled child. At other times it will not be so readily apparent, as in the case of the children of the depressed man or the grandparents of the troubled child. Usually it is useful to ask the patient, "Who are the people who are important to you and know you well?"

Often there will be resistance to involving some members of the family. The children of the depressed man may be considered too young. The parents of the troubled child may think the grandparents are too old. The therapist will have to assess each case to determine who should attend. Perhaps the children of the depressed man are too young. More likely, they are aware of their father's depression and would be relieved to learn that he is receiving treatment. Although their parents may not realize it, they may even have heard of his threats of suicide. Perhaps one set of grandparents are living in a distant city. But what about the other set who give their grandchildren their weekly allowance? In general, it is wise to be inclusive initially and to exclude family members only after having evaluated their contribution to the situation. Often, meeting with relevant subsystems of the family will be important, such as the couple, the siblings, or the father and the grandfather.

(2) *Form a therapeutic alliance with each member of the family.* Attempt to get to know each member of the family and especially to know their strengths. Do this by approaching them on an age-appropriate level. Talk to a child, for instance, while sitting on the floor. Look at things from each individual's perspective, realizing that each is doing his or her best. You have to be on each person's side, what Boszormenyi-Nagy has called multilateral partiality (Boszormenyi-Nagy and Ulrich, 1981). Try to find some quality of value in each member, especially in the ones who are devalued by the family. If the family blames the son's delinquency on the father's being alcoholic and unemployed for a year, develop an alliance with the father by learning that he was a skilled mason for many years.

The family members should feel that you care about each of them, that you have empathy for their positions. Saying to a child, "You must have felt scared to hear your father's talk of suicide," involves what Minuchin has called "joining" (Minuchin, 1974). It must be done in age-appropriate ways, you must fit in with their cultural and ethnic norms, and special efforts to involve fathers are often necessary.

(3) *Learn what each person thinks the problem is and what they think the strengths of the family are.* Usually the family will describe the problem as a symptom in an individual: "He has temper tantrums." Sometimes they will describe the problem as a symptomatic person: "She is disobedient." The latter differs from the former in that it implies an interaction, namely, she disobeys someone. The former operates independently of either individual control or family input. In family theory, symptoms are seen as possibly being the results of interaction between people or maintained by the interaction between people or both. Thus, the family perspective might reformulate the first description, "He gets enraged when his father tells him to clean up the kitchen," and the second, "She disobeys her mother."

Notice who appears to be involved and who appears to be uninvolved. Very often a seemingly uninvolved person is in fact a silent support or a mediator to an involved pair. As Bowen (1978) points out, a problem often involves a triangle, and as Minuchin (1974) says, a problem child often stands on the shoulders of a parent. Thus, the first description could again be reformulated, "He gets enraged when his father asks him to clean the kitchen, and his mother silently believes that his father should not ask him to do something that the father will not do himself." The second description could become, "She disobeys her mother because her father will take her side silently and when the mother leaves the room he will say, 'You know your mother really loves you.'"

(4) *Observe interaction.* Who sits where? Which child sits between the parents. Who speaks for whom? Does a mother answer questions addressed to her son? Who remembers for the family? Who checks with whom? Who controls the children's behavior? What are the alliances? Is there a coalition between the parents that governs the family, or is one parent allied with a child?

In questioning the family, the evaluator usually asks each person about individual perspectives and experiences. Focus the questions on significant history. "Can you tell me a little about your parents' marriage? What have been the key events in your family? What are your hopes, your expectations?" Not so common, but often quite useful, is to ask people about their views of others' experiences. Asking them to rank people may be especially useful. For instance, "Which of your siblings would you say is most likely to please mother? Who are her favorites, and in what order? What are you most worried about in this family?" Many siblings will have very clear beliefs about who is loved the most by their mother and by their father, often much to the surprise of the parents. Questions that compare often lead to answers which surprise the family members and lead to passionate discussions among them.

(5) *Do not overlook the sources of difficulties beyond those involved in problem interactions.* For instance, marital problems not infrequently arise from the depression or cyclothymic cycles of a member. In these instances, appropriate psychopharmacological treatment can have a major impact on the problematic marital interaction. Even when the depression of a family member is only partially the result of marital difficulties, that member will be better able to participate in the treatment if he or she is not so depressed.

Today it is not unusual for married individuals or adolescents to attribute their difficulties to their marriage or their family. Thus, the request for couples or family treatment can at times be a resistance to dealing with individual problems. A young adult who states that her family will not let her leave home may actually be afraid of peer relationships and heterosexuality in particular. This example points up the critical importance of the dialectic between dependence on the family and the ability to develop and maintain satisfactory peer relationships (Grunebaum and Solomon, 1980). A person cannot leave home if he or she cannot relate comfortably and intimately with peers. For instance, a successful executive with many colleagues but no close friends had no one to talk to when his only confidante, his wife, was unfaithful. His loneliness made him desperate. For this couple, a combination of couples and group psychotherapy was useful since the man's dependence on his wife had driven her away in the first place.

(6) *Evaluate to what extent the symptoms are the result of or maintained by the interaction between people.* Just as the individual psychodynamic theories maintain that symptoms are the result of internal forces, dynamics, and fantasies, the family theories maintain that symptoms are the result of or maintained by the properties of an interaction or the functioning of a family system.

The key task is to determine how much the individual or the family theory contributes to an understanding of the development and maintenance of the problem and, even more important, what approach is most likely to foster change. A purely physical symptom, such as postmyocardial infarct invalidism, can be maintained by the way family members treat the patient, not just by the individual's psychodynamics. Likewise, a problem such as difficulty in shared decision making can result more from individual dynamics than from interpersonal dynamics. If you decide that the family contributes to the problem, and if you believe that intervening with them may be productive of change, then discuss this with them and agree on a contract for meeting.

A GUIDE TO FAMILY INTERVENTIONS

While intervention begins during the evaluation process, it is best thought of separately. Remember that the family usually begins treatment with low self-esteem, believing they are seen as sick, incompetent, or blamed. The therapist must therefore comment favorably on any element of caring, warmth, reaching out, responsibility taking, or protecting that they demonstrate.

(1) *Direct the initial interventions toward problem behaviors.* Three types of problem behaviors require early attention: (a) those causing physical harm to one or more individuals; (b) those that entail parental inability to control children; and (c) those between overinvolved pairs. Later interventions will deal with more cognitive issues, such as problem-solving techniques, poor communication, feelings of injustice, and loyalties to the family of origin. Later interventions will also endeavor to provide new identifications and new experiences for families in which the emotional range is limited due to failures of development.

Some families and couples will require intervention of the initial type, and when problem behaviors cease, they will find they have no need for further help. Other families will present difficulties that are not easily framed behaviorally, such as poor communication or lack of affection. In such cases, initial therapeutic efforts should bypass a primarily behavioral focus.

(1a) *Prevent physical harm if present.* The single most important initial assessment and intervention involves the prevention of physical harm to the family members or to the therapist. Abused children, battered wives, and sometimes battered husbands, as well as abused grandparents, are all too common. The therapist must also be aware that violence directed toward therapists is not uncommon, particularly with patients who are angry, paranoid, alcoholic, or impulsive. Neither the family nor the therapist can work on other issues when they are afraid. Remember, too, that most families are afraid of psychotic individuals, even when there has been no violence or threat of it.

In these cases, the array of community resources must be considered and employed when appropriate. Encouraging family members to call the police when threatened, to seek shelter when abused, and to inform the appropriate authorities of child abuse should be regarded as the beginning of family therapy and as necessary for its success. Nothing can be accomplished when family members act from fear rather than from love or understanding.

(1b) *Strengthen the parental-marital coalition if the problem is in a child.** Depending on how one looks at it, the disturbed child either tends to split the parents, or the disturbance is a response to the parents' split. Do not work on marital issues early when the problem is in a child; this is a detour until parenting can be done jointly in a united way. Repair the parenting alliance by helping the parents to focus on behaviors, not on feelings or thoughts. It is important for parents to empathize with their children, but they should insist on appropriate behavior and agree on what appropriate means. Parents should also learn to be specific about what they expect: "If you wish to leave the hospital and come home, you must get up every morning

*Preceptor's note: Malone discusses this and the next intervention in his chapter.

and go to the day care center." The parents must "insist" as a unit and have worked out an agreement about what they expect.

Point out the positive aspects of behavior: "Your husband's silence allows you to be close to your son." Of the positive aspects of feelings, you might say, "His getting angry shows how much he cares." Of a child's symptoms, you might say, "Your not eating keeps your parents so busy that they never have time to argue with each other."

(1c) *Foster boundaries between overinvolved pairs.* Early interventions may also include the necessary step of extricating people from overly close units. This can mean strengthening the parental coalition by bringing in the uninvolved partner. The husband and wife may be asked to talk about what *he* can do with his son under *her* supervision, so that she will not have to worry so much about the boy. You could say to the parents, "Now talk it over and decide what you will expect of Jim when he comes home from the hospital." Or you might suggest, "I want father to control Billy and keep him from interrupting the grown-ups' conversation, and if he needs help he should ask mother what to do; otherwise, she will keep quiet."

Another technique is to insist that no one speak for anyone else. In this way, you can prevent an overly involved parent from speaking for a child. Similarly, you may prevent one child from acting parentally and taking excessive care of another child. You might insist that the couple plan some time for themselves and notice how the overinvolved child will act to disrupt their growing closeness.

All of this can be done during the session itself. As members of families are asked to behave appropriately to their generations and to maintain appropriate degrees of intimacy between the sexes, it will often be seen that one person finds the tasks increasingly anxiety provoking and difficult.

(2) *Observe and explore the reactions of the other family members to changes in the behavior of a member.* At this point the therapist is in the position of having to reevaluate the family, namely, its reaction to therapeutically induced changes. For instance, a husband who has always worked all the time, much to his wife's distress, greatly cuts down on this during the course of therapy and spends much more time at home. It then emerges that she finds it very difficult to share decisions with him, especially if she feels that he will not go along with her wishes. When she is asked why, she says that it would "require looking into a black hole in myself."

This is the time, in the presence of the husband, to explore certain of her internal fantasies. This can be carried out while simultaneously discussing the husband's reactions with him. While he appears to enjoy being home more and says he wants to be there, he cannot tell his wife he loves her. His fantasies about expressing love should also be explored. Both partners' fantasies very likely result from experiences in their families of origin.

(3) *Assess issues that may be interfering with family development and intervene appropriately.* Families often come to the attention of therapists when a single member has problems that can be traced to a failure to negotiate a family crisis.* They may come some time after the crisis event, even years later, rather than immediately. The unresolved issues

*Preceptor's note: In his chapter, Bloch discusses the family life cycle in greater detail.

often involve the loss or gain of a family member, a marked change in the situation of one or more members, and sometimes a normal developmental crisis. The task for the therapist is to mobilize the resources of the family to confront, share, and adapt to the change.

For instance, a ten-year-old boy was seen in a guidance clinic because of his fear of going to school. Evaluation revealed a family with many strengths and problems. Of special importance here, the family had never grieved the death of an older adult brother who had died in an accident involving a stolen car. This brother, while a hell-raiser outside the family, was a support, a teacher, and a companion to his younger siblings. After supervision, the initially nondirective therapist took charge of a session and insisted that the family discuss the loss. Much to the mother's surprise, the younger children were able to share their grief and their disappointment at not having been allowed to go to the funeral, but only to the wake. The family then agreed to make their first visit to the grave.

Regardless of significant coexisting difficulties or psychopathology, many families can be helped to return to their optimal levels of functioning with relatively simple interventions focused specifically on an issue which has not been faced. Simple rituals, such as visiting a grave, sharing "good thoughts" about a lost member, or having a wedding party for a member who eloped, are often useful.

(4) *Foster clear and open communication.* Families may have difficulties communicating with each other, as well as making clear what is troubling them. Helping them to express themselves is both necessary for conducting the therapy and potentially useful outside the session. What might be called English-to-English translation is often an important task of the therapist, who must often be quite active in ensuring clear communication.

Several ingredients of communication can be fostered by the therapy. First, family members can be helped to communicate verbally and to notice each other's nonverbal messages. Second, individuals can learn to *own* their own statements rather than having members speak for one another. Frequently one member of the family is given the task of speaking for the others, and this must be blocked if at all possible. But the gatekeeper may have to be dealt with carefully lest family balance be upset too early. If the therapeutic alliance is not strong enough, the family may leave treatment. A final and valuable way of helping with communications is to help family members clarify their statements. "He was very nice last night" may or may not communicate what the wife appreciated about her husband's behavior—bringing her a cup of tea, or leaving her to do her own work, or seducing her, or not losing his temper. It would probably be useful for the husband to know exactly which of these his wife meant.

(5) *Observe and listen carefully for the attributions and expectations of the family members.* Families usually assign specific attributions and roles to their individual members. When the "good" boy is bad, they might say, "Boys will be boys." But when the "bad" boy does the same thing, they may say, "He's a troublemaker and always was." Early experiences often will shape these attributions. If a husband does not hear what his wife says and respond immediately, and if that means to her that he deliberately is "not making an effort," she may be reacting to him as though he were her oblivious and sadistic father. For his part,

her husband is doing his best to be polite and attentive but is easily confused by her anger; he is still trying to placate his mother, who was determined that he should be polite at all times. Clarifying these attributions and their origins is useful to family members, for they can then test their validity in the present reality.

Family members, particularly spouses, have clear and often unexpressed expectations of one another. Thus, a husband will believe that he and his wife have an agreement that his enjoying his work is a key and shared value, which means to him that he can work as late as he needs to. On the other hand, she believes that their agreement is to have a jointly shared and fulfilling family life, which means to her that he should be home for supper. These so-called marital contracts have been discussed at length by Sager (1976) and are also discussed by Berman in her chapter. The contracts have several levels. Both partners know about the open agreements, such as, "We will bring our children up as Episcopalians." Some other agreements are also conscious, and each partner can verbalize them, but they may not have been discussed with the other. Finally, there are unconscious contracts between spouses. For instance, a couple may have the covert agreement that she will help him overcome his fears of sexuality, while he will keep her from being promiscuous. Delineating these contracts between spouses is often quite useful to them. It can help them explore the sources of current difficulties and revise their contracts to fit the present context more usefully.

(6) *Explore how mistaken attributions are rooted in the past.* As it becomes evident that mistaken attributions are leading to impaired communication and understanding, this is the time to look in greater detail at the families of origin of the couple. Family loyalties to parents and grandparents and to religious and ethnic groups, as Boszormenyi-Nagy and Spark (1973) discuss, are important here and cannot be overestimated. To have a marriage that is different from and better than that of one's parents is both sought for and feared. Conflicting loyalties may become apparent. For instance, a middle-aged physicist wanted to manage well the money his father had labored to accumulate, but remembered also that his father wanted him to succeed academically since he "had no head for money."

Often it will be useful to have parents or spouses develop a family genealogy (a genogram) in which intergenerational continuities become visible. Perhaps the women marry men who are "not religious enough," or the men all tend to desert their families, or the oldest daughters tend to fight with the fathers.

Sometimes having the grandparent generation present will be useful at this point in the therapy. Usually, much to everyone's surprise, the parents of adult children are forgiving of them and endeavor to free them from expectations which might once have been important to them.

(7) *Explore the balance of fairness and justice in the family.* All family members keep track of what they believe they have done for others and what they believe is owed to them. This important dimension of family life has been singled out by Boszormenyi-Nagy as a most powerful and influential familial reality (Boszormenyi-Nagy and Krasner, 1980). A middle-aged man, deserted by his wife and left with a small child, expects in vain that his devoted caring for the child will be taken

over by his second wife. Women owe him a debt. For her part, the second wife feels that she is owed a debt for caring for the motherless girl. Men owe her a debt.

Debts are also carried from one generation to another. For instance, the children of holocaust survivors may feel that there is no way that they can make it up to their parents for the losses of family, home, and livelihood, and for the suffering they have experienced. And, they believe, they are the only people who can pay the debt.

The therapist must recognize that it is often real acts which have been unfair or unjust and which have led to feelings of being owed. These are not unconscious sources of guilt which require exploration. They are actual events which require efforts to right the unfairness or injustice. The therapist can help the family to redress ethical imbalances. Just as the courts increasingly recognize a woman's claim to part of her husband's earnings if she has supported him during medical school, the family therapist must also help the couple to balance their accounts.

(8) *Foster changes in identification.* Family members commonly experience certain feeling states as alien. For instance, no matter how successful he is, a middle-aged husband and father feels driven to succeed as he thinks his own father wished. A wife and mother finds she cannot really enjoy sex, even though her husband has become as gentle and as forbearing as she could wish.

There are three possible sources of new identifications for such people. First of all, the exploration of the past may lead to a figure with whom an identification can be made. Thus, the woman became able to enjoy life more fully when she remembered the grandfather who had played with her and held her lovingly on his lap, unlike her rather puritanical parents. Second, it is often possible to foster a revision of an old identification. When the middle-aged man was seen in therapy with his father, the father told him that while he did want him to "succeed," this success should not be at the expense of his family. The father revealed that he had learned some new things as he himself had grown older. Third, it is sometimes possible to foster an identification with the therapist. Wrestling with a rebellious adolescent boy, Whitaker set an example for the father that one can sometimes set limits more effectively through actions than with words alone (Napier and Whitaker, 1978).

In some sense, the therapist cannot choose what identification will be made with him or her. Yet in certain ways identification is at the core of family therapy, just as it may be in any therapy. In a variety of ways the therapist provides an invaluable person for identification— by respecting the dignity and the views of each family member, young and old; by showing concern for the well-being of each person; by paying attention to those family boundaries which protect the weaker and which allocate appropriate responsibility to the parents; by believing in the importance of fairness to and between children and parents; and by believing in the value of relationships, in the continuity of the family, and in the ability of families to share and survive sorrows and to share and celebrate joys.

(9) *Aid family role assumption, education, and demythologization.* The therapist helps the family to test reality, to distinguish between what is actually going on and what is fantasy. This testing may be related to behavior, attitudes, or emotions and is not confined to

testing the reality of grossly psychotic family members. For example, one rural family needed this kind of help when the parents refused to allow the children to go to school for six months because of the possibility of an earthquake.

The therapist avoids any claim to omnipotence. As much as the case allows, the family itself does the work of changing, because the ultimate intent is to enable the family to solve its own problems. The more the family can do, without the therapist, the more autonomy it will develop.

As a model for identification, the therapist can provide an education in family living, roles, clear communication, emotional honesty, problem solving, and the realities of married life. The family learns from the therapist's speech and conduct. If the therapist plays the role of a more empathic spouse to a defensive wife, the family may see the possibility for an alternative set of transactions. If the therapist can focus on sexual issues in an open, direct, and mature manner, a sexually guilt-ridden, fearful family may be helped to come to terms with these issues. The therapist should be cautious about trying to remake the family in his or her own image, however. The family therapist may make use of advice and direction by trying first to identify and then to change maladaptive methods of coping. Family therapists also often indicate the importance of limit setting as a method to encourage change. Such a therapist might indicate, "I think your son should begin attending school within two weeks."

At times a more authoritarian style of treatment may be helpful. The therapist may occasionally need to assume the role of the all-knowing and all-powerful manipulator of the family's interactions and goals. People in some sociocultural settings are accustomed to such a directive style and would be left confused or unconvinced by an invitation to share authority and responsibility. This directive style may also be necessary with the most dysfunctional families, for it can aid them in becoming less chaotic and enable them to move to a more adequate level of functioning.

Therapists will often find themselves called on to function as demythologizers, or philosophers of family life. This usually means helping the family to experience and to make explicit covert family myths, but does not mean giving direct advice to the lovelorn or loveworn. Such myths might be expressed, "Father can't work," or "Neil is the stupid one in the family." The myths by which people live can serve as gratifying anchor points for stable relationships. But myths can also be incompatible with one another, particularly when they are extreme or relatively unrealistic. Moreover, they may not be accepted by all members of the family. In such instances, the mythical beliefs can cause disappointment and pain, and the family therapist will need to recognize the disruptive role that they are playing.

(10) *Make use of behavioral techniques adapted to the family problems.* Certain family problems, particularly those where a child manifests a single symptom like stealing or encopresis, respond well to behavior modification. Generally the technique should be based on positive reinforcement of more acceptable behaviors. The family should be helped to deal with the unacceptable behavior. They especially need to find a way not to reward the child with increased attention, including attention through punishment. Isolating the child or ignoring the problem behavior is often useful. Such

homespun remedies may, of course, have already been employed by the parents.

Other family problems such as sexual problems in a couple may require desensitization. A gradual approach to a feared sexual behavior is prescribed. The approach should occur in a nonpressured, pleasurable way, while the therapist investigates with the couple the fantasies and fears which may be involved in the symptom.

The straightforward behavioral approaches to family and marital problems are useful not only because they have particular merit for monosymptomatic cases, but also because they draw attention to the value of focusing on the complaint or what needs to change. Frequently a complaint is maintained because of the reinforcement provided. For example, a husband may be solicitous of his wife only when she is sick, or be affectionate only if rewarded by sexual relations. Such reinforcement contingencies are often easily delineated, and treatment can be the focused in an efficient and effective way.

Treatments focused on behavior can either be applied by parents when the problem is in a young child, or they can involve contracting between parents and older children or between spouses. The contracting procedure involves agreements where, in return for one person engaging in certain behaviors, the other person will engage in certain other behaviors.

Family therapists have found it valuable to have clearly defined goals whose achievement is both feasible and readily recognizable. "Better communication" is not such a goal, while "being home for supper five nights a week" is. Many families can define clear-cut therapy goals themselves and be pleased when they are achieved. Others will need more help, since their difficulties are vaguer and more complicated.

(11) *Deal carefully with family secrets.* Individual family members often have "secrets" that in most cases are known but not acknowledged by other family members. Secrets may involve overt behavior, such as marital infidelity, which one marital partner feels that he or she has been able to conceal from the other. Or they may involve thoughts, feelings, and attitudes that family members believe others are not aware of. For example, parents may not realize (or may deny) that children pick up the general emotional tone between mother and father. They may act as if their marital discord is hidden from their children and may want to keep that discord "secret."

Helping the family to bring these pseudosecrets into the open usually results in clearing the air and eventually leads to a sense of relief and greater mutual understanding. Interestingly, children commonly talk openly in the family sessions about what others thought was a secret. The therapist should be prepared to deal with acute shock waves when the secret first emerges. When a family member requests an individual session for the purpose of revealing a secret, the therapist will listen and then explore the consequences of discussing the issue within the family setting. If, for example, one spouse has an incurable illness and the other spouse does not know about it, the therapist would examine the reasons for the secrecy and encourage the spouse to share the information with the whole family. If the secret does not seem so crucial, the therapist might take a more neutral stance. The therapist must guard, however, against being trapped into becoming a repository of secrets.

In a variant on this theme, some family members may insist on total honesty. Either they are emotionally insensitive, or they actively seek to hurt another family member. For example, in the guise of honesty a parent might report to a child every negative feeling that crosses his or her mind. This clearly is not useful. Sometimes secrets are better kept secret. While sharing secret feelings of discontent with a partner may be useful, revealing an affair can be destructive. Decisions in this area require clinical sensitivity and empathy rather than rules.

A FINAL NOTE

Doing family therapy is very different from doing individual treatment. Therapists are usually apprehensive at first, but as they gain experience they are excited by the challenge and fascination of work with natural units. Many therapists find themselves uncomfortable doing family work and should not force themselves to undertake it. In some ways, the experience for the therapist is like sitting in the middle of the couple in *Who's Afraid of Virginia Woolf?* or the family in *Long Day's Journey into Night*, or like sitting in the middle of a three-ring circus. One has to pay attention not only to individuals in the family system, but also to the family unit, and at the same time be aware of one's own feelings toward the family. The task is to stay focused on the objective to be achieved with each family unit.

Chapter 14 # Family Systems Perspectives on the Management of the Individual Patient
by Donald A. Bloch, M.D.

INTRODUCTION

This chapter considers the relationship between family systems therapy and the therapy and management of the individual patient. It offers conceptual and practical guidelines for clinicians whose interests and primary skills are in individual psychotherapy, pharmacotherapy, and milieu management. Under each of these terms, there is, of course, a world of difference in both theory and practice, and generalizations about their possible relations must be put forward with extreme caution. Taking this caveat seriously, the author nevertheless believes that family systems perspectives can substantially add to the repertoire of the individually oriented practitioner.

An underlying assumption is that all clinicians will acknowledge that family patterns and events have at least some connection with the dysfunctional patterns of the individual. The family connection may be understood in many different ways: as helping to maintain the patient's malfunctioning in the present, as a resource and support system for the patient and the therapy, as a persistent and irritating hindrance to the conduct of the therapeutic work, as victimizing either the patient or the family, and as etiologic. Family may be understood in all these ways in various mixes, at various times. However the family is conceptualized, it is a plain fact that the family often initiates therapy and, as often, terminates it. The family frequently defines the problem and in many instances pays the bills. Whether central or peripheral to the problem and the therapy, family is almost always a part of psychiatric treatment in reality, and always in fantasy.

PERSPECTIVES AND PARADIGMS

This section outlines some of the major perspectives associated with family systems theory. Techniques of family psychotherapy vary as widely as do those of individual psychotherapy, and there are, of course, major differences among theoreticians as well. There are nonetheless some overriding concepts that distinguish family systems therapy from other approaches to psychiatric disorder. Some of these relate to the format and some to the paradigm.*

Format and paradigm are often confused, and this confusion causes much of the difficulty in properly understanding the differences between family and individual psychotherapy. Format simply means who is included in the treatment arrangement and what persons are explicitly involved in the conduct of the work. But issues of format are really secondary to paradigmatic issues. At first glance, for instance, one might conclude that if family members are physically present, then that defines the treatment as family systems therapy. If they are not, one might conclude, it is individual therapy. Although this view has a certain attractive simplicity, it is ultimately misleading and does not permit the full value of either approach to flower. The choice of format includes all of the arrangements of therapy, who is included, where it takes place, the frequency of contacts, and so forth. Almost any combination of these and other similar elements can occur and would be consistent with either an individual or a family systems perspective. It is quite possible to conduct family systems therapy in a one-to-one format where the therapist and the patient are the only persons in the consultation room. It is equally possible to conduct individual psychotherapy with the active physical involvement of other family members in the psychotherapeutic work.

As to the paradigmatic issue, the term *family systems therapy* is preferred here to the term *family therapy* because it more directly indicates the emphasis on therapeutic change in the family relational system. The perspectives of cybernetics and of general systems theory control the paradigm in family systems therapy. Most important is the view of a hierarchical organization of life in a *series of open systems* of increasing complexity. (All living systems are open in that they are constantly exchanging energy and information with their environments, across the system boundary.) Events at the cellular, organ, organism (individual), family, and societal levels of complexity are all of interest to psychiatrists. Disagreements as to etiology and treatment often reflect the clinician's preference for explanation and intervention at one rather than another of these levels. Such single-level orientations do have benefits, for it is heuristically useful to isolate the biological, psychological, or familial levels for analysis. However, living phenomena must also be understood in a holistic perspective, as has been eloquently set forth by numerous authors. Most recently and relevantly, Engel (1980) articulated this tenet in contrasting the biopsychosocial model in medicine to the biomedical model. For present purposes, it is sufficient to note that each of these levels of hierarchy is associated both with theory building and with intervention technology (and, one might add, with a political and economic territory).

*Preceptor's note: This distinction between paradigm and format is similar to the difference between family therapy as technique and family therapy as theory.

The systemic model offers a different formal view of such matters as cause (etiology) and change processes (therapy). Of principal importance is the matter of context. The systems perspective is that events can only be understood in terms of their contexts and that meaning derives from context. Family systems therapy thus would hold that psychological events in the individual—pain and malfunction—need to be understood and changed by modification of the significant context of which they are a part, the family system.*

This leads to yet another concept that is helpful in differentiating these two perspectives, the *locus of change*. Family systems therapists aim to produce change in the relational structure of the family. Individually oriented therapists aim to produce change in the psychological or biological organization of the individual. While it may be reasonably argued that one cannot occur without the other, quite different theories and clinical technologies flow from each starting point.

One more concept of central importance to the systems perspective is that of *equilibrium*. All living systems are maintained in a condition of dynamic equilibrium. Both pathogenic and healing events may be conceptualized as disturbing or restoring this equilibrium. Equilibrium is always dynamic and complex. Consider a circus performer working his way across a tightrope with a balancing pole. The performer is in constant motion, receiving information through many channels. His information comes from many sources, from his vision, from pressure on the pads of his feet on the wire, from shifting weight pressures from the balancing pole, from his muscles and joints, and from his vestibular apparatus, to mention some of the more important. Even the gasps of the audience, as balance or equilibrium appears endangered, are information. All of these signals are integrated, some reflexly and others at higher centers, and then translated into muscular acts that in turn correct (and somewhat overcorrect) the constant tiny errors. Note that the effects of the corrections are monitored and that they, too, become important information in the equilibrium-maintaining process. This is the dynamic equilibrium of a living system, always in motion, integrating vast and complex data flows, always monitoring its own performance, and always adjusting performance to approximate an internal comparison standard. For the tightrope walker, that standard includes staying on the wire, staying in control of body position, and more complexly, appearing sufficiently out of control at times so as to elicit awe and admiration from the audience. Even in this comparatively simple situation, the internal standard against which performance is measured is highly complicated and hierarchical. The situation with families is analogous. The difference lies in the complexity of the subsystems and the multiple levels at which information is first acquired and stored (in individual memory or through group organizational rules) and in how it later serves, in the aggregate, as a comparison standard against which behavior is judged. These comparison standards are in turn complex and often unknown, albeit profoundly influential.

A final point about the equilibrium model is that an event outside of the system can act to help maintain equilibrium or, oppositely, to unbalance the system. Living systems encounter a multitude of such

*Preceptor's note: Many family systems therapists would assert that while all human phenomena should be understood and evaluated in terms of their context, the decision as to how to intervene must be considered separately in terms of such factors as therapeutic alliance, effectiveness, and so forth.

external events moment by moment. Ordinarily they adapt and maintain balance easily and rapidly. Occasionally they do not. Then an escalating series of corrective moves takes place, leading finally to what is called a state change, a new equilibrium configuration.* It is useful to classify interventions broadly as to their equilibrium effects, noticing that almost all interpersonal acts have varying degrees of equilibrating and disequilibrating aspects. The therapeutic actions of a psychiatrist, for instance, are among the events outside the individual or family system that may act to maintain or disturb balance.

The sections that follow discuss two major classes of events from this perspective. A section on the family life cycle shows vividly how the family, moving through time, adapts (and fails to adapt) to the disequilibration produced by changes in its component parts—the birth, maturation, and death of family members. The section on families experiencing severe physical illness illustrates how this model helps to understand both pathogenicity and healing as functions of the family in dynamic equilibrium.

THE CLINICAL APPROACH

Earlier studies of the etiology of psychiatric problems and disorders unfortunately tended to view the psychiatric patient as a victim of his or her own family. The effort to find "causes" for "diseases" understandably has led in this direction, and this is one of the principal reasons that linear models of causality are misleading. From a systemic perspective, all persons in an interpersonal field are part of that field. The persons themselves make up the very context that provides them with the informational feedback which in turn maintains persistent maladaptive (or adaptive) patterns.

The systemic perspective leads to a different attitude toward family members. Since there are no victims, blame is inappropriate. Thus, generally speaking, family systems therapists assume a particular posture toward family members. The posture is optimistic, supportive and nonblaming, appreciative and neutral. These characteristics are emphasized in order to underscore the importance of avoiding their opposites. Families tend to feel blamed, oppressed, and beaten down and can therefore profit from a therapeutic posture which conveys both that they have a contribution to make and that they are entitled to a bit of justified hope as well. Thus, families are not invited to meet with the psychiatrist treating their family members in order to discover how they have caused the patient's difficulties. Nor are they to be blamed, subtly or otherwise. After all, as parents they have done as well as they could; they were children once, as indeed were their parents. Multigenerational fairness is called for, as well as neutrality in regard to competing interests at any given point in time.** The therapist's posture is not only neutral, but also appreciative, and it conveys the sense that everybody in the family has something to offer toward making things go better. Even when an individual patient is put in the center of the stage, the therapist values and acknowledges the potential for others

*Preceptor's note: In addition to encountering outside disequilibrating forces, human living systems can decide, consciously or unconsciously, to change. The analogy to the circus performer is strengthened if it is recognized that he or she can decide to change specialities, professions, or retire.

**Preceptor's note: The issue of fairness and justice between or among the generations is discussed in detail by Berman in her chapter.

in the family to help in the therapy. This is true no matter how difficult the immediate situation. Cautious optimism is called for whenever possible, although it should not fly in the face of dismal facts. In this overall posture, a therapist is in a good position to tap the many resources of the family and to permit them proper access to information about the patient and the therapy.

Relabeling and *reframing* are terms used to describe techniques that family therapists employ to reflect this attitude. Reframing and relabeling entail a cognitive restructuring of behavior to indicate its positive properties. While a therapist might acknowledge that an adolescent boy's misbehavior is irritating and self-damaging, he or she would also relabel the behavior as the boy's effort to provide an area of common interest and activity for two distant, alienated parents. The depressed wife provides her insecure husband with an opportunity to be useful to her by wanting his constant reassurance. The woman who has not separated from her mother helps her mother continue to feel needed by being dependent on her. The woman may also offer her difficulties in separating from her own daughter as proof of her loyalty to her mother. Reframing and relabeling are not dishonest or insincere. Rather, they are part of a different perspective. The systemic perspective organizes the data differently so that another structure for meanings becomes apparent.

THE INITIAL FAMILY INTERVIEW AND THE GENOGRAM

Two procedures widely used by family therapists are suitable for the individual therapist, since they require little in the way of special training and have immediate, visible clinical benefits. As they are used over time, they build family interviewing skills. These procedures, the initial family systems interview and the family genogram, are briefly outlined below.

The family systems interview is a diagnostic-therapeutic interview conducted over one or two sittings very early in the treatment process. Learning to conduct such an interview comfortably and effectively is a key to mobilizing the therapeutic benefits of family involvement. Families intuitively know that they are both affected by and influential in the patient's behavior. This reciprocity is widely acknowledged and in most instances can be assumed to be part of a family's sense of itself. Family members also tend to feel guilty and blameworthy. Less commonly they recognize that their valiant struggle to remedy the situation may indeed be contributing to the problem. Rarely do they recognize they have a positive contribution to make. For all of these reasons and especially in the early phases of the therapeutic work before strong alliances have been made, it is helpful to convene a family diagnostic-therapeutic meeting with the psychiatrist. The therapist lets the family members know that he or she is soliciting their views, ideas, and experiences with the problem at hand. They are invited to sit as a family, together with the psychiatrist, to review the situation, to share information, and to consider possible actions that might be supportive or beneficial.

The willingness of families to participate in such an interview seems to be directly related to the psychiatrist's own sense of ease with the idea and his or her conviction that it will have a high yield. If the therapist is accustomed to one-on-one interviewing formats, it is at first somewhat strange to be interviewing a group, particularly a family group which has spent a lifetime becoming accustomed to each other's ways. In the author's experience with trainees, conducting a half dozen such interviews will reduce the sense of unfamiliarity and generate increasing professional enthusiasm. Quite simply, the benefits to the therapeutic work are sufficient to confirm the value of the procedure.

This exploratory interview should be as flexible as possible, without a preconceived agenda. Nathan Ackerman (personal communication) has spoken of this as taking a "living history," meaning that the investigation of the past is keyed to the issues of the here and now. Standard clinical history taking often defines a set of events and categories about which data supposedly ought to be collected. Some of these are highly relevant to the matters at hand, and others are not. The therapist can use the initial family interview to augment his or her understanding of the presenting problem by taking a careful family history about the circumstances when the target behavior first appeared. A particular goal is to understand the contexts in which the symptomatic behavior is distinctively present or absent. What else is and was going on in the family? How do people respond to the target behavior? What strategies have been used to deal with it? Current history taking may, of course, lead naturally to issues more removed in time.

Of special value throughout the interview is the opportunity to observe the reactions of the family as various subjects are discussed. The observational field is rich and relevant—who speaks, who is silent, who has appropriate affect, who seems to experience painful affect, how the family operates to alter or reduce psychic discomfort. Most particularly, of course, the clinician is alert to the patient's involvement in the family pattern of psychic discomfort and to the part that his or her symptomatology may play in the pattern. Equally important is the direct observation of family strengths and healing capabilities—how people show affection and what functional areas are unimpaired. Again the focus is on family support for the patient.

A major benefit that accrues when the family meets a psychiatrist under these circumstances is that the therapist and the therapeutic process are demystified and rendered less awesome and strange. The patient's disabilities in turn are brought closer to the realm of the ordinarily comprehensible. Related to this, the complex emotional tie between the patient and the therapist and, for that matter, the tie between other family members and the therapist, are reduced in their intensity. For most forms of therapy, this is beneficial. Some therapists, however, count on what they term a hot transference and may feel that there are losses when this does not develop.

The gains from this diagnostic-therapeutic initial interview, of course, depend heavily on the techniques and style of the psychotherapist. Some will wish only to establish a clear contract and to agree on the nature of the commitment the family makes to the treatment, including such matters as fees, schedules, telephone calls, and so on. In all instances, the therapist is likely to gain valuable insights and a clearer first-hand sense of the experiential world in which the patient lives.*

*Preceptor's note: The value of interviews with relevant family members during the course of individual therapy should not be underestimated. For instance, seeing an individual patient who felt rebellious and different as a child, with her mother, a refugee from Russia, clarified the fact that the daughter as a second child was the first to be permitted and encouraged to be American by her mother and thus independent. The independence served her parents' need to acculturate but led to a feeling of being different from her conforming older sibling and her old-world parents.

The genogram is a simple procedure for representing graphically the history and the relationship structure of the family. Completing the genogram is a natural and easy part of the initial family systems interview. Essentially, the genogram is a family tree that lists the family of origin of each of the patient's parents. The chart can also include significant births, deaths, marriages, and divorces and changes in employment, geographical location, and health status. The result is an easy-to-use graphic representation that makes clear the connections between events and patterns. Families enjoy this simple procedure and intuitively recognize its usefulness. Making a genogram with a family frames the generational context in which present difficulties are embedded and of which they are often an expression. The information yield is often large and is obtained with economy.

The initial interview and the genogram can easily be done in two sessions of an hour to an hour-and-a-half each. Toward the end, the treatment plan can be put before the group, questions can be answered, and a contract can be agreed upon, allowing the work with the individual patient to proceed on a sound basis.

INDIVIDUAL AND FAMILY LIFE CYCLES

This section discusses the specific relations between family life-cycle issues and the management of an individual patient. All living systems have life cycles. As the individual is born and progresses through a series of developmental phases, each with its own distinctive characteristics, so does a family come into being, grow, and eventually die. The place of the individual patient in the family life cycle profoundly influences both the nature of the problems that will present to the psychotherapist and the use of family members in the treatment. Generally, the contribution that a family systems approach can make is based on the degree to which the symptomatic behavior appears to be context dependent, that is, the degree to which seemingly inappropriate behavior can be understood as an appropriate response to the situation in which the patient finds him- or herself. The less autonomous the person, the more likely it is that responses can be seen as context dependent. For example, there is considerable agreement that family methods are appropriate for dealing with the difficulties of children (see the chapter by Malone). The material that follows links suggestions about individual and family systems intervention to stages in the life cycles of both the individual and the family. The suggestions are intended to illustrate a general set of possibilities for family intervention, not to present possibilities that are exclusive to one age.

Adolescents

Family life-cycle issues associated with the adolescence of a family member depend on many factors. Is this the first or last of a sibling subset to be entering this phase? What sex is the youngster? How does the configuration of this family conform to, or differ from, the patterns of the families of origin of the parents? Where are the parents in their own lives? What is the nature and quality of their relationship? The movement of a child into adolescence profoundly stresses some parental relationships. It both raises dormant questions of sexuality and intimacy, and prefigures the problems of the postparental phase.

Since autonomy issues are so significant in adolescence, strong arguments are made for seeing the adolescent patient alone. Other age-related issues of adolescence also argue for a confidential dyadic relationship that does not permit information to flow back to the family. Young people certainly can benefit from the opportunity to explore their own love and sexual experiences with a knowledgeable, benign adult in a one-to-one relationship. The same applies to the rebellious risk-taking behavior often associated with adolescence. Drugs, sex, cars, politics, and peer relations may all need to be considered in a therapeutic environment where privacy is guaranteed, except, of course, when a clear and present danger arises in the form of self-destructiveness, damage to others, or the disabling of the treatment enterprise. All therapists working with this age group should feel free to breach confidentiality in the latter three circumstances, and they should make this explicit to their adolescent patients.

The individual therapist may also go beyond the one-to-one limitation in dealing with the adolescent's family. Although it is traditional to limit contacts with the family in order to encourage the intensity of the dyadic relationship with the therapist, this limitation can foster a situation in which "good" therapists and victimized adolescents are allied against "bad" parents. While the therapist may explicitly deny this as a fiction, refusing to see parents for an occasional consultation obstructs the goal of achieving a rounded, three-dimensional picture of the parents. When the therapist does see the parents, however, another danger looms. As the parents discuss their perspective and their concern with the adolescent patient, a scapegoating session may result, with the bulk of the discussion revolving around the difficulties that the child poses for the parents. Equally adverse is the self-blame position that some parents assume under these circumstances. It is no better to scapegoat one generation than another.

The therapist needs to avoid both situations and also needs to deal with the quite legitimate concerns of the parents. A generally successful procedure is to begin with an initial interview with the adolescent alone in order to establish the therapist's credibility as a potentially useful professional. This interview emphasizes understanding and clarifying the adolescent's experience and discovering his or her own agenda for improving things. During the interview, the therapist stresses that the rest of the family, including siblings, will be invited in so that the therapist can understand better what the patient has to deal with. The interview also establishes the notion of reciprocity of parent-child patterns. The therapist makes inquiries about how the adolescent's behavior can turn the parents' unwanted behavior on or off and suggests that part of the therapy may aim to give the patient greater power over these unwanted patterns. The adolescent is encouraged to sharpen his or her powers of observation in the forthcoming family interview. During the one-to-one interview, the therapist also defines the adolescent as someone who knows a great deal about the family, as someone who is indeed an expert on the family, having studied it for a lifetime, and as someone who can therefore coach the therapist on how things work in the family. The object here is to move the adolescent to an observing position. The implicit suggestion is that one does not simply suffer from, or participate in, patterns in the family, but can also stand outside them, gain distance from them, and ultimately have a measure of control over them. These goals are sufficiently attractive to most adolescents that they will suspend their fear of an interview with their parents.

Some adolescents will not agree even when they are reassured. In these instances the individual therapist should neither press the issue nor drop it completely. One might agree temporarily not to initiate interviews with the parents pending a greater degree of comfort about them, while insisting on some discussion of the source of the discomfort in the meantime. This discussion will open up many issues related to loyalty and fear of betrayal. Not unreasonably, the adolescent may believe that he who pays the piper calls the tune. The fact that the parents initiated the therapy and are paying for it implies that the parents have some goals to be achieved, and the patient thus questions the loyalty of the therapist. As good a response as any to such questions is to suggest that the youngster decide for him- or herself about the therapist's genuine neutrality by observing how the therapist actually deals with the family.

Young Adults

As adolescents grow into young adulthood and families move into the postparental phase of the family life cycle, the balance of autonomy and individuation is tilted further in the direction of separation from the family. With the young adult patient, while it may be useful to see the patient with the family, it may be unnecessary or impossible. Young adults are often separated from their families by considerable distance and are struggling with problems involved with completing the separation process. One conspicuous syndrome in this age group does, however, mandate a family approach. This occurs in the fused family where the young adult still retains a full position in the household as a child-in-residence. On occasion, economic circumstances may dictate such an arrangement. Frequently, though, the pattern is maintained by characteristics of the family system and is therefore very difficult to deal with without the family's involvement in therapy. Some families bind in and immobilize their members so strongly that the goal of one member to be free from the web of relationships cannot be attained until those relationships have been changed.

The individual psychotherapist, unless he or she sees the patient in the context of the family, will be limited to the view that the separation difficulties stem entirely from the psychological makeup of the young adult patient. Yet the author's experience is that the family system often depends for its equilibrium on the continuing presence of an unseparated adult child. This pattern is frequently associated with a failure of differentiation and separation in the prior generation. Parents themselves are still struggling with similar unresolved problems with their own parents. Indeed, sometimes the grandparents as well as the parents may need to be involved in treatment. While the individual therapist might not choose to make these interventions at the family systems level him- or herself, the therapist should have this kind of understanding so that the patient can be appropriately treated.

Further along in the developmental life cycle are those young adults whose parents are fully engaged in the postparental phase of the family life cycle and who are themselves attempting to set up a new family. For the parents, major shifts in work life are occurring. Women in traditional families are much less fully employed since domestic and child-care functions are receding. A similar shift in work definition is threatening the husband. The postparental house calls for a change in the relationship of the marital partners and creates a greater need for them to be resources to one another. Relationships may need to be renegotiated extensively. In these couples, a symptomatic picture in one partner, such as a depression in the wife or sexual impotence in the husband, is best understood in terms of the shift in the marital relationship. At such times the individual psychotherapist is well advised to consider working with the marital pair.

At the same time the young adult is making a concurrent shift into the early phases of new family formation. Difficulties associated with this developmental era are quite commonly couched in relationship terms. Generalized and poorly localized feelings of depression, unrelatedness, and inability to sustain commitments in intimate relationships are frequently seen, and these may be associated with the place of the young person in his or her family of origin. Direct contact with the family-of-origin system can help the individual therapist to comprehend better and to modify the patient's relationship pattern.

These days the problems in this age group are more often presented as family systems problems than as the problems of an identified patient. In cases of marital conflict, sexual incompatibility, or generational conflict, the patient is not an individual, but the relationship itself. The initial call to the therapist will tell of the breakdown in an essential relationship. "Our fights are escalating to the point where physical violence is a danger." "He has a problem with premature ejaculation, but I know there is some way I am contributing to it." "We are free adult children and competent in our own work but always screaming at each other when we are visiting our parents."

Strong clinical impressions and some hard data indicate that individual psychotherapy is inadvisable in some of these instances. In cases of marital conflict, psychotherapy for the individual marital partners can overemphasize the self-actualizing and individual growth needs of each partner and underemphasize the complementarity in the relationship and its positive contributions to each partner. A family systems level of intervention seems mandated when the initial complaint is couched in the terms of marital conflict.

Older Adults

The disorders of later years often require the involvement of family, particularly if physical or mental impairment begins to intrude on the coping capabilities of the individual. At this point, *family* means spouse and children. Here again, there may be an individual patient who is at the center of people's concerns, but family systems issues are so frequently connected to the problem, both positively and negatively, that the therapist must take them into consideration. Very often the parents' declining years present the opportunity to heal past wounds and mend earlier warps in the family fabric. The obvious practical arrangements required to provide adequate care for the older parents stir up dormant separation and abandonment issues for the adult children. To be abandoned by the death of a parent has a finality that cannot be renegotiated. Forgiveness and acceptance of the parents' limitations sets the stage for final partings that are appropriately painful but do not carry dysfunctional patterns to succeeding generations. Sibling struggles keyed to asymmetries in the family are much easier to reconcile while the parents are alive.

THE FAMILY WITH A PHYSICALLY ILL MEMBER

This section considers how family systems concepts and techniques can contribute to managing an individual patient with a severe physical disease. First, a brief theoretical discussion will show how family systems therapists conceive of the relationship between physical illness in a family member and events at the family level. The ideal theoretical model would allow for the consideration of at least three concepts.

(1) *Severe physical illness in a family member has profound effects on other family members and on the family as an operating unit.* Similar disease entities produce quite different responses from family to family. Significant psychosocial responses may be separated from the precipitating event by months or even years. For example, a myocardial infarction in a father may be temporally distant from a significantly related pattern, the delinquency of an adolescent boy. An unmourned death in one generation may likewise be distant from persistent malfunctioning in another. To be able to predict this variation and develop a typology of families and disease pictures that would predict these variations would be highly desirable.

(2) *Patterns of physical illness may be established, maintained, or intensified by family interaction patterns.* In some instances all of these effects occur. Such configurations have traditionally been known as psychosomatic illnesses.

(3) *The family is an essential component of the health care delivery system.* The family may be the only health care provider, it may be the provider of last resort (for the aged, chronically ill, or dying), or it may be an active partner with other elements of the health care delivery system (physicians, hospitals, or HMOs). Family characteristics may make the family a highly productive and effective partner in health care provision. But family characteristics may also be severely maladaptive. The problem of underutilization of services may arise when a family does not permit any of its functions to be taken over by outsiders. Overutilization may also occur, such as when a family member is delegated to seek outside assistance for family problems which have been redefined as physical in nature. Finally, noncompliance may develop when the treatment method proposed has disruptive consequences to the family relationship pattern or when healing itself is threatening or disruptive. When working with a physically ill patient, the clinician should ask two questions. How has this family system been disequilibrated by the illness event and by treatment? How do the illness event and treatment function to maintain the equilibrium of the family system? Equilibrium here means whatever pattern of stable adaptive relationships has existed. With this concept in mind and the foregoing considerations, some of the patterns of interaction between physical illness and the family system can be addressed in a rational, clinical approach.

Intuitively, physical disorder and disease seem most likely to be disequilibrating. There is, of course, no reason in nature for this necessarily to be so. Indeed, the counterintuitive notion is of perhaps even greater value—that a physical illness or the care it requires may help to maintain the equilibrium of a system. The idea that the illness and the treatment are equilibrating helps explain the often surprising ability of families to rally around a sick family member, to show unexpected strengths, and to endure objectively difficult burdens.

An example from the author's own family is illustrative. My father, in the last years of his life, became seriously disabled with multiple physical problems, including Alzheimer's disease, a broken hip, and mitral stenosis (he had survived two attacks of subacute bacterial endocarditis). As he was leaving the hospital with partial recovery from the broken hip, it seemed as if the only rational arrangement for him would be a nursing home. My sister and I had the good sense and good luck to agree that our mother should make the decision as to whether he came home or not. It was not a difficult decision for her. She decided that he should come home. In practical terms, the problems for our mother were enormous: to care in her own home for a senile, frequently incontinent, rarely but unpredictably rambunctious, old man. Financial resources were modest but adequate. Frail though our mother was, she was called on to do a good deal of the heavy lifting, but the decision was ego-syntonic for her and family-syntonic for our system, which included a small but meaningfully supportive kin network. My father survived for several years with benefits of consequence to himself, my mother, my sister, and me—and to a variety of third-party payers who would have been called on to support any institutional programs for him.

REMOTE CONSEQUENCES OF CRITICAL EVENTS

Family therapists are accustomed to seeing psychiatric symptomatology develop in families at some distance in space or time from the critical event associated with the symptoms. The language here is somewhat clumsy, since the author intends to avoid such a phrase as "caused by a critical event." One must be wary of committing the fallacy of *post hoc ergo propter hoc.* The simple fact that one thing happens after another does not mean that the two events are causally related. Nonetheless, the psychiatrist working with the individual patient should be alert to possible connections and be prepared to investigate those that look plausible. The key possibility is that the critical event has forced the family to reorganize itself in some new and dysfunctional pattern.

> When a tornado badly damaged a southern town, a movie theater was hardest hit. It was a Saturday afternoon, and many children were attending the matinee. A number were caught in the wreckage, and some lost their lives. The heroine of the disaster was a mother who had taken her own children and some neighbor children to the theater as a birthday treat. She had the quick wit to have them duck under the seats as the wall began caving in, and all were saved. Had they fled up the aisles, some would certainly have been killed.

This mother's position in the family system was that she was a leader, particularly of her husband who was characteristically in the position of taking advice from her. Because of shock, minor injuries, and the need for a recuperative period, the woman took to her bed following her rescue from the debris. Her husband then went into a depressive collapse, meanwhile urging his wife to be strong and complimenting her on her courage and quick wit. She was unwilling or unable to resume her strong position so soon. She needed, as she put it, "time to be sick." The two of them engaged in a symmetrical escalation for the position of the weakest and most needy family member.

The husband presented to the psychiatrist with a depressed, confusional state. He quickly responded to having his symptomatology relabeled as his efforts to help his wife heal herself and move back into her strong position. Alternative methods for achieving this desired outcome were suggested, and the family was soon back on track. It is interesting that the very pattern that saved the woman and the children, her strength, quick wit, and self-confidence, were associated with the difficulties that ensued after her rescue. Her need for a temporary respite could not be tolerated in this family system.

SUMMARY

A short chapter such as this could not explore the many implications of family systems for the management of the individual patient. We are living in times of rapid social change, and the practicing psychiatrist must deal with a varied and often bewildering array of human contexts. Ethnicity and economic and social class factors all interact with family systems in ways that are highly important. From the standpoint of the wide variety of individual patients, moreover, the very concept of family is manifold. It includes such varied arrangements and life-styles as the traditional nuclear family, the extended family network, the homosexual marriage, the single-parent family, and families at various stages of the divorcing process, to mention but a few of the most prominent subtypes. But regardless of the particular type of family arrangement, the problem that will come to the psychiatrist is at least somewhat related to the context both as to its etiology and maintenance, on the one hand, and as to its potential amelioration, on the other. A shift of attention onto these contextual issues is well within the technical grasp of the practicing psychiatrist. The family systems interview and the genogram provide tools with which it is easy to become familiar. Family support can often be rapidly gained by a non-blaming and hospitable attitude and many of the adverse reactions of families avoided from the very beginning. Finally, it should be noted that the perspectives and procedures discussed here are both safe and interesting. They add to and complement all other modes of working with patients, and they have an additional benefit of noteworthy import: they make the psychiatrist's work even more interesting.

Chapter 15 # The Treatment of Troubled Couples
by Ellen Berman, M.D.

INTRODUCTION*

The nature of psychiatric clinical practice today dictates that the clinician be able to evaluate and treat at least occasional couples. An increasing body of research indicates clearly that problems in couples are best treated by conjoint therapy sessions (see the chapter by Grunebaum and Glick in this Part, and also see Epstein, 1981). Over 50 percent of the individuals who come to psychiatrists present with some marital complaints (Sager et al., 1968), and with the publication in the lay press of such books as *The Family Crucible* (Napier and Whitaker, 1978), more and more patients are requesting couples therapy. The women's movement has also had a major impact, leading many women to insist that their husbands share equal responsibility for the well-being of the marriage.

*Editor's note: Dr. Berman does not discuss sex therapy or the sexual problems of couples in this chapter. Part I of *Psychiatry 1982* (*Psychiatry Update: Volume I*) deals with the psychiatric aspects of sexuality (pages 5–73).

Most psychiatrists have had only minimal training in couples work during residency training. Usually they learn through trial and error, extrapolating from individual therapy and common sense. Although this approach may produce some successes, it is often ineffective with more disturbed couples, and it can make the therapist feel frustratingly uncertain. Unfortunately for those seeking guidance from the literature, much of the theoretical work pertaining to families is published in the family-therapy literature, which has little crossover with the general psychiatric literature. In general, individually oriented psychiatrists who seek to incorporate marriage and family approaches confront two challenges—the theoretical switch to a transactional frame, which is often particularly difficult for experienced individual therapists (Wachtel, 1979), and an almost bewildering variety of new techniques. This chapter reviews the prevailing theoretical perspectives, the salient clinical issues, and some of the classes of intervention that pertain to couples therapy.

INDIVIDUAL AND MARITAL LIFE STAGES

Marriages and individuals have different needs at different stages. Certain periods in both individual and marital life are particularly likely to result in marital stress. A knowledge of the normative nature of these upheavals will decrease the anxiety of patients and the therapist and enable them to find appropriate coping techniques. Berman and Lief (1975), for instance, discuss correlations between individual life stages and marital issues. As an example, divorced individuals who begin new marriages later in their own life cycles are subject to a complex set of stresses beyond the stress of the new marriage.

In marital therapy clinics, the high points for seeking therapy are during the first two years of marriage and for couples in the 27- to 32- year age range who most commonly have been married about seven years (Berman et al., 1977). A developmental model suggests that as much of a couple's distress may stem from getting "stuck" at a particular stage as from any long-standing personality disorders.

Stages in the family life cycles of married couples are generally demarcated by the advent and ages of children: couple alone, couple with young children, couple with school-age children, and so forth (Carter and McGoldrick, 1980). No one has charted a specific set of life stages for childless couples. Major family transitions, notably the first one to two years of marriage, the birth of the first child, and the period of the child's adolescence, are times of particular stress for couples. Transitions in the grandparent generation, such as retirement or death, may also dramatically affect the couple.

Changes in the individual that result from life-cycle events may also produce marital stress. Vaillant's research, for example, indicates that intrapsychic defenses change and mature with age, producing a person who may be quite different at different points in time (Vaillant, 1977). Levinson describes transition periods at the end of each decade which produce stress and anxiety (Levinson et al., 1978). Certainly one's internal sense of time, one's idea of what is vital to one's existence and what is not, and one's perception of self are apt to change quite drastically over the course of adult life (Neugarten and Datan, 1974). Since marriage requires, among other things, some shared goals, needs, and wishes, individual developmental changes can produce considerable marital disruption if unaccompanied by similar changes in the spouse.

CONCEPTUAL MODELS FOR MARITAL THERAPY

Within the framework of a systems model, a wide variety of conceptual levels are possible.* Many different models have been created, some more focused on content issues of the different expectations and needs of couples, some based on a micro- or macroanalysis of structure and pattern. Using the concept of historical, interactional, and existential approaches, we find a variety of theories under each general category (see the chapter by Grunebaum and Glick). Although the major family therapy theories include dyadic functioning, certain models are especially well suited to the voluntary, single-generation marital dyad, as opposed to the larger kin-group structure of the family.

Historical Models

Historical models tend to focus on past events and conflicts which produce interacting sensitivities and demands in the present. The assumption is that people will struggle to reproduce some portion of their past in the marriage, not only their conflicts, but ego-syntonic patterns as well.

SAGER'S CONTRACT MODEL An excellent conceptual model for couples is Sager's contract model (1976). Sager's concerns are the needs, wishes, and expectations which the person brings to the marriage, which Sager calls the contract. Contract here refers to the set of assumptions and expectations of self and partner with which each person approaches the relationship, not to a legal, jointly agreed-on pact. Each person conceptualizes his or her individual contract in reciprocal terms (if I give x, I will receive y) and behaves as if the partner had explicitly agreed to this exchange. However, much of this contract is not shared with the partner, and in the case of certain intrapsychic needs, is not even conscious to the person making the contract. The possibilities for confusion are therefore considerable.

Sager describes a group of expectations drawn from past learnings, both familial and cultural, within which spouses choose their own behavior, and even more important, perceive and evaluate the other's behavior. There are usually several levels of expectations: (1) expectations of the marriage as an institution (*example:* marriage will provide financial security); (2) expectations of intrapsychic and biologic needs being met (*examples:* I need sex. I need to be in charge); and (3) external foci of problems (*examples:* life-style, number of friends).

These contracts come from various aspects of childhood development, cultural norms, needs and wishes of the family of origin, and internal, dynamically based needs. They may be verbalized (shared with the partner), secret (known only to the person imagining the contract), or "beyond awareness" (reflecting preconscious or unconscious needs) (Sager, 1976). The contracts a person makes depend on age, situation, previous experience, and partner. A person may form different contracts with different persons. From these individual contracts, couples join to form a system which has its own dyadic rules, the interactional contract.

Marital conflict, in this context, results from contracts that are incongruent or that cannot be fulfilled. Contracts may be incongruent between the partners, or an individual may be having an internal conflict

*Preceptor's note: Systems models are discussed in greater detail by Bloch in his chapter, and research on systems by Reiss in his chapter.

between the conscious contract and the one beyond awareness. The contract may be one which the particular partner cannot fulfill (expecting a schizoid person to be warm and expressive), or the person may change his or her needs over time (adult development).

This is a transactional model in that it depends on the interlocking needs and abilities of both persons. The complexity of marital dynamics and marital conflict is heavily related to that level of the contract which involves the person's intrapsychic needs and which is beyond awareness. A person's contract reflects only one portion of that person's own set of needs and is partly dependent on that person's perception of the other person and their dyadic interaction.

OBJECT-RELATIONS THEORY Sager's concept of the contract formed beyond awareness draws heavily from object-relations theory, originally described by Fairbairn (1967) and Klein (1959) and applied to marital relationships by Dicks (1967) and others (Framo, 1970). Object-relations theory describes the process by which the child handles conflicts with the parents by introjecting the relationship and dealing with it on an intrapsychic level. The child introjects both parts of the parent-child conflict, for example, both the helpless child and the critical parent. The child may also introject both halves of a parental conflict, for example, critical mother and passive father.* In projective identification, the person, as an adult, projects onto the partner an introjected part of the self which is repressed or repudiated.

Projective identification requires that the person retain some identification with the projected part. Otherwise he or she cannot continue the attempt to resolve the conflict. It also requires that the partner, because of his or her own needs, collude consciously or unconsciously in accepting the projection. For example, many men accept the role of the logical, unemotional spouse because it fits in with their intrapsychic needs and cultural expectations. Zinner has stated succinctly how this works in the marital sphere. "The projection of disavowed elements onto the spouse has the effect of charging a marital relationship with conflict that has been transposed from the intrapsychic sphere to the interpersonal" (Zinner, 1976, 296). In this light, object-relations theory becomes a transactional frame of reference.

The polarized relationships resulting from such projections have many problems. It becomes difficult to share feelings, to "own" one's own ambivalent feelings, or to produce collaborative behavior. In the extreme, people in such relationships demonstrate rigidly complementary behavior which appears sharply pathological to the observer. Such projective identification and collusion serve several needs: (1) defense (one does not have to struggle with one's own ambivalent wishes); (2) a mechanism for continued attempts at conflict resolution; and (3) restoration. These mechanisms may, for example, bring back to life the individual's original object in the form of the spouse. A passive woman with an angry, assertive mother may wish to reject identification with her mother, but may also need her, and so bring her back in the person of her husband.

*Preceptor's note: Rather than introjecting each of the two parents, the child may in fact learn (introject) a way of relating, for instance, what a marital relationship is supposed to be like. This may explain why, in different relationships, the style of relating remains the same but the individual behaves differently, critical in one relationship and passive in the other.

In general, such collusive relationships are tightly bonded, even if highly unpleasant, given that each one needs the other to carry the disavowed elements of the personality. The conscious perception of the partner as oppositional, ungiving, or "impossible" is painful in spite of the unconscious collusion. The struggle is between the conscious contract (we will be loving and open) and the unconscious contract (you will be weak and helpless so I can be strong and powerful, because I hate weakness).

INVISIBLE LOYALTIES The contract often has particular provisions that are related to invisible loyalties to a larger system. Here both historical and current interactional issues are involved. Boszormenyi-Nagy and Spark (1973) focus on concepts of loyalty, justice, and balance of merits. They see loyalty as the key linkage between generations and as involving integrity and certain things that are owed (Boszormenyi-Nagy and Spark, 1973). Caretaking, for example, might be owed in return for loyalty. While young, children are owed more than they owe back, and over time family members balance their accounts. Children eventually owe their parents, and ultimately their own children. Such concepts as loyalty and balance are multiperson considerations; that is, one must look at family members in relation to each other. They are also ethical and moral considerations, beyond pathology and beyond personality theory. Boszormenyi-Nagy and Spark see much of the central and intense nature of family relationships as residing in this "ontic dependency," that is, the existential dependency on the "other" of one's inner family circle. Loyalty ties are real, but there are no objective measures for evening out accounts. Each family member has his or her own sense of the balance of payments. In this model, families keep account ledgers of balance and imbalance, indebtedness and reciprocity. But the concept does not imply a constant moment-to-moment egalitarianism. Functional families have flexible ledgers, so that one may eventually pay back what one owes at an alternate time. Only pathological families have rigid and fixed imbalances, and these produce severe dysfunction.

Spouses may try to right family imbalances through the marital partner. For example, a businessman and his wife, raising children during the depression, work seven days a week, leaving little time for the children. Their daughter feels abandoned but loyal to her parents because "they couldn't help it." She attempts to balance her accounts by expecting someone else to pay her back, in this case, by marrying a man who "would make up for my lost childhood." This is a conscious, although secret, part of her contract. Severe marital stress follows his inability to live up to her contract.

One of the tasks of adulthood is rebalancing one's obligations to one's family and learning to balance old loyalties with new ones. One of the most common ways of balancing loyalty to one's parents is to become a parent, thereby giving to one's child what one has received. However, this is not a totally satisfactory solution. The grandparent generation may still demand, either in reality or in the person's fantasy, overwhelming loyalty.

Transformational Models

Transformational models examine the ways in which partners' present behaviors produce patterns and problems in functioning. At the extreme, these theories ignore internal, psychodynamically based data entirely. Two of these constructs, notably structural and strategic therapy, are described elsewhere in this Part (Malone discusses structural approaches, and McFarlane and his colleagues discuss strategic therapy, albeit briefly).

BEHAVIORAL ANALYSIS Behavioral analysis is a way of examining patterned behavior at the micro level, based on operant theory and social learning models of transactions. The basic assumption is that the most important determinants of behavior can be found in the external environment, although cognitions or attributions about the behavior are also relevant. By analyzing events which vary together with behavior, it is possible to make specific and accurate predictions about the recurrence of subsequent behavior.

At the level of individual transactions, behavioral analysis examines the presence and effects of reinforcers and punishers. A behavior which is reinforced or punished by the other will theoretically increase or decrease in the future. For example, if a greeting (behavior) is met with a smile from the other (reinforcement), greeting behavior will probably increase. Cognitive variables, particularly attribution of intent, are important, too, in that perception of a behavior is often central. For example, if a person perceives a smile but thinks, "He's only trying to manipulate me," that may be perceived as a punisher and communication may go down. Since a spouse's behavior in intimate relationships is viewed as a function of the consequences provided by the partner, one looks at chains of pleasing and displeasing behavior.

Spouses tend to reward and punish each other at approximately equal rates. Over time the collective outcome determines the tendency to further behaviors, that is, the partner's behavior develops freedom from control by the immediate consequences. For example, if a partner has received many positive and pleasing behaviors over the period of a week, a displeasing behavior (irritation expressed by the spouse) may increase the partner's lovingness and helpfulness, since the person perceives that he or she has been rewarded enough and that the other may now need taking care of. One may consider this model alone, but it may also be connected with a more historical point of view: what is seen as pleasing behavior may be determined by what one saw growing up.

A cognitive behavioral model yields a treatment method designed at the concrete level to help the couple increase pleasing behavior and decrease displeasing behavior. This treatment style assumes that couples would rather change their present dysfunctional pattern than continue with it for such reasons as invisible loyalties or projective identification. Skill training and communication training are emphasized (Jacobson and Margolin, 1979).

TECHNIQUES OF COUPLES THERAPY

General Issues

MARITAL PRESENTING STYLES Problem marriages tend to present in chronically conflicted, polarized states, demonstrating stereotypic, repetitive patterns. Usually each person is capable of much more flexibility outside the interaction. The broadest classification of dyadic patterns (Haley, 1963) divides couples into two groups: (1) symmetrical relationships in which people exchange the same type of behavior (advice, help, or criticism), and (2) complementary relationships, in which partners exchange different behaviors (one gives and one receives, one teaches and one learns, and so forth). In functional marriages, couples use both modes, depending on the circumstances. Dysfunctional symmetrical marriages become competitive and develop control struggles. A common example is the "sandbox marriage" in which both partners are struggling for control or demanding that they be the one who gets the most nurturance. Dysfunctional complementary marriages polarize in patterns where one partner becomes overadequate and overfunctioning and the other underadequate. Common variants include: (1) the husband appears overbearing, distant, overorganized, or paternal, and the wife seems childlike or "hysterical"; (2) the wife appears strong, angry, and in control, and the husband seems passive, overweight, or alcoholic; and (3) one member is ill, alcoholic, schizophrenic, or hypochondriacal, and the other is defined as a savior or a rescuer. Some dysfunctional complementary couples polarize primarily around the area of intimacy. One demands affection and closeness, while the other requests and demands more distance and progressively withdraws.

Once these patterns have been established, they tend to escalate due to each partner's attempt to solve the problem with more of the same behavior. For example, the overadequate partner, assuming that the other one will not do the job, takes over more and more responsibilities, while the underadequate partner becomes more and more helpless because all the responsibilities have been taken away. Whether one attributes such polarization to systemic issues totally, or sees them as also serving collusive intrapsychic functions, the goal of therapy is to allow each partner to stop putting out more of the same. This is usually done by working to reveal the hidden complementarity or underlying reversal of function. For example, the overadequate partner usually feels helpless, frightened, and undernurtured, while the passive partner has hidden strengths, and often a tremendous amount of hidden rage.

Depending on the therapist's conviction as to the source of such polarized behavior, the therapist may use insight-oriented therapy, specific behavioral tasks, or paradoxical interventions. The difficulty for therapists working with these couples is that they often see complementary couples as having one sick and one healthy partner, with the overadequate partner appearing at first to be without problems. It is the underadequate partner who will most often present first as an individual patient.

VALUES AND ETHICS A couples therapist faces a set of value questions which differs from the questions an individual therapist confronts. Existential real-life issues without easy answers are common. Should a person with small children leave an affectionless but functional marriage for a better relationship? Is this neurotic problem a systems issue or a life choice? How should the therapist begin to approach this couple? Facing these questions obviously brings up the issue of pathology versus real-life conflict, and it also calls forth the therapist's own values about divorce, the sanctity of marriage, and the needs of children.

A second set of value conflicts includes basic issues of who the patient is and of openness versus confidentiality. Can the therapist insist that both partners come in although one does not wish to? Where does the system need revelation of secrets, and where is the person's right to privacy? What if supporting the underadequate person causes stress to the overadequate person? For an excellent discussion of ethics, see Hansen (1982).

EVALUATION Because the science of normal family process is in its infancy (Walsh, 1982), evaluation varies according to the style of conceptualization the therapist is using. Almost all therapists evaluate the couple's ability to communicate clearly, the congruence of their goals, and their level of commitment to the relationship. Most therapists wish to have some sense of the origin of the problem, the extent of the couple's embeddedness in the family of origin, and the patterning of the system. Evaluation techniques range from the elaborate and careful paper-and-pencil assessment strategies developed by the behavioral therapists to the therapeutic probes and systems mapping of the transformational models.

Classes of Intervention

With a wide variety of techniques available corresponding to the variety of theories, the psychiatrist does best to start with techniques that fit his or her general frame and style of working. For example, a cognitive behavior-oriented psychiatrist will find a wide variety of techniques to apply to couples. A psychoanalytically oriented psychiatrist would be more comfortable with techniques which involve shared insights, mutual dream analysis, and so forth. A child psychiatrist may prefer to start with structural and strategic techniques. In general, psychiatrists working with couples should be familiar with the teaching of basic communication skills and problem-solving techniques, should have some method for directly helping couples to change their behavior patterns, and should adopt some comfortable method for dealing with family-of-origin issues, whether it be the family journey of Bowen (1978) or the family session of Framo (1981).

Over the last ten years, collaborative and concurrent modes of therapy for couples have given way to a conjoint model with occasional individual sessions and, to a lesser extent, couples groups. The same techniques which are useful with family groups are appropriate with couples. Couples sessions do tend to be more cognitively oriented than the family sessions, which include more action techniques and play.

Couples therapy differs from two-generation family work more in terms of issues than techniques.[1] Five issues specific to couples are particularly noteworthy. (1) Couples present a number of concerns about commitment and choice. (2) Symptomatology is less obvious, and dissatisfaction is vaguer ("we're not communicating"). Dissatisfaction must be clarified for treatment goals to be planned. (3) The prolonged marital time frame, in which couples attempt to stay together for many years in a situation of stable or increasing intimacy, creates potential problems such as boredom, changes in each partner due to adult development, and the possibility of storing up years of grudges. (4) Power relationships are less clear than in parent-child relationships. Couples may try a variety of styles from egalitarian to traditional, and culture

---

[1]Sex therapy is one technique that is especially designed for use with couples. It most commonly includes educational, exploratory, and behavioral components. The therapist must be certain to review the expanding body of information on sexual functioning before beginning treatment (Kaplan, 1979; LoPiccolo and LoPiccolo, 1978; Zilbergeld, 1978).

and role definition will influence these styles. (5) Since spouses play multiple roles with one another—lover, friend, business partner, coparent—possibilities for conflict or incompetence increase. Just as most therapists who start out working with a child soon discover that much of the work must be done with the family, most therapists working with couples find that the couples therapy at some point becomes family therapy. Either the children or the family of origin need to be brought into discussions or directly into treatment.

Although the major schools of family therapy tend to deride eclecticism as unfair and unscientific, most practitioners on the front lines eventually do develop a somewhat eclectic model based on a variety of techniques. Six classes of intervention will be briefly reviewed.

(1) *Clarifying history and feelings and reframing behaviors—perhaps the most commonly used technique in couples therapy.* Therapists may do this work themselves or, better yet, help the spouses clarify things for each other. "You're saying if she picks up your socks that's how you know she loves you. Are there any other ways that she can show you that she loves you?" "He is not getting quiet like this because he's angry at you. He is quiet because he learned in his family that's the way men behave when they're angry." Such clarification, based on the context and on historical issues, is designed to change the attributions that the other person makes about the spouse's behavior, and also to help the person admitting the behavior to understand its causes. Theoretical constructs such as those of Framo (1970; 1981) and Boszormenyi-Nagy (Boszormenyi-Nagy and Spark, 1973) are particularly useful in helping the couple to understand how they have gotten from there to here.

(2) *Teaching communications and problem-solving skills—a behavioral approach.* This is used when the couple has skill deficits or refuses to use communication skills that they have because they are angry at the partner. For a clear description of communication training, see Gottman et al. (1976) and Jacobson and Margolin (1979). Sager's description of helping couples restructure their contract has elements of both clarification and problem solving.

(3) *Giving tasks—a behavioral approach.* Behavioral tasks, given in conjunction with teaching communication and problem-solving skills, are designed specifically to decrease aversive control and to increase reciprocal reinforcement. These tasks are usually planned with the couple, and the couple decides which behaviors need to be targeted for change (Jacobson and Margolin, 1979).

(4) *Giving tasks—a systemic or strategic approach.* Tasks designed by the strategic therapist aim to restructure the system, to change the hierarchy, or in some way to upset the homeostatic balance. Tasks of this type are often paradoxical and are planned by the therapist alone (Madanes, 1981; Weeks and L'Abate, 1982).

(5) *Bringing in other members of the family system.* Couples therapists commonly find that when working with a couple alone is ineffective, bringing in either the children or the family of origin may allow the leverage needed for change. In these cases the focus may be primarily on reviewing and revising old alliances or identifications in the family, along the models of Bowen (1978) and Framo (1981), or on changing the structural alliances within the larger system.

(6) *The therapist as coach, role model, and celebrant—experiential approach.* The therapist may take many roles within ongoing couples therapy. Whether the therapist chooses to model behaviors actively or

to remain relatively distant from all members, he or she still functions as a role model for effective communication and at times functions as a supportive or challenging "uncle" or celebrant of the family's changes in state.

CASE EXAMPLE   Mrs. A., a married woman in her thirties with two children ages nine and seven, requested individual therapy for depression. Her complaints and anger seemed to be primarily related to her husband, whom she described as hostile and ungiving. Her mood was worse in the later afternoon and evening. She showed no vegetative signs of depression and functioned well at work. She noted that the depression had gotten markedly worse over the last year-and-a-half, but she was not sure why. Given that most of her complaints seemed to be related to her husband, evaluation of both together was indicated.

The woman who appeared sad and depressed alone in the office turned out to be an angry, bitter, accusing person with her husband present. Her husband responded with sullen silence and an occasional angry outburst. Both agreed that they argued all the time, that their sex was very poor, and that she was worse when he was home. He agreed that he had been working late recently and hadn't been home much, but said he couldn't stand coming home to listen to her complaints. She responded angrily that she was left with all the housework, as well as a job, and he never made her feel good. In addition, he had been spending more time in the last year with his mother, who had been widowed a year-and-a-half ago and who lived near them. The couple demonstrated a polarized complementary pattern; the husband was passive, and the wife was angry and overtly overcontrolling. Their communication style consisted predominantly of blaming, accusing, changing the subject, and attributing the other's behavior to malicious intent.

His personal history included a rather distant family style, which he disliked, with a cold but overcontrolling mother and a rather passive father. Her family in contrast was much warmer, but her mother also "ran the show." The couple stated that they would like to stay together and that so far the children did not seem to have been greatly disturbed by the increase in problems between them. Neither spouse was having an affair, which would make their commitment to therapy more tenuous.

The evaluation suggested that couples therapy was strongly indicated. The wife's symptomatology was directly related to the marital interaction, and had worsened since the husband's father died and his mother began putting more pressure on a poorly stabilized system. Both appeared at least moderately interested in changing the situation.

Most therapists faced with this couple would begin with the simplest moves first, that is, clarification and reframing behavior and some simple communication training. For example, one might accurately reframe her anger and depression as despair at being unable to get close to him. One might appropriately reframe his sullenness and withdrawal as helplessness in taking care of her, or as his attempt to be strong and not give in (both of which seem accurate). One might examine the homes they came from and their original contract. He wanted a warmer, more emotional climate than the one he grew up in, and she wanted a man who would not give in to her the way her father did. Of course, both were somewhat afraid of what they consciously wished for, and neither had the skills to engage successfully in the new behaviors. The therapist might point out the interlocking behaviors—how her attempts to get close to her husband and to be emotional become bitter and are read as overcontrol, producing more distancing, and how his attempts to avoid control by distancing produce more anger.

Although this reframing might help greatly, most therapists would also begin fairly quickly to teach the couple some direct communication skills. For example, the couple might be asked to have a conversation about some problem during the session. The therapist would help them stay on target and own their own feelings rather than accusing the other person and would encourage the woman to express her complaints more softly and the man to express his feelings more assertively. Since this couple did not know how nasty they often sounded, the therapist might use videotape playback, explanation, or modeling. To increase the couple's ability and skill with pleasing behaviors, a series of tasks might be devised by the therapist and the couple focused on what each would like from the other. The couple might negotiate an evening out together or replan their evenings so that the husband would come home earlier and the wife would arrange her time so they would have some quiet time together. Tasks such as this need to be clear, small, and agreed to by both members of the dyad. One common mistake in planning tasks is vagueness. "I'll be nicer to her this week" is not a clear behavioral task. Another mistake is choosing a task which is likely to lead to anger or failure. For example, the husband is likely to agree to come home a half hour earlier one or two days a week, but less likely, at least at first, to give up seeing his mother or to come home at 5:30 every night of the week.

Another approach to the couple might come from evaluating and working through the children, and there is no harm in having the children come in for an evaluation. Contrary to what the couple may wish, the children always know when there is something seriously wrong, and they are probably greatly relieved to find out that somebody is doing something about it. During this evaluation, even if the children have not been symptomatic, one commonly finds that one parent has become aligned with the children and that the other is peripheral. In the couple described above, the father has been abdicating his responsibility more and more, and the children had been ignoring him increasingly. Involving the father in pleasurable tasks with the children, such as going for ice cream, may not only remove some of the burden from the mother, but also allow him a way of moving back into the family. In addition, encouraging the couple to work together either around discipline issues or around having fun produces a structural shift in which the generational boundaries are clearer and a sense of effective partnership develops. Most of the work with many couples is done around parenting issues.

If these interventions do not change the couple's interaction, other possibilities come into play. A strategic approach would take the point of view that certain behaviors in both members of the couple are continuing the symptom, that the symptom serves a function in the relationship, and that problems might occur if the symptom remitted. Using such an approach, one might note that increased intimacy between husband and wife might remove the husband from his mother's orbit, which might make him anxious and guilty. In this case, a paradoxical task might be designed in which the system would be positively connoted and prescribed. A strategic approach is designed to deal with a target symptom, rather than all aspects of the relationship, and is principally designed for entrenched and resistant couples. Although not all strategic tasks are paradoxical, paradoxical tasks are often helpful for mobilizing the couple's wish to change. A minor paradoxical task which is often given in the course of relatively straightforward therapy is to predict or prescribe a relapse for the couple who has been doing very well. Encouraging slow change or a relapse allows the couple to go as fast as they wish and is a comfortable way of dealing with the resistance to rapid change.

Another intervention might entail bringing in the husband's mother. She was clearly having problems of her own and transmitting them to her son and through him to her daughter-in-law. A session with the son and mother together might deal more specifically with family loyalties and help the mother establish more independent functioning. In addition, since the husband's passivity and avoidance with women were presumably modeled on his relationship with his mother and father, learning to deal clearly with his mother and to set limits on the relationship could increase both his available energy and his freedom to deal more appropriately with his wife.

During the entire process of couples therapy, the therapist is acting as a model for identification. A generally supportive approach, treating both people as functional and potentially kind and giving, is one of the central factors in the therapist's success.

Some Common Problems in Couples Therapy

(1) *Differing agendas.* If agendas are incongruent, therapy cannot proceed. For example, if one spouse wants more closeness and the other is not interested, therapy will fail no matter how apparently worthy the goal. The therapist must help the couple find some common ground.

(2) *One or both members lack commitment to the marriage.* Deciding whether or not to remain in the marriage is almost invariably an issue with disturbed couples. When this is a central concern, the therapist must begin by clarifying the nature of the problem. A partner may be requesting specific relationship changes. Or he or she may be saying, "It doesn't matter what my spouse does or doesn't do. I want to be alone to explore the world." The therapist must then decide whether conjoint work is possible or whether an ambivalent partner needs time individually to think through the issues.

When it appears that the problems are based primarily on interaction problems, three possibilities emerge. First, the therapist can ask the couple to behave as if they were going to remain in the marriage for a given period (several weeks or months) and put their energy into working on changing the patterns. Second, the therapist could leave the question open and have the couple discuss the pros and cons of leaving or staying. Third, the therapist could help them consider the possibility of a trial separation. Although it is seldom wise for the therapist to recommend a separation, if the partners themselves make the decision to separate on a trial basis, the therapist can help with the planning. Here the therapist helps the couple structure how much time they will spend together, how they will work on the marriage, whether or not they will date, and how they will handle children, money, and so forth.

Although it may appear during the evaluation that one or both people may eventually need individual therapy, to send both members of the couple to individual therapists is unwise unless the initial couples therapist is the one who sees them individually. If the couple enters individual therapy with different therapists, it may well provide each with an ally and a "transitional object" and thereby facilitate divorce.

Such an approach could, however, occasionally be used as a tool to facilitate separation for a couple which has been unable to separate over a period of two to three years. During this ambivalent period some therapists see both members of the couple individually. If and when one person clearly decides to end the relationship, the therapist then must deal with issues of divorce.

(3) *Secrets*. The therapist who sees spouses individually during evaluation or during any point in treatment will eventually be privy to secrets. Most often these are sexual (affairs, homosexuality), but they may also be previous painful or embarrassing events such as jail terms or abortions. Although dealing with such secrets is difficult, most therapists prefer knowing them to the alternative of using only dyadic sessions and thereby losing crucial pieces of information. Therapists who use individual sessions therefore must make an overt contract with the couple beforehand as to the confidentiality of material discussed in individual sessions. Karpel (1980) has an excellent discussion of dealing with secrets. He distinguishes between secrets and private information, and he suggests that the distinction hinges on the relevance of the information to the unaware person. For example, an ongoing affair is a secret, whereas a traumatic but well-resolved event from childhood could well be considered private information.

Dealing with secrets is never easy. The therapist has several options—to reveal the secret him- or herself, to insist that the patient reveal the material, to encourage its revelation with the proviso that therapy will be terminated if the secret is not revealed, or to allow the material to remain secret, at least for a period of time. If the therapist determines that revealing the secret is necessary in order for him or her to remain trustworthy to both partners and for the therapy to be concluded successfully, it is best to work slowly toward disclosure with the holder of the secret. Although disclosure may not have to be immediate, when secrets such as ongoing affairs are undisclosed, long-term therapy is exceptionally difficult to conclude well. Many therapists feel that an affair which has ended is best kept secret.

SEPARATION AND DIVORCE

As separation and divorce become more common, specific knowledge of the stages of divorce and the options for treatment have increased. (See Kaslow [1981] for a general review.) Most researchers see the divorce process as having some similarities to the grief and mourning following a death. The common task is to renounce emotional ties and the sense of identity which partly depends on the partner. The feelings of confusion, anger, sadness, and obsessive concern with the absent partner, and the slow period of working through, are seen with both divorce and death of a partner. Divorce is, of course, complicated by the fact that the lost person is still available and contact is inevitable.

Bohannan's (1973) "six stations of divorce" is a helpful guide to the issues that the couple must confront. (1) Emotional divorce entails the loss of faith and involvement that precedes separation. (2) Legal divorce begins when the person moves out of the house and initiates the legal proceedings that lead to final termination of the relationship. This period can be greatly confused by the opposing goals of the therapist, the couple, and the attorney. (3) Economic divorce involves separating one's economic entanglements and dealing with reduced incomes for both spouses. (4) Coparental divorce relates to the parenting role. If there are children, the couple must negotiate the delicate transition to remaining parents while no longer being spouses. (5) The community divorce presents exceptionally difficult issues. Friendship networks are greatly reorganized by the divorce process, and the couple tends to lose most or all of their couple friends. Friends tend either to take sides with one or the other partner or to avoid both. A new life structure must be built. Kin may respond with anything from support to horror. The complicated relationships between divorcing spouses and their former in-laws, who are still the grandparents of their children, can confuse things even further. (6) Psychic divorce entails reestablishing autonomy and reorienting one's identity toward being a single person. Even for a relatively stable and well-functioning person, this process takes one to two years following the actual separation.

Therapeutic support for divorcing partners has become a subspecialty of marriage and family therapy in the last few years, and several different forms of therapy have been developed.

(1) *Individual therapy for the divorcing person.* This approach is usually supportive and reality oriented. Medication should be used very sparingly.

(2) *Counseling for the family around issues of parenting and separation or counseling for each parent separately with the children around establishing separate households.* Recently several specialized centers in family clinics have developed this approach.

(3) *Divorce groups.* Groups are best conducted as time-limited, same-sex groups with a task or educational focus rather than with an open-ended, process focus. Persons at various stages in the separating process can give each other enormous amounts of support.

(4) *Divorce mediation.* This is usually geared to helping the couple to resolve practical issues related to settlement, such as property division and custody. Divorce mediators generally do not use uncovering techniques, but encourage trust building, problem solving, and capping of feelings. An agreement that comes out of a divorce mediation process is then taken to both parties' lawyers for examination. This provides an excellent alternative to a legal adversary model, and many therapists and lawyers are becoming involved in divorce mediation.

Chapter 16 # Family Therapy and Childhood Disorder
by Charles A. Malone, M.D.

INTRODUCTION

Over the past quarter of a century, family therapy as a modality and the family systems conceptual model have had a far-reaching and growing impact on the field of child psychiatry. As a treatment modality, family therapy has added to the range, depth, and effectiveness of our capacity to diagnose and treat "childhood psychopathology" and to manage a variety of clinical tasks. Family therapy has also provided a data collection and research framework which enriches and modifies our understanding of developmental issues and the nature of symptoms and psychopathology. The family systems conceptual model has thus led to revisions and modifications in a number of clinical and conceptual issues in child psychiatry. Among these are the fundamental issues of who is the patient, what is the target of intervention, and what are the pathways of therapeutic change and repair.

The powerful impact of family therapy and the family systems conceptual model on child psychiatry has not been an unmixed blessing. Not only does family therapy present a number of problems and some disadvantages in clinical work (Malone, 1974), but the accompanying revisions of concepts and practice have generated controversy and conflict. This chapter both considers certain dimensions of this controversy and explores the usefulness of the family interactional model in child psychiatric clinical practice. Before discussing specific issues related to diagnosis, treatment, and clinical management, the chapter reviews some concepts central to the author's application of the family therapy model.

CENTRAL CONCEPTS OF THE FAMILY THERAPY MODEL

The first concept central to the treatment of children is the inseparability of internal and external: a child or an adolescent cannot be assessed accurately or treated successfully apart from or in isolation from the family life context. When the impact of family life is unknown, neither the child's developmental successes and failures nor his or her adjustments and maladjustments will be understood in their true light (A. Freud, 1972). As a consequence, intrapsychic dynamics and interpersonal transactions and the interventions related to them must be seen as interrelated and interdependent.

A second central concept involves the etiology of childhood disorders. Disenchantment increasingly surrounds those retrospective studies which have attempted without much success to trace a postulated underlying cause-and-effect connection between early trauma and later deviant outcome (Sameroff and Chandler, 1975). A range of later developmental difficulties does appear retrospectively to be related to pregnancy and perinatal complications. But the majority of infants who experience such complications have not been found to have later difficulties, and prediction of which infants will be adversely affected is difficult. Both socioeconomic and familial factors appear to have the potential of minimizing or maximizing the effects of perinatal complications, such as anoxia and low birth weight, or the effects of traumatic or depriving early childhood experience (Emde, 1981; Sameroff and Chandler, 1975).

Similarly, the investigation of environmental factors has failed to predict adequately the effects of disordered parent-child relationships and conditions such as child abuse, neglect, and failure to thrive. Very likely this is because these studies have been overly concerned with poor parenting and have as a consequence been almost exclusively focused on differentially characterizing the psychosocial environments of normal and deviant children. Recent research emphasizes the importance of the two-directional character of child-caretaker effects in predicting developmental outcome and suggests the value of a transactional model (Sameroff and Chandler, 1975; Sameroff, 1979; Malone et al., 1980). In this view, the constants of development are not some set of parental or child traits, but rather the processes by which these traits are maintained or altered in the transactions between parents and children over time. Here the child is seen as being in a state of continual active reorganization in which the child is shaped by and shapes parental care, which in turn shapes and is shaped by the child's qualities, behavior, and development. Once dysfunctional relationship patterns become a stabilized part of family structure, however, the patterns themselves exert a powerful influence on the child's development, depending, of course, on the level of the child's psychobiological vulnerability.

A third and final central concept in the author's family therapy approach is an organismic model of development. The resiliency and self-righting tendencies of the child are seen as such powerful forces toward normal development that protracted developmental disorders are typically found only in the presence of equally protracted and distorting familial or socioeconomic influences which in turn interfere with the child's reorganizing capacities. Thus, developmental continuities are usually the result of environmental continuities (Emde, 1981). This position argues that the present is as important as the past and that the experiences of the healthy infant and young child with its parents may not have long-lasting cumulative effects (Kagan, 1979). In this view, the plasticity of the child "allows for a great deal of leeway in early child rearing, and, in the end, provides a further opportunity for later development to supercede previous experiences" (Lewis, 1981, 194). This concept stresses the fact that important aspects of development may be discontinuous. For example, as the child moves from a sensorimotor mode of functioning to a conceptual mode, early deficits tend to disappear in the child's restructured cognitive functioning (Sameroff and Chandler, 1975; Kagan, 1979).

Transactions within the family play a critical role in determining what early experience endures and what opportunities for change prevail. Major changes in the environment can offer major compensation for early environmental deficits (Emde, 1981). Therefore, by countering dysfunctional patterns and introducing or discovering functional ones, family therapy removes distorting familial influences and allows the child's resiliency, reorganizing capacities, and self-righting tendencies to operate.

FAMILY THERAPY IN CLINICAL PRACTICE

The usefulness of family therapy in child psychiatric clinical practice can be illustrated and categorized in three areas: (1) the advantages which it provides in diagnosis; (2) the advantages which it offers in treatment; and (3) the ways in which it contributes to the management of clinical tasks.

Diagnostic Advantages

Within the diagnostic process are three perspectives from which one can view and understand families (Grunebaum and Chasin, 1980; Malone, 1980): (1) a historical-developmental perspective (Brown, 1980; Zilbach, 1974);* (2) an interactional-social learning perspective (which is emphasized in this chapter); and (3) an existential perspective.

*Preceptor's note: For a discussion of the historical-developmental perspective and intergenerational loyalty and projective identifications, see the chapter by Berman.

As the author has discussed elsewhere in relation to diagnosis (Malone, 1979), family interviews which elicit interaction and reveal family structure and functioning enable us to assess how a child's symptoms or dysfunctions are influenced by and influence the family system. The interview provides an opportunity to observe both the family reactions and contributions to the problem and also the balance of capacity and motivation for or against family change (Skynner, 1976). This allows us to identify and ensure the involvement of all of the psychologically relevant family members who are contributing to the problem and to avoid an interminable treatment working with only part of the relevant family. While family interviews help us to assess a child's general functioning in the family context, they are particularly useful in determining the dysfunctional family patterns and especially the non-verbal patterns. The interviews can reveal how these patterns contribute to a child's impulsivity and poor behavior control, modes of expressing and monitoring affect, overstimulation or understimulation in relation to drives, response to parental demands and prohibitions, defensive and coping processes, identifications, and the quality of his or her intra-familial relationships. Determining the contribution of nonverbal communication is especially helpful because family members are generally not aware of the presence or influence of nonverbal factors. Knowledge of the presence and influence of nonverbal communication factors is often not available in the symbolic representational memory of family members. They may therefore not report such factors in the process of history taking. Here the lack of report does not stem from resistance, mistrust, or guardedness, but from unawareness.

Finally, family interviewing enables us to identify *structural imbalance*, patterns of projective identification, and underlying marital, parental, and family-of-origin problems. The value of family interviews in identifying and treating structural imbalance in families deserves particular emphasis and can be illustrated by considering three commonly found patterns of structural imbalance: role reversal, alliance and splitting, and scapegoating.

ROLE REVERSAL: THE PARENTAL CHILD　　In all families there are times when parents need the help of older children to carry out the tasks of daily living. Commonly this involves leaving the younger children temporarily in the care of the oldest child who is, for that short period of time, given the parents' authority. Such arrangements are most common and necessary in single-parent families, in families which are large, and in families where both parents work. Depending on the age of the oldest child, the amount of responsibility involved, whether the delegation of authority is clear and explicit, and the frequency and duration of the allocation of parental authority, this can work out well. The parent or parents receive needed assistance or respite, the younger children are cared for, and the oldest child has an opportunity to demonstrate responsibility and competence in caring for his or her siblings.

The arrangement can become problematic for the parent-child structure if it exceeds the oldest child's ability and becomes a chronic family pattern in which child and parent(s) reverse roles and if the oldest child is given too much responsibility and control. In such situations the parental child may feel burdened by demands that exceed his or her ability to cope. The parental role often interferes with childhood needs and the youngster may feel threatened by his or her adultlike role in relation to the parent(s). Because of immaturity the parental child may use authority harshly or in the service of rivalrous wishes. Frequently the structural imbalance is complicated by the fact that the parental child stands between the parent(s) and the other children, interfering with their need for direct access to their parent(s).

This type of pattern is readily identified in family interviews. The therapeutic tasks then are to counter the structural imbalance and realign the family by: (1) reducing the parental child's authority and responsibility to a manageable age-appropriate level where he or she can still help the parent(s); (2) moving the parental child out of the go-between role and returning him or her to the sibling subsystem and to age-appropriate peer group activities; and (3) supporting the increased authority and responsibility of the parent(s) and the parental child's direct access to and interaction with the other children.

ALLIANCE AND SPLITTING: THE INEFFECTIVE PARENTAL COALITION Various dysfunctional patterns occur in families when the parental coalition is weak, ineffective, or nonfunctional. The development and maintenance of an effective parental coalition is the most powerful structure in stabilizing family life, especially during periods of stress. The parental coalition becomes particularly important during times of marital discord. When the parental coalition is ineffective, we often see one parent, usually the mother, becoming dominant in parenting activities and forming a coalition with one or all of the children. In such a pattern, the other parent, usually the father, has a marginal role, appears split off from the family, may be regarded as ineffectual, and is often difficult to engage. The children may overtly or covertly ally themselves with their powerful mother and then experience loyalty conflicts vis-à-vis their apparently powerless father, or they may rebel and struggle against the mother's dominance. A clinical example illustrates this problem.

The B. family was concerned about the delinquent behavior and the school difficulties of their two young adolescent sons. The mother was an attractive, verbal, assertive person. She brought the boys in, seated them next to her, and began to tell the therapist about the problems which had brought them to the clinic. The father, on the other hand, sat quietly on the far side of the room, literally with his hat in his hand. The pattern of the mother's centrality and dominance and the father's isolation became immediately clear. The sons sat close to the mother listening to her detailed portrayal of their misbehavior and ignoring their father.

After observing this pattern for a while, the therapist attempted to shift the pattern by ignoring the pathway of the mother as an informant. He turned to one of the boys and asked a question. The boy hesitated for a moment, and the mother answered for him. Without paying attention to the mother's answer, the therapist asked the boy how old he was. After a short exchange about what it was like to be 14, the therapist again addressed a question to the boy, and again his mother answered. Once more the therapist did not respond to the mother's answer, but instead began talking to the boy and his brother about his surprise that at 14 the boy did not answer for himself. The therapist pointed out that the boy's hesitation and looking at his mother seemed to be cues for her to take over. He sympathized with the mother's overworked and overburdened position in having to answer for boys who would not speak for themselves. Needless to say, the boys could speak for themselves, and very competently at that. As the boys became involved in talking actively about their current life situation, the father, who had appeared so peripheral, watched the exchange with increased interest. After a while he moved his chair in closer and soon thereafter began to join the group. The therapist not only listened to him, but exhibited his interest in and his agreement with the valuable points that the father was making.*

The initial treatment approach with this family focused on increasing the father's involvement with the boys and his role in parenting. As it turned out, an important focus of the work with this family also involved the marital relationship and the task of increasing Mr. B.'s role in providing satisfaction for his wife. Because she did not have such satisfaction, Mrs. B. had been displacing her needs onto her parenting role and had become overinvested in it. In effect, she was seeking gratification from her sons, while they were attempting to protect themselves through rebellious and delinquent behavior.

CONFLICT DETOURING: THE FAMILY SCAPEGOAT   In well-adjusted families, stress in a marital, parent-child, or sibling subsystem is usually negotiated within that subsystem rather than being expressed through another subsystem in the family. In dysfunctional and disturbed families, however, conflict is often detoured from one subsystem to another. This is most commonly seen when parents use a child as scapegoat to deflect or diffuse their marital conflict. In this situation, the couple develops an equilibrium by minimizing both their contact with each other and their expressions of affect, particularly their strongly felt hostility, in order to be able to live together and maintain the marriage (Vogel and Bell, 1960). In this type of family children learn that they must maintain a scapegoat role to ensure family integrity (Gherke and Kirschenbaum, 1967). In view of the finding among non-patient populations of a high incidence of controlled but pervasive conflict among married couples (Cuber and Harroff, 1965) and a large number of marriages which are stable but devitalized and unsatisfactory (Lewis, 1980), many families seem to ensure family integrity and functioning by avoiding the expression of marital discord. And this may be done by conflict detouring and by scapegoating a child. Conflict detouring can take two forms: the parents may define the child as sick or defective and unite to protect him or her, or they may define the child as the cause of the family problems and then attack their scapegoat. This case illustrates the latter form.

Mr. and Mrs. D. were concerned about the underachievement, unruliness, and oppositional misbehavior of their 11-year-old son Carl. In the initial family session Mr. D. encouraged Carl to recount a discussion they had had the night before, and Carl proceeded to criticize his mother as being unfair and favoring his brother. Mrs. D. ignored Carl's criticism and launched into an angry description of his misbehavior during the past week. Soon Mr. D. took up his wife's complaints, and they both condemned Carl's irresponsibility (a trait which both parents had and found offensive in themselves and each other). Later in the interview the therapist drew attention to some disagreement and annoyance that Mr. D. developed toward his wife. Carl immediately started an argument with

*Preceptor's note: Much of the effectiveness of family therapy may result from the fact that efforts are made to engage the father as a parent to participate actively in the treatment. Gathering the family together is often a problem. It may be important for the therapist to call reluctant members personally to insist that both parents be present at intake. Approaching the father-husband through the mother-wife is often likely to be ineffective. He should be dealt with as a parent in his own right.

his younger brother, deflecting attention away from the conflict between the parents. Despite the conflict-detouring pattern, it was possible to determine that Mr. D. was generally unhappy with his wife's inconsistency with Carl and with her aloofness from him. He had found, however, that if he cooperated with his wife in criticizing Carl, he could keep the burden of problems away from himself. Thus he joined with his wife, projected his own difficulties and problems onto Carl, and dealt with them as Carl's problems rather than as his own.

Scapegoating involves the phenomenon of *triangulation*, in which a dyad within the family preserves its stability and viability by focusing its threatening hostility on a third person (Bowen, 1978a; Ackerman, 1961). Unfortunately, this pattern is a common means of maintaining homeostasis in all social groups; its most malignant form is racial or religious prejudice. In addition to scapegoating a child, the detouring of marital conflict and triangulation can take two other forms: loyalty conflicts and the formation of a parent-child coalition against the other parent. In the first form, each spouse attempts to get the child to side with him or her against the other parent. The child is caught in a no-win situation. Either the child allies with one parent and suffers from guilt, or the child is paralyzed because any movement toward either parent is an attack on the other parent. In the second form, one parent, usually the more permissive mother, has succeeded in forming a coalition with a child who then becomes the particular focus of the other parent's anger and restrictiveness. This form of marital conflict detouring has been found in girls to be associated with a lack of control and in boys to be associated with destructiveness, oppositional noncompliant behavior, and aggression (Hetherington et al., 1981).

Therapeutic Advantages

The usefulness of family treatment is very broad, providing the therapist employs a flexible approach that allows for combining family therapy with individual or marital treatment (Ackerman, 1958; Malone, 1974). It has both general and specific advantages (Malone, 1979). Family therapy increases the clinician's ability to recognize and counter the secondary gain which the child's symptoms provide for parents, siblings, and the child him- or herself. It offers more direct therapeutic access to acting-out and symptomatic behavior. It keeps responsibility for problem solving within the family so that, when progress occurs, everyone can change accordingly and a new equilibrium can be reached (Skynner, 1976). Finally, family therapy increases therapeutic potential by offering a means of identifying and enlisting healthy members or aspects of the family.

Family therapy also has specific therapeutic advantages, particularly in the same areas in which family interviews have diagnostic advantages (Malone, 1979). Hence, family therapy is especially useful in treating developmental delays and behavior disorders; in dealing with separation-individuation problems or unmourned losses; in modifying structural imbalances; in countering scapegoating; in dispelling myths, divisive secret keeping, and other chronic intrafamilial communication problems; in working with families dominated by projective identification; and in working with families in which marital, parental, or family-of-origin problems underlie the child's presenting problem (see Table 1). A discussion of two commonly referred clinical problems, separation-individuation problems and intergenerational family-of-origin problems, illustrate the specific advantages of family therapy.

Table 1. Indications for Family Therapy

Developmental Delays and Behavior Problems in a Child
(1) Excessive aggressiveness, behavior problems, or poorly socialized behavior
(2) Overactivity and impulsive behavior
(3) Excessive separation anxiety
(4) Excessive sibling rivalry
(5) Delayed urinary and bowel control
(6) Failure to develop effective speech

Certain Family Presenting Problems
(1) Separation-individuation problems (except age-appropriate individuation)
(2) Structural relationship and role imbalances (ineffective parental coalition, parent-child role reversal, confused generational boundaries)
(3) Scapegoating (use of a child's symptom or dysfunction for detouring marital or parental conflict)
(4) Chronic communication difficulties
(5) Unmourned losses or family crises
(6) Chronic problem families
(7) Families with several symptomatic or dysfunctional children
(8) Families dominated by projective identification
(9) Families in which family-of-origin, parental, or marital conflict underlies the child's presenting problems

Acting Out in Children and Adolescents
(Ego-syntonic character disorders of "delinquents" who act out parental impulses)

Family Adjustment or Adaptation Issues Related to Chronic or Life-Threatening Illness
(Particularly when the child has moderate to severe secondary emotional disturbance or developmental interference)

Certain Psychosomatic Illnesses
(Such as anorexia nervosa, asthma, and diabetes; not severe cases unless collaborating closely with pediatric care)

SEPARATION-INDIVIDUATION PROBLEMS Separation-individuation problems are among the most frequently identified reasons for recommending family treatment. It is therefore not surprising that many family therapists conceptualize their approach to family therapy in separation-individuation terms. With individual variations, these therapists speak of assisting family members to break pathological symbiotic and dependency ties and to separate and differentiate themselves from family enmeshment so that they can achieve effective independent functioning (Ackerman and Behrens, 1959; Bowen, 1978b; Paul and Grosser, 1965). In more seriously disturbed families, complementary interlocking patterns of projective identification are involved (Wynne, 1965; Zinner and Shapiro, 1972). These patterns interfere with differentiated independent functioning of family members, and they create varying degrees of individual and interpersonal problems, pathological family enmeshment, and concomitant problems related to separation anxiety. In less seriously disturbed families, separation-individuation problems are less pervasive and occur at particular family and individual developmental junctures such as adolescence. The case which follows illustrates these points.

Mr. and Mrs. J. consulted the therapist about their oldest child, 14-year-old Helen, because of her increasing angry outbursts, hostile, disrespectful attitude, and provocative, defiant behavior. Although they had no evidence, they were concerned about drug use and sexual activity because of the "wildness" of some of Helen's friends. When seen with her parents, this attractive, full-bodied girl was indeed explosively angry, provocative, and antagonistic with her parents, especially her mother. On the other hand, the parents, particularly Mrs. J., were extremely overcontrolling and overinvolved with Helen and frequently got into angry arguments with her. Excessively anxious about and focused on Helen's actual or potential misbehavior, Mr. and Mrs. J. "crowded" her by attempting to know about, monitor, and be responsible for even the smallest details of her life. For her part, Helen contributed to the enmeshment by inviting parental involvement through her provocative and defiant behavior.

Family therapy initially focused on helping Helen to negotiate with her parents around activities with friends and responsibilities at home and on helping the parents to pull back from their overinvolvement. As Helen's provocativeness and defiance decreased, the parents began to allow her to take more responsibility and to become more independent. As Helen got more involved in social activities, however, the parents returned to their former restrictive overcontrol, and the family battles reappeared. In exploring this resistance, Mrs. J. realized that much of her anxiety came from concern that Helen would repeat the still-regretted sexual wildness of her own early adolescence. Mr. J. realized that he was vulnerable to Helen's "challenges" of his authority because he was not her biological father. Interestingly, when Mr. and Mrs. J. successfully changed their approach to Helen's "demands" for independence, Helen's underlying feelings of inadequacy and fears about growing up, particularly in regard to sexuality, became more evident. At times Helen attempted to reexternalize her conflicts about growing up through provocative attempts to induce her parents into angry arguments and restrictiveness. Her parents' ability to avoid induction helped her to focus on and deal with her own concerns about becoming independent.

INTERGENERATIONAL FAMILY-OF-ORIGIN PROBLEMS

Ever present in the conceptualizations of many leading family therapists, regardless of their theoretical orientation, are themes involving the family of origin (Brown, 1969; Kramer, 1968; Boszormenyi-Nagy, 1965). From their families of origin, parents can carry over into their own nuclear family life unresolved conflicts and losses, organizing views of self and others, identifications, and roles. These ghosts from the past can affect or dominate marital choice (Dicks, 1967), the character of a marriage, parental functioning, and parent-child and family interactions. This is illustrated in the following example.

Mr. and Mrs. A. consulted the therapist about the increasing number of serious family "upsets" over the last few years centering around their daughter Mary, age ten. Mary was stubborn and balky and avoided or refused to do what was expected of her. She was easily upset or frustrated and given to angry outbursts and tantrums. Most distressing of all for the parents was the "lying" and deception Mary engaged in to avoid responsibility or the consequences of misbehavior. When seen with her family, Mary appeared subdued and unhappy. She made "grouchy" faces which brought giggles from her older brother and sister and angry glares from her mother. Her speech and behavior were quite immature compared with that of her siblings. Despite her siblings' efforts to protect her by talking about general family problems and their own misbehavior, Mary managed to demonstrate her position as the troublemaker and the odd person out in the family. Contrasted with their delight with the older children, the parents' anger and impatience with Mary were abundantly evident. Exploration of family patterns revealed that a significant portion of the family upsets with Mary occurred in the evening around homework versus TV and in the mornings around getting ready for school. Mary was in danger of flunking the fourth grade because of her failure to do or turn in homework, which infuriated her parents and especially her mother.

Family therapy focused on countering Mary's devalued position in the family and the dysfunctional interactions between her and her parents, particularly her mother. Exploration of the parents' resistance to these restructuring efforts revealed critical underlying issues. Repeatedly identifying how devalued and inadequate Mary felt as the family "unfavorite" stimulated Mrs. A. to remember, in bits and pieces, how devalued she herself had felt as a child and especially her feeling that she was not smart enough. Her underachieving daughter Mary represented and reminded her of this painful, unacceptable part of herself (projective identification). Identifying the parents' repeated exaggerated anger around Mary's "misbehavior" led to their realizing how threatened they were by Mary's "defeating" them in their parenting. Mr. and Mrs. A. had invested a great deal in being good parents (in sharp contrast with their own parents). They had, in fact, been extremely successful in raising all their children *except* Mary. As the parents were able to put these issues into perspective, they were able to change their approach to Mary. After some back-and-forth movement, Mary became able to deal more openly with her feelings of inadequacy. She began to do her school work, even though that in turn revealed her actual learning deficits and further exposed her to feeling inferior compared with her siblings.

DISCUSSION   The two clinical examples of Helen J. and Mary A. illustrate how family therapy leads to modifications and revisions of well-established psychiatric concepts. Internalization and externalization, for instance, have always been viewed as individual psychological mechanisms or defenses. Internalized unresolved conflict and painful handicapping feelings about the self have always been regarded as indicators of a kind of personal suffering that requires individual psychotherapy. Externalization, on the other hand, has usually been regarded as a defense mechanism for which individual psychotherapy is more difficult, because the person experiences conflict and pain as being outside and therefore as not being the responsibility of the self. When we consider Helen J. and Mary A., however, we have to modify these concepts considerably.

Initially, Helen presented as a young teenager who externalized and viewed her problems as the fault of her overcontrolling, angry, and restrictive parents. Indeed, Helen easily externalized her tensions, painful affects, and conflict with her provocative behavior, which in turn quickly brought angry, restrictive, and overcontrolling behavior from her anxious, threatened parents. Ultimately it emerged that a significant part of Helen's conflicts about growing up and becoming independent did, in fact, come from her parents' anxious distortions and projections, in other words from *their* externalizations. The fact that Helen did have her own inner anxiety and conflict about growing up (probably stimulated by or the result of internalizing her parents' and especially her mother's concerns) could only be determined when her parents later changed their dysfunctional patterns of interaction with her.

Similarly, Mary at first presented as an unhappy, maladjusted child, who had strong feelings of inadequacy and conflict over her rivalry with her siblings and over her hostile feelings toward her mother. Mary's internal conflict and painful feelings, however, were strongly influenced by her mother's projective identification and by the fact that her parents were angry and devaluing toward her. In effect, Mary was defeating her parents in their determined effort to be different from their own parents. In addition, because they felt they had failed Mary as parents, Mr. and Mrs. A. would often accept Mary's angry externalizing accusations. They felt they were to blame for the things that went wrong and for the upsets that occurred in relation to her.

These abbreviated examples of family therapy also illustrate how family treatment involves the use of multiple models (Grunebaum and Chasin, 1980; Malone, 1979; 1980). In the cases described above treatment involved a structural approach (restructuring by modifying dysfunctional patterns), an insight-understanding approach (uncovering underlying conflict and painful childhood experience), and an experiential-modeling approach (corrective relationship). In addition, these cases show the interplay between treatment approaches. In each case the initial therapeutic effort involved restructuring—disembedding Helen from family enmeshment by countering the parents' overinvolvment and countering Mary's devalued position. At the same time, the therapist served as a corrective model for identification, demonstrating how to negotiate age-appropriate responsibility by talking with an angry, provocative adolescent and modeling empathy for Mary's painful feelings and devalued "unfavorite" position in her family. In both cases the turning point occurred when explorations of resistance to restructuring led the parents to gain insight into the roles which their own childhood experiences and conflicts played in their current difficulties with their daughters. Interestingly, although both families initially accepted and responded to restructuring efforts, resistance quickly appeared, and the parents were able to change their patterns only when they understood their own underlying conflicts. An important aspect of each case was that the child herself was able to begin facing her own inner conflicts and painful feelings only when the complementary dysfunctional patterns of interaction with the parents had changed in a sustained way.

Finally, these clinical examples illustrate the central concepts that underlie family therapy and some of the pathways to therapeutic change that family therapy clears. Restructuring by modifying dysfunctional patterns and introducing or discovering new patterns offers several pathways of change for a family. It destabilizes chronic patterns and promotes reorganization, which then allows resiliency and self-righting tendencies to come into play. As alternative family patterns begin to operate, family members activate alternative patterns or learn new ways of functioning. This leads to new ways of experiencing the self and others within the family, and these new ways can become personal-interpersonal corrective experiences. These experiences, in turn, enhance self-esteem and alter the dynamics of available models of the self and others. Quite frequently, as in the examples given, restructuring efforts have an initially positive response and then meet with parental resistance. Exploration of resistance usually leads to underlying conflict and painful childhood experience. More lasting structural change then results from successful removal of the interfering influence of these underlying issues, usually through insight and understanding.

Management of Clinical Tasks

The therapeutic power of the family systems approach is not confined to family therapy. Family interventions involving several interviews or a time-limited series of family interviews can be extremely valuable in the management of specific clinical tasks. Such tasks include assisting families through painful transitions, helping families to adjust to acute nonrecurrent stresses, and providing consultation in medical settings. Transitions at times of significant family life change, such as a job change, family relocation, or an adolescent going to college, offer important opportunities for brief preventive intervention. Acute nonrecurrent family stresses, such as marital separation or divorce, the loss of home or job, or the death of a family member, are critical times in the life of a family. They usually require some type of family intervention to identify issues, needs, and resources, and if possible to prevent pathological outcomes. Many acute nonrecurrent family stresses and crises occur in relation to illness, hospitalization, or events like the birth of a handicapped child, and these can be addressed through consultation. In the author's experience, the present-oriented, problem-focused quality of family interventions tends to be more readily understood and accepted by medical colleagues than other psychiatric orientations.

In the management of many of these clinical tasks, the model of family crisis intervention has proved extremely valuable (Malone, 1979). At times of marked stress or crisis, family interviews can help identify the life-style and values of the family and its patterns of coping and problem solving as they relate to the situational stress. The crisis can be evaluated in terms of the emotional strain on each family member, the mobilization of both intrapsychic and interpersonal problems, and the intrafamilial, extended family, and social network resources available for meeting and resolving the crisis. Family interviews offer an opportunity for members to share information, to ventilate feelings, and to clarify affective and cognitive confusion or distortion about the event itself. The interview can reduce the possibility of family members acting out their guilt and anxiety with provocative behavior and with such mechanisms as projection, displacement, and scapegoating. Since these crises involve both actual and threatened losses, a crucial aspect of the clinical work involves facilitating a grieving process. Family interviews encourage this process by countering avoidance and the institution of massive defense and by assisting family members to face and master the painful personal-interpersonal feelings involved.

THE INDIVIDUAL-VERSUS-FAMILY-THERAPY DILEMMA

Ironically, at the same time that family therapy increasingly demonstrates its usefulness for addressing children's clinical needs, disagreements prevail in the field of child psychiatry regarding the use of family therapy. These disagreements are manifest in such issues as the indications-contraindications controversy and the individual-treatment-versus-family-therapy dilemma. The effects of these issues and their resolution could be far-reaching. McDermott (1981), for example, recently stated that the degree to which family therapy comes together with child psychiatry or remains apart will depend on whether the indications-contraindications controversy is resolved.

The controversy is primarily conceptual. The medical diagnostic model is a linear conceptual model which attempts to establish links between cause and effect. In this model indications-contraindications guidelines are necessary so that treatment can be pinpointed at removing specific underlying causes. On the other hand, many forms of family therapy are based on the conceptual model of family systems. In this model the child's symptoms are viewed as having a function for the family system, and pathology is viewed as being located in the family interactions that generate and support the child's disturbed behavior.* Indications versus contraindications are not addressed, because one should always direct treatment to the dysfunctional family system.

Unfortunately, the indications-contraindications controversy is often accompanied by the individual-versus-family-treatment dilemma. Disagreements around these issues are somewhat inevitable not only because of inherent conflict between the relevant conceptual models, but also because of the complexity of many child-family clinical problems. On the other hand, making an issue over the choice between individual and family therapy is often spurious and even misleading, precisely because the clinical problems are so complex. Paradoxically, even some family therapists who employ the systems model in diagnosis and treatment do not construe the clinical issues in a systems framework. They fail to conceptualize the presenting symptoms and dysfunctions of the identified patient as involving complex, often interdependent, interrelationships between systems within the family at many or all levels—individual, marital, parent-child, and family, including extended family.

In the author's experience, the complexity of many child-family problems actually requires a flexible combination of individual, subsystem, and family perspectives and interventions (Malone, 1982). Clinicians working with families are familiar with the ways in which presenting problems can mask or defend against other levels of conflict within the family system. They are familiar with the family problems which screen underlying parent and child problems, with the marital problems which are related to disorder, defect, or chronic illness in a child, and with the unresolved parental or marital conflict which can underlie the presenting dysfunctions of children and adolescents. Clinical experience also demonstrates that pathological patterns often involve different interrelated systems or subsystems.

The example of conflict detouring, which was discussed earlier, is illustrative. In conflict detouring marital discord contributes to dysfunction in the child, and the child often becomes a family scapegoat. In such families the parents, the siblings, and the identified patient often collude to maintain the integrity of the family and to guard against uncovering the marital conflict. In these families it is not unusual to see the scapegoated child actually seeking the scapegoat role, particularly at times when marital tension is high. This phenomenon is a part of the complementary pattern which the family uses to divert attention from marital conflict. Often, however, closer examination reveals that the scapegoated child provokes and uses the family scapegoating process to avoid facing or to defend against internal or external conflict. For example, the child provokes the parents or siblings into fights, and these become a means of avoiding school work, which in turn defends against painful feelings of inadequacy related to a learning disorder. As the clinical process unfolds, still closer examination may reveal that marital discord is at times specifically related to the child's failures at school or that one parent cannot face and deal with the child's learning disorder

---

*Preceptor's note: Recent research on the systems function of symptoms is discussed by Reiss in his chapter.

because it is too painful a reminder of the parent's own childhood difficulties.

In understanding and treating child-family problems, one must often disentangle symptoms occurring on the individual intrapsychic level from dysfunctional patterns and structural imbalance in the family. Sometimes this involves disembedding an individual from family enmeshment, as in the dependence-independence struggles of an adolescent (as seen in the J. family). Sometimes it involves differentiating and treating separately the individual problems of a parent and a child who are engaged in a highly dysfunctional dyadic relationship and at the same time countering the family contributions to these dyadic parent-child difficulties (as partly seen in the A. family). Sometimes the clinical task is to uncover and treat family contributions to a child's dysfunction and then to determine whether the child's difficulties clear up in a sustained way or persist in the form of continuing developmental interferences or symptoms.

In carrying out these clinical tasks, the issue is not and should not be whether individual treatment or family therapy is indicated. The issue is how to combine family, subsystem, and individual interviewing in order to explore effectively the interplay between levels within the family system and to determine whether family, subsystem, and individual treatment are indicated separately or in combination, at one time or in stages over time. Accomplishing any of these tasks in the family context may lead to sustained improvement in the child or to a clear indication for individual psychotherapy. In either case, the family context of the child's symptoms will have been clarified and treated where indicated. Moreover, the child's treatment, should that be indicated, will not be undermined by family defenses and resistance, by conflict detouring, by complementary patterns which allow the child to externalize conflicts, or by ongoing dysfunctional patterns which sustain the child's problems.

This leads to a final important consideration: the structuring and timing of treatment interventions. Since the presenting problem often obscures or serves as a detour from other levels of conflict in the family system, this consideration is particularly critical at the outset of treatment. The clinician must fully appreciate how the family's focus on the identified patient both expresses and hides underlying marital or family-of-origin conflict and the ways in which family problems both reflect and obscure individual child and parent pathology. Otherwise, treatment plans and related interventions run the risk of reinforcing pathological patterns and structures. Plans and interventions developed without this full appreciation are therefore either antitherapeutic or doomed to fail because they meet with powerful resistance in the family system or the individual patient. Children and adolescents, for instance, may not be able to respond to a treatment which inadvertently sides with one parent against the other in a bitter marital or postdivorce conflict or one that allies with one generation against another in an intense multigenerational family struggle. Similarly, a child may not respond to individual psychotherapy before patterns of conflict detouring or projective identification have been clarified or countered. Even though individual psychotherapy is indicated, it may have a distorted antitherapeutic meaning in the child's family context. If any intervention is to succeed, therefore, its structuring and timing must take into account a variety of possible complications.

Chapter 17

New Developments in the Family Treatment of the Psychotic Disorders

by William R. McFarlane, M.D., C. Christian Beels, M.D., M.S., Stephen Rosenheck, M.S.W.

FAMILY THERAPY AND SCHIZOPHRENIA: OLD AND NEW VIEWS*

Family therapy for schizophrenia has undergone a dramatic change in the last few years. Once a uniform treatment based on the assumption that the family is an important cause of the illness and therefore needs treatment, family therapy for schizophrenia now uses the varied approaches of supportive group, rehabilitative, and educational programs, and the programs are based on empirical research. That research has supported the view that the family, far from causing the illness, is a major source of structure and strength on which to base the treatment of schizophrenia. This positive partnership between treatment organization and family is the principal revolution which has taken place in the field.

The original assumption that the family was a cause of schizophrenia stemmed from the work of Lidz, Jackson, Bateson, Bowen, and Fromm-Reichmann. Contributing to the recent eclipse of this assumption, a new wave of family investigation failed to confirm the theories put forth in the earlier work. Rather, these investigations demonstrated, with their more rigorous research methods, that the families of schizophrenics were distinguished by more circumscribed problems. Singer, Wynne, and Toohey (1978) found that schizophrenics' parents showed "communication deviance," a tendency toward a fragmented or amorphous conversational style. In a laboratory setting, Reiss (1975) documented parents' difficulties in jointly solving cognitive problems. Evidence for higher degrees of marital discord seemed substantial (Mishler and Waxler, 1975). However, the researchers did not claim a causative role for these factors. Likewise, Brown, Birley, and Wing (1972) identified a factor called expressed emotion (EE), excessive criticism of and overinvolvement with the patient by a family member, which significantly predicted relapse. They concluded that it seemed to be a factor contributing to the course of a presumably biologic illness, but not a cause.** A second major challenge to the early theories was the finding that nonspecific family techniques, which implicitly blamed the family, did not even seem to alleviate symptoms, let alone produce a cure (Massie and Beels, 1972). On the other hand, multiple family therapy, in which several families met together, did seem to be moderately effective, apparently because it provided family support, improved morale, and established a shared perspective at the same time that it promoted improvements in family interaction.

Emerging from these various trends was the tentative conclusion that families are affected *by* schizophrenia in one of their members and that

*Editor's note: In Part II of *Psychiatry 1982* (*Psychiatry Update: Volume I*), recent research advances in understanding the family and social context of the schizophrenic disorders and research on family treatment are discussed in the chapters by Dr. Samuel J. Keith and Ms. Susan M. Matthews (pages 172–174) and by Dr. Robert Paul Liberman (pages 97–112).
**Preceptor's note: This research is discussed in greater detail by Reiss in his chapter.

their responses to the illness can become secondary contributors to its worsening course. This message was implicit in the EE research, and many other findings could be seen in the same way. A number of innovative family approaches to schizophrenia are now based on this idea, and judging from the available data on their efficacy, they may eventually play a vital role in the optimal treatment for the disorder.

THE NEW FAMILY THERAPIES FOR SCHIZOPHRENIA

Core Elements

Although no one of the new therapies can be fully described here, their common features can be summarized. All have as their goal the amelioration of the course of the illness, not its cure. Most aim to reduce relapse frequency beyond that achievable with good pharmacologic management, and most specifically attempt to enhance the psychosocial functioning of the patient. The medical model therapies assume that the effects of drug and family therapy will reinforce each other. Kopeikin, Marshall, and Goldstein (1983) have provided an elegant confirmation of that assumption: they demonstrated that adequate drug treatment significantly enhances patient response to family therapy, in some patients by reducing hostility, and in others by fostering concentration. At the same time, their family intervention seemed to orient the patient and the family members toward the rationale for drugs, thereby enhancing compliance.

The means to achieve these goals include a small group of seemingly essential, specific, and targeted interventions, designed either to compensate for identifiable deficits in the patient (tendencies toward hyperarousal or attentional deficits) or to reverse common iatrogenic or culture- or illness-induced phenomena in the family.

(1) *Joining with family members.* Most of these new approaches begin with efforts to join empathically with family members, validating their despair, fears, confusion, and exasperation, while mobilizing their concern and energy for the ensuing rehabilitation effort. The objective is the creation of a strong, task-oriented organization among staff, family, and patient. Issues of blame are discussed openly, and assurances are given that there is little evidence to substantiate a parental responsibility for the illness. In fact, family members are usually recruited explicitly to become vital partners in the treatment.

(2) *Family education.* Most of these therapies have education of family members at the core. Ranging from orientation to the seriousness of the acute psychotic episode to lectures on neurochemistry and the mechanism of action of neuroleptics, these educational programs have a variety of functions. They attempt to demystify symptoms, to clarify various aspects of the treatment process, and to sensitize the family to the reality of the patient's subjective experience and the validity of his or her immediate postpsychotic inability to function. They also teach the family how their behavior can have positive or negative effects on the patient's overall condition and course. In most families this kind of information raises morale, relieves guilt, enhances cooperation, and elicits true sympathy for the patient's predicament.

(3) *Interactional change.* As the family acquires a clear concept of basic schizophrenic phenomena, they become prepared to accept a few crucial interventions directed at family interactions. These have three highly specific foci: (1) recognizing prodromal signs and symptoms and

taking early action to forestall relapse; (2) reducing expressed emotion, especially criticism and overinvolvement; and (3) correcting common and symptom-reinforcing patterns of family communication. These interventions are central to the capacity of these therapies to prevent relapse, because they directly address the most common and well-documented sources of recidivism. Combined as they are with education, they have the quality of training rather than psychotherapy.

(4) *Family structural intervention.* Perhaps nothing more clearly illustrates the differences between the old and the new approaches than the way in which power is optimally distributed. While the old concept put the therapist at the service of the patient to rescue him or her from the destructive influences of the family, the new therapies strongly validate the relatives as co-therapists and caretakers, and the patient is temporarily placed in a structurally subordinate and age-inappropriate position. This strategy is a matter of principle for Haley (1980) and Madanes (1981). For the medical model therapies, it is a matter of common sense and pragmatism, a natural implication of the illness-based orientation. In practical terms it means that the family must take charge of the patient in order to implement the rest of the treatment package and to reduce organizational confusion and emotional intensity in the family environment. Ultimately, this strategy also puts the family in a position to foster the patient's gradual and controlled resumption of responsibility.

(5) *Multiple family meetings.* The value of bringing affected families into contact with one another has been suggested both by research on the role of social support in reducing morbidity (Beels, 1981) and by the apparent effectiveness of multiple family groups. As has been noted, the families of many schizophrenics have constricted social networks (Brown et al., 1972). Multiple family, relatives', and self-help groups all expand the availability, variety, and flexibility of social supports for participating families. Perhaps the primary rationale for fostering relationships between families is the time-tested value of banding together to cope with major chronic illnesses and traumatic events. This is particularly true in schizophrenia where stigmatization, real or self-perceived, commonly drives families into isolation. Beyond providing social support and empathy, families also are quite adept at pointing out to each other the obvious interactional problems and holding each other responsible for making the necessary corrections.* For all these reasons, many of the new therapies include multiple family meetings, which serve as the preferred format for altering interaction, providing education, or enhancing family socialization. In addition, the meetings seem to be effective in their own right in reducing relapse, are economical, and are enthusiastically accepted by families (McFarlane, 1983). They seem inevitably to foster the staff, family, and patient partnership that is so central to all the new therapies.

The discussion now turns to the new therapies themselves, reviewing how each incorporates these five elements and how each is carried out.

*Preceptor's note: The groups facilitate a process of grieving, for these families, like the parents of retarded children, suffer from chronic unacknowledged grief. The groups foster exploration of the parental denial, hypercontrol, intrusiveness, and inability to maintain distance which threaten their marriages, friendships, and employment. (See McLean CS, Grunebaum, H: Parents' response to chronically psychotic children, unpublished paper presented at the American Psychiatric Association Annual Meeting, May 1982.)

They are separated into medical model and communication therapies, on the basis of their originators' views of schizophrenia.

Medical Model Therapies

FAMILY CRISIS THERAPY Goldstein and his colleagues at UCLA were the first to report a new family treatment and outcome data to support its effectiveness (Goldstein and Kopeikin, 1981). Their approach is crisis oriented and begins in the immediate posthospital period, usually for patients having their first episode (69 percent of 104 patients) or their second episode. Its goal is to reduce short-term relapse. Therapy is carefully sequenced and limited to six weekly sessions. Four treatment objectives are introduced, and each is completed before undertaking the next. A preliminary phase helps the family to accept that a major and very serious event, an acute psychosis, has occurred for one of their members and that it can recur unless everyone makes an effort to avoid a repetition. Then the four objectives are addressed. (1) The therapist leads the family in an exploration of the stressful events or charged interactions that immediately preceded the acute episode. (2) Specific, detailed plans are worked out as to how the family might reduce or eliminate these stressors. (3) Those tactics that can be implemented immediately are evaluated and modified in light of the family's experience with them. (4) All family members, especially the patient, are then asked to devise plans for implementing these new coping tactics should unsettling events recur. As may be apparent, this approach applies well to most forms of psychosis and is not limited to schizophrenia. Outcome data from this and other treatments are summarized in Table 1.

PSYCHOEDUCATIONAL FAMILY THERAPY Anderson, Hogarty, and Reiss (1980) are in the middle of an evaluation of their ambitious and carefully designed psychoeducational treatment program for chronic schizophrenia. They hypothesized that high EE in families precipitates relapse by overloading the patient's limited capacities to

Table 1. Outcome of Family or Individual Treatment with All Patients on Drugs

| | Months of Exposure | | | Relapse Rate | |
Study[1]	To Therapy[2]	To Risk[2]	N	Family Therapy	Individual Therapy
Goldstein and Kopeikin (1981)[3]	1.5	6	49	0/25 (0%)	4/24 (17%)
Anderson et al. (1980)	12	12	57	2/28 (7%)	10/29 (34%)
Leff et al. (1983)	9	9	24	1/12 (8%)	6/12 (50%)
Falloon and Liberman (1983)	9	9	36	1/18 (6%)	8/18 (44%)

[1]Families in Goldstein and Kopeikin's study were presumably mixed high and low EE. The others involved *only* high-EE, high-risk families.

[2]Risk and therapy intervals are concurrent. Risk is usually defined by the patient's having been included in the study.

[3]Moderate-dose patients only

handle stimulation, which in turn leads to hyperarousal and impairment of attentional processes. They created a family therapy to reduce EE, because they assumed that much of the family's overinvolvement derives from misconceptions about what is actually helpful to the patient and that their hypercriticism arises inevitably from frustration in the face of their failure. Thus, Anderson et al. see high EE partly as a response to the disorder, as well as a negative influence upon it.

Their psychoeducational family therapy is a four-stage procedure. In Phase I, shortly after the patient's admission, the therapist establishes an empathic, ombudsman-like connection with the family. Family responses to the latest relapse are elicited and validated, after which the therapist mobilizes their concern and secures their commitment to collaborate in preventing a recurrence. Phase II, the most innovative aspect, is a daylong "survival skills workshop." Explicit information about the technical and subjective aspects of schizophrenia are presented to a group of families with the attention-arousal model as the center-piece (see Appendix 1.) Then the workshop presents a clear set of family interactional guidelines that will reduce stimulation and foster a slow, but more predictable and complete recovery. Phase III consists of up to two years of weekly, then biweekly, single family sessions that focus on applying those guidelines in each specific family. Phase IV consists of conventional family therapy dealing with deeper and more long-standing family problems and is offered to those who request it. Bimonthly multiple family meetings are held throughout the course of treatment; they have increasingly become well-attended social events, widening the network of supports for each family.

RELATIVES' GROUPS Leff, Berkowitz, and Kuipers (1983) have developed and tested an economical, relatively simple, and theoretically sound treatment that, like that of Anderson et al., is focused on reducing EE. Leff and his colleagues intervene in two ways: (1) they educate family members about schizophrenia in their own homes, with the goal of reducing criticism engendered by excessive expectations and by misunderstanding about negative symptoms; and (2) they form groups of relatives only, in which high-EE relatives are encouraged to adopt the low-EE relatives' coping methods and styles. The biweekly groups concentrate on information, management, and emotional responses to and social distance from the patient. After nine months, EE ratings had fallen to normal levels in most of the high-EE group. Those patients whose relatives did improve had no relapses at all, compared with the 50 percent relapse rate in the control (high-EE) group. A two-year follow-up study is now underway.

BEHAVIORAL FAMILY THERAPY AND SOCIAL SKILLS TRAINING Falloon and Liberman (1983) have devised a wide-ranging, complex, long-term, and highly specific treatment program. Like the strategies of the Anderson and Leff groups, their approach aims to reduce EE and relapse rates through education, multiple family interaction, medication, and family training in preferred behavioral patterns. It goes even further by using behavior therapy techniques to alter family communication dysfunction and to change specific patient behaviors through "social skills training." They assume that the patient behaviors, if they are sufficiently bizarre or maladaptive, can predispose the family to resurgent dysfunction.

Their rigorous family behavioral assessment looks for high EE, communication problems, and symptom-reinforcing investment in the illness. Next they provide educational workshops and nine months of weekly problem-solving sessions in the family's home. Afterwards, these sessions either continue at monthly intervals or are replaced with multiple family groups at the clinic, for a total of two years. Meanwhile, as a separate intervention, the patient receives social skills training.

Given the strong association of schizophrenia and communication deviance (Singer et al., 1978; Doane et al., 1981), Falloon and Liberman's techniques for correcting dysfunction in this area could become as significant as their own and others' work on EE. Their communication guidelines for the family are simple but have many salutary effects on the patient's and the family's well-being. Guidelines include listening respectfully, emphasizing positive reactions, reducing criticism, and asking for behavioral change specifically, directly, and calmly. Because the context is one of a technical approach to the problem, rather than a blame-inducing family therapy, families seem to accept such suggestions readily. Their results are most impressive, both with respect to relapse and with respect to psychosocial functioning.

Communication Therapies

STRATEGIC FAMILY THERAPY Haley (1980) and Madanes (1981) have created a therapeutic approach that is nominally antimedical. Strategic family therapy is a general therapy for severe problems of late adolescence, regardless of diagnosis. Their approach therefore does not focus on schizophrenia per se. Its dominant developmental theme is the separation-individuation of parents and offspring. The goal is to enable successful, normative leave-taking of the young person and parents, without the intervention of such agents of social control as psychiatric hospitals.

For Haley and Madanes, the common dysfunction in all failures of separation is a hierarchical incongruity in the family. The parents are supposedly in charge of the patient, and because he or she has been defined as ill, the parents are responsible for his or her welfare; at the same time, in terms of overt power, the patient is in charge of the parents through symptomatology or intimidation or both. The strategic approach assumes first that the parents must regain the *actual* hierarchically dominant position, and then that they must use that position to expect or even demand normal role functioning of their disturbed offspring, much as would the rest of society.

The techniques that Haley and Madanes use to achieve this goal are remarkably simple and straightforward, at least on paper. The therapist emphatically joins with the parents and helps them establish a set of household rules and a timetable for the young person to resume responsibility. Consequences for failure are agreed upon. The therapy protocol assumes a near relapse shortly after this intervention as a test of the parents' newly regained authority. At this critical moment, the therapist supports the parents in their doing whatever is necessary to contain the young person's behavior, except to hospitalize him or her. Once this struggle is won, the process usually leads to a higher level of patient functioning and an eventual physical separation.

SYSTEMIC FAMILY THERAPY Selvini-Palazzoli, Boscolo, Cecchin, and Prata (1978) have devised a number of systemic approaches to cases which they describe as schizophrenic, but which do not generally appear to meet strict diagnostic criteria. Their techniques, many of which are paradoxical, are important because they have been so much discussed and so widely copied. The essence of the method seems to be a radical neutrality of therapeutic attitude, in which the family system is in various ways redefined as working for its own best interests in its apparent dysfunction. Particular aspects of that dysfunction are reframed as a conservative avoidance of change which might be even more threatening.

Discussion

Evaluating the communication therapies is difficult because their proponents eschew diagnostic and outcome criteria. In any case, the proponents have reported only a few cases that seem to be schizophrenic. In the authors' opinion, these approaches are best viewed as ways of dealing with certain family characteristics. Strategic therapy may be useful with severe parental abdication of authority, and systemic therapy may be useful with highly resistant, defiant, illness-invested families. Neither seems applicable to any particular diagnostic entity. From that perspective, two of the authors have suggested that they may have specific therapeutic roles when medical model approaches fail (McFarlane and Beels, 1983). (See also Appendix 2.)

A final point about the medical and nonmedical approaches is that we do not know enough about their long-term effects. Medical model programs emphasize improving the course of chronic illness by strengthening the organization of those who support the patient and by giving them a common philosophy of the illness. As Estroff (1981) has so eloquently argued, this approach provides social support, but it also imposes social control. The medical model may limit the patient's opportunity to find some other way of life, one that is not dependent upon the medical service system. We have all known people who manage not to be patients by being beggars, perpetual students, monastics, itinerant marginal workers, addicts, and so on. Those who direct medical programs assume that, given the same diagnosis, their charges do better than those who pursue these other types of careers. If they do not do better, they assume that the diagnosis must be different. We cannot be sure of either of these assumptions.

Several nonmedical treatment systems encourage other life-styles. Mosher and Menn's Soteria project is a nonfamily example (Mosher et al., 1975), as is the Mental Patients' Liberation Movement. At Soteria medication and formal professional services are renounced in favor of peer support, and the family is kept at a friendly distance. Haley and Madanes's family treatment intends leaving home for a life definitely free of hospitals, medication, and psychiatrists. All of these programs see the patient career as the dead-end victimization of a person who might otherwise have better chances. Some successes have been claimed for these nonmedical approaches, and the Soteria project has documented the superior social and occupational adjustment of its graduates (Mosher et al., 1975). At the very least, we do need to know which patients in which group, medical or nonmedical, eventually cross over into relatively independent careers.

The importance of this point for the education of families is clear. Families devote hard work to programs such as those of the Anderson and Falloon groups and the home-leaving therapy of Haley and

Madanes, and they do this with the limited prospect of short-term effectiveness. But parents are ultimately concerned about how their offspring will live after the struggles of youth are over. We are just now coming to a position where we can collect some data on the long-term question. For the first time, we now have a patient generation which has spent most of its life outside the hospital in a variety of careers and treatment programs.

FAMILY APPROACHES TO AFFECTIVE DISORDER

Bipolar Affective Disorder

The research literature on family therapy and manic-depressive disease is far more recent, smaller, and less robust than the schizophrenia and family literature. For example, none of the work compares with the work on EE to demonstrate conclusively a relation between family factors and the course of manic-depressive illness. Nor does any of the research suggest as strongly that family intervention can forestall relapse beyond the effects of medication.

A partial compensation for this relative underdevelopment, however, is that in the actual treatment of bipolar disease, rigid application of a pure family therapy model has been less of a problem than it has in schizophrenia. One reason for this difference is that manic-depressives are less socially impaired than schizophrenics and are more often married. Consequently, mental health professionals generally have less opportunity during a hospitalization for mania to convey blame to the family of origin. Their primary contact is with the spouse rather than the family of origin.

Another reason for the difference is that a distinctive family theory of the etiology of bipolar disorder never emerged within the mental health professions. Purely psychogenic etiologies were advanced by analysts during the 1940s and 1950s, but these were compromised by the advent of lithium. In their place and almost immediately emerged a tentative, multilevel causal model, much like that which is coming to dominate the field of schizophrenia today.

As a result, when a literature on family intervention in bipolar disease did begin to develop during the 1970s, it included from the start a healthy respect for two aspects of what we find in the new approaches to schizophrenia: (1) basic education in the nature and treatment of the disease and (2) practical coaching in crisis management (Fitzgerald, 1972; Greene et al., 1976). This literature shows an almost continuous agreement that families which are threatened by or are experiencing a hospitalization for mania should have short-term therapeutic support that pays attention not only to family dynamics, but also to these more practical elements. (In writing about manic-depressive disease, "pure" family therapists have, if anything, been rather on the defensive [Keith, 1980].)

Basic education about bipolar disorder should, at a minimum, explain that it is a distinct, diagnosable disease. This helps relieve the patient of feeling that he or she is "bad" and the family of feeling that they are victims of willful mistreatment. Discussions with the family should also provide a full introduction to lithium maintenance so that the family experiences itself as a respected, informed participant in its own therapy, rather than as a passive recipient of mysterious instructions.

Practical coaching for crisis management should address the obvious necessities that families commonly ignore. In a manic crisis they need to make sure that relatives and friends are informed and available to provide support and to set up a bank account solely in the name of the well spouse in order to assure the continued availability of cash for daily necessities.

Short-term family intervention involving a combination of education, management, and therapy has been found highly effective in the short-run with schizophrenic patients, but of diminishing value over the longer term (Goldstein and Kopeikin, 1981). In contrast, for a significant proportion of bipolar patients, this kind of treatment alone is sufficient. Impressive evidence already demonstrates that with lithium maintenance many bipolar patients do not suffer lasting social impairment and can resume normal lives (Carlson et al., 1974; MacVane et al., 1978; Dunner and Hall, 1980). All writers agree, however, that in some families where manic depression occurs, short-term intervention alone will not be sufficient and something more will be required. Unfortunately, the proportion of families who fit this category and the optimal way of helping them are at present imperfectly understood.

The one systematic study available on this issue is that which the Davenport group conducted at the National Institute of Mental Health (NIMH) (Davenport et al., 1977). They tested the outcome of therapy in a couples group homogeneous for bipolar disorder against both medication maintenance at NIMH and follow-up in the home community. The results are at once intriguing and ambiguous. Patients in the couples group were divorced less and relapsed less. But methodological problems make it hard to interpret the high divorce rate of couples not in the group or how much the apparent effect of the group in preventing relapse was actually a function of medication maintenance. (Medication maintenance, of course, is a significant achievement in itself, but a regular couples group is not necessarily the only or the most efficient way to achieve it.)

The limitations in this study are important not only in themselves, but also because they are symptomatic of a general deficiency in current knowledge about an aspect of manic depression that is crucial for family therapy: the level of social and marital adjustment among remitted bipolar patients maintained on lithium. The group working at NIMH has reported evidence of substantial dysfunction among this population. One frequently cited follow-up study of 53 bipolar patients, for example, found that one third suffered from substantial impairment (Carlson et al., 1974). Contrary to the notion that manic-depressive illness is a benign, remitting illness, the researchers concluded that it, too, has a variable prognosis. Outcomes ranged from complete recovery to a chronicity as devastating in its own way as any other chronic, severe illness. The NIMH group has also published several clinical papers specifically describing severe marital dysfunction in this population (Ablon et al., 1975; Davenport et al., 1979). On the other hand, several other groups have reported no significant difference at all between remitted bipolar patients on lithium and individuals with no psychiatric history (Dunner and Hall, 1980; MacVane et al., 1978; Donnelly et al., 1976). Researchers on both sides acknowledge the possibility of sampling bias in their work. None claim that all remitted bipolar patients are well or that all are impaired.

The practical implication of this uncertainty is that clinicians cannot know what to expect from bipolar patients for whom short-term intervention proves insufficient. If chronic disability is likely, a long-term multiple couple or family format like that used at NIMH (Davenport et al., 1977) may very well be the most appropriate form of treatment. If not, conventional marital therapy with the couple alone may be indicated. The former mode is usually easiest to organize in a clinic setting, while the latter can occur in a private office. At present, this decision must be left to individual clinical judgment, since empirical research provides no reliable guide. Indeed, the research is particularly unreliable because many of the bipolar families studied came from the transitional generation who are now stabilized on lithium but who had endured years of travail before it was introduced. The findings thus may not apply to the new phenomenon of bipolar marriages where lithium has been used from the initial onset.

Given the present uncertainty about prognosis, the most one can do is anticipate the treatment issues that are likely to occur no matter which way the long-term course develops. The issues are threefold.

(1) As soon as a manic or depressive episode is over, the patient frequently wants to resume normal relations immediately. After the ordeal that the spouse has just been through, however, he or she is frequently not ready to do so, and an atmosphere of conflict results. The therapist must thus be prepared to frame this issue for the couple and to help them work it through.

(2) Dysfunctional patterns frequently arise around the issue of dependence (Davenport et al., 1979; Mayo, 1979). Probably most common is the situation in which the spouse and patient collude to keep the patient in an underfunctioning, incompetent role, resulting again in mutual resentment. Interactions regarding medication provide a common example. Immediately after the patient has been discharged, family members, encouraged by mental health personnel, are often active in ensuring medication compliance. While it is appropriate for a time, continued too long such activity becomes dysfunctional and deprives the patient of the chance to assume full responsibility for his or her own well-being.

This systemic enforcement of a dependent position is found in virtually all families where one member suffers from a disabling condition. Often it can be seen as a response to the crisis through which the family members have all just passed. Clinicians have described a subcategory of families with a bipolar member, however, where the dynamic seems far more deeply rooted. They describe marriages that are deeply symbiotic, in which the bipolar patient is continuously, irritably, and omnipotently demanding, and massively denies anyone's attempt to point this out. (There is some evidence, in addition, that this character trait is related to a history of early object loss, which renders the patient brittlely intolerant of frustration and disappointment.) Spouses in these marriages are described as simultaneously resentful, compliant, and controlling. Such families are often isolated and highly enmeshed. As a result, they seem to be good candidates for treatment in a multiple family format.

(3) Family members, consumed with worry about the onset of another episode, are on edge and find danger in virtually any expression of anger or sadness on the part of the patient. (Such behavior can be

overdetermined, of course, and can spring from a preexisting family dynamic as well.) Its effect is to reinforce the patient's dependent position and also to disqualify virtually all of his or her emotional expression. The therapist must intervene both by elucidating any underlying family dynamic and by training the family to distinguish between genuine prodromal signs and ordinary emotional expression.

Unipolar Depression

Remarkable though it seems, there is virtually no literature on the family treatment of unipolar depression.* The one exception is an elegant study by Friedman (1975) that tests the efficacy of psychopharmacology or marital therapy alone vs. psychopharmacology and marital therapy combined. Though the results of this study are highly interesting and favor a combined approach, the paper is solely concerned with outcome and says nothing whatsoever about clinical method and technique. The absence of a clinical literature probably means that once the antidepressants have been administered and done their work, nothing special differentiates the family therapy of unipolar depression from family treatment in general.

The prudent approach is to administer medication, wait until the depression clears, and then see if there are important family issues to address. While waiting for the medication to take effect, it is best to restrict oneself to management and not to attempt anything more ambitious. During the acute phase, everyone in the family is generally too preoccupied by the overt symptomatology to address other issues. At this stage, in other words, the primary need is for crisis management, not the excavation of family conflict.

SUMMARY

A review of contemporary approaches to the family of the severely ill adult is much like looking at the proverbial half-filled glass. Several of the new family therapies seem effective and are based on more comprehensive views of the illnesses themselves. Especially in relation to schizophrenia, they assume (1) that the forms of the illnesses, patient types, and family dynamics are heterogeneous; (2) that contributing factors are to be found at several levels of the social system—biological, psychological, family, and social network; and (3) that an effective treatment must address quite specifically each of those factors and levels. Further, the originators of these methods have advanced the view that the therapist must establish a new treatment team of staff, family, and patient in order to realize the full potential of modern treatments for these severe conditions.

The glass seems half empty only when one considers that the outcome evaluation of the new approaches is only partially complete. Conclusive, longer-term results will not be available for a few years. Thus, it may be too soon to be fully assured that these reasonable and seemingly well-designed therapies will continue to be effective. Moreover, longitudinal studies should examine the possibility that the medi-

*Preceptor's note: There is, however, ample evidence for the importance of marital and family problems in the etiology of unipolar depression, strongly suggesting that attention to these problems may have significant therapeutic implications.

cal model approaches may close off opportunities for other life-styles for chronic patients or foster excessive degrees of underfunctioning.

What does seem well supported is the general principle that the family of the mentally ill adult has an untapped therapeutic potential. This potential can be realized if family members are approached with the proper attitude and technique, and the probability is good that there will be an improvement in the course of illness and that a more stable, knowledgeable, and resilient family will result in the long term. At this time, the results of these therapies are sufficiently positive that judicious application in clinical practice seems well justified. Even incremental improvements in these disorders, if achieved economically, are worth the effort, given that a more definitive treatment still seems frustratingly beyond our grasp.

APPENDIX 1.
TOPICAL OUTLINE FOR
PSYCHOEDUCATIONAL WORKSHOPS

For the reader who would undertake psychoeducational workshops for the families of schizophrenic patients, the authors have prepared a topical outline. It is derived from published work of Anderson et al. (1980), Goldstein and Kopeikin (1981), Falloon and Liberman (1983), and from survival skills workshop notes graciously shared by Dr. Anderson. One of the authors (W.R.M.) has used this outline in several presentations and has found it useful.

At present, what would be an optimal format for family education sessions is not known. The authors' experience suggests that the one which Dr. Anderson uses has the greatest advantages. The leaders meet with several families in a group early in the course of an acute episode, without the patients present and with ample opportunity for contact between families during coffee breaks, lunch, question-and-answer periods, and so on.

Part 1. Basic Information about Schizophrenia
Introduction
    Definition
    Brief history of ideas and treatments
Symptom description
    Prodromal
    Acute
    Chronic: negative vs. positive symptoms
Etiology
    Biochemical and genetic abnormalities
    Psychological dysfunction (attentional disorder, susceptibility to stimuli, reality testing, affective flattening)
Interpersonal difficulties
    Social withdrawal, problems with social ambiguity and social learning, inability to tolerate pressure
Course of illness
    Best possible (good premorbid, reactive type)
    Worst possible (untreated, unsupported process type)
    Factors influencing course (medication, supportive psychotherapy, occupational and social rehabilitation, family support, and special types of interaction)
Role of research and present areas of investigation

Part 2. Management of Schizophrenia

Professional treatment
    Goals and rationale
Medication
    Types
    Action (in relation to biochemical and psychological dysfunction, i.e., dopamine blockade, enhanced attentional processes, and reduced arousal)
Psychosocial therapies
    Individual supportive psychotherapy
    Milieu therapy
    Family and multiple family therapy
    Group socialization, social rehabilitation, and social skills training
    Occupational rehabilitation
    Inpatient and partial hospitalization
Family management
    Family as a power in influencing course of illness
    Encouragement about medication and psychosocial therapies
    Avoiding over- and understimulation of patient
    Diffusing intensity at home
    Creating boundaries at home ("psychological space")
    Distancing from patient without rejecting
    Setting limits on bizarre and destructive behavior
    Dealing with irrational fears and paranoid delusions
    Fitting expectations to phase of recovery
    Finding optimal level of expectations in stable periods
    Normalizing daily routine
    Maintaining attention for other family members
    Noticing and handling prodromal symptoms
    Anticipating effects of upsetting life events
    Crisis avoidance and crisis management
    Encouraging social involvement by patient
    Keeping up communication with therapist and agencies
    Avoiding hopelessness and resignation
Family communication
    Rationale (patient's difficulty in processing complex and/or ambiguous information)
    Helpful rules
    1. Keeping conversations at a *moderate* level of specificity
    2. Listening with empathy
    3. Differentiating description from evaluation or judgment
    4. Accepting responsibility for one's own statements and vice versa
    5. Expressing acknowledgment and warmth; emphasizing positive and supportive messages
    6. Requesting behavioral change directly, instead of through criticism
Family's concern for self
    Orientation to schizophrenia as a possibly lifelong problem
    Reorganizing family's functioning after an acute episode
    Having patience in middle phase of recovery (with oversleeping, etc.)
    Avoiding domination of family life by the patient and the illness

Enlisting support from friends and relatives
Developing other resources (social programs, self-help groups)
Need for enjoyable contact with others and/or gratifying work
Sharing problems with families of other patients
Importance of a balanced concern in maintaining capacity to cope
with and be helpful to the patient in the long term

APPENDIX 2.
A DECISION-TREE APPROACH TO CHOOSING
FAMILY TREATMENTS FOR THE PSYCHOTIC PATIENT

Given the variety of available family treatments for schizophrenia, some question arises about their interrelationship. While one might first assume that they are essentially competitive and then attempt to study which is more effective, an alternative strategy is to arrange them in a hierarchical sequence based upon their apparent indications. Two of the authors have speculatively attempted the latter elsewhere (McFarlane and Beels, 1983). A summary of this decision-tree approach is presented in Figure 1.

A number of assumptions come into play in such an endeavor. Space does not allow their full explication here, but the principal points are as follows:

(1) Family therapy for patients having an initial psychotic episode of uncertain diagnosis should be different from that for chronic schizophrenics.

(2) The major risks in the medical model interventions appear to be long-term underfunctioning or reduction of life-style options or both. The communication therapies (strategic and systemic) seem to carry risks of short-term dropout or clinical deterioration or both. The former should therefore precede the latter in a given case.

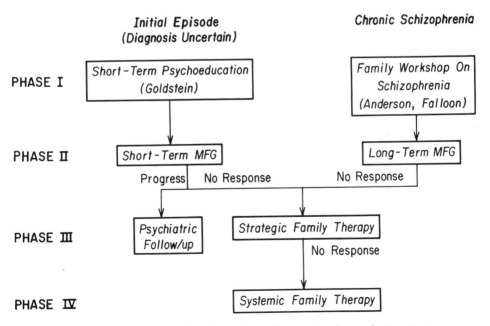

Figure 1. A decision-tree method for combining family therapies for the psychotic patient

(3)   The communication approaches seem best suited to resistant families, in which the members are either lacking in authority (an indication for strategic therapy) or are invested in the patient's illness (an indication for systemic therapy). These families will be identified by their failure to respond to the medical model strategies.

(4)   The follow-up phase of the medical model approaches may be adequately accomplished by working on their specific content in multiple family groups, which have the added benefit of reducing social and ideological isolation.

From these assumptions emerges the schema shown in Figure 1. Family therapies are offered to various patients based on considerations of risk, family resistance, and degree of chronicity. Two forms of multiple family group (MFG) are suggested. The short-term MFG emphasizes the application of the points in the Goldstein therapy (Kopeikin et al., 1983) with additional attention to family communication and structural problems and high EE. The long-term MFG would stress application of the approaches of Anderson et al. (1980), Leff et al. (1983), and Falloon and Liberman (1983), while building a social support network for the participating families.

References for the Introduction

Gurman A.S., Kniskern D.P.: Family therapy outcome research: knowns and unknowns, in Handbook of Family Therapy. Edited by Gurman A.S. and Kniskern D.P. New York, Brunner/Mazel, 1981.

Richmond M.E.: Social Diagnosis, 1917. New York, The Free Press, 1965.

Sullivan H.S.: The Interpersonal Theory of Psychiatry. New York, W.W. Norton, 1953.

Annotated Bibliography for the Part

Journals

Family Process, Bloch D.A. (ed.). 149 East 78th St., New York, N.Y. 10021.
   An old, superior, and sophisticated journal. Theory, clinical material, and research on marital and family therapy.

Journal of Marital and Family Therapy, Gurman A.S. (ed.). American Association for Marriage and Family Therapy, 924 W. 9th St., Upland, CA 91786.
   Official journal of the AAMFT. Clinical and research topics. Rapidly becoming excellent.

Journal of Sex and Marital Therapy, Kaplan H.S., Sager C.J., Schiavi R.C. (eds.). Brunner/Mazel, 19 Union Square West, New York, N.Y. 10003.
   Good basic clinical and research articles. Especially helpful for sex therapy.

American Journal of Family Therapy, Sauber S.R., (ed.). Brunner/Mazel, 19 Union Square West, New York, N.Y. 10003.
   A new and rapidly improving journal.

Books

Introductions

Glick I.D., Kessler D.R.: Marital and Family Therapy, 2nd ed. New York, Grune & Stratton, 1980.
   An excellent introduction to the field covering all areas, but not in depth.

Grunebaum H., Christ J. (eds.): Contemporary Marriage: Structure, Dynamics, and Therapy. Boston, Little, Brown & Co., 1976.
   This is still probably the most useful, short introduction to the treatment of couples and the problems of marriage and their evaluation and treatment.

Bloch D.A. (ed.): Techniques of Family Therapy, New York, Grune & Stratton, 1973.
   Still a useful collection of articles.

Edited Volumes—Surveys of the Field

Gurman A.S., Kniskern D.P.: Handbook of Family Therapy. New York, Brunner/Mazel, 1981.
   Most comprehensive. A chapter on almost everything, many chapters very good.

Paolino T., McCrady B.S.: Marriage and Marital Therapy, New York, Brunner/Mazel, 1978.
   Specific attention to psychoanalytic, behavioral, and systems perspectives on marriage.

Sholevar G.P. (ed.): Handbook of Marriage and Marital Therapy. New York, Spectrum Medical & Scientific Books, 1981.
   Good collection of articles on marital therapy.

Seminal Papers

Ackerman N.W.: The unity of the family. Archives of Pediatrics 55:51–62, 1938.
   A pioneering paper.

Bateson G., Jackson D.D., Haley J., et al.: Toward a theory of schizophrenia. Behavioral Science 1:251–264, 1956.
   The beginnings of communication and strategic approaches. Still important.

Bell J.E.: Family Group Therapy. Public Health Monograph #64, U.S. Dept. of Health, Education & Welfare. Washington, D.C., U.S. Government Printing Office, 1961.
   An early clinical approach to families with troubled children.

Bowen M.: Toward the differentiation of a self in one's own family, in Family Interaction. Edited by Framo J.L. New York, Springer Publishers, 1972. Also in Bowen M.: Family Therapy in Clinical Practice. New York, Jason Aronson, 1978.
   The first description by a family therapist of his work with his own family. Created a sensation when given and is still a useful summary of Bowen's ideas.

Framo J.L.: Family of origin as a therapeutic resource for adults in marital·and family therapy: you can and should go home again. Fam. Process 15:193–210, 1976.
   A very useful discussion of family interviews during the course of individual psychotherapy.

Wynne L., Ryckoff I., Day J., et al.: Pseudo mutuality in the family relations of schizophrenics. Psychiatry 21:205–220, 1958.
   The first paper on the therapist's experience of working with schizophrenics and their families. Still invaluable.

Books on Particular Aspects of Family Psychiatry

Family Therapy

Boszormenyi-Nagy I., Framo J.L. (eds.): Intensive Family Therapy. New York, Harper & Row, 1965.
   This early book is still a fascinating discussion of family therapy.

Boszormenyi-Nagy I., Spark G.: Invisible Loyalties. New York, Harper & Row, 1975.
   Not an easy book to read, but very rewarding and very important.

Hoffman L.: The Foundations of Family Therapy. New York, Basic Books, 1981.
   An excellent discussion of the systems approach to family therapy. Clear and comprehensive.

Minuchin S.: Families and Family Therapy. Cambridge, MA., Harvard University Press, 1974.

Minuchin S., Fishman H.C.: Family Therapy Techniques. Cambridge, MA., Harvard University Press, 1981.
   A very useful pair of books which provide a good introduction to structural family therapy and structural techniques.

Napier C.A., Whitaker C.: The Family Crucible. New York, Harper & Row, 1978.
   This is a uniquely accessible book on family therapy for both professionals and clients.

Papp P. (ed.): Family Therapy, Full Length Case Studies. New York, Gardner Press, 1977.
   A fascinating collection of case reports.

Marital Contract Theory

Sager C.J.: Marriage Contracts and Couple Therapy. New York, Brunner/Mazel, 1976.
   A useful discussion of marriage as a contract.

Behavioral Marital Therapy

Jacobson N.S., Margolin G.: Marital Therapy. New York, Brunner/Mazel, 1979.

Separation and Divorce

Kaplan, H.S.: The New Sex Therapy, Active Treatment of Sexual Dysfunction. New York, Brunner/Mazel, 1974.
   The best introduction to an integrated approach to the treatment of sexual problems in marriage.

Visher E.B., Visher J.S.: Stepfamilies. New York, Brunner/Mazel, 1979.
   An excellent basic book on problems of remarriage. Patients like it, too.

Wallerstein J.S., Kelly J.B.: Surviving the Breakup. New York, Basic Books, 1980.
   Major research on how children fare in separation and divorce.

Weiss R.S.: Marital Separation. New York, Basic Books, 1975.
   The experience of separation. A good book to give to patients.

Family Life Cycle

Carter E., McGoldrick M.: The Family Life Cycle. New York, Gardner Press, 1980.

References for Chapter 12

Family Studies: Reframing the Illness, the Patient, and the Doctor

Brown G.W., Birley J.L.T., Wing J.K.: Influence of family life on the course of schizophrenic disorders: a replication. Br. J. Psychiatry 121:241–258, 1972.

Doane J.A., West K.L., Goldstein M.J., et al.: Parental communication deviance and affective style. Arch. Gen. Psychiatry 38:679–685, 1981.

Duff R.S., Hollingshead A.B.: Sickness and Society. New York, Harper & Row, 1968.

Gershenson J., Cohen M.S.: Through the looking glass: the experiences of two family therapy trainees with live supervision. Fam. Process 17:225–230, 1978.

Goldstein M., Rodnick E.: The family's contribution to the etiology of schizophrenia: current status. Schizophr. Bull. 14:48–63, 1975.

Gurman A.S., Kniskern D.P.: Research on marital and family therapy, in Handbook of Psychotherapy and Behavior Change: An Empirical Analysis, 2nd ed. Edited by Garfield S.L., Bergin A.E. New York, John Wiley & Sons, 1978.

Hauser S.T.: Physician-patient relationships, in Social Contexts of Health, Illness, and Patient Care. Edited by Mishler E.G., Amarasingham L.R., Hauser S.T., et al. New York, Cambridge University Press, 1981.

Jacob T.: Family interaction in disturbed and normal families: a methodological and substantive review. Psychol. Bull. 18:35–65, 1975.

Lewis J.M.: The family matrix in health and disease, in The Family: Evaluation and Treatment. Edited by Hofling C.K., Lewis, J.M. New York, Brunner/Mazel, 1980.

Lief H.I., Fox R.C.: Training for "detached concern" in medical students, in The Psychological Basis of Medical Practice. Edited by Lief H.I., Lief V.F., Lief N.R. New York, Harper & Row, 1963.

Liem J.H.: Family studies of schizophrenia: an update and commentary. Schizophr. Bull. 6:429–455, 1980.

Minuchin S., Rosman B.L., Baker L.: Psychosomatic Families: Anorexia Nervosa in Context. Cambridge, MA., Harvard University Press, 1978.

Mishler E.G.: The social construction of illness, in Social Contexts of Health, Illness and Patient Care. Edited by Mishler E.G., Amarasingham L.R., Hauser S.T., et al. New York, Cambridge University Press, 1981.

Osherson S.E., Amarasingham L.R.: The machine metaphor in medicine, in Social Contexts of Health, Illness, and Patient Care. Edited by Mishler E.G., Amarasingham L.R., Hauser S.T., et al. New York, Cambridge University Press, 1981.

Patterson G.R.: A performance theory for coercive family interaction, in The Analysis of Social Interactions: Methods, Issues and Illustrations. Edited by Cairns R.B. Hillsdale, N.J., Lawrence Erlbaum Associates, 1979.

Reiss D.: The family and schizophrenia. Am. J. Psychiatry 133:181–185, 1976.

Reiss D.: The Family's Construction of Reality. Cambridge, MA., Harvard University Press, 1981.

Scott R.A.: The Making of Blind Men. New York, Russell Sage, 1969.

Stanton M.D.: Drugs and the family. Marriage and Fam. Review 2:1–10, 1979.

Steinglass P., Robertson A.: The alcoholic family, in The Biology of Alcoholism, vol. 7: Psychosocial Pathogenesis of Alcoholism. Edited by Kissin B., Beglieter H. New York, Plenum, in press.

Straker G., Jacobson R.: A study of the relationship between family interaction and individual symptomatology over time. Fam. Process 18:443–450, 1979.

Vaughn C.E., Leff J.P.: The influence of family and social factors on the course of psychiatric illness: a comparison of schizophrenic and depressed neurotic patients. Br. J. Psychiatry 129:125–137, 1976.

Wolin S.J., Bennett L.A., Noonan D.L., Teitelbaum M.A.: Disrupted family rituals: a factor in the intergenerational transmission of alcoholism. J. Stud. Alcohol 41:199–214, 1980.

Zabarenko R.N., Zabarenko L.M.: The Doctor Tree: Developmental Stages in the Growth of Physicians. Pittsburgh, University of Pittsburgh Press, 1978.

Zuk G.H.: The go-between process in family therapy. Fam. Process 5:162–178, 1966.

Annotated Bibliography for Family Studies: Reframing the Illness, the Patient, and the Doctor

Doane J.A., West K.L., Goldstein M.J., et al.: Parental communication deviance and affective style. Arch. Gen. Psychiatry 38:679–685, 1981.
   These are among the best data on the role of the family in eliciting or shaping the schizophrenic syndrome.

Gurman A.S., Kniskern D.P.: Research on marital and family therapy, in Handbook of Psychotherapy and Behavior Change: An Empirical Analysis, 2nd ed. Edited by Garfield S.L., Bergin A.E. New York, John Wiley & Sons, 1978.
   Although there have been several important studies of the outcome of family therapy published since this review, this contribution is the most thoughtful and comprehensive in the field. It describes the major methodologic and clinical issues involved in the careful, quantitative, and controlled assessment of the efficacy of family therapy.

Liem J.H.: Family studies of schizophrenia: an update and commentary. Schizophr. Bull. 6:429–455, 1980.
   This is a particularly thoughtful review of family studies in the field of schizophrenia. After reviewing the recent literature, it suggests how basic social science studies of the family can be integrated into clinical investigations.

Minuchin S., Rosman B.L., Baker L.: Psychosomatic Families: Anorexia Nervosa in Context. Cambridge, MA., Harvard University Press, 1978.

This surely is one of the most impressive descriptions of a set of family therapy techniques. Although the authors also make an effort to integrate some exploratory research with their clinical presentations, systematic research is somewhat overshadowed by descriptions of innovative clinical interventions.

Reiss D.: The Family's Construction of Reality. Cambridge, MA., Harvard University Press, 1981.

This book describes a theory and a series of methods for analyzing indigenous family cultures. Data are presented to support a notion that each family is, in part, organized by *paradigm*, a unique shared conception of the social world in which the family lives.

References for Chapter 13

The Basics of Family Treatment

Ackerman N.W.: Treating the Troubled Family. New York, Basic Books, 1966.

Alexander J.F., Parsons H.V.: Short-term behavioral intervention with delinquent families: impact on family process and recidivism. J. Abnorm. Psychol. 81:219–225, 1973.

Anthony E.F.: Is child psychopathology always family psychopathology? Yes, no, and neither: the views from Freud to Laing, in Controversies in Psychiatry. Edited by Brady J.P. and Brodie H.K.H. Philadelphia, Saunders, 1978.

Avallone S., Aron R., Starr P., et al.: How therapists assign families to treatment modalities: the development of the treatment method choice set. Am. J. Orthopsychiatry 43:767–773, 1973.

Beck D.F.: Research findings on the outcomes of marital counseling. Soc. Casework 56:153–181, 1975.

Beels C.C.: Family and social management of schizophrenia. Schizophr. Bull. 1:97–118, 1975.

Boszormenyi-Nagy I., Spark G.M.: Invisible Loyalties: Reciprocity in Intergenerational Family Therapy. New York, Harper & Row, 1973.

Boszormenyi-Nagy I., Krasner B.: Trust-based therapy: a contextual approach. Am. J. Psychiatry 137:767–775, 1980.

Boszormenyi-Nagy I., Ulrich D.N.: Contextual family therapy, in The Handbook of Family Therapy. Edited by Gurman A.S., Kniskern D.P. New York, Brunner/Mazel, 1981.

Bowen M.: Family Therapy in Clinical Practice. New York, Jason Aronson, 1978.

Boyd W.H., Bolen D.W.: The compulsive gambler and spouse in group therapy. Int. J. Group Psychother. 20:77–90, 1970.

Clarkin J.F., Frances A.J., Glick I.D.: The decision to treat the family: selection criteria and enabling factors, in Group and Family Therapy: 1981. Edited by Aronson M.L., Wolberg L.W. New York, Brunner/Mazel, 1981.

Fleck S.: General systems approach to severe family pathology. Am. J. Psychiatry 33:669–673, 1976.

Glick I.D., Kessler D.R.: Marital and Family Therapy, 2nd ed. New York, Grune & Stratton, 1980.

Goldstein J.M., Rodnick E.H., Evans J.R., et al.: Drug therapy and family therapy in the aftercare treatment of acute schizophrenia. Arch. Gen. Psychiatry 35:1169–1177, 1978.

Greenberg I., Glick I.D., Match S., et al.: Family therapy: indications and rationale. Arch. Gen. Psychiatry 10:7–24, 1964.

Greene B.L., Lee R.R., Lustig N.: Treatment of marital disharmony where one spouse has a primary affective disorder (manic-depressive illness): I. General overview—100 couples. J. Marr. Fam. Couns. 1:39–50, 1975.

Gross A.: Marriage counseling for unwed couples. New York Times Magazine, April 24, 1977, pp. 52–68.

Group for the Advancement of Psychiatry (GAP): The Field of Family Therapy, vol. 7. New York, Mental Health Materials Center, 1970.

Grunebaum H., Christ J., Neiberg N.: Marital diagnosis for treatment planning, in Current Psychiatric Therapies, vol. 2. New York, Grune & Stratton, 1971.

Grunebaum H. Chasin R.: Thinking like a family therapist, in The Challenge of Family Therapy. Edited by Flomenhaft K., Christ A.E. New York, Plenum Press, 1980.

Grunebaum H., Chasin R.: Thinking like a family therapist. J. of Marital and Family Therapy, in press.

Grunebaum H., Solomon L.: Towards a peer theory of group psychotherapy: I. On the developmental significance of peers and play. Int. J. Group Psychother. 30:23–49, 1980.

Gurman A.S.: Some therapeutic implications of marital therapy research, in Couples in Conflict. Edited by Gurman A.S., Liss D.G. New York, Jason Aronson, 1975.

Gurman A.S.: Contemporary marital therapies: a critique and comparative analysis of psychoanalytic, behavioral and systems therapy approaches, in Marriage and Marital Therapy. Edited by Paolino T.J., McCrady B.S. New York, Brunner/Mazel, 1978.

Gurman A.S., Kniskern D.P.: Deterioration in marital and family therapy: empirical, clinical and conceptual issues. Fam. Process 17:3–20, 1978a.

Gurman A.S., Kniskern D.P.: Research on marital and family therapy, in Handbook of Psychotherapy and Behavior Change: An Empirical Analysis, 2nd ed. Edited by Garfield S.L., Bergin A.E. New York, John Wiley & Sons, 1978b.

Haley J.: Leaving Home: The Therapy of Disturbed Young People. New York, McGraw-Hill, 1980.

Hurvitz N.: Marital problems following psychotherapy with one spouse. J. Consult. Psychol. 31:38–47, 1967.

Kaplan S.: Structural family therapy for children of divorce: case reports. Fam. Process 16:75–83, 1977.

Langsley D.G., Pittman F.S., Machotka P., et al.: Family crisis therapy: results and implications. Fam. Process 7:145–158, 1968.

Liebman R., Minuchin S., Baker L.: The use of structural family therapy in the treatment of intractable asthma. Am. J. Psychiatry 131:535–540, 1974.

Minuchin S.: Families and Family Therapy. Cambridge, MA., Harvard University Press, 1974.

Minuchin S., Rosman B., Baker L.: Psychosomatic Families: Anorexia Nervosa in Context. Cambridge, MA., Harvard University Press, 1978.

Napier C.A., Whitaker C.: The Family Crucible. New York, Harper & Row, 1978.

Newman L.: Treatment for the parents of feminine boys. Am. J. Psychiatry 133:683–687, 1976.

Offer D., Vanderstoep E.: Indications and contraindications for family therapy, in The Adolescent in Group and Family Therapy. Edited by Sugar M. New York, Brunner/Mazel, 1975.

Sager C.J.: Sexual dysfunctions and marital discord, in The New Sex Therapy. Edited by Kaplan H.S. New York, Brunner/Mazel, 1974.

Sager C.J.: Marriage Contracts and Couple Therapy. New York, Brunner/Mazel, 1976.

Satir V.: Conjoint Family Therapy. Palo Alto, CA., Science & Behavior Books, 1967.

Schomer J.: Family therapy, in Handbook of Treatment of Mental Disorders in Childhood and Adolescence. Edited by Wolman J., Egan J., Ross A. Englewood Cliffs, N.J., Prentice-Hall, 1978.

Shapiro R., Harris R.: Family therapy in treatment of the deaf: a case report. Fam. Process 15:83—96, 1976.

Skynner A.C.R.: Systems of Family and Marital Psychotherapy. New York, Brunner/Mazel, 1976.

Steinglass P.: Experimenting with family treatment approaches to alcoholism: a review. Fam. Process 15:97—123, 1976.

Toomin M.: Structured separation with counseling: a therapeutic approach for couples in conflict. Fam. Process 11:299—310, 1972.

Wynne L.C.: Some indications and contraindications for exploratory family therapy, in Intensive Family Therapy. Edited by Boszormenyi-Nagy I., Framo J.L. New York, Harper & Row, 1965.

References for Chapter 14

Family Systems Perspectives on the Management of the Individual Patient

Bloch D.A.: Family therapy, in The Family, Evaluation and Treatment. Edited by Hofling C.K., Lewis J.M. New York, Brunner/Mazel, 1980.

Bloch D.A. (ed.): Techniques of Family Therapy. New York, Grune & Stratton, 1973.

Carter E.A., McGoldrick M. (eds.): The Family Life Cycle: A Framework for Family Therapy. New York, Gardner Press, 1980.

Engel G.L.: The clinical application of the biopsychosocial model. Am. J. Psychiatry 137:535—544, 1980.

Framo J.L.: Family of origin as a therapeutic resource for adults in marital and family therapy: you can and should go home again. Fam. Process 15:193—210, 1976.

Hoffman L.: Foundations of Family Therapy. New York, Basic Books, 1981.

Kaplan H.S.: The New Sex Therapy: Active Treatment of Sexual Dysfunction. New York, Brunner/Mazel, 1974.

Minuchin S., Fishman H.C.: Family Therapy Techniques. Cambridge, MA., Harvard University Press, 1981.

Scheflen A.E.: Susan smiled: on explanation in family therapy. Fam. Process 17:59—68, 1978.

Simon R.M.: Family life cycle issues in the therapy system, in The Family Life Cycle: A Framework for Family Therapy. Edited by Carter E.A., McGoldrick M. New York, Gardner Press, 1980.

von Bertalanffy L.: General Systems Theory, Foundations, Development, Applications, revised ed. New York, George Braziller, 1968.

References for Chapter 15

The Treatment of Troubled Couples

Berman E.M., Lief H.I.: Marital therapy from a psychiatric perspective: an overview. Am. J. Psychiatry 132:583—592, 1975.

Berman E.M., Miller W.R., Vines N., et al.: The age 30 crisis and the 7-year itch. J. Sex. Marital Ther. 3:197—204, 1977.

Bohannon P.: The six stations of divorce, in Love, Marriage and Family: A Developmental Approach. Edited by Casswell M.E., Casswell T.E. Chicago, Scott, Foresman & Co., 1973.

Boszormenyi-Nagy I., Spark G.M.: Invisible Loyalties: Reciprocity in Intergenerational Family Therapy. New York, Harper & Row, 1973.

Bowen M.: Family Therapy in Clinical Practice. New York, Jason Aronson, 1978.

Carter E.A., McGoldrick M. (eds.): The Family Life Cycle, New York, Gardner Press, 1980.

Dicks H.V.: Marital Tensions. New York, Basic Books, 1967.

Epstein N.B., Vlok L.A.: Research on resulting psychotherapy, summary of evidence. Am. J. Psychiatry 138:1027—1035, 1981.

Fairbairn W.R.D.: An Object Relations Theory of Personality. New York, Basic Books, 1967.

Framo J.L.: Symptoms from a family transactional viewpoint, in Family Therapy in Transition, vol. 7. Boston, Little, Brown & Co., 1970.

Framo J.L.: The integration of marital therapy with sessions with family of origin, in Handbook of Family Therapy. Edited by Gurman A.S., Kniskern D.P. New York, Brunner/Mazel, 1981.

Gottman J., Notarius C., Gonso J., et al.: A Couple's Guide to Communication. Champaign, IL., Research Press, 1976.

Haley J.: Strategies of Psychotherapy. New York, Grune & Stratton, 1963.

Hansen J.C. (ed.): Values, Ethics, Legalities and the Family Therapist. Rockville, MD., Aspen Publications, 1982.

Jacobson, N., Margolin G.: Marital Therapy. New York, Brunner/Mazel, 1979.

Kaplan H.S.: Disorders of sexual desire, in The New Sex Therapy. Edited by Kaplan H. New York, Brunner/Mazel, 1979.

Karpel M.A.: Family secrets. Fam. Process 19:295—307, 1980.

Kaslow F.: Divorce and divorce therapy, in Handbook of Family Therapy. Edited by Gurman A.S., Kniskern D.P. New York, Brunner/Mazel, 1981.

Klein M.: Our Adult World and Its Roots in Infancy. London, Tavistock, 1959.

Levinson D., Darrow C., Klein E., et al.: The Seasons of a Man's Life. New York, Little, Brown & Co. 1978.

LoPiccolo J., LoPiccolo L.: Handbook of Sex Therapy. New York, Plenum Press, 1978.

Madanes C.: Strategic Family Therapy. San Francisco, Jossey-Bass, 1981.

Napier C.A., Whitaker C.: The Family Crucible. New York, Harper & Row, 1978.

Neugarten B., Datan N.: The middle years, in American Handbook of Psychiatry, 2nd ed., vol. 1. Edited by Arieti S. New York, Basic Books, 1974.

Sager C.J.: Marriage Contracts and Couple Therapy. New York, Brunner/Mazel, 1976.

Sager C.J., Gundlach R., Dremer M., et al.: The married in treatment. Arch. Gen. Psychiatry 19:205—217, 1968.

Stuart R.: Helping Couples Change: A Social Learning Approach to Marital Therapy. New York, Guilford Press, 1980.

Vaillant G.: Adaptation to Life. Boston, Little, Brown & Co., 1977.

Wachtel E.F.: Learning family therapy: the dilemmas of an individual therapist. J. Contemporary Psychotherapy 10:122—135, 1979.

Walsh F.: Normal Family Processes. New York, Guilford Press, 1982.

Weeks G., L'Abate L.: Paradoxical Psychotherapy. New York, Brunner/Mazel, 1982.

Zilbergeld B.: Male Sexuality. Boston, Little, Brown & Co., 1978.

Zinner J.: The implications of projective identification for marital interaction, in Contemporary Marriage: Structure, Dynamics, Therapy. Edited by Grunebaum H., Christ J. Boston, Little, Brown & Co., 1976.

References for Chapter 16

Family Therapy and Childhood Disorder

Ackerman N.W., Behrens M.L.: The family group and family therapy, in Progress in Psychotherapy. Edited by Masserman J.H., Mareno J.L. New York, Grune & Stratton, 1959.

Ackerman N.W.: The Psychodynamics of Family Life, New York, Basic Books, New York, 1958.

Ackerman N.W.: Prejudicial scapegoating and neutralizing forces in the family group, with special reference to the role of family healer. Int. J. Soc. Psychiatry, Special Edition, 2:90–96, 1961.

Boszormenyi-Nagy I.: A theory of relationships, in Intensive Family Therapy, Edited by Boszormenyi-Nagy I., Framo J.L. New York, Harper & Row, 1965.

Bowen M.: Family Therapy in Clinical Practice, New York, Jason Aronson, 1978a.

Bowen M.: The use of family therapy in clinical practice. Compr. Psychiatry, 7:345–374, 1978b.

Brown S.L.: Diagnosis, clinical management and family interviewing, in Science and Psychoanalysis. Edited by Masserman J.H. New York, Grune & Stratton, 1969.

Brown S.: The developmental cycle of families: clinical implications. Psychiatr. Clin. North Am. 3, No. 3, 1980.

Cuber J.F., Harroff P.B.: The Significant Americans: A Study of Sexual Behavior Among the Affluent. New York, Appleton-Century, 1965.

Dicks H.V.: Marital Tensions, New York, Basic Books, 1967.

Emde R.N.: Changing models of infancy and the nature of early development. J. Am. Psychoanal. Assoc. 29:179–219, 1981.

Freud A.: The child as a person in his own right. Psychoanal. Study Child 27:621–625, 1972.

Gherke S., Kirschenbaum J.: Survival patterns in family conjoint therapy. Fam. Process 6:67–80, 1967.

Grunebaum H., Chasin R.: Thinking like a family therapist, in The Challenge of Family Therapy. Edited by Flomenhaft K., Christ A.E. New York, Plenum Press, 1980.

Hetherington E.M., Cox M., Cox R.: Effects of divorce on parents and children, in Nontraditional Families. Edited by Lamb M. Hillsdale, N.J., Lawrence Erlbaum Associates, 1981.

Kagan J.: The form of early development. Arch. Gen. Psychiatry 36:1047–1054, 1979.

Kramer C.H.: Psychoanalytically oriented family therapy. The Family Institute of Chicago, 1968 (mimeographed).

Lewis J.M.: The family matrix in health and disease, in The Family: Evaluation and Treatment. Edited by Hofling C.K., Lewis J.M. New York, Brunner/Mazel, 1980.

Lewis J.M.: Child psychiatry perspectives. J. Am. Acad. Child Psychiatry, 20:189–199, 1981.

Malone C.A.: The treatment of low-income families. Presented at Family Therapy Society Meeting, Boston, 1968 (mimeographed).

Malone C.A.: Observations on the role of family therapy in child psychiatry training. J. Am. Acad. Child Psychiatry 13:437–458, 1974.

Malone C.A.: Child psychiatry and family therapy: an overview. J. Am. Acad. Child Psychiatry, 18:4–21, 1979.

Malone C.A.: The theoretical perspective in teaching family therapy: discussion of Dr. Grunebaum's and Dr. Chasin's paper, in The Challenge of Family Therapy. Edited by Flomenhaft K., Christ A.E. New York, Plenum Press, 1980.

Malone C.A., Drotar D., Negray J: Failure to thrive: a model of family oriented intervention. Paper presented at Evanston Hospital and New York Medical College, 1980 (unpublished).

Malone C.A.: The family interactional perspective in research and clinical practice. Presented at the Harvard Medical School Course on Family Therapy, Boston, 1982 (unpublished).

McDermott J., Jr.: Indications for family therapy. J. Am. Acad. Child Psychiatry, 20:409–419, 1981.

Paul N.L., Grosser G.H.: Operational mourning and its role in conjoint family therapy. Comm. Ment. Health J. 1:339–345, 1965.

Sameroff A.J., Chandler M.J.: Reproductive risk and the continuum of caretaking causality, in Review of Child Development and Research. Edited by Horowitz, F.D. Chicago, IL., University of Chicago Press, 1975.

Sameroff A.J.: The etiology of cognitive functioning. Edited by Kearsley R.B., Siegel I.E. New York, John Wiley & Sons, 1979.

Skynner A.C.R.: Systems of Family and Marital Psychotherapy. New York, Brunner/Mazel, 1976.

Vogel E.F., Bell N.W.: The emotionally disturbed child as the family scapegoat, in A Modern Introduction to the Family. Edited by Bell N.W., Vogel E. Glencoe, IL., Free Press, 1960.

Wynne L.C.: Some indications and contraindications for exploratory family therapy, in Intensive Family Therapy. Edited by Boszormenyi-Nagy I., Framo J. New York, Harper & Row, 1965.

Zilbach J.J.: The family in family therapy. J. Am. Acad. Child Psychiatry 13:459–467, 1974.

Zinner J., Shapiro R.: Projective identification as a mode of perception and behavior in families of adolescents. Int. J. Psychoanal. 53:523–529, 1972.

References for Chapter 17

New Developments in the Family Treatment of the Psychotic Disorders

The references marked with an asterisk are those which describe the treatment protocols discussed in the text. Each also contains an ample bibliography with which to enlarge the reader's understanding of any particular approach.

Ablon S.L., Davenport Y.B., Gershon E.S., et al.: The married manic. Am. J. Orthopsychiatry 45:854–866, 1975.

*Anderson C.M., Hogarty G., Reiss D.J.: Family treatment of adult schizophrenic patients. Schizophr. Bull. 6:490–505, 1980.

Beels C.C.: Social support and schizophrenia. Schizophr. Bull. 7:58–72, 1981.

Brown G.W., Birley J.L.T., Wing J.K.: Influence of family life on the course of schizophrenic disorders: a replication. Br. J. Psychiatry 121:241–258, 1972.

Carlson G.A., Lotin J., Davenport Y.B., et al.: Follow-up of 53 bipolar manic-depressive patients. Br. J. Psychiatry 124:134–139, 1974.

*Davenport Y.B., Evert M.H., Adland M.L., et al.: Couples group therapy as an adjunct to lithium maintenance of the manic patient. Am. J. Orthopsychiatry 47:495–502, 1977.

Davenport Y.B., Adland M.L., Gold P.W., et al.; Manic-depressive illness: psychodynamic features of multi-generational families. Am. J. Orthopsychiatry 49:24–35, 1979.

Doane J., West K.L., Goldstein M.J., et al.: Parental communication deviance and affective style. Arch. Gen. Psychiatry 38:679–685, 1981.

Donnelly E., Murphy D., Goodwin F.K.: Cross-sectional and longitudinal comparisons of bipolar and unipolar depressed groups on the MMPI. J. Consult. Clin. Psychol. 44:233–237, 1976.

Dunner D.L., Hall K.: Social adjustment and psychological precipitants in mania, in Mania: An Evolving Concept. Edited by Belmaker R., Van Praag H.N. New York, Spectrum Publications, 1980.

Estroff N.: Making It Crazy. Berkeley, University of California Press, 1981.

*Falloon I.R.H., Liberman R.P.: Behavioral family interventions in the management of chronic schizophrenia, in Family Therapy in Schizophrenia. Edited by McFarlane W.R. New York, Guilford Press, 1983.

Fitzgerald R.: Mania as a message: treatment with family therapy and lithium carbonate. Am. J. Psychother. 26:547–555, 1972.

Friedman A.S.: Interaction of drug therapy with marital therapy in depressed patients. Arch. Gen. Psychiatry 32:619–637, 1975.

*Goldstein M.J., Kopeikin H.S.: Short-and-long-term effects of combining drug and family therapy, in New Developments in Interventions with Families of Schizophrenics. Edited by Goldstein M.J. San Francisco, Jossey-Bass, 1981.

Greene B.L., Lustig N., Lee R.R.L.: Marital therapy when one spouse has a primary affective disorder: Am. J. Psychiatry 133:827–830, 1976.

*Haley J.: Leaving Home: The Therapy of Disturbed Young People. New York, McGraw-Hill, 1980.

Keith D.: Family therapy and lithium deficiency: J. Marital Family Ther. 6:49–53, 1980.

Kopeikin H.S., Marshall V., Goldstein M.J.: Stages and impact of family crisis therapy in the aftercare of acute schizophrenia, in Family Therapy in Schizophrenia. Edited by McFarlane W.R. New York, Guilford Press, 1983.

*Leff J.P., Berkowitz R., Kuipers L.: Intervention in families of schizophrenics and its effects on relapse rate, in Family Therapy in Schizophrenia. Edited by McFarlane W.R. New York, Guilford Press, 1983.

MacVane J.R. Jr., Lange J.D., Brown W.A., et al.: Psychological functioning of bipolar manic-depressives in remission. Arch. Gen. Psychiatry 35:1351–1354, 1978.

*Madanes C.: Strategic Family Therapy. San Francisco, Jossey-Bass, 1981.

Massie H.N., Beels C.C.: The outcome of the family treatment of schizophrenia. Schizophr. Bull. 6:24–37, 1972.

Mayo J.: Marital therapy with manic-depressive patients treated with lithium. Compr. Psychiatry 20:419–426, 1979.

*McFarlane W.R.: Multiple family therapy in schizophrenia, in Family Therapy in Schizophrenia. Edited by McFarlane W.R. New York, Guilford Press, 1983.

McFarlane W.R., Beels C.C.: A decision-tree model for integrating family therapies for schizophrenia, in Family Therapy in Schizophrenia. Edited by McFarlane W.R. New York, Guilford Press, 1983.

Mishler E.G., Waxler N.E. (eds.): Family Processes and Schizophrenia. New York, Jason Aronson, 1975.

Mosher L., Menn A., Matthews S.: Evaluation of home-based treatment of schizophrenia. Am. J. Orthopsychiatry 45:455–467, 1975.

Reiss D.: Individual thinking and family interaction, II, in Family Processes and Schizophrenia. Edited by Mishler E.G., Waxler N.E. New York, Jason Aronson, 1975.

*Selvini-Palazzoli M., Boscolo L., Cecchin G., et al.: Paradox and Counterparadox. A New Model of the Therapy of the Family in Schizophrenic Transaction. New York, Jason Aronson, 1978.

Singer M.T., Wynne L.C., Toohey M.L.: Communication disorders and the families of schizophrenics, in The Nature of Schizophrenia. Edited by Wynne L.C., Cromwell R.L., Matthysse S. New York, John Wiley & Sons, 1978.

IV

Bipolar Illness

Bipolar Illness

Authors for Part IV

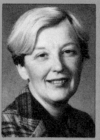

**Paula J. Clayton, M.D.,
Preceptor**

Professor and Head
Department of Psychiatry
University of Minnesota
    Medical School

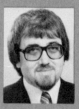

Hagop Souren Akiskal, M.D.
Professor of Psychiatry
Director of Affective
    Disorders Program
University of Tennessee
    College of Medicine

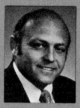

David L. Dunner, M.D.
Chief of Psychiatry
Harborview Medical Center
Professor, Department of Psychiatry
    and Behavioral Sciences
University of Washington

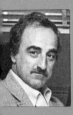

Robert F. Prien, Ph.D.

Chief, Affective Disorders Section
Pharmacologic and Somatic
    Treatments Research Branch
National Institute of Mental Health

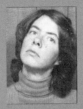

Kay R. Jamison, Ph.D.

Associate Professor and Director
UCLA Affective Disorders Clinic
Department of Psychiatry
UCLA School of Medicine

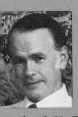

Frederick K. Goodwin, M.D.

Scientific Director
National Institute of Mental Health
National Institutes of Health

Introduction

by Paula J. Clayton, M.D.

Mania is derived from a Greek word meaning "to be mad." The history of its use in medical and psychiatric nosology is instructive. Karl Menninger (1977), in *The Vital Balance,* presents a detailed history of psychiatric nomenclature. He credits Hippocrates, who lived from about 430 to 377 B.C., with introducing psychiatric diagnoses into medical nomenclature. Two of the six diagnoses that Hippocrates proposed were mania and melancholia. Mania referred to acute mental disorders without fever and melancholia to a wide variety of chronic mental disturbances.

In the first century A.D., Aretaeus noted that depression and excitement often alternated in the same person and might therefore represent different aspects of the same illness. Although it is difficult to know how pervasive this idea of cycling became in the centuries thereafter, the term mania remained prominent in all classifications. For hundreds of years, the diagnosis of mania seems to have been based primarily on the acuteness of onset and on a mood of merriment or rage or fury.

Kraepelin synthesized the various approaches to nosology bequeathed to him from the preceding century by such notable predecessors as Falret, Kahlbaum, Morel, Wernicke, and Krafft-Ebing. Beginning in 1883, he published nine editions of his textbook of psychiatry. It was Kraepelin, of course, who separated dementia praecox from manic-depressive illness, using clinical descriptions and the natural history of the illnesses.

If we can assume that names are given to illnesses in an attempt to organize clinical observations, then it must be said from the long history of the term mania that the recognition of mania, and probably the occurrence of mania, were much more apparent to clinicians throughout history than the latecomer to classification, schizophrenia. Particularly in America, schizophrenia rather than manic-depressive psychosis became the focus of attention during the first fifty years of the twentieth century. The epitome of this trend is exemplified in the saying, "A touch of schizophrenia in anyone is schizophrenia." With the advent of treatments such as antipsychotics, antidepressants, and lithium, a reemphasis on separating the specific psychiatric diagnoses developed. Thus, one outcome of psychopharmacologic treatment was that it changed the theory and practice of psychiatry.

Leonhard (1957) was the first to suggest that bipolar and unipolar forms of affective illness may be different, separate illnesses. Perris (1966) and Angst (1966) confirmed Leonhard's evidence on this point. The first American researchers to place emphasis on this distinction were Winokur, the Preceptor, and Reich (Winokur, Clayton, and Reich, 1969). Although bipolar illness was initially separated from unipolar illness on the basis of differences in age of onset, course, family history, and response to treatment, this separation may not in the end prove valid. Data are beginning to accumulate which suggest that the two illnesses are different forms of the same disorder. It now appears that bipolar illness is a more severe and earlier-onset form and that unipolar illness is a later-onset and less severe form. This returns us to the view of Kraepelin, who placed both illnesses in the same family of disorders.

The original hope in separating the two illnesses was that through a better delineation of patients suffering from bipolar affective disorder, we would come to understand better the basic pathophysiology of this disorder. To date, however, this goal has not been achieved. Because of this, the Part contains no detailed description of biochemical hypotheses based on the bipolar-unipolar dichotomy. In the next Part, which deals with the topic of depression, Dr. Elliot S. Gershon describes genetic hypotheses and findings regarding affective disorders. Also in that Part, Drs. Myrna M. Weissman and Jeffrey H. Boyd present a systematic, quantitative comparison of epidemiologic studies throughout the world.

This Part begins with a comprehensive discussion by Dr. Hagop S. Akiskal of the classification of the bipolar disorders, including bipolar I, bipolar II, unipolar II, and cyclothymia. This chapter also reviews in detail the clinical diagnosis of the various forms and manifestations of bipolar illness and the differential diagnosis of bipolar illness from organic affective disorders, nonbipolar major depression, personality disorders, and schizophrenic disorders.

In the next chapter, Dr. David L. Dunner discusses the pharmacologic treatment of the acute manic syndrome. Dr. Dunner also discusses diagnosis, but he uses a somewhat different vantage point from that of Dr. Akiskal. A major emphasis in this chapter, of course, is on the use of lithium, its clinical efficacy in the control of manic episodes, its side effects, and its administration, alone or in combination with antipsychotic medications.

Dr. Robert F. Prien then reviews the prophylactic treatment of recurrent bipolar affective disorder. His chapter focuses on the long-term efficacy and administration of lithium and other pharmacologic agents for the particular purpose of preventing recurrent episodes. In the course of his discussion, he considers a number of clinical management issues, including the role of psychotherapy, the duration of drug treatment, dosage levels, and patient compliance.

Drs. Kay R. Jamison and Frederick K. Goodwin have prepared the final chapter for the Part, a review of the psychotherapeutic issues in treating bipolar illness. While their discussion does cover a number of the general psychological factors that arise in psychotherapy with patients who have bipolar illness, it particularly highlights the psychotherapeutic issues connected with lithium treatment. In a review of some of their own very recent research, they present findings concerning patients' and clinicians' opinions on the effectiveness of lithium and psychotherapy and patients' reasons for not complying with the pharmacologic regimen.

Some material in this Part is presented more than once, but this is purposeful, for it points up a central issue—the importance of proper diagnosis. Adolescents with symptoms of schizophrenia or drug abuse may have an underlying bipolar illness. Blacks with paranoid schizophrenia may be manic. As we become more sensitive to the diagnosis of bipolar affective disorder, it will appear to become more prevalent. A recent study by Egeland (1982) of a total population of Amish found the ratio of bipolar to unipolar affective disorder to be almost one to one, much higher than in incompletely sampled populations.

The Preceptor hopes that after reading this Part, others will come to the same conclusion that nosologists over the centuries have reached—mania and melancholia are fundamental elements in the psychiatric nomenclature.

Chapter 18

The Bipolar Spectrum: New Concepts in Classification and Diagnosis
by Hagop Souren Akiskal, M.D.

INTRODUCTION

Recent advances in the epidemiology, psychobiology, and pharmacotherapy of manic-depressive conditions have led to a greater recognition of this illness in all of its varieties (Clayton, 1981). The lifetime risk for manic-depressive conditions is at least 1.2 percent (Weissman and Myers, 1978), which makes them somewhat more common than schizophrenic disorders. A higher percentage of acute psychiatric hospital admissions are now being assigned to the category of manic depression (Baldessarini, 1970), and subtle outpatient forms of the illness are increasingly being recognized (Akiskal et al., 1979a). According to Winokur's review of the literature (1980), reported ratios of bipolar to unipolar illness range from 1:10 to 1:4. However, Gershon and Liebowitz (1975) noted that 45 percent of the affectively ill in Jerusalem suffered from bipolar illness, and Bazzoui (1970) had reported similar findings in Iraq. Egeland's recent investigation (1982) among the Amish in the United States showed that bipolar illness was about as common as unipolar depression. While the data from these studies may not be generalizable to all populations, bipolar illness is apparently much more common than previously suspected.

For several reasons, the current focus is on the entire diagnosable range of manic-depressive conditions or what Egeland (1982) has aptly termed "the bipolar iceberg." Diagnostic practice in medicine often follows the availability of effective treatment modalities (Lehmann, 1970). Thus, the discovery of chlorpromazine in the 1950s led to the increased diagnosis of schizophrenic disorders. North American psychiatrists-in-training were for several decades tacitly encouraged to elicit subtle degrees of formal thought disorder from their patients in order to bring them the benefits of this new class of drugs. This trend was so pronounced that by the early 1970s schizophrenia had become more or less synonymous with psychosis (exclusive of organic brain syndrome). The advent of lithium carbonate reversed this trend. In DSM-III the concept of schizophrenia is largely restricted to a core group of deteriorating psychotic disorders, whereas Affective Disorders have been broadened to include even those with mood-incongruent features (American Psychiatric Association, 1980). Furthermore, milder degrees of Bipolar Disorder, subsumed under the rubrics of Atypical Bipolar Disorder and Cyclothymic Disorder, are now categorized under the general heading of Affective Disorder rather than being grouped with neurotic or personality disorders.*

The current practice of giving precedence to the diagnosis of affective disorders is not merely due to therapeutic fashion, however. Medico-legal considerations necessitate avoiding the risk of tardive dyskinesia in misdiagnosed manic-depressive patients (Baldessarini et al., 1980), especially in light of the documented relative specificity of lithium carbonate for bipolar illness (Dunner and Fieve, 1978). Even more influential than these considerations are the criteria which have been developed to ascertain the membership of a given syndrome in the group of affective disorders (Feighner et al., 1972; Akiskal, 1980). These criteria include characteristic age of onset, sex ratio, and other demographic features, family history, natural and treated outcome, and, in the last few years, laboratory tests. This chapter presents data which document the existence of a spectrum of bipolar disorders in accordance with these validating nosologic principles, and it also provides clinical and laboratory guidelines for diagnosing and clas-sifying the bipolar disorders.

BIPOLAR AND UNIPOLAR AFFECTIVE STATES

Kraepelin's concept of manic-depressive insanity (1921) brought to-gether the entire domain of endogenous affective psychoses and affec-tive temperaments. He enunciated this concept in the opening passage of his monograph on the subject:

> Manic-depressive insanity . . . includes on the one hand the whole domain of so-called *periodic and circular insanity*, on the other hand *simple mania*, the greater part of the morbid states termed *melancholia* . . . Lastly, we include here certain slight and slightest colorings of *mood*, some of them periodic, some of them continuously morbid, which on the one hand are to be regarded as the rudiment of more severe disorders, on the other hand pass without sharp boundary into the domain of *personal predisposition*. In the course of the years I have become more and more convinced that all the above-mentioned states only represent manifestations of a *single morbid process*. (Kraepelin, 1921, 1).

In recent years, four groups of independent workers (Leonhard, 1957; Perris, 1966; Angst, 1966; Winokur and Clayton, 1967) chal-lenged Kraepelin's unitary concept and proposed making a sharp distinction between the unipolar form of affective disorder (depressions only) and the bipolar form (elevated periods required). The reported differentiating characteristics of these two forms of illness have been reviewed by Goodwin and Bunney (1973), Akiskal and McKinney (1975), Depue and Monroe (1978), Gershon (1978), and Dunner (1980). In addition to the presence of mania or hypomania, bipolar illness compared with unipolar is reportedly characterized by the following: an equal sex ratio; an earlier age of onset; more retarda-tion and hypersomnia during depressive episodes; higher genetic loading for affective disorder (both unipolar and bipolar) in consecutive generation pedigrees; shorter but more frequent episodes; "augmentor" status with the average-evoked-potential technique; low platelet mono-amine oxidase (MAO) activity; tendency for lower excretion of urinary

*Editor's note: In his chapter in Part V, Klerman discusses the DSM-III classification of Affective Disorders in greater detail and also elaborates on the relationships of earlier categorizations and terminologies to the DSM-III groupings.

3-methoxy-4-hydroxyphenylglycol (MHPG, the central metabolite of norepinephrine) during depressive episodes; lowered threshold for developing hypomania during antidepressant treatment; and response to lithium carbonate during both elevated and depressed phases. Gershon's review (1978), however, concluded that none of these differences was sufficiently compelling to argue for a biologic separation of unipolar and bipolar disorders. His conclusion remains essentially unchallenged by biologic markers introduced since he undertook his review. The dexamethasone suppression test (DST) is positive in both unipolar and bipolar depressions (Carroll et al., 1981), although the proportion of nonsuppressors is somewhat higher among bipolars (Schlesser et al., 1981). Likewise, REM latency, the time elapsed from sleep onset to the first REM period, is considerably shortened in both unipolar and bipolar depressions (Kupfer et al., 1978). Finally, in tests of the thyroid-stimulating hormone (TSH) response to thyrotropin-releasing hormone (TRH), some but not all investigators have reported blunted responses in unipolar depressives and normal responses in bipolar depressives (Van Praag, 1982).

Recent evidence indicates that the family histories of unipolar and bipolar probands are more similar than dissimilar (Gershon et al., 1975; Smeraldi et al., 1977; Taylor and Abrams, 1980) and that a spectrum of atypical bipolar disorders forms a phenomenological bridge between unipolar and bipolar disorders (Akiskal et al., 1979a; Klerman, 1981). Indeed, Gershon et al. (1975) have suggested that bipolar illness is the more severe or penetrant of the two disorders, which may explain the earlier age of onset, the high frequency of episodes, and the lowered threshold for hypomanic and manic decompensation. With the currently broadened definitions of depression (Spitzer et al., 1978), some of the reported unipolar-bipolar differences may well be due to the contamination of the unipolar illness category with dysphoric anxiety states, as well as nonendogenous conditions like neurotic and social misery, demoralization, and personal unhappiness. When endogenous depressions are studied (Taylor and Abrams, 1980), unipolar-bipolar differences are apparently minimized, because non-specific dysphoric states are least likely to occur in this population. In this sense, the distinction between bipolar and unipolar affective states has to some extent been the distinction between affective and nonaffective disorder, or the distinction between affective illness and the nonspecific dysphoria common to a variety of nonaffective disorders (Roth and Barnes, 1981).

All of these considerations suggest that the pendulum may be swinging back to Kraepelin's model. Indeed, recent experience has shown that many patients with recurrent primary depressive disorders develop mild and short-lived hypomanic episodes either spontaneously or upon pharmacologic challenge with tricyclic antidepressants (Akiskal et al., 1978; 1979b). These patients can be mistakenly classified as unipolar, because they usually experience hypomania as pleasant and therefore seldom report it. Skillful phenomenological questioning and close personal follow-up using observational criteria can help to document hypomania in such cases. Questioning will often also reveal that these patients have family histories that are positive for bipolar illness (Akiskal et al., 1982b). On the other hand, there is no reason to include all depressions, especially those with late onset and a low frequency of episodes, in the manic-depressive spectrum. There are probably many nonfamilial phenocopies of unipolar depression that, because of low genetic risk, have a predictably low frequency of episodes.

A spectrum of genetic risk may exist for affective disorders, proceeding from infrequent-episode unipolar (low risk), to recurrent unipolar, to bipolar (highest risk). Within this spectrum there are probably at least two varieties of unipolar illness (Kupfer et al., 1975; Winokur, 1980; Akiskal, 1981a): (1) a pure depressive form with unipolar but no bipolar family history and with a relatively low frequency of episodes (unipolar I) and (2) depressions with a high frequency of episodes and with bipolar family history, i.e., a phenotypic expression of bipolar genotype (unipolar II).

When unipolar II disorders are treated with tricyclic antidepressants, one can expect short-lived hypomanic responses or a transformation of the depressive state into a dysphoric-irritable mixed state. This is why lithium is often considered to be a better treatment for these unipolar depressions (Kupfer et al., 1975; Bowden, 1978). Personal follow-up will eventually provide evidence for spontaneous brief hypomanic episodes in the course of these recurrent depressions (Akiskal et al., 1978). In other words, unipolar II depressives have considerable overlap with the bipolar II depressives described by Fieve and Dunner (1975). They have depressions severe enough to warrant hospitalization and also have hypomanic periods of subclinical intensity, but they are distinct from the bipolar I or classic manic-depressives who have full-blown manic episodes of psychotic proportions. In summary, many recurrent depressions probably belong to the bipolar spectrum, and bipolar II disorder is an intermediary phenomenological type that lies between unipolar II and bipolar I disorders (see Table 1).

Table 1.   Relationship between Bipolar and Unipolar Affective Subtypes

1.	Recurrent Mania:	No evidence for clinical depression
2.	Bipolar I:	Mania and depression
3.	Bipolar II:	Depression and spontaneous hypomania
4.	Unipolar II:	Recurrent depressions with bipolar family history; may switch to hypomania with pharmacologic challenge
5.	Unipolar I:	Depressions with low frequency of episodes and no bipolar history

Source: summarized from Akiskal (1981a).

CLASSIFICATION

Bipolar Disorder

The DSM-III concept of Bipolar Disorder overlaps with that of bipolar I. An unequivocal history or current episode of full-fledged mania is the diagnostic sine qua non. However, neither psychosis nor hospitalization for mania is required in DSM-III.* In the author's opinion, the term *mania* should be restricted to elevated periods where the illness is of such severity that pleasant euphoria can alternate with or

*Preceptor's note: Table 1 in Dunner's chapter summarizes the DSM-III criteria for mania.

give way to irritable belligerence, where judgment is impaired and social or financial catastrophies are imminent, and where grandiosity is of delusional proportions. This approach takes cognizance of the fact that excitement meeting the syndromal criteria for mania can explode rapidly into such a disastrously psychotic state that most clinicians will elect to hospitalize the patient. Although the majority of patients with excited periods of such severity eventually develop many episodes of major depression (circular bipolar disorder), up to 10 percent may suffer no depressions of syndromal depth (so-called unipolar manias, Leonhard, 1957).

Atypical Bipolar Disorder

Kraepelin (1921) introduced the concept of hypomania to apply to nonpsychotic and ambulatory forms of psychomotor excitement which lasted for a few days or weeks or sometimes for many months or which might even fluctuate over a lifetime. In other words, Kraepelin observed that many manic-depressives experienced milder elevated periods for which they were not hospitalized. Still others were hospitalized only for depression and developed occasional periods of mild excitement that did not require clinical attention. This latter group is included in bipolar II (Fieve and Dunner, 1975) and is labeled Atypical Bipolar Disorder in DSM-III. The term *atypical* can imply statistical rarity and therefore appears an unfortunate choice for what seems to be a very common outpatient presentation for depression (Akiskal et al., 1979a). Indeed, in the Weissman and Myers epidemiologic survey (1978), it accounted for 50 percent of bipolar cases.

Cyclothymic Disorder

Cyclothymic Disorder is a bipolar condition with an even lesser degree of severity than bipolar II disorder, in that neither the hypomanic nor the depressive periods reach the clinical threshold for hospitalizable episodes (Akiskal et al., 1977). Typically, affective oscillations last only a few days and occur on a subsyndromal plane of intensity. However, full-fledged depressive episodes of longer duration are not uncommon complications (transition to Atypical Bipolar Disorder), and occasionally manic periods supervene (transition to full-blown Bipolar Disorder). Four other sets of evidence argue for classifying cyclothymia in the bipolar spectrum: (1) phenomenological overlap between the two disorders; (2) the ready mobilization of hypomania by tricyclic antidepressant treatment; (3) family pedigrees indistinguishable from those seen in classic manic-depressive illness; and (4) response to lithium carbonate in about 60 percent of cases.

Dysthymia as a Bipolar Variant

Recent evidence (Akiskal et al., 1981) indicates that some dysthymic patients belong to the bipolar spectrum. This work has shown that the DSM-III concept of Dysthymic Disorder is too broad. Incompletely remitted late-onset depressions pursuing a low-grade chronic course should be differentiated from characterological depressions which have exhibited a low-grade intermittent course since their beginnings in late childhood or adolescence. Studies at the University of Tennessee (Akiskal et al., 1980; Rosenthal et al., 1981) have further identified a thymoleptic-responsive dysthymic disorder within the early-onset group. This condition is characterized by miniepisodes of endogenous depression occurring intermittently and lasting for days to weeks, and it is often complicated by superimposed major depressions, very much like the "double depressions" described by Keller and Shapiro (1982).

The author and his colleagues have argued that thymoleptic-responsive dysthymia represents a true subaffective disorder, i.e., an attenuated phenotypic variant of primary affective disorder. They have based this idea on several observations. Depressive phenomenology tends to be hypersomnic-retarded. Brief hypomanic responses can be pharmacologically mobilized in about one third of patients. Family history is often positive for both unipolar and bipolar affective disorder. Finally, REM latency is shortened in many cases, even when the patient is not in a state of major depression. These findings, coupled with an even sex ratio and positive therapeutic response to lithium, suggest kinship between dysthymic and cyclothymic disorders (Akiskal et al., 1980; Rosenthal et al., 1981). That some dysthymic conditions might represent phenotypic variants of bipolar affective psychosis has also been suggested by recent genetic work (Turner and King, 1981).

Indeed, subaffective disorders can be classified into four overlapping subtypes along a dysthymic-cyclothymic continuum (Akiskal, 1982c), as depicted in Figure 1. In the least common expression of these disorders, hypomanic periods predominate (see top of figure). Hyperthymic individuals are highly driven, ambitious, and successful. They

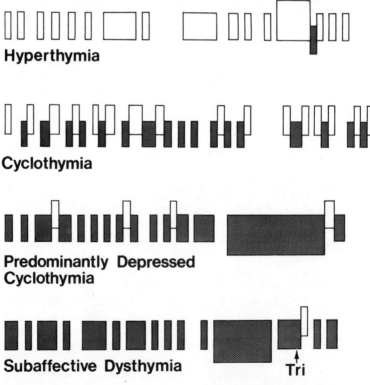

Hyperthymia

Cyclothymia

Predominantly Depressed Cyclothymia

Subaffective Dysthymia

Tri

Figure 1. White rectangles represent hypomanic periods and gray rectangles, depressive swings. The arrow indicates hypomania elicited during tricyclic antidepressant administration.

rarely present for psychiatric treatment but may be seen in sleep disorders centers, where they seek help because of insomnia (Akiskal, 1982d). A second group includes patients with the "purest" form of cyclothymia. They have about equal numbers of depressive and hypomanic periods. In a third group, predominantly depressed cyclothymics, depressive periods outnumber hypomanias. Finally, the patients designated subaffective dysthymic (see bottom of figure) suffer from lifelong, intermittent, and short-lived episodes of depression, sometimes of full syndromal depth. These patients do not spontaneously develop hypomanic periods unless pharmacologically challenged by tricyclic antidepressants.

Secondary Mania

Mania is most commonly expressed as a phase of circular bipolar disorder, which has strong genetic determinants (Mendlewicz and Rainer, 1977). Available evidence does not permit separating unipolar mania as a distinct nosologic entity from these circular forms (American Psychiatric Association, 1980). Some preliminary data (Winokur, 1981) do suggest that postpartum mania without depression is distinct from familial bipolar disorder, where both depressive and manic episodes can occur in the postpartum period. But the evidence for a distinct puerperal manic disorder is not compelling. However, a recent review (Krauthammer and Klerman, 1978) has documented that phenocopies of mania occur in the context of medical disorders. Family history is seldom positive in these cases, suggesting a low genetic risk and hence a lowered risk for recurrences.

Less well-defined phenocopies of mania are the so-called reactive manias or maniacal grief reactions (Racamier and Blanchard, 1957). Personal loss or bereavement are described as antecedents (Ambelas, 1979), and the reaction is essentially conceptualized in psychodynamic terms as a denial of loss. While such explanations may be plausible in individual cases, no systematic data are available to suggest that these

Table 2. Selected Precipitants of Mania

Pharmacologic factors:	Steroids
	Levodopa
	Amphetamine
	Methylphenidate
	Cocaine
	Monoamine oxidase inhibitors
	Tricyclic antidepressants
Medical factors:	Influenza
	Tertiary syphilis
	Thyrotoxicosis
	Systemic lupus erythematosus
	Rheumatic chorea
	Multiple sclerosis
	Diencephalic and third ventricular tumors
Chronobiologic factors:	Sleep deprivation
	Seasonally increased exposure to sunlight
Psychological factors:	Object loss

Source: summarized from Akiskal (1982a). © 1982 Merck & Company, Inc. Used with permission.

patients differ in family history from other manics. This also applies to the elevated periods of depressed patients who switch to mania subsequent to antidepressant drug treatment or sleep deprivation (Bunney, 1978). With these patients, a bipolar diathesis is usually manifest, either in family history for mania or in spontaneous hypomanic periods during prospective observation (Akiskal et al., 1979b; 1982b). Although skeptics remain (Lewis and Winokur, 1982), the cumulative evidence suggests that bipolar switches commonly occur during the first one or two weeks of antidepressant treatment. Table 2 presents a host of pharmacologic, medical, chronobiologic, and psychological factors which can be considered precipitants of mania.

Summary

Mania, like depression, appears to be a syndrome rather than a disease entity. It is the final common pathway of many etiologic factors, both biologic and psychological. At this time, biologic factors, especially familial-genetic predisposition, are the best-established causes. But while genetic predisposition is a necessary substrate, it needs to be activated by environmental precipitants. These environmental causes are not always obvious, which then gives the appearance of endogenous mood swings. Moreover, environmental factors alone (including interpersonal factors) rarely account for manic states, with the possible exception of medically induced secondary mania.

Manic-depressive illness is expressed in a spectrum of phenotypes ranging from subaffective temperamental deviations (cyclothymia and dysthymia) to recurrent depressions with infrequent hypomanias, to full-blown bipolar psychosis (Akiskal, 1981a). Many patients do not make the transition from one form to another, but transitional forms occur frequently enough to suggest a psychopathological process that is common to the entire spectrum, as originally hypothesized by Kraepelin (1921) and as Klerman (1981) recently elaborated. Probably only those manic states induced by medical disease should be left out of this spectrum.

CLINICAL DIAGNOSIS

The Manic Syndrome

Cross-sectional diagnosis of mania, especially in its psychotic form, is customarily considered unreliable, since it shows considerable overlap with such conditions as schizophrenia and drug-induced psychoses. However, some recently developed operational definitions (Feighner et al., 1972; Spitzer et al., 1978) have produced good to excellent interrater reliabilities, ranging from 0.82 to 0.93 (Spitzer et al., 1975; Helzer et al., 1977). These definitions are now incorporated into the DSM-III concept of mania. DSM-III requires (1) a distinct period which represents a break from premorbid functioning, (2) a duration of at least one week, (3) elevated or irritable mood, (4) at least three to four classic manic signs and symptoms, and (5) absence of any toxic factors that could account for the clinical picture. Extreme psychotic manifestations, including mood-incongruent delusions and hallucinations, are permissible so long as they occur in the midst of the full affective syndrome.

The DSM-III definition acknowledges three features of mania which until recently were not widely accepted. First, it recognizes that mania as a syndrome is sometimes secondary to medical or toxic factors and that these need to be excluded when diagnosing the more commonly occurring manic states as part of bipolar disorder. Second, while elation is common in mania, DSM-III recognizes that a broader range of affects also occurs, including depression, irritability, and hostility. Third, DSM-III acknowledges that severe psychotic disorganization is not incompatible with the diagnosis of mania, provided it occurs in the setting of the manic syndrome. The first point has already been discussed; the second and third require further elaboration.

A number of clinical observations over the years (Campbell, 1953; Kraines. 1957; Winokur et al., 1969; Carlson and Goodwin, 1973; Pope and Lipinski, 1978; Akiskal and Puzantian, 1979) have reconfirmed the classic descriptions of mania (Kraepelin, 1921). In addition to elation, euphoria, and ecstasy, the manic patient experiences labile mood, characterized by alternation of euphoria with irritability and depression and sometimes with irritable and angry periods which in the extreme may explode into destructive rage. The labile mood, especially in its irritable-angry coloration, reflects manic and depressive admixtures characteristic of a mixed state and is a common presentation of mania (Himmelhoch et al., 1976). Manics, not paranoid schizophrenics, are the most hostile patients encountered in psychiatric practice (Blackburn, 1974). Thus the mood in mania, far from being invariably pleasant, is frequently dysphoric. This is one reason why family and friends are often alienated from the patient.

Recent studies have also shown that mood-incongruent psychotic pictures are not uncommon in mania (Clayton et al., 1965; Carlson and Goodwin, 1973; Abrams et al., 1974; Taylor et al., 1974; Pope and Lipinski, 1978; Berner, 1980). There is now convincing evidence that Schneider's first-rank symptoms are not pathognomonic for schizophrenia and may occur in as many as one fourth of all manic-depressives (Carpenter et al., 1973). Furthermore, Andreasen's systematic work (1979a) has documented that most types of formal thought disorder are common to both schizophrenic and affective psychoses. Only poverty of speech content (vagueness) emerges as significantly more common in schizophrenia (see Table 3). Finally, even certain catatonic features like posturing, negativism, and others have been shown to occur in mania (Abrams and Taylor, 1976). Although not specifically mentioned in the DSM-III definition, confusions, even pseudodemented presentations, can occur in mania (Clayton, 1981).

Retarded Depression

DSM-III criteria for clinical depression require (1) a distinct period of illness which represents a break from premorbid functioning, (2) dysphoric mood or anhedonia, (3) at least four classic signs or symptoms of depression, (4) sustained duration of several weeks, and (5) absence of any toxic factors that could account for the clinical picture.

The Pittsburgh group (Detre et al., 1972; Kupfer et al., 1975) has convincingly argued that the uncomplicated depressive phase of bipolar illness is typically manifested by hypersomnia and psychomotor retardation. When mixed states supervene, either spontaneously or in the context of sedative and alcohol abuse, agitation and insomnia appear (Himmelhoch et al., 1976). Thus, the diagnosis of the depressive phase of bipolar illness requires a special emphasis on these aspects of the syndrome.

Table 3. Thought, Language, and Communication Disorders in Patients with Schizophrenia and Affective Psychoses[1]

	Schizophrenic Patients (N=45)	Manic Patients (N=32)	Depressive Patients (N=36)
Negative formal thought disorders			
Poverty of speech (laconic speech)	29	6	22
Poverty of content of speech (vagueness)	40	19	17
Positive formal thought disorders			
Pressure of speech[2]	27	72	6
Tangentiality (oblique replies)	36	34	25
Illogicality (non sequiturs)	27	25	0
Derailment ("looseness," "slippage")[2]	56	56	14
Incoherence (word salad)	16	16	0
Others			
Circumstantiality ("long-winded")	4	25	31
Perseveration	24	34	6
Distractibility	2	31	6
Clanging	0	9	0
Neologisms	2	3	0
Echolalia	4	3	0
Blocking	4	3	6

[1] Expressed in percentages
[2] Combination gives rise to "flight of ideas."
Source: data from Andreasen (1979b). Arch. Gen. Psychiatry 36:1325–1330, © 1979 American Medical Association. Used with permission.

Not surprisingly, the depressive phase of bipolar illness, which is the prototype of an autonomous genetic disorder in psychiatry, is characterized by melancholic features. This is supported by positive results on the DST in as many as 95 percent of bipolar probands (Schlesser et al., 1981). Psychotic features, including an occasional Schneiderian symptom, have also been described in the depressive phase, but they are not as common as in the manic phase. Stupor, on the other hand, is not an uncommon mode of psychotic presentation of bipolar illness. This is especially true in adolescents and young adults where the mistaken diagnosis of catatonic stupor is often made (Akiskal et al., 1982b). Pseudodemented "organic" presentations have been described in the elderly (Cowdry and Goodwin, 1981).

Other common expressions of bipolar depression are periodic anergia, hypersomnolence, and weight gain. The patient will not ordinarily complain of hypomania because it is experienced either as rebound relief from depression or as pleasant short-lived ego-syntonic moods (Jamison et al., 1980). Expert questioning is often required in the diagnosis of these conditions. When in doubt, direct clinical observation of hypomania (not uncommonly elicited by tricyclic pharmacotherapy) will provide definitive evidence for the bipolar nature of the disorder. However, in some cases depressive and hypomanic periods are not easily discerned because of superimposed caffeinism (Neil et al., 1978).

Mixed States

Momentary tearfulness, depressed mood, and even suicidal ideation are not uncommon at the height of mania or during transition from mania to retarded depression (Kotin and Goodwin, 1972). Another common manifestation is racing thoughts in the context of a retarded depression. These labile and transient mixed periods, which occur in at least two thirds of bipolar patients, must be contrasted with totally mixed attacks.

These less common mixed bipolar episodes are characterized by dysphorically elevated moods, severe insomnia, psychomotor agitation, racing thoughts, suicidal ideation, grandiosity, and hypersexuality, as well as persecutory delusions and auditory hallucinations (Himmelhoch et al., 1976). Mixed states are often misdiagnosed as unipolar depression and, worse, as atypical or neurotic depression, while severely psychotic forms of the illness are misdiagnosed as paranoid schizophrenia. Correct diagnosis, often supported by a positive DST, is mandatory for proper management, because both tricyclics and MAO inhibitors when used singly may further contribute to the mixed pathology of these patients, and both minor and major tranquilizers will generally be ineffective. Lithium carbonate alone or in combination with antidepressants is usually required for producing satisfactory remissions in the nonpsychotic group, while ECT may be required in the psychotic group.

Subtle Forms of Bipolar Disorder

Clinical studies in ambulatory settings (Akiskal et al., 1977; Wold and Dwight, 1979; Depue et al., 1981; Dunner et al., 1982) have verified the existence of a spectrum of relatively mild and subtle bipolar disorders. In this spectrum, disturbances are more often manifested in the psychomotor, interpersonal, and vocational spheres and in substance abuse, rather than in mood swings per se.

The clinical presentation of *cyclothymic disorder* has been described in some detail elsewhere (Akiskal et al., 1979a). Generally, the *onset* is in the teens or early adulthood. The disorder may present as a personality disorder, since the patient is often unaware of moods per se. Cycles are *short*, usually lasting a few days, and they recur in an irregular fashion, with infrequent euthymic periods. While the disorder may not attain full syndromal status for depression and hypomania during any one cycle, *the entire range of affective manifestations* does occur at various times. Patients experience *endogenous mood changes* (e.g., patients often awaken with a mood). The *biphasic course* of cyclothymia has a number of prominent features. Hypersomnia alternates with decreased need for sleep, although intermittent insomnia can also occur. Shaky self-esteem manifests in alternations between a lack of self-confidence and a naive or grandiose overconfidence. Periods of mental confusion and apathy alternate with periods of sharpened and creative thinking, and patients experience marked unevenness in the quantity and quality of productivity, often associated with unusual working hours. A final biphasic feature is uninhibited people seeking, which may lead to hypersexuality and which alternates with introverted self-absorption. *Behavioral manifestations* of cyclothymia include: irritable-angry-explosive outbursts that alienate loved ones; episodic promiscuity and repeated conjugal or romantic failure; frequent shifts in line of work, study, interest, or future plans; resort to alcohol and drug abuse as a means for self-treatment or for augmenting excitement; and occasional financial extravagance.

In subaffective *dysthymic disorders*, hypomanic periods are even more subtle, and they are not evident unless pharmacologically mobilized. Elsewhere the author has detailed his suggestions for identifying this thymoleptic-responsive subgroup of dysthymia (Akiskal, 1982d). To summarize the criteria, subaffective dysthymic disorders have an *indeterminate onset*, but cardinal manifestations usually appear before age 21. The *course fluctuates* over many years, but typically the patient is not free of depressive manifestations for more than a few weeks at a time. Usually *the symptom profile* is subsyndromal, although the full range of depressive symptoms occurs at various times and may even crystallize into superimposed syndromal episodes. Patients manifest at least two of the following melancholic features: psychomotor inertia, hypersomnia, anhedonia, and/or diurnal variation (worse in A.M.). They are habitually introverted, but brief periods of extraversion are sometimes seen in relatively "well" periods. At least five of the seven Schneiderian depressive personality items are present in these patients. Patients are (1) quiet, passive, and indecisive; (2) gloomy, pessimistic, and incapable of fun; (3) self-critical, self-reproaching, and self-derogatory; (4) skeptical, hypercritical, and complaining; (5) conscientious and self-disciplining; (6) brooding and given to worry; and/or (7) preoccupied with inadequacy, failure, and negative events to the point of morbid enjoyment of their failures. The final criterion is that the patient not have any *diagnosable nonaffective disorder* that appears on the Washington University list of validated psychiatric disorders. The one exception is that the patient may manifest sedativism (alcohol and drug abuse), for this may mask affective manifestations in the early course of the disorder.

VALIDATION OF THE BIPOLAR TYPOLOGY

Such a broadly enlarged concept of bipolar spectrum disorders may cause some questions about the validity of the concept.* At the psychotic border, it overlaps considerably with schizophrenia, and at the nonpsychotic end of the spectrum, with character disorders. Course, family history, and recently developed laboratory tests can be used to examine this question.

Course was Kraepelin's well-known validating principle for distinguishing the affective from the schizophrenic psychoses. Since his pioneering distinction at the turn of the century, course as a distinguishing principle appears to have been upheld in essentially all studies. Classified on the basis of a gradient of affective symptoms, psychotic patients show a distinct pattern in rates of recovery. Thus, over a thirty- to forty-year follow-up, 54 percent of manic-depressives, 44 percent of schizoaffectives, 22 percent of patients with schizophreniform illness, and only 8 percent of patients with process schizophrenic psychoses show full recovery (Coryell and Winokur, 1980). It is also remarkable that in patients initially manifesting the full manic syndrome, a 93 percent stability of diagnosis is shown at forty-year follow-up. (This is why DSM-III diagnostic rules are explicit about excluding schizophrenia from diagnostic consideration when a sustained and full affective syndrome occurs.) Regarding the course of cyclothymic and related disorders, not a single instance of schizophrenic breakdown has appeared in a Memphis study of 46 cyclothymics, while one out of three developed superimposed elevated or major depressive episodes (Akiskal et al., 1977).

Family history has been another powerful validating principle. For instance, it is well known that in the families of patients with primary

---

*Preceptor's note: For further discussion of the breadth of the concept, see the chapter by Dunner in his review of diagnostic considerations.

Table 4. Illness in First-Degree Relatives of Affective Probands

Diagnosis of Probands	N	Diagnosis of Relatives[1]			
		Schizoaffective	Bipolar I	Bipolar II	Unipolar
Schizoaffective	83	6.2	10.9	6.2	14.7
Bipolar I	548	1.1	4.3	4.1	14.0
Bipolar II	191	0.6	2.6	4.5	17.3
Unipolar	166	0.7	1.5	1.5	16.6

[1] Expressed in percentages
Source: Gershon et al. (1982).

affective disorders, the morbid risk for serious affective illness is significantly raised above population expectations (5 to 6 percent), while for schizophrenia it is the same as in the general population (1 percent). The reverse holds true for the families of schizophrenic patients. Data such as these argue for a discontinuity between primary affective and schizophrenic disorders (Coryell and Winokur, 1980). Studies conducted by Gershon et al. (1982) have shown that in addition to bipolar I illness, schizoaffective and bipolar II as well as unipolar disorders occur in the families of bipolar I probands (see Table 4). These data argue for a continuum from severe schizoaffective and bipolar I disorders to milder bipolar II and recurrent unipolar disorders.

Finally, the inclusion of border conditions into the affective spectrum has been validated with laboratory techniques. For instance, the DST has been shown to be positive in a high proportion of psychotic, mixed, and atypical bipolar depressives (Carroll, 1982). Essentially similar findings have emerged with the REM-latency technique (Kupfer et al., 1978; Akiskal et al., 1982a).

THE EFFECT OF AGE

Childhood

Recent evidence indicates that while rare before puberty, hypomanic and manic episodes are not unknown in children (Campbell, 1953; Kestenbaum, 1979; Davis, 1979; Orvaschel et al., 1981). Although cases of children meeting the usual (adult) criteria for hypomania and mania have sporadically appeared in the literature, the similarity or lack of similarity between bipolar disorder in childhood and bipolar disorder in adulthood has not yet been fully determined. Davis (1979) has offered the following criteria for diagnosing bipolar disorder in children: (1) affective storms, (2) hyperactivity, (3) sleep disturbances, (4) absence of sustained formal thought disorders, and (5) positive family history for affective disorders. While the clinical criteria for diagnosing bipolar illness in prepubertal children still need considerable refinement, many psychotic or behaviorally disturbed children from families with bipolar history do respond to lithium carbonate (Youngerman and Canino, 1978; McKnew et al., 1981).

Adolescence

Winokur et al. (1969) reported that in a third of their adult manic-depressive probands, onset was during the second decade. Other authors (Loranger and Levine, 1978), who also used retrospective chart review, have come to the same conclusion. Studies at UCLA (Strober and Carlson, 1982) have documented prospectively that depressive as well as manic psychoses are not uncommon between ages 13 and 16 and that when rigorous operational criteria are used, misdiagnosis of bipolar psychosis as schizophrenia can be avoided. These studies have also shown the feasibility of applying the usual (adult) criteria to teenage affective disorders (Carlson and Strober, 1978).

In a recently completed Tennessee study (Akiskal, 1982b), the offspring or younger sibs of adult manic-depressives were observed within one year after the onset of their own symptoms. The results, tabulated in Table 5, show that depressive onsets (both major and dysthymic) are the most common and that insidious onsets (temperamental plus polydrug abuse) are almost as common as episodic onsets. Another interesting finding was that the reasons for psychiatric presentation in these adolescents were essentially the same as the reasons for adult bipolar affective probands (see Table 6).

Table 5.   Types of Onset in the Children and Younger Siblings of Bipolar Patients

TYPES OF ONSET	N (TOTAL = 68)	PERCENT
Affective onset (N = 57)		
Episodic (N = 35)		
Major depressive episode	24	35.3
Manic episode	8	11.8
Mixed state	3	4.4
Intermittent (N = 22)		
Dysthymic disorder	12	17.7
Cyclothymic disorder	10	14.7
Undiagnosed at onset		
Polydrug abuse	11	16.2

Source: summarized from Akiskal (1982b).

Table 6.   Clinical Presentation of Adolescent- and Adult-Onset Bipolar Patients[1]

Clinical Presentation	Adolescents (N = 68)	Adults (N = 68)
Psychosis	16.2	16.2
Alcohol and drug problems	10.3	10.3
"Moody"	11.8	16.2
Suicidal ideation/attempt	8.8	10.3
Academic (job) failure[2]	8.8	10.3
Philosophic brooding	7.4	5.9
Obsessional brooding	7.4	4.4
Somatic complaints	7.4	5.9
School phobia (staying at home)[2]	7.4	10.3
"Hyperactivity"	5.9	5.9
Stupor	5.9	4.4
Flagrant antisocial behavior	2.9	1.5

[1] Expressed in percentages within groups
[2] Items in parentheses refer to equivalent clinical presentation in adult.
Source: summarized from Akiskal (1982b).

In summary, onset of bipolar illness with cyclothymia, dysthymia, and polydrug abuse is common in adolescence, and depressive onsets outnumber nondepressive onsets. Major affective disorders meeting adult criteria, as well as affective psychoses (often misdiagnosed as schizophrenia), are far more common in adolescence than previously suspected. Finally, the existing data do not seem to support the prevalent clinical opinion that adolescents are more likely than adults to manifest affective disturbances in antisocial acting out or substance abuse.

Late Life*

Although depressive states are the most frequent mode of bipolar illness in the teens, hypomanic and manic episodes also make their appearance relatively early in the course of the illness (Coryell and Winokur, 1980). A first episode of mania after the age of 65 is rare (Roth, 1955; 1976; Post, 1962; 1982), but when bipolar illness has begun in early life, a late-life transformation of depression to mania is not unknown (Shulman and Post, 1980; Akiskal et al., 1982b).

Angst et al. (1973) have shown that depressive attacks become more common with age and that the interval between affective episodes shortens. Grof et al. (1974) have argued that while such recurrence is common, after many years patients may reach a threshold beyond which the illness burns out, but this interesting claim remains unproven.

Chronic forms of bipolar illness are not unknown. One pattern involves what has been termed chronic mania. Not only do patients fail to experience full remissions, but they may intermittently harbor grandiose delusions (Wertham, 1928; Batchelor, 1969); Kraepelin described this severe denouement as manic dementia. Deterioration is often profound, raising questions of differentiation from schizophrenia or superimposed cerebral pathology. Schizophrenia is an unlikely explanation, since the early course of these patients is ordinarily like that of other bipolars. Nor have cerebral factors been conclusively established as etiologic in these chronic manic excitements (Spicer et al., 1973).

In summary, it appears that with advancing age many bipolar patients experience more episodes, especially of a depressive nature, and that a small subgroup undergo a chronic denouement. While the introduction of lithium has certainly improved the short-run prognosis of manic-depressive illness, how lithium has influenced the long-term prognosis of the illness remains uncertain.

SEQUELAE

Social Advantages

Bipolar disorder has major social consequences. On the positive side, those with predominantly hypomanic temperament are ambitious, driven, and enterprising. They climb on the social ladder of success and assume leadership positions (Ostow, 1980). The most conclusive evidence linking bipolar illness and creativity has come from Andreasen's work with creative writers (Andreasen and Canter, 1974).

*Editor's note: For further review of affective disorders in late life, see the chapter by Friedel in Part II of this volume.

The inconsistently reported association between bipolar illness and upper social class (Gagrat and Spiro, 1980) is probably due to the cultural advantage conferred to the bipolar individual by virtue of recurrent periods of mild psychomotor activation. Furthermore, bipolar women tend to marry men of higher social status (Winokur, 1981). However, more severe bipolar excitements and the paralyzing inertia of the depressive phase, especially when episodes occur at a frequent rate, eventually give rise to serious interpersonal and vocational disability in 30 to 45 percent of cases (Braftos and Haug, 1968; Welner et al., 1977). Despite these liabilities, the moodiness and tempestuous life-style associated with bipolar illness seem to have an inherent interpersonal charm.

Interpersonal Complications

Explosive and unpredictable mood swings often cause bipolar individuals to sustain repeated object losses, most clearly evident in their high divorce rate (Brodie and Leff, 1971). According to Gershon et al. (1973), bipolar men tend to marry women with depression (assortative mating), which may be another factor in conjugal instability. The tendency to promiscuity and financial extravagance, as well as instability in work, also contribute to the alienation of loved ones. Some bipolars are dilettante in academic and related pursuits, beginning a given line of study or project with great enthusiasm, but seldom bringing it to full fruition (Akiskal et al., 1979a). In many of these bipolar individuals, personality disturbances are so flagrant that the underlying affective disorder goes unrecognized. These patients are at risk of being labeled character disorders and being denied specific treatment, contributing to further deterioration in their social status.

Substance Abuse

It is a common clinical observation that polydrug and ethanol abuse are frequent complications in bipolar illness. This is especially true of sedativism to self-treat insomnia and dysphoric psychomotor excitement (Reich et al., 1974). Such abuse does not necessarily have a dipsomaniacal or episodic pattern, but it may occur on a more or less chronic basis. The increased risk for substance abuse is particularly common in the forms of bipolar illness that have a high frequency of episodes, such as cyclothymia and bipolar II disorder (Akiskal et al., 1977; Dunner et al., 1982). Actually, substance abuse may precede the full-blown manifestations of bipolar illness in as many as 50 percent of cases. This conclusion is based on a finding by the National Institute of Mental Health Collaborative Study on the Psychobiology of Depression (Robert Hirschfeld, personal communication, March 1982). The study has found that almost one half of bipolar cases were classified as chronologically "secondary" to alcoholism and, to some extent, drug abuse. While the risk for excessive drinking does appear elevated in bipolar conditions, it is uncertain whether alcoholism as a disease (as defined in the Feighner criteria, 1972) is more common than would be expected by chance (Morrison, 1974).

Mortality

Suicide in untreated patients remains the major risk of bipolar illness, and it tends to occur relatively early in the course of the illness (Miles,

1977). Among the affectively ill, 15 percent commit suicide, compared with 0.01 percent of the general population. The rate is probably slightly higher for bipolar compared with unipolar disorders (Dunner, 1980). Mortality, largely from cardiovascular causes, also appears modestly increased in bipolar illness (Petterson, 1977; Weeke, 1979), but the reasons for this are not entirely clear.

DIFFERENTIAL DIAGNOSIS OF BIPOLAR DISORDER

Organic Affective Disorders

The need to distinguish bipolar from organic affective disorders arises in connection with secondary manic states which are symptomatic of a medical disorder or drug intoxication (see Table 2). Before ascribing mania to putative medical or toxic causes, it is necessary to document that the organic factor has clearly preceded the affective state and that this factor is of sufficient severity, virulence, or dosage to account for the affective state. Even when a medical or toxic factor is implicated, appropriate treatment of the medical disorder may not terminate the manic psychosis, and instituting lithium carbonate or a neuroleptic treatment may be necessary. Family history for bipolar illness is typically absent in organic affective disorders (Krauthammer and Klerman, 1978), premorbid personality is neither hyperthymic nor cyclothymic, and previous episodes of retarded depression are uncharacteristic. Unless the patient is exposed again to the toxic substance or has a recurrence of the medical disorder, further manic attacks and bipolar course are not ordinarily expected. Systemic lupus erythematosus might be the major exception to this rule. With this disease, manic and stuporous depressive psychoses can recur, giving the semblance of a bipolar course (Guze, 1967; Ganz et al., 1972).

Nonbipolar Major Depressions

Most depressions, especially ambulatory forms, involve neither a melancholic quality nor retarded psychomotor activity. Consequently, few problems develop in differentiating them from bipolar disorder. In adolescents and young adults, however, subtle depressive manifestations are often the precursors of mania (Akiskal et al., 1982b), so the question arises whether the subsequent occurrence of mania can be prospectively predicted in the course of depression.

A transformation to mania does occur in 4 to 33 percent of depressives (Clayton, 1981). Higher rates of transformation are found in recurrent depressions (Akiskal et al., 1979b), endogenous depression (Rao and Nammalvar, 1977), and in long-term follow-up studies (Winokur et al., 1982). Even mild or so-called neurotic depressives experience change in polarity in as many as 18 percent of cases (Akiskal et al., 1978).

Some authors (Dunner et al., 1976) have reported that the interval from first depression to first mania is one to two years. However, recent evidence (Rao and Nammalvar, 1977; Shulman and Post, 1980) indicates that it may be as late as a decade or longer, with a mode of five to six years (Akiskal et al., 1982b). Table 7 lists predictors identified in a cohort of depressives where the onset of depression ranged from age 12 to 65 years. An especially high risk for developing mania exists among young adults who have psychotic depression, particularly postpartum or stuporous psychotic depression. A high risk

Table 7. Diagnostic Performance of Variables Significantly Associated with Bipolar Outcome

Variable	Sensitivity (%)	Specificity (%)	Predictive Value (%)
Onset of depression before age 26	71	68	69
Hypersomnic-retarded depression	59	88	83
Psychotic depression	42	85	74
Postpartum onset	58	84	88
Pharmacologic hypomania	32	100	100
Bipolar family history	56	98	94
Loaded pedigrees	32	95	87
History of affective illness in family for consecutive generations	39	83	72

Source: summarized from Akiskal et al. (1982b).

also exists in anergic-hypersomnic depressions that quickly brighten up with noradrenergic tricyclics. A family pedigree loaded with affective illness also leads to a high risk of developing mania. Significantly, hypomania and mania typically develop in primary depressions and are rare in the context of depressions that are secondary to a validated psychiatric illness such as an anxiety disorder, schizophrenia, sociopathy, or somatization disorder.

Personality Disorders

Recent evidence suggests that personality disturbance in nonpsychotic bipolar disorders is sometimes so flagrant that it effectively masks the affective basis of the disorder. Thus, in a study of cyclothymic and bipolar II disorders, the author and his associates (Akiskal et al., 1977) found that such personality diagnoses as borderline, emotionally unstable, or hysterical were given to bipolar patients. Reasons for these personality diagnoses included the patients' repeated marital failure or romantic breakups, episodic promiscuous behavior, alcohol and drug abuse, uneven work and school record, geographic instability, and dilettantism. It would appear that some patients who were in the past considered to be emotionally unstable characters (Rifkin et al., 1972), hysteroid dysphorics (Liebowitz and Klein, 1979), or borderline (DSM-III), actually belong in the bipolar realm (Akiskal, 1981b). Furthermore, London and Taylor (1982) have recently documented that bipolar patients are not uncommon in prison populations, where they are mistakenly diagnosed as either sociopathic or schizophrenic.

The error of diagnosing bipolar illness as personality disorder occurs as a result of the clinical lore that considers bipolar patients to be warm, pleasant, ambitious, and socially successful. This view tends to disregard the morose and irritable moods that alienate loved ones and co-workers and the frequent episodes of illness that prevent proper ego maturation or ego stability. Three sets of clinical characteristics are useful in distinguishing cyclothymic and related temperaments from personality disorders (Akiskal et al., 1979a). (1) Periods of elevation and depression which typify the affective disorders tend to be endogenous. They come out of the blue, with little external provocation (e.g., patients often awaken in one state or another). (2) Diurnal variation with morning worsening is characteristic. (3) The disturbances of the cyclothymics are typically biphasic. They alternate between psychomotor acceleration and deceleration, hyposomnia and hypersomnia, and so forth. Changes in mood, when not accompanied by such observable behaviors, are unreliable as diagnostic indicators. In addition, recent evidence has shown that REM latency is often shortened during both dysthymic and hypomanic phases of illness (Akiskal et al., 1980; Akiskal, 1982d).

Schizophrenic Disorders

Differentiating bipolar disorder from schizophrenia is not as difficult in practice as diagnostic staff conferences in academic centers would suggest. Predictably, these conferences attract the most controversial cases. The following points are useful in differential diagnosis.

(1) Longitudinal course, characterized by periods of relatively normal or "supernormal" functioning, favors bipolar illness. Such history, which should be routinely obtained from family informants (Braden et al., 1980), carries greater diagnostic weight than a one-time cross-sectional observation of mental status.

(2) A bipolar course in past history is generally incompatible with a schizophrenic disorder (Sovner and McHugh, 1976; Shopsin, 1979; Clayton et al., 1981).

(3) Psychotic symptoms in affective illness typically occur at the height of mania (Carlson and Goodwin, 1973) or at the depth of melancholia, and they seldom persist beyond periods of syndromal mania or depression. Furthermore, the presence of a manic or a melancholic *syndrome* argues against the diagnosis of schizophrenia.

(4) The more reliable Schneiderian symptoms have not been shown to be pathognomonic for schizophrenia (Carpenter et al., 1973). An occasional Schneiderian symptom, especially delusions of somatic passivity (Clayton et al., 1965) or "voices arguing" (Mellor et al., 1981), carries little diagnostic weight for schizophrenia. However, after excluding a concurrent organic psychosis like alcoholic hallucinosis or other drug psychosis, the presence of *multiple* Schneiderian symptoms argues in favor of schizophrenia (Mellor, 1970; Akiskal and Puzantian, 1979). The less reliable Bleulerian signs are more useful when unequivocally present on repeated mental status examination, i.e., persistent incoherence, especially with poverty of content (Andreasen, 1979b), or severe affective flattening (Andreasen, 1979a).

(5) Dramatic response of a psychotic illness to lithium, deterioration when lithium is withdrawn, and remission upon lithium reinstitution favor a bipolar diagnosis. Unequivocal response of a psychotic depression to a tricyclic antidepressant, which occurs more commonly than recorded in the literature (Akiskal and Puzantian, 1979), also favors an affective diagnosis.

(6) Both the DST and the REM-latency test are positive in the depressive and mixed phases of bipolar psychosis (Carroll, 1982; Kupfer et al., 1978). Whether mania can be distinguished from schizophrenia by a blunted TSH response to TRH (Extein et al., 1982) will require further study.

Difficulties in the differential diagnosis for schizophrenia (Akiskal and Puzantian, 1979) arise when bipolar illness develops in mentally retarded individuals (where bizarre excited states commonly occur), in introverted personalities (where psychotic elaborations tend to be

Table 8. Common Errors that Lead to Mislabeling Affective Psychoses as Schizophrenia

TYPE OF ERROR	N(TOTAL = 100)[1]
Unusual premorbid characteristics	
Belief that the premorbid personality of manic-depressives is always cyclothymic, extroverted, friendly, and warm	3
Failure to recognize an affective psychosis in a mentally retarded individual because of hostile belligerence, frenzied agitation, and marked "regressive" tendencies	1
Variation in course	
Belief that affective psychoses are invariably episodic, and the corollary belief that all chronic functional psychoses must belong to the schizophrenic group	25
Lack of familiarity with the phenomenology of mixed affective states and rapid cycling, which may both give rise to unpredictable, unstable, and tempestuous progression of the clinical course	19
"Atypical" clinical manifestations	
Difficulty in distinguishing severe anhedonia from emotional blunting	4
Difficulty in distinguishing flight of ideas from formal thought disorder	30
Failure to appreciate the extent to which the manic patient could become irritable, hostile, cantankerous, and even violent	30
Associating paranoid ideation with schizophrenia	30
Failure to recognize affectively based hallucinations and delusions	100
Heavy reliance on incidental Schneiderian symptoms	10
Equating "bizarre" ideation with schizophrenia	20
Superimposed or epiphenomenal features	
"Organic"-type hallucinations secondary to sleep deprivation and metabolic disturbances	10
Schizophreniform clinical picture due to concomitant drug-induced or drug-withdrawal psychosis	10

[1] Number of affective patients in whom error led to a schizophrenic diagonsis. The total adds up to over 100, because each patient exhibited several of the features listed.
Source: Akiskal and Puzantian (1979).

autistic), or in those with extensive substance abuse (where super-imposed amphetamine psychosis or alcoholic hallucinosis may occur). These and other common errors in the diagnosis of bipolar affective psychoses are summarized in Table 8.

Although blacks have at least the same rate of bipolar illness as whites (German, 1972; Clayton, 1981), they are at some risk for being misdiagnosed as schizophrenic (Adebimpe, 1981), probably because of the higher prevalence of psychotic symptoms in hospitalized black psychiatric patients (Welner et al., 1973).

THE QUESTION OF SCHIZOAFFECTIVE PSYCHOSIS

In DSM-II schizoaffective states were subsumed under schizophrenia (American Psychiatric Association, 1968). DSM-III created a Schizoaffective Disorder category distinct from both the Affective and the Schizophrenic Disorders, but DSM-III did not provide any operational criteria for this diagnosis. This apparent solution to the problems presented by undiagnosed cases of acute psychosis with both affective and schizophrenic syndromes reflects the current uncertainty regarding the nosologic status of these conditions.

Hypotheses regarding schizoaffective states include the following four. (1) They are a variant of schizophrenic disorders. (2) They are a variant of affective disorders. (3) They result from hybrid affective and schizophrenic heredity. (4) They represent a third and distinct psychosis. Because the evidence for hypotheses (3) and (4) has been largely inconclusive to date (Tsuang, 1979; Fischer and Gottesman, 1980), one must conclude that they do not account for the most commonly observed forms of this behavior.

With regard to hypotheses (1) and (2), the cumulative evidence, based on such external validators as family history and course, has tended to favor hypothesis (2), which calls for including schizoaffective states under the affective psychoses (Procci, 1976).* This is particularly true for schizoaffective states which are bipolar in course or have had a manic episode at some point in time (Clayton et al., 1981). In the Schlesser et al. study (1981), 91 percent of bipolar schizoaffectives were DST-positive in their depressive phases, compared with a rate of 52 percent in unipolar (depressed) schizoaffectives. In other words, patients labeled bipolar schizoaffective are as likely as patients with bipolar affective psychoses to have positive DST results, suggesting that they are neuroendocrinologically indiscriminable.

If one studies schizoaffective depressives without regard to polarity, only 24 percent will yield positive DST results (Greden et al., 1981), suggesting that heterogeneity exists among schizoaffectives, especially nonbipolar schizoaffectives. But even within the limits of this heterogeneity, the sleep EEGs of schizoaffectives are not much different from those of patients with affective psychoses (Kupfer et al., 1979). This suggests that the proportion of schizoaffectives who would not fall within the affective psychosis category is very small.

Why then, one may ask, has there been such confusion about the nosologic status of schizoaffective psychoses? The author believes that this rubric has been unnecessarily used for apparent depressions occurring in the context of well-established schizophrenic illnesses. In this light, it is redundant to invoke the concept of schizoaffective disorder for these schizophrenia-related "depressions." These conditions have several different underlying mechanisms (Donlon et al., 1976; Siris et al., 1981; Johnson, 1981; Knights and Hirsch, 1981).

Depressive symptoms in a schizophrenic patient can be caused by neuroleptic medication, in which case the term pseudodepression would be most appropriate. In another mechanism, the nonspecific vegetative signs associated with schizophrenic relapses can combine with such well-known schizophrenic features as low self-esteem and a sense of incompetence and powerlessness to lead to a mistaken diagnosis of clinical depression. Another underlying mechanism involves the existential suffering and personal anguish that schizophrenic patients, particularly the young and intelligent, experience as a result of having

*Editor's note: In the early part of his chapter in Part V, Gershon discusses the evidence from family studies of the relatives of schizoaffective probands.

a mentally crippling illness. These are truly reactive depressions and may develop the syndromal criteria for a major depression. In this case, the disorders warrant *separate* schizophrenic and major depressive diagnoses. Finally, when schizophrenia develops in the context of an attention deficit disorder, certain manifestations of the latter disorder may mimic clinical depression. The situation is further confused because this disorder may respond favorably to imipramine (Cole, 1980).

The conditions described above represent manifestations, correlates, or complications of chronic schizophrenia and do not constitute a separate schizoaffective entity. The author has also demonstrated that bipolar schizoaffective states are best considered to be bipolar affective psychoses with mood-incongruent features. Judging from DST data, acute nonbipolar schizoaffective states are heterogeneous: some are related to major depression (and should be categorized as major depression with mood-incongruent psychotic features), while others cannot be so characterized. In the author's view, the concept of schizoaffective disorder as a distinct category, neither schizophrenic nor affective, should be restricted to this residual group of nonbipolar, nonorganic acute psychoses which cannot be classified under psychotic major depressive disorder. Defined in this way schizoaffective psychosis would become a rare disorder which somewhat overlaps with the concept of cycloid psychosis (Perris, 1974). This disorder has six distinguishing characteristics (Akiskal et al., unpublished data). (1) Onset is acute. (2) Confusion and disorientation occur commonly. (3) Affective and schizophrenic syndromes coexist during the same episode. (4) Schizophrenic symptoms are apparent at the onset of psychosis. They are not a transient mood-incongruent phase at the height of a psychotic illness. (5) Full recovery is typical. (6) Course is nonbipolar, in that all episodes are similar in kind.

SUMMARY

Recent clinical research experience has considerably broadened the concept of bipolar illness to incorporate a spectrum of disorders very similar to Kraepelin's original description of manic-depressive illness. The spectrum has five major categories. The first category includes bipolar schizoaffective and many unipolar schizoaffective psychoses (i.e., affective disorders with mood-incongruent psychotic features). A second category is made up of bipolar I disorder, characterized by at least one episode of full-fledged mania. Bipolar II disorder makes up the third category, and it is characterized by anergic-hypersomnic major depressive episodes and brief hypomanic periods of subclinical intensity. The fourth category is made up of unipolar II disorder, which includes recurrent endogenous depressions with bipolar family history. A fifth and final category consists of cyclothymic disorder and also subsumes overlapping affective temperaments ranging from hyperthymia to subaffective endogenous dysthymia.

With the exception of manic states secondary to medical and toxic factors, bipolar affective illness appears to be a distinct psychopathological disorder. While it is heterogeneous in clinical phenotypes, separate genetic subtypes of the disorder have yet to be delineated. It is understandable why Kraepelin hypothesized that a single morbid process lay behind these polymorphic manifestations.

Chapter 19

Drug Treatment of the Acute Manic Episode
by David L. Dunner, M.D.

This chapter discusses the treatment of acute manic disorders. Since diagnosis is the key to treatment, the chapter first discusses certain problematic aspects of the differential diagnosis of acute manic disorders. Following this is a discussion of the setting for treating acute mania, and particularly whether the patient should be hospitalized. Next the chapter reviews the evidence for the efficacy of lithium carbonate in treating acute manic disorders and the principles involved in lithium therapy. The use of lithium combined with antipsychotic medication is then discussed. Finally, the chapter reviews some complications of treatment and special considerations.

The ravages of acute manic disorders were described well in a classic article by Pollock (1931). This article described the course of acute mania in the hospital during an era that predated modern treatment. These severe illnesses resulted in prolonged hospitalization, often of several months' duration and often with considerable mortality. In contrast, modern treatment of bipolar disorder is preventative. Maintenance therapy with lithium carbonate has served largely to prevent rehospitalization for manic episodes in patients with recurrent bipolar affective disorder.

It is often easier to diagnose bipolar affective disorder during subsequent attacks than during an initial episode. The differential diagnosis of an initial attack must include a variety of mental as well as medical syndromes. Even for the initial episode, however, consideration of mania in the differential diagnosis of acute psychotic episodes will often lead to proper diagnosis and treatment.

DIAGNOSTIC CONSIDERATIONS

The United States-United Kingdom study (Cooper et al., 1972) revealed that American psychiatry needed to amplify and clarify the diagnosis of manic-depressive and other affective disorders. Cases of mania diagnosed by British-trained psychiatrists were diagnosed in various other ways by American-trained psychiatrists. The American psychiatrists had been trained largely in a diagnostic methodology which equated psychotic symptoms with a diagnosis of schizophrenia. Furthermore, studies by the Washington University group (Winokur et al., 1969) pointed to a separation of mania from other affective disorders on the basis of familial data. The diagnostic criteria developed by these researchers (Feighner et al., 1972) form the basis for the current DSM-III diagnostic nomenclature (American Psychiatric Association, 1980). DSM-II had employed a broad concept of schizophrenia, and DSM-III considerably narrows this concept. Moreover, the triage style of diagnosis reflected in DSM-III forces clinicians toward a diagnosis of bipolar affective disorder if the symptoms of mania are present. The DSM-III criteria for the diagnosis of mania are illustrated in Table 1. The DSM-III criteria consist of inclusion criteria and exclusion criteria. The inclusion criteria relate to the duration of symptoms and the number

Table 1. DSM-III Criteria for Mania

A. [A period of] elevated, expansive, or irritable mood . . .

B. Duration of at least one week . . . [and] three of the following symptoms (four if the mood is only irritable)
   (1)   increase in activity . . .
   (2)   more talkative than usual or pressure to keep talking
   (3)   flight of ideas or subjective experience that thoughts are racing
   (4)   inflated self-esteem (grandiosity, which may be delusional)
   (5)   decreased need for sleep
   (6)   distractibility . . .
   (7)   [impulsivity,] excessive involvement in activities which have a high potential for painful consequences

C. Neither of the following dominate the clinical picture when an affective syndrome (i.e., criteria A and B above) is not present, that is, before it developed or after it has remitted:
   (1)   preoccupation with a mood-incongruent delusion or hallucination . . .
   (2)   bizarre behavior

D. Not superimposed on either Schizophrenia, Schizophreniform Disorder, or a Paranoid Disorder.

E. Not due to any Organic Mental Disorder, such as Substance Intoxication.

Source: American Psychiatric Association (1980).

of symptoms required to establish the diagnosis. Exclusion criteria distinguish bipolar disorder from other illnesses.

The application of DSM-III criteria will increase the diagnosis of mania in American psychiatry, and this will address some of the problems revealed by the United States-United Kingdom study. On the other hand, the DSM-III criteria may encourage an unnecessarily broad concept of bipolar disorder. The DSM-III criteria differ from the Feighner et al. (1972) criteria in that the Feighner et al. criteria have a primary-secondary distinction, while DSM-III does not. Manic symptoms occurring in a patient with another preexisting psychiatric disorder would thus be diagnosed as a secondary affective disorder in the Feighner et al. system, but not in the DSM-III system. Krauthammer and Klerman (1978) have discussed secondary mania, manic episodes which occur in the course of other psychiatric or medical illness.* Since DSM-III does not separate disorders into a primary-secondary format, such cases would be included in bipolar affective disorder, and this could unnecessarily widen our concept of the condition.

Much of the research on manic disorder in the United States in the 1960s and 1970s dealt with patients who had been hospitalized specifically for mania. The author and his colleagues termed such patients bipolar I patients when they had primary affective disorder and had been hospitalized specifically for mania (Dunner et al., 1976b). Patients who were hospitalized for depression and had histories of hypomania were classified as bipolar II. The Research Diagnostic Criteria, a forerunner of DSM-III, attempted to differentiate patients with depression and mania from patients with depression and hypomania, corresponding to the earlier concepts of bipolar I and bipolar II affective disorders. However, the final formulation of DSM-III somewhat obscured this dis-

*Preceptor's note: In the preceding chapter, Akiskal reviews this concept in greater detail.

tinction. Cases of bipolar II affective disorder would presumably be classified as Atypical Bipolar Disorder in DSM-III. However, many patients with bipolar II affective disorder will reportedly meet criteria for Bipolar Disorder in DSM-III because their hypomanic symptoms are sufficient to meet the DSM-III criteria for mania (Dunner et al., 1982). Although the DSM-III criteria will make for greater interrater reliability among clinicians in the diagnosis of manic-depressive illness, and manic episodes in particular, the application of DSM-III will not be totally concordant with prior research studies involving manic patients. However, since most of the research on treatment of acute mania used hospitalized patients, it should be assumed that such patients would meet DSM-III criteria for Bipolar Disorder.

Clinical Issues

Although the typical euphoric manic may be relatively easy to diagnose, the affect of some manic patients is irritable (Murphy and Beigel, 1974). Patients with an irritable manic syndrome are often more difficult to diagnose than the euphoric manic.

Another clinically apparent diagnostic problem is that the patient who has a relapsing illness with good to normal interim functioning between episodes can fail to meet inclusion criteria for mania during the acute episodes. For example, in their study of reactive psychosis, McCabe and Strömgren (1975) noted that these patients had familial factors which were similar to those in patients with affective disorder and patients with schizophrenia. They concluded that a reactive psychosis represented a disorder which was neither manic-depressive illness nor schizophrenia, although some of their patients were rediagnosed as bipolar on readmission.

The pendulum of diagnosis for mania may have swung from the point of underdiagnosis to the point of overdiagnosis. Many clinicians now feel that any episodic disorder is a form of manic-depressive illness, even if the patient has not evidenced the inclusion criteria for manic symptoms. Although maintenance treatment (with lithium carbonate) may be clinically indicated for such patients, the evidence that this treatment is beneficial for them is lacking in comparison with the benefits shown for strictly defined bipolar patients. The evidence for using lithium carbonate for treating such patients' acute episodes is also lacking.

An additional problem for clinicians is the patient who has a history of both affective disorder and hallucinogen use. Some patients describe a manic syndrome years after the extensive use of hallucinogenic drugs. These patients are often clinically diagnosed as bipolar because they describe transitory elations and depressions and they have histories of impulsive behavior. This group of patients probably fits the concept of secondary mania, and a DSM-III diagnosis of Organic Affective Disorder may be more appropriate for them than a diagnosis of Bipolar Disorder.

The author and his colleagues reviewed the course of development of mania in patients who had diagnosed bipolar illness and found that in approximately 80 percent of cases mania was present at the onset of the psychiatric disturbance (Dunner et al., 1976a). Thus, many patients with bipolar I affective disorder will be hospitalized for mania as their first psychiatric contact or will be hospitalized for depression and abruptly develop mania. It is unusual for patients to have either a long course of recurrent depression or a long course of treatment for other psychiatric symptoms prior to the development of a manic syndrome. The usual age of onset for bipolar I disorder is in the 20s, although 5 percent of patients with bipolar I affective disorder have a history of psychiatric treatment before the age of 15, and about 5 percent of patients have their initial psychiatric treatment after the age of 50. Bipolar I disorder has an earlier onset compared with bipolar II disorder and unipolar depression, as determined from data from the Lithium Clinic of the New York State Psychiatric Institute (see Table 2).

As a clinical guide, mania should be diagnosed in patients who have no prior psychiatric diagnosis and who develop a syndrome with manic inclusion symptoms. The DSM-III criteria allow the clinician to include patients with mood-incongruent delusions in a bipolar diagnosis, and data support this inclusion (Rosenthal et al., 1980). In contrast, mania should not be diagnosed in patients who have an acute psychosis without manic inclusion symptoms or who have other preexisting psychiatric disorders or medical illnesses of the type that may be accompanied by manic syndromes. Although DSM-III does not provide for a diagnosis of secondary mania, such a diagnosis may be clinically appropriate in certain cases. Etiologic considerations should lead to a fairly extensive medical work-up, including thyroid studies and evidence for other hormonal disturbances, recent use of stimulant medication or caffeine, infections, neoplasms, and epilepsy (Krauthammer and Klerman, 1978).

In summary, euphoric and grandiose patients who meet the criteria for bipolar illness remain relatively easy to recognize and diagnose within the framework of bipolar affective disorder. Patients whose mania may be characterized as irritable can also have bipolar illness but continue to present diagnostic problems. On the other hand, the DSM-III criteria probably define manic syndromes too broadly: they lead to including cases of secondary mania and to overincluding milder forms of hypomania. The considerable amount of data regarding treatment of mania was obtained through the study of a core group of typical manic patients. When clinicians cannot achieve the treatment responses that would be expected from the literature about manic patients, they may

Table 2.   Age of Onset of Bipolar I, Bipolar II, and Unipolar Depression

| Age | Cumulative Percentage Receiving Treatment at Age Indicated | | |
	Unipolar (N = 50)	Bipolar II (N = 90)	Bipolar I (N = 159)
15	2.0	2.2	5.0
19	10.0	10.0	20.2
25	20.0	28.8	46.2
29	30.0	41.1	56.0
35	42.0	58.8	71.1
39	52.0	73.3	79.2
45	62.0	83.3	89.3
49	78.0	85.6	95.6
55	90.0	94.4	98.7
59	94.0	95.6	99.3
65	98.0	100.0	100.0
69	98.0		
75	100.0		

Source: data from the Lithium Clinic, New York State Psychiatric Institute.

be treating an atypical patient or a patient with secondary mania in whom the response to treatment may be less predictable.

The foregoing applies mainly to diagnosing mania in patients who have not previously been diagnosed as having a bipolar illness and who in general are not undergoing maintenance therapy with lithium carbonate. The effects of lithium maintenance treatment are to decrease the frequency and severity of recurrent manic episodes (Stallone et al., 1973). However, such episodes may occur in spite of lithium maintenance treatment. These manic relapses may pose diagnostic difficulties for the clinician because the manic symptoms may occur in an unusual form. For example, a patient undergoing lithium maintenance therapy may present with only part of his or her usual manic syndrome (such as diminished need for sleep and somewhat impulsive behavior), and not with full-blown manic psychosis. Other patients have brief periods of rapid thoughts and grandiosity without the full constellation of symptoms typical of mania. As a clinical guide, a manic (or hypomanic) relapse should be considered if the behavior of the lithium-maintained bipolar patient becomes unstable. Symptoms that are particularly helpful in this consideration seem to be disturbances in sleep and social activity.

WHERE THE PATIENT SHOULD BE TREATED

For most manic episodes aside from relapses during lithium maintenance treatment, the patient should be treated in a hospital setting. The usual course of mania includes such an escalation in behavior that hospital treatment becomes necessary. Moreover, manics often stop their treatment when it is attempted on an outpatient basis. Hospitalization is thus necessary both to effect continuation of treatment and to protect the manic patient from the physical and social consequences of the episode. Prior to lithium treatment, most of the relapses of bipolar patients involved mania, and most of these relapses resulted in hospitalization (Dunner et al., 1979a). Thus, knowledge of the natural course of illness is helpful in designing a treatment plan.

Manic patients are at times assaultive and dangerous to others, and their assaultiveness may lead either to hospitalization or to incarceration. Parenthetically, in the criteria for bipolar I affective disorder, being jailed for manic episodes or being otherwise confined aside from in a hospital (as with hospital-type care in the home) is considered equivalent to being hospitalized. The manic patient may become physically exhausted from sleeplessness, hoarse from overtalkativeness, or grandiose and may attempt feats which are not physically possible. Socially unacceptable behavior may also escalate during mania. Such behaviors may include sexual promiscuity and overspending the family's resources. For the most part, patients who are hospitalized for mania show clear evidence of at least one of these factors. They are hospitalized essentially for their own protection as well as for the protection of their family members. In the hospital, patients can be controlled within a physical space and can have access to telephones limited. Generally they can be prevented from spending money, although one patient once spent an inordinate amount of money in the hospital gift shop. Furthermore, patients can be observed in a controlled situation, and medication can be more effectively administered within the hospital setting.

On the other hand, some relapses during lithium treatment and certain hypomanic episodes can be effectively treated in an outpatient setting. This is especially true when treatment is begun early in the course of the hypomanic disorder and when the patient is agreeable to taking medication and following through with frequent outpatient appointments. Support from the patient's family is often quite helpful in effecting such treatment.

The hypomanic episodes characteristic of bipolar II patients rarely require treatment (Dunner et al., 1976b). About 20 percent of patients diagnosed as bipolar II receive outpatient treatment for mania. This is because psychosis is not present during their episodes and because many patients diagnosed as bipolar II are productive or creative during their hypomanic periods.

EVIDENCE FOR THE EFFICACY OF LITHIUM CARBONATE IN ACUTE MANIA

Since the time that Cade (1949) reported that lithium was an effective antimanic drug, several well-conceived and well-controlled studies have demonstrated the efficacy of lithium carbonate in acute mania. Studies comparing lithium carbonate with placebo were performed by Schou et al. (1954), Maggs (1963), Bunney et al. (1968), Goodwin et al. (1969), and Stokes et al. (1971) (see Table 3). These were generally two-week studies, and they demonstrated that lithium was considerably more effective than placebo in the treatment of acute manic excitement. Most of the studies had either a randomized design or a crossover design. Notably, Bunney et al. (1968) used a placebo substitution technique with two patients, and random substitution of placebo for lithium carbonate resulted in an increase in the mania ratings of both patients while they were receiving placebo.

Lithium has also been compared with other antipsychotic drugs, particularly chlorpromazine and haloperidol. In most studies lithium was at least as efficacious as the antipsychotic agents. When Prien et al. (1972b) separated patients into more actively and less actively manic groups, they found that chlorpromazine seemed to be more efficacious in the more actively manic patient, while lithium carbonate was more efficacious in the less actively manic, hospitalized patient. Shopsin et al. (1975) compared the effects of lithium, haloperidol, and chlorpromazine in manic patients. They found that lithium was more efficacious than the other two drugs for the treatment of acute mania.

In addition to the several well-controlled studies that indicate the efficacy of lithium salts for acute mania, over one hundred published reports support the use of lithium in the acute manic phase of manic-depressive illness. In a review of these papers, Prien (1979) notes that

Table 3. Studies Comparing Lithium Carbonate with Placebo Treatment for Acute Mania

Source	Number of Patients	Duration of Treatment	Result
Schou et al. (1954)	30	2 weeks	Lithium better than placebo
Maggs (1963)	18	2 weeks	Lithium better than placebo
Bunney et al. (1968)	2	Longitudinal	Increase in mania with placebo substitution
Goodwin et al. (1969)	12	2 weeks	66 percent response to lithium
Stokes et al. (1971)	38	10 days	Lithium better than placebo

the controlled and uncontrolled studies involve over 3,000 patients in twenty countries.

Studies generally indicate that approximately 80 percent of patients with acute mania will respond to lithium treatment, but it should be noted that most of the studies were two or three weeks in duration. The placebo-controlled studies were generally two weeks in duration, and most of the studies comparing lithium with other antipsychotic drugs lasted for three weeks. Notably, Takahashi et al. (1975) found that several patients who had not responded to lithium within a two- to three-week trial did respond by five weeks. Since the natural history of mania may include a several-month illness, the failure of patients to respond within a short period of time should not necessarily be taken as evidence of an incorrect diagnosis.

PRINCIPLES OF LITHIUM THERAPY

The principles of lithium therapy involve the medical preparation of the patient and the monitoring of lithium concentration in the serum (Dunner, 1981). Lithium is a potent medication and has numerous side effects, particularly cardiac, antithyroid, and renal effects. The patient must therefore have a good medical work-up prior to the institution of lithium treatment. The work-up should include a physical examination, tests for thyroid function, for kidney function (such as blood urea nitrogen and creatinine), and for white blood count (lithium may increase the white blood count), and for patients over 40, an electrocardiogram. In addition, the patient should have a relatively normal electrolyte picture, and the use of medications such as diuretics which may interfere with the excretion of lithium carbonate should be noted. Once lithium therapy has begun, the patient should be assessed daily or more frequently for the presence of side effects such as nausea, vomiting, diarrhea, or tremor, as well as for manifestations of lithium toxicity, such as confusion, hyperactive reflexes, and choreiform movements. Lithium levels should be monitored frequently, at least two or three times in the first week of lithium treatment and at least weekly thereafter. Lithium plasma or serum levels should always be obtained after doses of lithium have been increased and when the patient's clinical picture changes. The author and his colleagues prefer that the dose of lithium be increased somewhat gradually in order to keep side effects to a minimum and safety at a maximum. By using this approach, satisfactory blood levels can be obtained within five to seven days after beginning treatment.

At least two tests have been proposed for predicting a maintenance dose for treatment (Cooper et al., 1973; Chang et al., 1979). These tests involve first administering a fixed dose of lithium carbonate and then obtaining a blood lithium level at a timed interval after that dose. The blood lithium concentration obtained at that interval is then used to predict the milligrams of lithium carbonate per day needed to achieve a satisfactory blood level, based on the relationship of blood level to dose calculated from other patients' data. In the author's experience, these tests should be avoided. Many patients loaded with lithium in this fashion develop severe gastrointestinal side effects. At least two patients have shown lithium neurotoxic symptoms because the physicians using the test were overly confident that the recommended dosage was all that was required and that lithium levels need not be followed closely.

Frequent adjustment of the dose and frequent clinical monitoring of the patient are imperative for successful treatment of the acute manic episode with lithium carbonate. The dose usually needs to be lowered when the episode abates and the patient begins a post-manic-depressive phase. The author has avoided noting "therapeutic" blood lithium levels in this chapter. Although it is important to monitor blood lithium concentration frequently, the patient's clinical condition, age, state of hydration, and medical condition are all factors in determining dosage. Thus, in some patients the reduction of manic symptoms may require inducing briefly (for a few hours) a mild state of lithium toxicity. In other patients, particularly older patients and those who have underlying renal disease, blood lithium levels should always be maintained at the lower limits of the so-called therapeutic range.

THERAPY WITH LITHIUM AND ANTIPSYCHOTIC MEDICATION

Several studies have compared lithium with antipsychotic medication in the treatment of acute mania (see Table 4). Of particular note is the previously cited study by Prien et al. (1972b) which indicated that chlorpromazine was of greater efficacy than lithium in the more agitated manic patient while lithium was better for the less agitated patient. The studies of Johnson et al. (1968; 1971), Spring et al. (1970), Platman (1970), Takahashi et al. (1975), and Prien et al. (1972b) all employed chlorpromazine as the reference drug, and lithium treatment was at least equivalent in efficacy to chlorpromazine. Shopsin et al. (1975) also studied haloperidol, and they concluded that lithium was better than chlorpromazine or haloperidol for the treatment of acute mania, although the number of subjects (thirty) was small. Prien (1979) concluded that all three drugs have proven efficacy in treating manic behavior but that there was disagreement as to their comparative efficacy. In his review of these studies, Kocsis (1981) noted methodological problems in all. He recommended using lithium alone for the treatment of most acutely manic patients, since research regarding the efficacy of combined treatment (lithium with antipsychotic medication) is lacking.

Table 4. Studies Comparing Lithium with Antipsychotic Medication Treatment for Acute Mania

Source	Number of Patients	Duration of Treatment	Comparison Drug	Result
Johnson et al. (1968)	28	3 weeks	Chlorpromazine	Remission: lithium 78% and chlorpromazine 36%
Platman (1970)	23	3 weeks	Chlorpromazine	Lithium better
Spring et al. (1970)	12	3 weeks	Chlorpromazine	Remission: chlorpromazine 3/5
Johnson et al. (1971)	21	3 weeks	Chlorpromazine	Remission: chlorpromazine 6/7
Prien et al. (1972)	225	3 weeks	Chlorpromazine	Chlorpromazine better with highly active Lithium better with mildly active
Shopsin et al. (1975)	30	3 weeks	Haloperidol, Chlorpromazine	Lithium best, then haloperidol, then chlorpromazine
Takahashi et al. (1975)	77	5 weeks	Chlorpromazine	Moderate improvement: lithium 68% and chlorpromazine 47%

Most clinicians do not use lithium alone for the treatment of acute mania but combine lithium with an antipsychotic drug. The choice of antipsychotic drug should be predicated on the severity of the mania as well as on the willingness of the patient to take medication. For example, if the patient is unwilling to take medication orally and requires intramuscular injections to control the mania in the initial few days, then lithium carbonate cannot be prescribed. If the patient is showing irregular compliance with taking pills, then lithium can be given in liquid form. If the patient is severely manic, high-potency intramuscular neuroleptics, such as haloperidol or thiothixene, in addition to lithium may be indicated for the control of acute manic excitement in the initial few days of treatment. If the patient's mania is more moderate, the author recommends using a less potent but more sedating antipsychotic medication, such as thioridazine or chlorpromazine. The latter drugs are usually given at bedtime, perhaps with additional medication for sleep. In general the author and his colleagues find that the manic illness will be controlled after the patient can be made to sleep regularly at night.

Some evidence suggests that in some patients combined therapy, particularly lithium with haloperidol, results in brain damage. The initial report concerned four patients who had neurological syndromes from the combination (Cohen and Cohen, 1974), but they may have represented instances of prolonged and untreated lithium toxicity. However, sporadic reports do continue to suggest that this combination of medication results in neurological symptoms. Recently, Thomas et al. (1982) reported that patients treated with haloperidol and lithium showed greater verbal-performance discrepancies on the WAIS than did patients treated with chlorpromazine and lithium. They suggested taking care in prescribing haloperidol with lithium.

The author suggests paying careful attention to the hydration status of patients who are treated with combined therapy. It is possible that such patients are at greater risk for developing lithium neurotoxicity (on the basis of their impaired hydration) than are patients treated with lithium alone.

COMPLICATIONS OF TREATMENT

Lithium toxicity is the most serious complication of lithium therapy. Neurotoxic effects include confusion, ataxia, choreiform movements, seizures, coma, and death. Although lithium is usually measured in the serum, lithium toxicity should be viewed as an intracellular phenomenon wherein lithium ions accumulate within cells and disrupt normal homeostatic intracellular mechanisms. The first treatment measure for lithium toxicity is to prevent its occurrence through careful monitoring of patients. When lithium toxicity develops, the general principles are to discontinue lithium therapy and to rehydrate the patient with fluids and electrolytes. Potassium administration is often critical, because intracellular hypokalemia frequently results from lithium toxicity.

Older patients are prone to develop lithium toxicity much more frequently than younger patients (Dunner et al., 1979b). This is due to many factors, including the compromised renal function in older patients and their frequent medical need for other medications which have effects on lithium metabolism. Thus lithium should be cautiously increased in older patients.[*]

*Editor's note: For further discussion of the use of lithium with older patients, see the chapter by Friedel in Part II of this volume.

It is generally safer to begin lithium with a patient who is already taking a diuretic than to add a diuretic with a patient who is already taking lithium. Changes of sodium metabolism during lithium treatment may lead to an increase in lithium reabsorption by the kidney and result in lithium toxicity. Thus, once lithium therapy is instituted, administering diuretics and reducing sodium in the diet should be avoided.

An initial diuresis usually accompanies lithium treatment, but patients are unlikely to develop severe polyuria during the treatment of acute mania. However, some patients who have been treated with lithium in the past and who have shown evidence of polyuria may develop a diabetes-insipidus-like syndrome during treatment of acute mania. Indeed, one patient in the author's experience urinated approximately ten liters a day during treatment of acute mania with lithium carbonate. When the lithium was discontinued, her mania became worse, and her thirst also increased. Thus, she urinated almost twice that amount when taken off lithium. Other authors have also noted an increase in thirst and urine output during mania. Polyuria during lithium treatment for acute mania should therefore not necessarily be taken as evidence of lithium nephrotoxicity.

Complications of combined treatment with antipsychotic medication include the usual side effects of these medications, such as dry mouth, blurring of vision, and orthostatic hypotension. Parkinsonian reactions may occur during treatment with antipsychotic medication, and the patient may require treatment with an antiparkinsonian medication. Dosage of the antipsychotic medication should be regulated so as to minimize side effects.

Finally, the manic patient creates an interpersonal toll on those caring for him or her. Those stressed by being with the manic patient include family members as well as staff. Often, reviewing the excellent paper by Janowsky et al. (1976) with relatives and staff can help to alleviate interpersonal tension.

SPECIAL CONSIDERATIONS

The use of electroconvulsive therapy has not been studied as well as the use of lithium or antipsychotic agents. McCabe and Norris (1977) analyzed data from a retrospectively collected group of manics treated with chlorpromazine and electroconvulsive therapy. On follow-up they noted similar outcomes in the two groups.

Schizoaffective disorder presents special complications, since the criteria for the disorder have not been stated to the point of facilitating a high degree of interrater reliability. While the diagnosis is listed in DSM-III, criteria for the diagnosis are not. Many clinicians use the schizoaffective category to refer to patients who have a manic syndrome complicated by Schneiderian first-rank symptoms or bizarre delusions. As pointed out earlier (Rosenthal et al., 1980), approximately one third of manic patients will have bizarre psychotic symptoms during the course of mania. Carlson and Goodwin (1973) also demonstrated that many otherwise typical manic patients will demonstrate such psychotic symptoms. Prien et al. (1972a) reported that excited "schizoaffective" and manic patients had similar responses to lithium and chlorpromazine. The more active patients responded best to chlorpromazine, and the less active patients responded best to lithium. Most clinicians faced with a patient who has a manic syndrome complicated by psychotic features would opt for treatment with an antipsychotic drug in combination with lithium treatment. When such patients have a remitting psychiatric disorder, they often show an excellent response to combined treatment.

Rapid-cycling bipolar patients present particular treatment difficulties, since the treatment should be directed both toward the acute manic relapse and toward preventing future cycles (maintenance treatment). The author and his colleagues reported that rapid-cycling bipolar patients did show benefits from lithium therapy (Dunner et al., 1977). In general, antidepressants should be avoided in such patients, and treatment with lithium carbonate and low doses of antipsychotic medication may be helpful (Dunner, 1979). The thyroid status of rapid cyclers should be carefully assessed, since these patients seem to be very sensitive to the antithyroid effects of lithium (Cho et al., 1979). Recently, thyroid hormone has been reported to be of benefit to such patients (Stancer and Persad, 1982). The anticonvulsant carbamazepine has also been beneficial to rapid cyclers (Ballenger and Post, 1980).

Patients who are being treated with lithium maintenance therapy and who have mild manic relapses can sometimes be treated as outpatients. Often, increasing the lithium dose and adding a small dose of an antipsychotic medication at bedtime to assist sleep will suffice to treat the relapse. However, such patients should be seen frequently on an outpatient basis, because their condition may escalate and hospitalization may be required or they may develop side effects from medication.

SUMMARY

Important principles in the treatment of acute mania include diagnosis and determination of medication, either lithium carbonate alone or in combination with antipsychotic medication. The medical health of the patient should be assessed carefully prior to instituting treatment. Dosage of medication and the clinical state of the patient should be monitored carefully during treatment. Psychosocial aspects of treatment must also be considered, with careful attention paid to interactions of the patient with his or her family and with the treatment staff.

The diagnosis of mania in this country was once problematic. It is now routine. Lithium therapy for acute mania was once controversial. It is now accepted. These advances in knowledge have resulted from years of careful research into a most fascinating clinical state—manic-depressive illness.

Chapter 20 # Long-Term Prophylactic Pharmacologic Treatment of Bipolar Illness
by Robert F. Prien, Ph.D.

INTRODUCTION

During the past 15 years, clinical and research interest in the affective disorders has shifted from the treatment of acute episodes to treatment over the long term. This shift stems not only from the availability of effective pharmacologic treatments, but also from a greater knowledge of the longitudinal nature of the affective disorders. Interest in the long-term treatment of affective illness has been most evident in the area of bipolar disorder. Bipolar illness has a strong tendency for recurrence, and only a minority of untreated patients can expect to escape with but one or two episodes. Surveys indicate that approximately 80 percent of patients experiencing an initial manic episode will have subsequent episodes of mania or major depression (Winokur et al., 1969; Nystrom, 1979). According to a survey developed by the Department of Health and Human Services (1979), the average female experiencing an onset of bipolar disorder at age 25 can expect to lose approximately 9 years of life and 14 years of major life activity (work, school, keeping house) if the illness goes untreated. Bipolar disorder is therefore a highly legitimate focus for long-term pharmacotherapeutic approaches.

This chapter deals with the research findings and the issues and strategies that pertain to the long-term preventive drug therapy of bipolar disorder. Before beginning this review, several definitions are necessary. The term *long-term preventive therapy* here refers to pharmacologic treatment which is administered over long periods of time for the purpose of preventing future episodes or reducing their severity and duration. Long-term preventive therapy differs from *continuation maintenance therapy* which is administered following the initial control of acute symptomatology for the purpose of maintaining control over the episode. These two types of maintenance therapy, though distinguishable in theory (Quitkin et al., 1976), are often blurred in clinical practice. It may be extremely difficult to determine when continuation therapy ends (i.e., when the episode is over) and when preventive therapy begins. As a rule of thumb, either six months of symptom-free behavior or a return to usual functioning after pharmacologic control of acute symptomatology is considered evidence that the episode is over (Klerman, 1978). It is recognized, of course, that with some patients the interval between episodes may be considerably shorter than six months.

Some researchers have subdivided the bipolar classification into bipolar I and bipolar II. Bipolar I patients have a history of at least one manic episode. Bipolar II patients have a history of hypomanic episodes and depression, but no history of mania. It is unclear whether the bipolar II classification represents a separate diagnostic category or whether it should be included in the bipolar or unipolar categories. The only preventive therapy trial separately identifying unipolar, bipolar I, and bipolar II patients suggests that in terms of therapeutic response the bipolar II classification corresponds more closely to the unipolar than to the bipolar I classification (Dunner et al., 1976b). In this chapter, the term *bipolar* is used only where patients had a history of mania.

Reports on the effectiveness of long-term maintenance therapy with lithium first appeared in the early 1960s (Hartigan, 1963; Schou, 1963; Baastrup, 1964). It was not until several years later that long-term maintenance treatment attracted widespread attention. In 1967 Baastrup and Schou compared the course of illness before lithium therapy against the course of illness during lithium therapy in a large sample of patients. They concluded that "lithium is the first drug demonstrated as a clear-cut prophylactic agent against one of the major psychoses" (Baastrup and Schou, 1967, 172). This report prompted well-publicized rebuttals (Blackwell and Shepherd, 1969) and generated questions and issues that have been partially, but not entirely, resolved by subsequent placebo-controlled trials.

This chapter addresses several of the critical questions that may be asked of long-term preventive drug therapy: (1) Who should receive treatment? (2) What drug should be used? (3) How effectively will the drug modify the course of illness? (4) How long should treatment be administered? (5) Is psychotherapy of value to a long-term preventive drug therapy program? (6) What dosage should be employed?

WHO SHOULD RECEIVE TREATMENT

Several factors should be considered in determining whether to start long-term preventive drug therapy: the likelihood of a recurrence in the near future; the severity and abruptness of previous episodes and the potential impact of a subsequent recurrence on the patient, family, job, and therapeutic relationship; the patient's willingness to commit himself or herself to a program of indefinite maintenance treatment; the presence of possible medical contraindications to long-term treatment; the patient's response to prior antimanic or antidepressive regimens; and the family's insight into the illness and capacity to recognize and report the first signs of a recurrence.

Most clinicians feel that a patient should have had at least two or three well-defined episodes requiring psychiatric treatment before being treated with long-term preventive pharmacotherapy. Patients who have had only a single attack, who have had only mild attacks, or who have had a long interval between episodes (i.e., over five years) should probably not receive long-term treatment. An exception is the patient for whom a second episode would be life threatening or highly disruptive to career or family functioning. For patients with regular seasonal episodes, preventive drug treatment might be considered only for vulnerable periods (Ban and Hollender, 1981).

Supportive data indicate the rationale for using long-term preventive therapy after two episodes. Angst et al. (1973) conducted a survey on the natural course of affective illness at five European centers and clearly demonstrated the relationship between episode frequency and risk of recurrence in bipolar illness. As shown in Table 1, cycle length (the period

Table 1.   Relationship between Episode Number and Mean Cycle Length

Number of Episodes	Mean Cycle Length (Months)
1	33
2	21
3	16
4	13
5	11
6	11
7	10
8	11
9	9
10	8

Source: Angst and Grof (1976).

between the onset of one episode and the onset of the next, including the period of the first episode) tends to decrease with successive episodes through the first four or five episodes and then plateaus. Average cycle lengths range from 33 months for the first episode to 21 months for the second to 11 months for the fifth. The progressive decrease in cycle length is attributed to a shortening of the intervals in between the episodes, rather than to any change in the lengths of the episodes themselves. These findings, combined with those of other surveys, suggest that patients with two or more episodes are at risk for an early recurrence and might be suitable candidates for preventive pharmacotherapy.

Factors other than frequency of prior episodes may also affect the risk of recurrence. The frequency of recurrences tends to increase with increasing age. Zis and Goodwin (1979) calculated the probability of a recurrence within the two years following the initial episode as a function of the patient's age. As shown in Table 2, the older patient at the onset of first illness, the greater the likelihood of an early recurrence. The risk of recurrence for bipolar patients who suffer their first episode after age 30 is estimated to be twice as high as the risk for patients with an earlier onset.

Using survey data to determine the risk of recurrence for individual patients does have limitations. Many of the surveys of the course of affective illness have focused exclusively on episodes requiring hospitalization (Zis and Goodwin, 1979). In their aforementioned study, Angst and associates (1973) recorded both inpatient and outpatient episodes, but since they selected all the patients from hospital records, the patients had to have had at least one episode severe enough to require hospitalization. How accurately one can generalize from these populations to populations with less severe episodes is a matter for speculation. In addition, the group statistics presented in many survey reports fail to reflect the tremendous variability in the course of illness among individual patients. Some patients may remain episode free for many years after the initial episode, while others may have their second episode within a few months. Even patients who have had two or three episodes within a two-year period are not necessarily doomed to a recurrence during the following two years. Grof and associates (1979) examined the relationship between the frequency of prior episodes and the risk of recurrence for patients not treated with maintenance medication. Whenever the patient met the criterion of having had two

Table 2.   Probability of a Recurrence within 24 Months following the First Episode

Age at First Episode	Probability of Recurrence
Under 20	0.2
20 through 29	0.2
30 through 39	0.5
40 through 49	0.5
50 through 59	0.6
60 and over	0.8

Source: Zis and Goodwin (1979).

episodes within two years, they counted the number of episodes the patient had in the successive two years. The investigators found that 35 percent of the bipolar patients did not have a recurrence. When they extended the criterion to three episodes within a three-year period, this reduced the percentage of patients who failed to have a recurrence during the following two years to 31 percent.

In conclusion, to determine whether the patient will benefit from long-term drug therapy, the physician must still rely upon information specific to the individual case, e.g., the potential consequences of a subsequent episode, the patient's prior response to medication, and the attitudes of the patient and family toward the maintenance program. Knowledge of the general principles governing the natural course of affective illness can, however, be a valuable aid in supplementing the information gained from the individual history.

CHOICE OF DRUG

The clinician's choice of medication for long-term preventive therapy in bipolar illness is relatively limited. Only six treatments have been evaluated in controlled long-term studies: lithium, imipramine, imipramine plus lithium, carbamazepine, flupenthixol, and placebo. Controlled trials are summarized in Table 3. All but one of the trials used lithium as one of the treatments.

LITHIUM VERSUS PLACEBO   Six studies have compared lithium with placebo (Baastrup et al., 1970; Coppen et al., 1971; Cundall et al., 1972; Stallone et al., 1973; Prien et al., 1973a; Prien et al., 1973b). In all six, lithium was significantly superior to placebo in reducing the frequency of recurrences (statistical significance is based on the $p = .05$ level, as determined by Fisher's Exact Probability Test.) Summed across studies, 33 percent of the lithium-treated patients had a recurrence, compared with 81 percent of the placebo-treated patients. These findings were the basis of the 1974 decision by the Food and Drug Administration to approve use of lithium for the long-term maintenance treatment of bipolar disorder.

When one looks separately at manic and depressive recurrences, the picture is less clear. The studies conclusively demonstrate that lithium is more effective than placebo in reducing the occurrence of manic episodes. Lithium-treated patients had fewer manic episodes than placebo controls in all studies; in only one study did the difference between treatments fail to reach statistical significance. While the studies also suggest that lithium is superior to placebo in reducing the occurrence of depressive episodes, the evidence is not as conclusive as it is for manic episodes. Lithium-treated patients had fewer depressive episodes in all studies, but in only one was the difference between treatments statistically significant. One problem in interpreting the data on depressive recurrences is that most of the treatment failures on placebo had a manic rather than a depressive episode, leaving a relatively small data base from which to establish statistical significance for depressive recurrences.

LITHIUM VERSUS IMIPRAMINE   The Veterans Administration-National Institute of Mental Health (VA-NIMH) Collaborative Study of Lithium Therapy (Prien et al., 1973b) found lithium to be significantly

Table 3. Controlled Trials of Long-Term Pharmacologic Treatment

Investigators	Design	Trial Period (mos.)	Treatment	N	Total Failures	p	Manic Failures	p	Depressive Failures	p
Baastrup et al. (1970)	Outpatients previously on lithium; half switched to placebo. *Criterion for failure:* episode requiring hospitalization or use of nonstudy drugs.	5	Lithium	28	0 (0%)	<.001	0 (0%)	<.01	0 (0%)	<.01
			Placebo	22	12 (55%)		7 (32%)		6 (27%)	
Coppen et al. (1971)	Patients randomly assigned to two treatments. *Criterion for failure:* no major improvement over pre-study global clinical state.	14	Lithium	17	3 (18%)	<.001	Not Reported		Not Reported	
			Placebo	21	21 (100%)					
Cundall et al. (1972)	Outpatients previously on lithium: half switched to placebo, with crossover after 6 months. *Criterion for failure:* same as for Baastrup et al.	6	Lithium	12	4 (33%)	<.05	1 (8%)	<.05	3 (25%)	n.s.
			Placebo	12	10 (83%)		9 (75%)		5 (42%)	

Study	Description	N	Treatment	n	(%)	p	n (%)	p	n (%)	p
Stallone et al. (1973)	Outpatients (some previously on lithium) randomly assigned to two treatments. *Criterion for failure:* episode requiring nonstudy drugs.	28	Lithium	25	11 (44%)	<.001	5 (20%)	<.02	7 (28%)	n.s.
			Placebo	27	25 (93%)		15 (55%)		13 (48%)	
Prien et al. (1973a) (VA-NIMH-I)	Patients randomly assigned to two treatments after hospitalization for acute mania. *Criterion for failure:* same as for Baastrup et al.	24	Lithium	101	43 (43%)	<.001	32 (32%)	<.001	16 (16%)	n.s.
			Placebo	104	84 (80%)		71 (68%)		27 (26%)	
Prien et al. (1973b) (VA-NIMH-II)	Patients randomly assigned to three treatments after hospitalization for acute depression. *Criterion for failure:* same as for Baastrup et al.	24	Lithium	18	5 (28%)	Note[1]	2 (11%)	Note[2]	4 (22%)	Note[3]
			Imipramine	13	10 (77%)		7 (54%)		4 (31%)	
			Placebo	13	10 (77%)		5 (38%)		8 (62%)	
Kane et al. (1981)	Patients euthymic for 6 weeks randomly assigned to two treatments. *Criterion for failure:* episode meeting RDC for major depression, mania, minor depression (4 weeks or more), or hypomania (1 week or more).	18–24	Lithium	38	8 (21%)	n.s.	4 (11%)	n.s.	4 (11%)	n.s.
			Lithium + Imipramine	37	12 (32%)		9 (24%)		3 (8%)	

Table 3. (Continued)

Investigators	Design	Trial Period (mos.)	Treatment	N	Total Failures	p	Manic Failures	p	Depressive Failures	p
Ahlfors et al. (1981)	Patients randomly assigned to two treatments. *Criterion for failure:* not defined.	18	Lithium	14	.60	n.s.[4]	Not Reported		Not Reported	
			Flupenthixol	19	Note[4] .64					
Okuma et al. (1981)	Patients randomly assigned to two treatments. *Criterion for failure:* marked decrease in frequency, severity, or length of episodes over prestudy state.	12	Carbamazepine	10	4 (40%)	n.s.	4 (40%)	n.s.	Not Reported	
			Placebo	9	7 (78%)		7 (78%)			

[1]Lithium vs. imipramine: p = .02; lithium vs. placebo: p = .02; imipramine vs. placebo: n.s.

[2]Lithium vs. imipramine: p = .02; lithium vs. placebo: n.s.; imipramine vs. placebo: n.s.

[3]All comparisons: n.s.

[4]Mean number of episodes per patient per year (difference between treatments: n.s.)

more effective than imipramine in preventing manic episodes and equally as effective as imipramine in preventing depressive recurrences. Preliminary findings from the ongoing five-hospital NIMH Collaborative Study of Maintenance Drug Therapy in Affective Disorder (Prien, unpublished data) also demonstrate that lithium is significantly superior to imipramine in reducing the frequency of manic episodes. In both studies, approximately 55 percent of the imipramine-treated patients developed a manic episode, compared with 11 percent of the lithium-treated patients in the VA-NIMH study and 30 percent in the five-hospital collaborative study. It is not possible to determine whether this high incidence of manic recurrences on imipramine resulted from imipramine-induced mania or from the failure of imipramine to prevent naturally occurring manic episodes. Although much has been written about the tendency for tricyclic antidepressants to precipitate manic attacks or to cause a switch from depression into mania (Bunney, 1978; Lewis and Winokur, 1982), this phenomenon has not been demonstrated in long-term controlled studies. The VA-NIMH study showed no major difference between imipramine and placebo in the incidence of mania. But regardless of what interpretation one chooses regarding the high incidence of manic recurrences in imipramine-treated patients, imipramine is not recommended for the long-term preventive treatment of bipolar disorder.

LITHIUM VERSUS LITHIUM PLUS IMIPRAMINE The rationale for combining lithium and imipramine is that lithium will protect the patient against manic recurrences and imipramine will provide protection against depressive recurrences. In the only controlled trial evaluating the combination, Kane and associates (1981) reported that 32 percent of patients treated with lithium plus imipramine had a recurrence, compared with only 21 percent of those who received lithium alone. The difference between treatments was due almost entirely to the higher incidence of manic recurrences on the combination.

LITHIUM VERSUS FLUPENTHIXOL Flupenthixol decanoate is an antipsychotic drug that may also possess antidepressant properties (Kielholz et al., 1979). The drug's long-term effectiveness in bipolar illness was evaluated by Ahlfors and associates (1981). Comparing flupenthixol with lithium in 33 patients, they found no difference in the incidence of recurrence between the two groups, and neither group showed significant improvement over the prestudy course of illness. The lack of effect with lithium was attributed to a "prognostically negative" selection of patients. In an uncontrolled trial of flupenthixol in 85 bipolar patients (Ahlfors et al., 1981), the results suggested that the drug may warrant further study in patients whose disorder is dominated more by manic than depressive recurrences. Flupenthixol is not marketed in the United States.

CARBAMAZEPINE VERSUS PLACEBO Carbamazepine is an anticonvulsant used extensively in temporal lobe epilepsy. The drug has been reported to have significant antimanic properties (Ballenger and Post, 1978; Okuma et al., 1979). The long-term efficacy of carbamazepine has been evaluated in only one small-sample study.

Okuma and associates (1981) reported that carbamazepine was more effective than placebo in reducing the incidence of both manic and depressive recurrences; however, the difference between treatments failed to reach statistical significance at the p = .05 level. Uncontrolled trials (Okuma and Kisimoto, 1977; Post, 1982) suggest that carbamazepine may be effective for cases not responding to lithium.

IMIPRAMINE VERSUS PLACEBO The only study comparing imipramine with placebo found no significant difference in frequency of recurrences between the two treatments (Prien et al., 1973b).

OTHER DRUGS Unquestionably, lithium must be considered the drug of choice for the long-term maintenance treatment of bipolar illness. However, before attaching too much significance to this claim, note that, with the exception of imipramine, lithium is the only drug that has been adequately evaluated in this disorder. It is possible that tricyclic antidepressants such as nortriptyline or amitriptyline may be more effective than imipramine in preventing depressive recurrences and may involve less risk of mania. Newer antidepressants such as amoxapine, buproprion, maprotiline, mianserin, and trazodone also require careful evaluation of their effectiveness as long-term preventive treatments. Precursor amines such as L-tryptophan or L-5-hydroxytryptophan may be of use in protecting against depressive recurrences. Carbamazepine, which offers promise as a useful alternative to lithium for both acute mania and long-term treatment, also needs further study. Other antiepileptic drugs such as valproic acid may be similarly effective. Finally, neuroleptics, alone or in combination with lithium, may be beneficial for selected patients. A long-term trial with neuroleptics would appear most justifiable with patients who develop severe manic recurrences while receiving lithium.

EFFECTS ON THE COURSE OF ILLNESS

Both the clinician and the patient must have realistic expectations about the benefits and risks of long-term preventive drug therapy. This section deals only with lithium since other drugs have not been carefully evaluated for their long-term efficacy in bipolar illness.

Clinical Efficacy

Lithium is far from a panacea for bipolar disorder. Failure rates for lithium in long-term preventive trials average 30 to 40 percent. (In most studies, failure is defined as the appearance of an episode requiring either hospitalization or treatment with a psychopharmacologic agent other than lithium.) The failure rate tends to increase significantly where the patient has a history of rapid cycling, poor compliance in taking medication, or atypical features such as formal thought disorder or mood-incongruent delusions or hallucinations (Dunner and Fieve, 1974; Prien, 1980). Patients with an underlying characterological disorder or "neurotic" personality also tend to respond less positively to lithium therapy (Coppen et al., 1982).

With patients who are responsive to lithium, the question arises whether the drug actually prevents the occurrence of major episodes or whether it merely dampens an emerging episode sufficiently to prevent a full attack. Research findings suggest that the drug may act in both ways, depending upon the individual case (Kukopulos et al., 1975; Schou and Thomsen, 1975). Despite the differing opinions about how lithium modifies the course of illness, most do agree that only a minority of patients show complete normalization of the disorder during lithium treatment. Schou (1980) has reported that only about one fifth of the patients who are suitable candidates for lithium treatment can be expected to have a complete cessation of recurrences. The remaining four fifths will manifest varying frequencies and severities of recurrences, ranging from rare and mild attacks to frequent and severe episodes.

Some patients who show complete cessation of episodes may show unusual mood stability. DePaulo and associates (1982) have reported that episode-free lithium-treated patients tend to show significantly less day-to-day mood variability than do normal control subjects. This mood stability may be a mixed blessing to the patient, for the patient may perceive the stable state as an unpleasant constriction of mood (see below regarding adverse reactions).

A source of disagreement is the question of whether a patient who has a moderate to severe episode during lithium treatment should be reinstated on the drug after the episode has been resolved. The literature reflects three positions on this question. (1) Patients who fail once on lithium are at high risk for a subsequent failure and should not be continued on the drug (Prien et al., 1973a; Dunner et al., 1976a). (2) Recurrences that occur early in treatment should be tolerated since the full prophylactic effect of lithium may be achieved only gradually. Episodes may occur during the first months or even the first year of treatment, but they will become shorter and less severe and eventually disappear (Schou, 1980). (3) Success or failure of lithium therapy must be evaluated against the course of illness before treatment (Angst and Grof, 1976). Accordingly, a patient who suffers a recurrence every one to two years during lithium therapy is considered a treatment success if he or she had more frequent or severe episodes before treatment.

Perhaps the strongest argument for continuing long-term lithium therapy after an initial recurrence is that no well-tested alternative to lithium therapy exists in this situation. It would be much easier to discontinue lithium if there were something appropriate to offer in its place. On the other hand, lithium is not an innocuous treatment, and continuation of therapy without reasonable expectation of benefit may needlessly expose the patient to the risk of adverse reactions.

In sum, until more data are available, the decision to continue or discontinue lithium treatment after a recurrence must be determined on an individual basis, taking into account factors such as the prelithium course of illness, the patient's tolerance to lithium, and the adequacy of dosage.

Adverse Reactions

Lithium produces adverse reactions in a large proportion of patients during long-term treatment. The most prevalent are fine hand tremor, polyuria and polydipsia, and weight gain. Vestergaard and associates (1980) recorded side effects in 237 patients during long-term lithium therapy and found that 70 percent had polydipsia, 45 percent developed hand tremor, 25 percent complained of nycturia, 20 percent had a weight gain exceeding ten kg, 20 percent complained of periodic "troublesome" diarrhea, and 10 percent had edema, usually in the feet and ankles. Less frequent side effects included dermatologic problems, hypothyroidism with or without goiter, and muscle weakness. Nine tenths of the patients had one or more of the adverse reactions. A control group of manic-depressive patients about to start long-term treatment reported none of the aforementioned effects. Other studies (Schou et al., 1970) have reported similar incidences of side effects.

During the past few years, considerable attention has been focused on the long-term effects of lithium treatment on renal structure and function. Renal biopsy studies have revealed structural changes (interstitial fibrosis, tubular atrophy, and glomerular sclerosis) in some lithium-treated patients (Hestbech et al., 1977; Davies and Kincaid-Smith, 1979; Rafaelson et al., 1979). The significance of these changes is not known. A number of recent studies have failed to confirm a significant relationship between lithium treatment and renal damage (Braden et al., 1981; Ramsey and Cox, 1982). Furthermore, the relationship between the morphological damage and functional impairment is not clear. The issue is unlikely to be settled until the results of ongoing prospective studies are available. Reports also suggest that lithium-induced nephrogenic diabetes insipidus may persist for months after cessation of lithium treatment (Rabin et al., 1979; Bucht and Wahlin, 1980). It is not known to what extent this condition is irreversible, slowly reversible, or rapidly reversible. Existing studies have not ruled out the possible contributions of factors such as other psychopharmacologic agents and concurrent medical illness (Coppen et al., 1980).

Since the studies available to date are not definite and at worst suggest that a small minority of patients develop significant renal insufficiency, fear of renal effects should not deter the clinician from employing lithium for appropriate clinical indications. The clinician should, however, monitor renal function carefully to detect possible impairment in glomerular filtration rate and renal concentrating capacity. Vestergaard, Schou, and Thomsen (1982) offer a reasonable approach to monitoring renal functioning during long-term treatment. They believe that elaborate determinations of glomerular function such as creatinine clearance are unnecessary in physically healthy patients who have no history of renal disorder. They do recommend serum lithium and serum creatinine determinations every two to four months. Serum creatinine levels should be closely observed for increased values within the normal range as well as for raised absolute abnormal values. The authors also suggest that thyroid-stimulating hormone (TSH) levels be obtained every six months to detect thyroid complications. For further discussion of baseline tests and monitoring schedules, see Vestergaard (1980), Galenberg (1981), and DePaulo (1981).

Teratogenic effects of lithium may pose special risks in the case of a woman in her childbearing years. A register of pregnancies exposed to lithium in the first trimester suggests that babies born to lithium-treated mothers have a higher incidence of congenital heart disease (e.g., Ebstein's anomaly) than the general population (Weinstein, 1980). It is usually advisable to stop lithium treatment with patients who plan to become pregnant. If the patient becomes pregnant during lithium treatment, the drug should be discontinued, at least in the first trimester, unless the evidence is convincing that withdrawal would seriously endanger the mother or the pregnancy (Schou, 1980).

Mental functioning may also be affected by lithium. Some patients report feelings of mild depression, tiredness, lethargy, inertia, and constriction of mood during long-term lithium treatment (Schou, 1980). Patients may also experience difficulties in memory and concentration (Ghose, 1977; Kjellman et al., 1980). It is not clear whether these reactions are the direct effect of lithium or whether they are due to an unrecognized mild depressive recurrence or an underlying characterological disturbance. Lithium-treated bipolar patients are particularly susceptible to feeling blunted emotion, impaired creativity, and loss of productivity when hypomanic episodes are flattened.

The impact of even mild side effects on patient compliance should not be underestimated.* A survey of patients receiving long-term lithium therapy (Jamison et al., 1979) identified lethargy, tremor, decreased coordination, and "dulling of senses" as the most aversive and upsetting side effects of lithium. The physician's failure to acknowledge and address these reactions, however mild they may appear, may adversely affect patient compliance and the success of the therapeutic program.

DURATION OF TREATMENT

A critical decision facing the practitioner is how long to continue long-term maintenance drug therapy. There is no evidence that long-term preventive drug therapy cures bipolar illness. There is evidence, however, that recurrences may cease spontaneously after many years of illness. A survey by Angst and Grof (1979) indicated that one of eight bipolar patients over 65 years of age stops having episodes. This suggests that patients who have had a long duration of illness and who have been free of abnormal mood swings for several years may no longer require medication. But the only way to determine whether a patient still needs long-term preventive therapy is to discontinue treatment and to follow the patient carefully for signs of a recurrence.

In deciding whether to discontinue treatment, the physician and the patient should consider the likelihood and potential consequences of a new episode and balance these considerations against the risks involved in continuing medication. When the patient has a history of attacks characterized by suicide attempts, need for hospitalization, or serious disruption of career or family life, medication should not be discontinued unless the physician and the patient are reasonably sure that subsequent episodes can be detected early enough to prevent serious symptomatology from developing. Some clinicians recommend an arrangement in which the physician and patient agree to continue drug treatment for a specific period such as five years (Schou, 1980). After this period, they discuss whether treatment should continue, taking into account the course of illness before and during treatment and any adverse effects that the medication may have had on the patient's social, mental, and physical functioning. In discussing the risks of discontinuing medication, the physician should explain carefully that several studies of patients who had maintenance medication withdrawn after years of treatment found a high incidence of recurrences within the six months following withdrawal (Baastrup et al., 1970; Bialos et al., 1982).

*Preceptor's note: This topic is a major focus of the following chapter by Jamison and Goodwin.

OTHER CLINICAL MANAGEMENT ISSUES

Drugs and Psychotherapy

The combined use of psychotherapy and drugs for the long-term treatment of bipolar disorder has not been studied well. Although patients with bipolar disorder have traditionally been considered poor candidates for psychotherapy, some promising results have emerged when psychopharmacologic and psychotherapeutic approaches were combined. Long-term group psychotherapy or structured psychological support may enhance drug compliance and acceptance of long-term drug therapy programs (Shakir et al., 1979). Psychotherapy may also help to ameliorate the social, family, and daily coping impairments that can result from frequent and severe manic and depressive recurrences (Davenport et al., 1977; Jamison, 1982). Jamison and Goodwin discuss these areas of treatment further in the next chapter.

Other Factors Affecting Treatment Outcome

Two factors that can have a particularly adverse impact on the outcome of long-term therapy are inadequate dosage and poor compliance in taking medication.

DOSAGE No well-defined dosage strategy exists for long-term preventive therapy with bipolar illness, even for a drug studied as well as lithium. The maintenance dose guidelines specified in the lithium package insert (for maintaining serum levels at 0.6 to 1.2 mEq/l) are based primarily on the trial-and-error experiences of individual investigators. Most practitioners seek to maintain serum levels at the lower end of the range, typically 0.6 to 0.9 mEq/l (Prien and Caffey, 1977). However, the threat of renal complications and other adverse reactions with long-term lithium treatment have caused some clinicians to recommend even lower maintenance doses (0.4 to 0.6 mEq/l) (Brown, 1973; Jerram and McDonald, 1978; Hullin, 1980).

Two studies warrant examination. In a trial designed to determine minimum effective plasma levels for long-term maintenance therapy, Jerram and McDonald (1978) found that levels below 0.5 mEq/l were just as effective as levels exceeding 0.7 mEq/l. A follow-up study with the same patients (Hullin, 1980) indicated that the relapse rate did not increase until plasma levels fell below 0.4 mEq/l. The author and his colleagues obtained markedly different results from the VA-NIMH study (Prien and Caffey, 1976): levels above 0.7 mEq/l were associated with significantly fewer recurrences than levels below 0.5 mEq/l.

The difference in results from the two studies may be due, at least in part, to differences in the respective patient populations. The VA-NIMH study treated a high-risk group of patients who had just recovered from a severe manic or depressive episode and followed them for 24 months. In the Jerram and McDonald study, the patients were lithium responders who had been on a stable lithium maintenance dose for at least 6 months and in most cases for a period of years. This study followed patients for a period of 12 months after adjusting the dosage. Thus, it would appear that the Jerram and McDonald study used a group at lower risk for an early recurrence than the VA-NIMH study, and it may have missed some recurrences due to the shorter follow-up period. Nonetheless, the findings from the Jerram and Mc-

Donald study are provocative in that they suggest that the established dose guidelines for lithium may be higher than necessary for some patients. This may be particularly true for patients who have been clinically stable for a number of years. The results from the VA-NIMH study have equally strong implications. Doses of less than 0.6 to to 0.7 mEq/l may not provide adequate protection for bipolar patients who are just starting on lithium maintenance treatment following a severe episode, and some patients may require levels of 0.8 mEq/l or higher.

Even more uncertainties surround the question of dosages of antidepressants. No established dosage guidelines or plasma-level ranges exist for long-term preventive therapy with the tricyclics or other classes of antidepressants. In general, clinicians tend to employ tricyclic doses on the very low end of the therapeutic range (100 mg/day or less) to avoid anticholinergic side effects and toxicity and to reduce the risk of a manic attack (Giller et al., 1979).

Careful dose-response studies of long-term preventive treatment with lithium and other appropriate treatments are clearly needed.

PATIENT COMPLIANCE A critical, but frequently neglected factor affecting the success of any program of maintenance drug therapy is patient compliance. Without the cooperation and support of the patient and the family, even the most carefully titrated medication regimen is destined to fail. Noncompliance is a common problem with patients on long-term maintenance treatment programs. For example, surveys suggest that 25 to 50 percent of patients receiving long-term lithium therapy discontinue medication, reduce dosage, or otherwise fail to take medication as prescribed (Van Putten, 1975; Ban, 1979; Jamison et al., 1979; Jamison, 1982). Many suffer recurrences as a result. Patients may refuse to continue long-term preventive drug therapy for a variety of reasons. Patients who are feeling well and have no symptoms to remind them of their illness may see no need to continue medication. They may also miss the productivity associated with hypomanic periods. Patients may experience annoying or embarrassing side effects such as fine hand tremor. Some patients may equate lifetime need for treatment with the stigma of incurable illness and may attempt to test or deny the presence of mental illness by stopping treatment. Patients with manic symptomatology may have an exaggerated sense of well-being and discontinue medication. In the next chapter, Jamison and Goodwin elaborate on patients' reasons for noncompliance and ways of improving acceptance of the treatment program and adherence to the medication schedule. Suffice it to say here that increased emphasis on techniques for improving patient compliance may significantly increase the success rate with lithium and other treatments.

Plasma-level measures of both lithium and antidepressant drugs may be useful for evaluating patient compliance in taking medication. Loo and associates (1980) obtained the plasma levels of several antidepressants over a 3- to 26-month period. They reported that good response was associated with small fluctuations in plasma levels over time, while poor response was associated with large fluctuations which were usually due to poor patient compliance. Thus, the variations of plasma levels over time may be useful for identifying patients who are at high risk for poor response because of their noncompliance.

SUMMARY

Controlled studies of long-term preventive drug therapy provide information on six treatments: lithium, imipramine, lithium plus imipramine, carbamazepine, flupenthixol, and placebo. These studies have had four major findings. First, lithium is significantly superior to placebo in reducing the occurrence of manic episodes. Studies also suggest that lithium is more effective than placebo in reducing the occurrence of depressive episodes, but the evidence here is less conclusive than it is for manic episodes. Second, lithium is superior to imipramine by virtue of its greater effectiveness in protecting against manic recurrences. Third, the combination of lithium and imipramine provides no advantage over lithium alone. And fourth, carbamazepine appears to be more effective than placebo, but this finding requires confirmation.

Among the treatments evaluated, lithium must therefore be regarded as the drug of choice for the long-term treatment of bipolar disorder. But the need to evaluate other drugs is clear. Lithium is not a panacea; approximately one third of patients treated with lithium in controlled studies are classified as treatment failures. They develop an episode severe enough to require either hospitalization or treatment with psychopharmacologic agents other than lithium. Whether treatments other than those reviewed are equally effective or more effective than lithium has not yet been determined.

Other gaps remain in our knowledge of how best to treat the long-term course of bipolar illness. Relatively little information exists on the effectiveness of long-term therapy with patients who have a history of mild or infrequent episodes. We have no comprehensive dose-response studies to guide the practitioner in adjusting dosage. We do not know how long an effective long-term drug therapy program should be continued. Even more important, we cannot yet predict accurately how the individual will respond to long-term therapy. In the case of lithium therapy, the evidence indicates that patients who have a history of rapid cycling, atypical features, poor compliance in taking medication, and poor therapeutic response to lithium do not do well on long-term preventive lithium therapy. However, there is no evidence that these patients respond any better to other agents. Even among lithium responders, we cannot predict specifically how the drug will modify the course of illness. While some patients may show a reduced frequency of episodes, others may have less severe or shorter episodes. In general, good response to lithium appears to be the result of an admixture of good patient selection, proper drug administration, and the patient's acceptance of the program and adherence to the medication schedule. It is difficult to fit these variables into a formula that will predict success or failure for the individual patient. For the time being, the clinician must continue to rely on empirical trials to determine responsiveness to lithium and other treatments.

In conclusion, although many unresolved issues remain concerning the long-term preventive drug treatment of bipolar illness, there is no question concerning the ability of drugs such as lithium to reduce significantly the considerable recurrent morbidity associated with the disorder. Further research will be necessary before we can refine the treatment programs to gain the maximum benefit for the largest group of patients.

Chapter 21

Psychotherapeutic Issues in Bipolar Illness†

by Kay R. Jamison, Ph.D. and Frederick K. Goodwin, M.D.

INTRODUCTION

Psychoanalytic Perspectives

Biological assumptions about the etiology of bipolar illness (and, of course, clinical pragmatism) long ago determined the dominance of organic therapies in the treatment of this illness. Thus, physicians, ancient and modern, have sought cures not through talking and listening, but through direct actions of control: mineral baths, bloodletting, herbs, chains, vapors, bromides, opiates, warm waters, cold waters, and physical and chemical restraints. For quite obvious reasons, psychotherapy has never been an integral or comfortable part of the treatment of bipolar illness. Clearly the "psychotic" disorders and their empirically derived remedies long predate psychological treatments. Both history and necessity have embedded bipolar illness in medicine, much more so than the "neurotic" disorders. Unipolar depressions, on the other hand, have had an easier alliance with psychotherapy. In part this is because they generally constitute a wider spectrum of psychopathology that shows a range of milder syndromes with prominent psychological factors. Because depression encompasses a relatively normal spectrum of emotions and feelings, it has traditionally stimulated counsel from priests, physicians, and friends.

How then was "manic-depressive illness" perceived by the pioneers in the field of psychotherapy, the psychoanalysts? Patients suffering from manic-depressive illness did not fare particularly well with most psychoanalytic writers as potential candidates for psychoanalytic treatment. Fromm-Reichmann (1949) characterized manic-depressives as lacking in "complexity and subtlety;" Abraham (1927) described them as "impatient, envious, exploitive, and with dominating possessiveness;" and Rado (1928) felt them to be continually involved in a "raging orgy of self-torture." As analytic patients, manic-depressives were generally compared with schizophrenics and found to be lacking in introspection and too dependent and "clingy" (Fromm-Reichmann, 1949), disconcertingly able to find vulnerable spots in the therapist (Fromm-Reichmann, 1949; Janowsky et al., 1970), and often able to elicit strong feelings of countertransference in the analyst (Rosenfeld, 1963; English, 1949).

Thus, prior to the availability of lithium, limited enthusiasm for treating bipolar illness is easy to understand. One can imagine the frustration of attempting to treat psychotherapeutically a hypomanic or manic patient, or in fact trying to get or keep such a patient in the office, let alone trying to engage him or her in a meaningful therapeutic endeavor. Likewise, any clinician can appreciate the different kind of frustration involved in treating a profoundly depressed patient. The natural history of the illness carries an exceedingly high spontaneous remission rate which no doubt encouraged therapists in some cases to

---

†This chapter is a revised and shortened version of a chapter in *Manic-Depressive Illness*, by Goodwin, F.K. and Jamison, K.R. New York, Oxford University Press, 1983.

attribute changes to their therapeutic interventions. Conversely, therapists in other cases would tend to assume responsibility when no change or a relapse occurred.

Why emphasize what the analysts have had to say about manic-depressive illness? If the biological substrate and its treatment is so clear, why go back so far in time and science for attitudes and impressions? First, and as always, the psychoanalysts provide a source of clinically descriptive information, virtually all of it from unmedicated patients. This is all the more important because present medical ethics discourage the psychotherapeutic treatment of unmedicated patients with bipolar illness. Second, the psychoanalytic school continues to have a profound effect on clinical thinking about bipolar illness. Not only are most psychotherapists strongly influenced by psychoanalytic conceptions of the illness, but so are many of those who contribute to the biological and pharmacological literature.

The Influence of Lithium on Psychotherapy

In the three decades since Cade's discovery (1949), lithium has moved from a position of therapeutic promise to an extensively studied treatment of choice in bipolar affective disorders. Marketing firms and pharmaceutical companies estimate that more than 120,000 Americans are currently taking lithium (Garth Graham, Smith Kline & French Laboratories, personal communication). These figures are consistent with Jenner and Eastwood's (1978) estimate that one person in 2,000 in the United Kingdom is now receiving lithium.

Lithium treatment is now well established. Patients now remain in remission for long enough periods of time to make psychotherapy a viable adjunctive treatment and long enough to enable therapists to see the underlying personality-character structure emerge as the chaotic mood changes are abated. Consequently, it is timely to reexamine the role of psychotherapy with patients on lithium. Johnson (1980) has discussed the fact that studies of the combined use of lithium and psychotherapy are lacking in the psychiatric and psychological literature. Yet, as he states, the needs for therapy are varied and considerable. Among the more important needs are: (1) analysis of maladaptive behavior patterns which patients acquire during their illnesses and which remain unaffected by lithium treatment, but are amenable to psychotherapeutic intervention; (2) the resolution of interpersonal problems following successful lithium therapy; and (3) support for a long-term prophylactic medication regime.

Characteristics of the illness create certain problems which invite psychotherapeutic intervention. Bipolar illness is chronic, serious, and potentially life threatening. Denial is a natural response. The personal, interpersonal, and social sequelae of the illness are often severe, and they can create catastrophic reactions in patients experiencing recurrent manic and depressive episodes. Suicide, violence, alcoholism, and hospitalization are but a few of the well-established correlates of the illness. Although biological variables predominate in etiology and in much of the symptomatic presentation, the primary manifestations are behavioral and psychological, with profound changes in perception, attitudes, personality, mood, and cognition. Psychological interventions can be of unique value to the patient undergoing such devastating changes in self-perception and the perception of others.

Finally, the fact that bipolar illness is effectively controlled by a chemical treatment makes certain problems particularly difficult to manage *without* psychological interventions. Medication is the central treatment, not an adjunctive one, and from time to time lithium non-compliance is a major theme in the therapy of many patients. Confusion often arises because both lithium and the illness can affect cognition, perception, mood, and behavior. Concerns about being on medication in general and specific concerns about lithium are substantive psycho-therapeutic issues. As the chapter later discusses, these concerns about lithium derive both from the direct effects of lithium on the illness (it deprives some patients of much sought-after highs and energy) and from the side effects of the drug.*

General Issues

From a more general perspective, what are the potential advantages and disadvantages of combining psychotherapy with pharmacotherapy? For relevant studies we must turn to the related but in many respects very different field of drug-psychotherapy interactions in the treatment of unipolar depression; these studies are discussed in more detail else-where in this volume (see the chapter by Cole and Schatzberg in Part V). No comparable controlled studies exist for bipolar illness. In part the reasons mentioned earlier account for this (easier alliance of depression with verbal treatments, less need for restraints, and so forth), and in part the lack of studies stems from the longer period that the tricyclic antidepressants as opposed to lithium have been clinically available in the United States (roughly twenty years instead of ten). Although lithium has been available for a far longer time in Europe, virtually all of the drug-psychotherapy studies have been conducted in the United States.

Klerman (1975) has outlined several potential negative and positive drug-psychotherapy interactions. Particularly relevant to the treatment of bipolar patients would be the hypothesized positive effects of drug treatment on psychotherapy, including increased accessibility of the patient and psychotherapeutically useful symptomatic changes such as increased memory, improved sleep, enhanced verbal skills, decreased distractibility, and so forth. Also relevant are the positive effects of psychotherapy on drug treatment, which include more reliable patient attendance and increased compliance with the drug regimen. Weissman (1978) reviewed the controlled studies of antidepressants alone and in combination with psychotherapy and came to two pertinent con-clusions. First, in ambulatory, unipolar depressed outpatients, the combination of antidepressant medications with psychotherapy (group, individual, or conjoint) was more efficacious than either treatment alone. Second, there were no negative drug-psychotherapy interactions (findings further documented by Rounsaville et al., 1981).

Analogous studies of the treatment of bipolar illness do not exist. Thus, the discussions which follow are limited to more hypothetical issues, supplemented by a few noncontrolled clinical investigations.

*Preceptor's note: As the authors later point out, and as Prien discusses in the preceding chapter, lithium's effectiveness should not be overestimated, and some of its physical side effects warrant careful consideration, particularly with older patients and women who are planning to become pregnant or who are already pregnant.

Several modalities of psychotherapy are available to the clinician wishing to work with patients on lithium. Informal psychological treatments include the supportive role of the physician in medication management, educational models that convey medical information about manic-depressive illness and lithium through lectures, handouts, films, or information-giving groups, and self-help groups modeled on Alcoholics Anonymous and run by patients for themselves. A wide range of theoretical orientations govern more formal psychological treatments such as individual, group, family, and conjoint psychotherapy or some combination of these.

Very little is known about the appropriateness of any of these modalities or orientations for a particular patient or type of presenting problem. For example, we do not know if cognitive-behavior therapy is more effective for lithium compliance problems or if psychodynamic therapy is more appropriate for the interpersonal sequelae of bipolar illness. Likewise, we do not know if group therapy is more useful for problems of illness denial and self-esteem or, relatedly, if individual therapy is more appropriate for short-term crisis intervention in such problems as suicidality or for the long-term treatment of idiosyncratic, intrapsychic problems. There has been no research addressing these issues.

CLINICAL REPORTS ON COMBINED PSYCHOTHERAPY AND LITHIUM TREATMENT

The available clinical reports on combined lithium treatment and psychotherapy are summarized in Table 1. None of these studies focused on the interaction of individual psychotherapy with lithium. Only one of the studies used comparison groups for the analysis of analyzing treatment outcome (Davenport et al., 1977), and only two of the remaining studies, one a continuation of the other (Shakir et al., 1979; Volkmar et al., 1980) used pre- and posttest measures. While the substantial methodological shortcomings in all of these investigations make interpretations virtually impossible, the clinical observations made by the therapists conducting the studies are conceptually very useful.

A recent doctoral study by Cochran (1983) has examined the effect of a modified form of Beck's cognitive therapy on lithium compliance.* In her research Cochran compared 13 patients who received individual short-term cognitive therapy with 13 patients who received standard clinical care at the UCLA Affective Disorders Clinic. The immediate posttreatment phase was admittedly a short follow-up period (six weeks), but was clinically very significant for lithium compliance. During this phase Cochran found a significant ($p < .05$) positive effect of cognitive therapy on increasing lithium compliance. Although the six-month follow-up data are not yet complete, the trend appears to be in the same direction. Compliance was determined by ratings of blind judges (81 percent exact agreement) who examined self-reports, physician ratings, reports by significant others, serum lithium values, and chart notations.

*Editor's note: Kovacs discusses cognitive therapy in some detail in her chapter in Part V of this volume.

COMMON PSYCHOTHERAPEUTIC ISSUES

Overview

Lithium is a unique drug in psychiatry: it is prophylactic, it is both an antimanic and an antidepressant agent, and paradoxically, at high blood levels it can produce signs of both depression (lethargy, slowed speech, impaired cognition, apathy) and, more rarely, mania (a neurotoxicity-induced organic brain syndrome which can mimic or trigger mania). Finally, lithium is a maintenance medication which to date remains relatively free of the unfortunate side effects associated with the use of the phenothiazines and butyrophenones.

Ironically, because lithium is such a highly effective medication, many therapists tend to minimize their own therapeutic role and the role of psychotherapy generally in the treatment of bipolar illness. Although the topic has received little research attention, patients themselves find that psychotherapy is a highly useful adjunct to lithium treatment. In one study (Jamison et al., 1979), twice as many patients as therapists thought that psychotherapy was valuable as an adjunct to lithium treatment.

Without question, the competent and compassionate psychotherapy of bipolar illness is predicated upon a solid knowledge of the illness. Kraepelin's injunction to his turn-of-the-century medical students is still compelling. "It is one of the physician's most important duties to make himself, as far as possible, acquainted with the nature and phenomena of insanity" (Kraepelin, 1904, 3). A solid knowledge of bipolar illness encompasses phenomenology, the natural history of the illness (including its cyclicity and degree of predictability), biological aspects of the illness (including drug responses in mania and depression), biological theories of etiology, and mechanisms of action of the drugs used in its treatment. A good scientific grasp of phenomenology and biology generally increases therapeutic self-assurance, while it decreases two problems common in less comprehensively trained therapists. First, some therapists manifest biological overdeterminism due to their being well-grounded in biological theories but poorly trained in psychological studies such as personality theory and development, perception, motivation, and learning theory. A second problem is the tendency of other therapists to ignore or downplay or, conversely, to overemphasize the biological substrate because of an inadequate understanding of it.

The psychotherapy of bipolar illness requires considerable flexibility in style and technique. Flexibility is necessary because of patients' changing moods, cognitions, and behaviors and the fluctuating levels of dependency that are intrinsic to the illness. In the therapeutic relationship a "long-lead" approach is often useful to maximize the patient's sense of control over his or her behavior. It is important not to overcontrol the patient and not to allow lithium to become the focus of a power struggle. The symbolic value of lithium is enormous, and its role as a projective device is also extremely important (discussed below in greater detail). A thin line exists between overly extensive therapeutic control, which can lead to increased dependency, decreased self-esteem, decreased compliance, and increased acting out, and too little control, which occasionally leads to feelings of insecurity, unnecessarily tenuous holds on reality, and feelings of abandonment. Thus, firmness and consistency in ordering routine lithium levels or tests of thyroid

Table 1. Clinical Reports on Combined Lithium Treatment and Psychotherapy

Author/ Year	Type of Therapy/ Therapeutic Orientation	Study Design/ Treatment Format	Patients	Results	Clinical Observations
Fitzgerald (1972)	*Family Therapy and Lithium.* Eclectic: educational, emphasis on communications, playback of video tape session	Clinical study; no comparison group	N = 25 bipolar, index hospitalization for mania	No systematic follow-up	Family therapy can help manic patients: (1) continue to take lithium, (2) help prevent relapses, and (3) improve verbal communication within family system (i.e., replace the role of mania in the expression of anger and frustration)
Davenport et al. (1977)	*Couples Group Therapy and Lithium.* Psychodynamic	Group I—Couples group therapy four times weekly	N = 12 bipolar patients	No rehospitalizations; no marital failures	Family interactions and social functioning best in couples group therapy; family interaction better in NIMH maintenance group than in community-referred; no significant difference between latter two groups on social functioning
		Group II—NIMH outpatient department lithium maintenance four times monthly; crisis treatment as needed	N = 11 bipolar patients	2 rehospitalized; 5 marital failures	Strong recommendation for co-therapist model
		Group III—Referral back to community—community clinic or private care *Note:* Marriages intact at time of discharge from index hospitalization for all patients; follow-up period variable for all groups (2–10 years posthospitalization)	N = 42 bipolar patients	16 rehospitalized; 10 marital failures; 3 suicides	Marital dynamics: (1) fear, by both partners, of recurrence, (2) sense of helplessness, (3) need to control all affect and defend against closeness, (4) use of massive denial, and (5) themes related to early parental loss and failure to grieve

Study	Type of therapy	Design	Sample	Follow-up	Group themes/comments
Shakir et al. (1979)	*Group Therapy* and Lithium. Interpersonal, interactional, here and now	Clinical study; compared group means of patients' pre- and posthospitalization records. 75 minutes weekly. Lithium dispensed during last 30 minutes of group	N = 15 bipolar patients; 13 men, 2 women; mean age: 43, range: 19–63; mean mo. on lithium prior to group: 21	*Pregroup:* 16 wks/yr. in hospital *Postgroup:* 3 wks/yr. in hospital Two-year follow-up	Group themes: (1) initial skepticism about lithium and group therapy, (2) complaints of loss of well-being due to lithium, (3) denial of problems, (4) projection of responsibility for lithium deficiency onto psychiatrists, (5) concerns: fears about recurrence, illness chronicity, social adjustment, and social acceptance
Rosen (1980)	*Group Therapy* and Lithium. Directive	Clinical study; no comparison or pre- or posttest measures. 90 minutes 4 times a week for 4 weeks	N = 25 patients with mixed diagnoses; 12 men, 13 women; mean age: 36, range: 25–57	No systematic follow-up; over $2\frac{1}{2}$ years 8 patients remained in group	Group themes: (1) lithium, (2) concerns about manic-depressive illness, (3) lowered morale when a group member hospitalized. Described lively group atmosphere where "therapist works not so much to stimulate interaction as to moderate it"
Volkmar et al. (1980)	*Group Therapy* and Lithium. Interpersonal, interactional, here and now	(Continuation of group therapy outlined in Shakir et al.)			Group themes as reported in Shakir et al., above. Additional comments: Cessation of lithium use results from denial of illness, lack of information about lithium, lack of support from family and friends. "It is not clear whether the high rate of compliance is secondary to the effects of group therapy *per se* or to the close follow-up the patients received or to the inter-action between the two"

Source: Goodwin and Jamison (1983).

and kidney functioning may be interpreted as caring, but undue emphasis on precise medication patterns, e.g., not allowing for some degree of self-titration, may result in unnecessary power struggles and compliance problems. Collaborative aspects of management through self-ratings, chartings, and patient and family education (using films, lectures, books, or handouts) are also integral parts of good clinical care. Finally, the therapist must be able to use hospitalization as an occasionally necessary adjunct to outpatient care and must not regard hospitalization as a rejection or punishment of the patient or as an indication that the therapist has failed in his or her therapeutic endeavors.*

Review of the Specific Issues

LOSSES ASSOCIATED WITH LITHIUM (1) *Realistic losses* are realistic in the sense that the drug can produce alterations not desired by the patient. Such alterations include decreases in energy level, loss of euphoric states, increased need for sleep, possible decreases in productivity and creativity, decreased sexuality, and so on (Jamison et al., 1979; Polatin and Fieve, 1971; Schou and Baastrup, 1973; Schou, 1980; Van Putten, 1975).

A recent study of patients who were in remission suggested that many patients felt their bipolar illness had made positive contributions to their lives in one or more important ways, specifically through increased sexuality, productivity, creativity, and sociability (Jamison et al., 1980). Attributions of this kind are important for several reasons. From a clinical perspective, the therapist needs to realize the meaning, nature, and value of positive as well as negative behavior and mood changes for an individual patient. From a learning-theory point of view, altered states of consciousness can be highly potent reinforcers during euthymic or depressed periods, and in some patients they create a potentially strong, variable reinforcement schedule, with significant benefits on the one hand and the risk of severe emotional and pragmatic problems on the other.

Treatment management under such circumstances is not an altogether straightforward matter. For example, compliance with a therapeutic lithium regime has at best a tenuous and delayed relationship with the alleviation of dysphoric features of bipolar illness, and this competes with a highly positive, intermittent reinforcement schedule, an exceedingly difficult behavior pattern to modify. In some ways the illness itself is analogous to a drug self-administration paradigm in which a highly pleasurable and often immediate state can be obtained. Thus, for some patients the illness may represent an endogenous stimulant addiction. Clinical experience suggests that patients may attempt to induce mania by discontinuing lithium not just when they are depressed, but also when they have to face problematic decisions and life events. Because the negative consequences accrue only later, it is understandable that the patient may not clearly see how the costs of noncompliance outweigh the benefits.

Thus, the clinician must be aware of the positive features of mood swings in order to understand the nature of affective disorders better. Thereby the clinician can be more effective therapeutically, particularly

*Editor's note: In their chapter in Part III, McFarlane, Beels, and Rosenheck discuss family therapy with bipolar patients, and they emphasize the value of educating the family about the illness and coaching them on crisis management.

with lithium maintenance. The subtle and powerful clinician-patient alliance possible in lithium therapy is predicated upon a thorough understanding not only of the benefits of lithium to the patient, but also of the realistic and unrealistic fantasies of loss that many patients have at some point before or during lithium treatment. These fantasies often focus on missing the highs and cannot effectively be understood through the simplistic formulation that the patient is shortsighted, regressive, or escapist. Effective therapy with bipolar patients, whether it uses drugs alone or combines drugs with psychotherapy, must address the reality of the patient's positive perceptions of the illness, as well as addressing the altered state of perception that phases of the illness induce.

Other realistic losses include alterations in the patient's cognitive, perceptual, physical, emotional, or social spheres which come about as a result of lithium side effects and social sequelae such as self-labeling or social stigma. The most significant side effects from a psychotherapeutic point of view are those detailed by Schou and Baastrup (1973) and Schou (1980): decreased energy, decreased enthusiasm, and sexuality (occasionally a factor in increased marital problems), curbing of activities, and the common perception that life is flatter and less colorful. Again, of course, it may be difficult to separate lithium side effects from the medication's impact on symptoms of the illness.

(2)   *Symbolic losses* can include a loss of perceived omnipotence and independence. Also, due to the learned associations that pair lithium with dysphoric states, lithium may come to symbolize a certain loss of innocence from prepsychotic to postpsychotic consciousness. In this context lithium noncompliance can represent an attempt to recapture an earlier prepsychotic existence, one not yet spoiled by mania or depression.

(3)   *Unrealistic losses* include circumstances where lithium and psychotherapy come to symbolize the patient's personal failures. In addition to the normal difficulties patients have in adjusting to the need for treatment, patients occasionally project all of their other life failures, thwarted ambitions, and inadequacies onto lithium. Under such circumstances lithium can become the psychological whipping boy and represent a rationalization for other failures which predate the onset of an affective disorder.

FEARS OF RECURRENCE   Fears of recurrence are almost endemic in patients with bipolar illness. Some patients become so preoccupied with such fears that they are almost phobic about the illness. They become unduly self-protective and hyperalert for signs of an impending episode. These concerns are often reflected in the process of learning to differentiate normal from abnormal moods and states. A related concern is a perceived decreasing tolerance for affective episodes. This is usually secondary to the stress of the illness and the large amounts of psychological energy consumed by earlier bouts of depression and mania. Patients often express fears about the decreasing tolerance in their families and friends for such recurrences. Bipolar illness also takes a severe toll in its cumulative effects. Thus, Lowell wrote "but the breakage can go on repeating once too often" (Lowell, 1977, 113). And Logan described in his autobiography a certain weariness: "I was only forty-five years old, but I felt exhausted by this last experience, hollowed out, as though I were a live fish disemboweled" (Logan, 1976, 388).

DENIAL OF THE ILLNESS   Denial of the illness, of its severity, of the possibility of recurrence, and occasionally of its very existence are frequent clinical themes in bipolar illness. In some instances, the cognitive impairments in depression are sufficiently pronounced that they alone account for some problems in recollection. More often repression and psychological and temporal distance cause the depression to pale into relative insignificance. The severity and nature of the manic episode is frequently minimized or "forgotten." Again, this can be due to several factors: the relatively clearer perception of the earlier and more enjoyable stages of mania, amnesia secondary to the organic features of manic psychosis, repression, and finally the sheer volume of cognitions, perceptions, and behaviors during mania that make good recall unlikely.

Denial of the illness has been seen as crucial in lithium noncompliance by many researchers (Cade, 1949; Schou et al., 1970; Polatin and Fieve, 1971; Van Putten, 1975; Jamison et al., 1979). In a study discussed further below, the authors and a colleague surveyed the attitudes of fifty clinicians, each of whom had treated at least fifty lithium patients, and they found that 64 percent of the clinicians felt that lithium noncompliance was a result of patients acting out their denial of serious lifelong illness (Jamison et al., 1979).

LEARNING TO DISCRIMINATE MOODS   Problems in learning to discriminate normal from abnormal moods are common throughout the psychotherapy of bipolar patients maintained on lithium. Many bipolar patients, because of the intensity of their emotional responses, fear the escalation of a normal depressive reaction into a major depressive episode and, less commonly, fear the escalation of a state of well-being into hypomania or mania. Of course, many emotions range into several mood states, spanning euthymia, depression, and hypomania. For example, irritability and anger can be a part of normal human existence; alternatively, they can be symptoms of either depression or hypomania. Tiredness and lethargy can be due to normal circumstances, medical causes, or clinical depression; so, too, can sadness and pessimism. Feeling good, being productive and enthusiastic, and working hard can be either normal or pathognomonic of hypomania. These overlapping emotions can be confusing, and they arouse anxiety in many patients. These patients question their judgment and become unduly concerned about recurrences of their affective illness. Occasionally patients become conservative or excessively conforming. Benson noted that bipolar patients "tend to be more conservative and more conforming to others' attitudes because they are afraid that their ideas are the result of their misperception" (Benson, 1976, 6).

Therapy often consists of helping the patient to discriminate normal from abnormal affect and teaching him or her to live within a narrower range of emotions, while using those emotions with greater subtlety and discrimination. Closely related to the discrimination of moods is the slow, steady process of learning to unravel what is normal personality from what has been superimposed upon it in terms of turbulence, impulsiveness, lack of predictability, and depression. Of course, it takes a long time before adjustment, stabilization, and insight occur.

DEVELOPMENTAL TASKS Developmental tasks previously over-shadowed by the bipolar illness often become issues for the euthymic patient. Ironically, bipolar illness can act in some ways as a protection against many of the slings and arrows of fortune that people encounter in normal life. Because late adolescence and early adulthood are the highest-risk periods for the onset of the illness, many of the developmental tasks of these periods are impaired or temporarily halted, including individuation, interpersonal intimacy, romantic involvements, hurts and rejections, and career development. Once the illness is in remission or under control, patients often have to deal with these problems within the therapy, as well as with problems of a more general existential nature.

CONCERNS ABOUT FAMILY Concerns about effects of the illness on a family system can be profound. Patients often report feeling guilty about the things they have done in mania and those they have left undone in depression. The most frequently voiced concerns center on the interpersonal sequelae of the illness, generally the effects felt by spouses, family members, and friends. Mayo et al. (1979) studied the families of 12 patients with manic-depressive illness and have described the tremendous impact of the illness on the family system.

CONCERNS ABOUT GENETICS Concerns about the genetic component of bipolar illness are considerable for many patients. Such concerns relate to guilt over possible transmission of the disorder to children, overidentification and problems with individuation when a close family member, particularly a parent, has the illness, and occasionally guilt over receiving lithium, an effective treatment which was not available to an afflicted parent. This latter phenomenon, although not common, is particularly striking in those patients with a parent who either committed suicide or was hospitalized for long periods of time. A similar guilt is sometimes seen in those patients who are successfully treated with lithium but whose siblings or parents refuse treatment.

Countertransference

As discussed earlier, many psychoanalysts who worked in the pre-lithium era found it frustrating to treat bipolar patients. Countertransference issues were openly discussed, and anger at such patients for their seeming inconstancy and lack of insight (or desire for insight) was described in some detail. English said succinctly what others have said at great length. "The manic-depressive rejects you because he seems to be unsure that he needs you at all" (English, 1949, 126). Although many aspects of therapeutic work with manic-depressives have radically changed as a result of lithium, such patients continue to elicit strong countertransference feelings. Therapists who work with bipolar patients are often frustrated by the inconsistencies that patients show during different mood states in their behavior and attitudes toward self, therapist, therapy, and lithium. Their various moods can also result in fluctuating levels of intimacy and trust within the therapeutic relationship, both from patient to therapist and from therapist to patient.

Anger and frustration can also be engendered in the therapist when the patient rejects an effective treatment. Patient omnipotence can confront therapist omnipotence (reinforced by a highly potent medication) in a classic power struggle. Often the basis of such encounters is the therapist's lack of comprehension about what the illness means to the patient, as well as the patient's lack of understanding, usually secondary to denial, about the consequences of rejecting such a treatment regimen. Greenson (1967) emphasized that the therapist should have a broad and rich background for empathy. A breadth of fantasy is particularly relevant and useful to the therapist who deals with psychotic patients, where the emotions and ideas that the patient alludes to are often not from the same experiential base as that of the therapist. In addition to having the kind of personal background advocated by Greenson, a therapist can reduce the feelings of being excluded from the patient's experience by having a solid grounding in phenomenology.

Therapists often experience anger and feelings of impotence when the patient's denial and omnipotence lead to lithium noncompliance and result in rehospitalization for manic or depressive episodes, suicide attempts, or exacerbations in hostile and aggressive behaviors. Feelings of inadequacy and failure when illness recurs can develop even when the patient is compliant. Such feelings occur often when therapists treat patients who are depressed, suicidal, or hypomanic (Fromm-Reichmann, 1949; Janowsky et al., 1970). For example, when hypomanic a patient may show a special sensitivity to vulnerabilities in the therapist. Such awareness of and tuning in to the therapist's "jugular" is the core of many patients' acute and intense feelings of rage and violation. Although this pattern of interaction is most likely to occur during hypomania and mania, it is not uncommon during the depressive phase when the patient's defenses are down and his or her level of paranoia, irritability, and hopelessness have increased. Patients under such circumstances are often exquisitely tuned in to feelings of frustration, annoyance, and impotence in the therapist. The anger and hopelessness a patient expresses at such times often have a large impact on the already vulnerable therapist. In such instances, of course, recognizing and coping effectively with countertransference feelings are vital so that the repercussions will be minimal for the depressed patient.

Yet another problem with countertransference potential centers on misinterpretation of resistance in bipolar patients. The authors have already discussed such patients' difficulties in differentiating normal from pathological mood states and their fears of recurrence. Therapists occasionally assume that a patient's depression is a reaction to a particular environmental, interpersonal, or therapeutic event, and they therefore attribute problems in discussing and handling the depression to resistance. Often such depressions represent mild breakthrough cycling in the illness, something which the patient senses but cannot articulate. The therapist's tendency to link such feelings with external events can be problematic. Even when the depressions are not really endogenous, patients are often frightened by the similarity between such affects and cognitions and earlier severe major depressive episodes. A therapist needs to use a delicate approach in order both to help the patient differentiate types of feelings and also to recognize his or her own possible need to deny recurrence or to see psychological causality when little exists.

Another area of potential countertransference problems can develop when the therapist acts out through the patient. The therapist is in an unusual position for influencing the patient by unconsciously encouraging both lithium noncompliance and the behaviors linked to affective states. Also relevant here is the special appeal of the illness in general and hypomania and mania in particular. The potential exists for envy, projective identification, and seduction, as well as guilt over depriving patients of a special state. This latter potential is heightened when patients resist lithium and proclaim that they miss the highs. Unconscious collusion in medication resistance is not uncommon. Likewise, the seductive aspects of hypomania are often impossible to ignore, and a therapist's seduced response can be illustrative of the reasons why patients miss their highs in the first place. Moods are obviously contagious, and occasionally the loss of a patient's hypomania results in a corresponding, albeit lesser, loss reaction in the therapist as well. A certain number of psychotherapists espouse a set of attitudes about psychosis which the authors term the Equus-Laingian view of madness. This refers to a romanticization or eroticization of madness, and it can range on the one hand from a tendency to overvalue the positive aspects of bipolar illness while minimizing the negative, painful ones to a conviction on the other hand that all psychopharmacological interventions in such patients are oppressive and contraindicated.

LITHIUM COMPLIANCE ISSUES

Review of the Literature

With a growing number of patients receiving lithium therapy, problems with compliance have become common. No data exist on how many patients actually stop taking lithium against medical advice, for what reasons they stop, for how long, and at what point in their therapeutic regime or mood cycles, and whether or not there are sex and age differences in the incidence of and reasons for noncompliance or incomplete compliance. Very little systematic research has been done on patients' perceptions of the positive and negative consequences of taking the drug regularly and the effect of these perceptions on actual patterns of lithium use.

The published reports on lithium noncompliance are anecdotal and include some proposed explanations for the phenomenon. Polatin and Fieve (1971) emphasized that patients often attribute decreases in creativity and productivity to lithium, and these authors also stressed the role of the patients' lithium noncompliance in their denial of a chronic, serious illness. Fitzgerald (1972) speculated that refusal to take lithium stemmed from intolerance of reality-based depressions, preference for a hypomanic life-style, or provocation by a spouse or other family member who also missed the patient's hypomanic episodes. Van Putten (1975) also stressed the importance of patients and their family members missing hypomania, and in addition he has noted the importance of lithium side effects and lithium-induced dysphoria, characterized by a driveless, anhedonic condition (Theodore Van Putten, written communication, 1977). Along with Schou et al. (1970), Van Putten has also cited depressive relapse or the tendency to feel well and to see no further need for medication as significant variables. Kerry (1978) suggested that the social stigma associated with bipolar illness may lead patients to reject the medication, the most concrete symbol of the illness.

The UCLA Study

In a preliminary exploration of these and related questions, the authors pursued two obvious sources of information and experience, the attitudes of patients themselves (47 lithium patients from the UCLA Affective Disorders Clinic) and, independently, the attitudes of clinicians well experienced in the use of lithium (50 physicians). Each of the physicians had treated at least 50 patients with lithium, and many had treated hundreds more. Remarkably, nearly one half (47 percent) of the patients reported having stopped lithium at some time against medical advice; of those, 34 percent said that they stopped taking lithium more than once. Of those who reported that they had never stopped, over 90 percent stated that they had never even considered stopping. This suggests the possibility of two distinct subgroups of patients, a distribution perhaps more bimodal than continuous in nature.

OVERVIEW OF FINDINGS No significant differences existed in sex, age, education, or income between the group of 22 patients who reported that they discontinued lithium treatment against medical advice and the group of 25 patients who reported they had not. Patients with a prior history of mania (bipolar I) tended to be less compliant than those with a prior history of hypomania (bipolar II). The number of months on lithium was the only variable that significantly differentiated the groups; more patients reported discontinuing lithium during long-term treatment. These preliminary data do not allow further inference about the increasing tendency to discontinue lithium over time. They may reflect only the effect of increasing the period at risk for noncompliance.

Both groups of patients reported that lithium was highly effective in preventing recurrences of mania but less so in preventing recurrent depressions, and patients perceived that lithium was more effective in preventing depressions than the clinicians did. Interestingly, while 96 percent of the clinicians had found lithium an extremely effective or very effective treatment for mania, 73 percent of the patients evaluated it as such. No significant relationship existed between perceived effectiveness and reported compliance. Both the compliant and noncompliant patient groups indicated that a fear of depression was a stronger reason for staying on lithium than a fear of mania. The clinicians concurred in this perception.

While 50 percent of the patient group considered psychotherapy to be "very important" in lithium compliance, only 27 percent of the clinicians, most of whom were practicing psychotherapists, regarded therapy as very important. This may indicate a tendency for clinicians to value the potency of an effective medication so highly that they underestimate psychological aspects both of the illness and of medication compliance. Over half the clinicians (59 percent) indicated that they almost always encouraged patients to seek adjunctive psychotherapy.

SIDE EFFECTS Clinicians rated side effects as more important factors in noncompliance than did the patients who reported discontinuing lithium therapy. Both patients and clinicians viewed lethargy, impairment in coordination, and lithium-induced tremor as the most important side effects in noncompliance. While patients reported that dulling of senses was relatively important, clinicians emphasized weight gain.

Female patients considered that lethargy and dulling of senses were significantly more problematic than did male patients. Women may be more sensitive to or bothered by these effects for psychosocial reasons, or hormonal changes may produce subtle changes in women's lithium retention, resulting in more subtoxic episodes of symptom exacerbation.

GENERAL REASONS FOR NONCOMPLIANCE Table 2 lists in rank order of importance the reasons cited by the entire patient sample, by the group which had reported noncompliance, and by the clinicians. (When patients reported that they had always complied, they were asked to give reasons that might cause them not to comply.) From the patients' perspective, the four most important reasons for noncompliance were (1) a dislike of the idea that their moods were controlled by medication, (2) being bothered by the idea of having a chronic illness, symbolized by the necessity of lithium therapy, (3) feeling depressed, and (4) side effects, particularly lethargy, decreased coordination, and dulling of senses. A considerable agreement existed between patient and clinician perceptions, with a few significant exceptions. Patients were much more bothered by the idea that their moods were controlled by medication than the clinicians perceived them to be. Those patients who reported discontinuing lithium were also significantly more likely to report missing highs and the hassle of taking medications as important reasons for noncompliance. On the

Table 2.   Rank Orders of General Reasons for Noncompliance: UCLA Study

Rank Order	Total Patient Sample (N = 47)	Patients who Reported Discontinuing Lithium Treatment (N = 22)	Independent Clinician Sample (N = 50)
1	Bothered by idea that moods are controlled by medication	Bothered by idea that moods are controlled by medication	Felt well, saw no need for lithium
2	Felt depressed	Missed highs[1]	Missed highs
3	Bothered by idea of chronic illness	Felt depressed	Bothered by idea of chronic illness
4	Felt less attractive to spouse	Bothered by idea of chronic illness	Felt less creative
5	Felt well, saw no need for lithium	Felt well, saw no need for lithium	Felt less productive
6	Hassle to take medications	Hassle to take mediations[1]	Bothered by idea that moods are controlled by medication
7	Missed highs	Felt less attractive to friends	Hassle to take medication
8	Felt less creative	Felt less creative	Felt less attractive to friends
9	Felt less productive	Felt less productive	Felt depressed
10	Felt less attractive to friends	Felt less attractive to spouse	Felt less attractive to spouse

[1]p < .05. Patients who actually discontinued lithium rated these reasons significantly more important than did those patients who did not stop lithium.
Source: Jamison et al. (1979).

other hand, all patients generally perceived that decreased productivity, creativity, and attractiveness to spouse or friends were not very important reasons for discontinuing lithium. This finding contrasts with several prevailing notions about reasons for noncompliance, and it also suggests that most patients do not necessarily equate highs with creativity or productivity. From the clinicians' point of view, the three most important reasons for lithium noncompliance were that (1) the patient felt well and saw no need to continue the medication, (2) the patient missed the highs of hypomania, and (3) the patient was bothered by the idea of having a chronic illness.

Although this relatively small sample showed no overall significant differences in scores between men and women on general reasons for noncompliance, women were more likely to mark "missing highs" and "bothered by the idea of moods being controlled by medication" as very important. One could speculate that women may perceive more desirable benefits from their highs than do men due to more extensive changes from women's baseline experience in areas such as hypersexuality, increased energy, and productivity. Some corroborating evidence for this hypothesis has been presented (Jamison et al., 1980). Furthermore, women may be accustomed to accepting extremes of moods and emotions as being within the bounds of normal feminine and culturally sanctioned experience, and consequently they may be more upset than men by the idea of external control. As a result of the natural history of bipolar illness, women may also experience more frequent "miniepisodes," leading to further accommodation to mood swings, if not actual acceptance and learned modulation.

Men, on the other hand, may regard fluctuating moods as aberrant and thus more legitimately subject to external or medical control. Although not systematically studied, the legal and financial sequelae may be more extensive for men than for women. This in turn may be due to differences in men's cultural expectations and their actual phenomenology of the illness, for example, their higher ratio of mania to depressive episodes, their more aggressive and destructive behavior when manic, and their greater physical strength. In short, the cost-benefit ratio for lithium compliance is probably different for men and women.

PSYCHODYNAMIC ISSUES More than one half the physicians (64 percent) felt that lithium noncompliance was "somewhat" or "very" related to patients acting out their denial of having a serious life-long illness. Thirty-five percent of the clinicians felt that by not complying patients were acting out psychodynamic factors in therapy. Approximately one fourth (26 percent) felt that patient anger at the therapist or at a significant other was an important reason for patients stopping lithium against medical advice.

From these findings and those of others, it is clear that incomplete compliance with lithium is a major clinical problem and one that brings with it a substantially increased risk of personal and interpersonal chaos, hospitalization, and suicide. Approximately one half of the patients in this study reported discontinuing lithium treatment against medical advice at least once. On the basis of extensive clinical experience, the physicians in the sample estimated that one third of those patients taking lithium would stop taking it against medical recommendations. These figures are consistent with other reports in the literature. In his review, Van Putten (1975) summarized available statistics and concluded that 20 percent to 30 percent of patients with manic-depressive illness discontinue their lithium treatment against medical advice. Again it is interesting that of the thousands of lithium citations in the scientific literature only a few papers have focused on the psychological or psychotherapeutic aspects of lithium treatment.

The UCLA-Columbia Study

One of the authors and colleagues (Jamison, Litman-Adizes, and Fieve, unpublished data) extensively examined 71 bipolar manic-depressive patients from two very different geographic and social class settings. A group of 31 came from Dr. Fieve's private practice, located in East Side Manhattan, one of the wealthiest areas in the world, and the remaining 40 came from the UCLA Affective Disorders Clinic, a public university clinic located in Los Angeles. Although it is not the purpose here to detail the geographic and social class differences which emerged, it is of interest that despite significant differences between the two samples, the overall comparisons were far more impressive for their similarities than for their differences.

All patients in the study were bipolar, but a significantly higher proportion of the Los Angeles sample was bipolar I ($p < .05$). There was no significant difference in mean age for the samples or number of months in lithium treatment; the combined samples had a mean age of 37.7 years and a mean length of treatment of 36.0 months. Mean incomes, not surprisingly, were strikingly different. The New York patients had a mean income of $64,000, while the Los Angeles group had a mean of $16,000. In the discussion which follows, patients from both samples are combined.

OVERVIEW OF FINDINGS   Two patient variables were significantly related to lithium compliance: older patients were more compliant ($p < .05$), and women were far more compliant than men ($p < .007$). There was no significant relationship between compliance and IQ, ethnicity, marital status, income, or religious background.

The UCLA study did not examine the relationship between illness variables and lithium compliance, although one might expect results here. The UCLA-Columbia study found that the numbers of both depressive episodes ($p < .05$) and manic ($p < .05$) episodes were significantly related to compliance. An important if not surprising finding was that the more affective episodes a patient had, the more likely he or she was to report compliance. This finding is even more impressive in that the more episodes a patient had, the longer the time period available for noncompliance. Almost certainly, this reflects an early high-risk period for noncompliance and a tendency for many patients to have to experience recurrences of their illnesses before their initial denial is meaningfully altered. The study showed no relationship between compliance and polarity of the first episode, type of mania or hypomania (euphoric, dysphoric, mixed), or the extent of perceived positive aspects of hypomania. There were no differences in the rates of compliance between bipolar I and II patients.

In terms of treatment attitudes, noncompliant patients felt more than compliant ones that psychotherapy was important to them in complying with a lithium treatment schedule ($p < .02$). Noncompliant patients were also more likely to give as an important reason for stopping lithium that they felt well and saw no further need for it (p < .01). They also perceived lithium as far more of a hassle to remember than did compliant patients (p < .02). On a semantic differential test of attitudes toward lithium, antidepressants, and psychotherapy, there were no significant differences. Interestingly, there were also no differences between the groups on their experience of lithium side effects.

The following psychological measures revealed no significant differences between the compliant and noncompliant groups: Beck Depression Inventory, Manic-Depressive Scale, Eysenck Personality Inventory, Breskin Rigidity Test Aesthetic Preference Scale, Sensation-Seeking Scale, Internal-External Locus of Control, and the Jenkins Activity Survey, a measure of Type A or cardiac-prone behavior.

SIDE EFFECTS   The UCLA study had neglected to include memory problems in the listing of lithium side effects, reflecting the fact that cognitive effects are generally not mentioned in the lithium literature. But since the authors were impressed by such complaints from patients, the UCLA-Columbia study included it. Memory problems, in fact, were evaluated by patients as the most important problem in considering stopping lithium against medical advice. Fully one third of the patients found memory problems very important, compared with only 18 percent who felt polyuria would be a significant contributor to noncompliance. Ironically, polyuria is the lithium side effect that is most studied, while changes in memory functioning are studied the least. Weight gain and problems with coordination and tremor were also cited as quite problematic. The authors' questioning about side effects has varied from that of other authors. Questions are tied to a behavioral base (e.g., "How important is the side effect in question to your decision making about continuing to take lithium?") rather than a presence-or-absence-of-the-symptom format. This may result in differences in findings across studies.

GENERAL REASONS FOR NONCOMPLIANCE   Table 3 outlines several reasons for lithium noncompliance. In the case of those who did stop lithium, the question focused on why they did. In the

Table 3.   Rank Orders of Reasons for Lithium Noncompliance: UCLA-Columbia Study

Rank Order	Reasons for Noncompliance (Total Sample, N = 71)
1	Side effects
2	Indefinite intake/chronicity of illness
3	Less creative
4[1,2]	Felt well, saw no need to take lithium
5	Less productive
6	Missed highs
7	Less interesting to spouse
8	Disliked idea of moods being controlled by medication
9[3]	Hassle to remember to take medication
10	Felt depressed, thought mood would improve

[1]Males > females, p < .05
[2]Those who stopped lithium > those who did not, p < .01
[3]Those who stopped lithium > those who did not, p < .02
Source: Jamison et al. (1982).

case of those who did not, the question asked what would be important factors in why they eventually might. The results vary somewhat from the UCLA study. The perception of decreased creativity ranked as more important in the UCLA-Columbia study, and the disliking for being on medication ranked as less important. These differences may be due to sampling or, in the case of dislike for being on medication, differences in social attitudes over the past several years.

REINFORCEMENT ISSUES

One more relevant detail should be mentioned in the context of psychotherapy, lithium, and compliance: the reinforcement issues that are intrinsic to lithium treatment. Lithium is a drug with a delayed therapeutic action, five to seven days for an antimanic effect and three to five weeks for an antidepressant effect. Lithium also has no known reinforcing qualities, either immediate or delayed. The onset of the initial lithium treatment is often paired with highly aversive emotional states such as depression, mania, or dysphoria. If the initial lithium is prescribed for a manic episode, the natural history of the illness predicts that any given patient is at significant risk for a substantial postmania depression, further pairing the onset of lithium treatment with dysthymia. On the other hand, the cessation of lithium is often accompanied by relatively immediate positive experiences, due either to the disappearance of side effects or to breakthrough hypomania, which is often a contributing factor in lithium noncompliance. Another problem is that patients are expected to stay on the drug for indeterminate periods of time, and most of this time they are in a euthymic state and therefore without symptomatic motivation. Moreover, if a patient stops the medication, the negative consequence of noncompliance, i.e., recurrence of the affective illness, is almost always delayed a long time, and the patient therefore has no immediate negative reinforcer. These issues challenge the psychotherapist to contend with a singularly difficult set of problems in the treatment of bipolar illness.

References for the Introduction

Angst J. Zur Atiologie und Nosologie endogener depressiver Psychosen. Monographien aus dem Gesamtgebiete der Neurologie und Psychiatrie. Berlin, Springer Verlag, 1966.

Egeland J.: Bipolarity: the iceberg of affective disorders? Paper presented at the Annual Meeting of the American Psychiatric Association. Toronto, Canada, May 1982.

Leonhard K.: Aufteilung der endogenen Psychosen. Berlin, Akademie-Verlag, 1957.

Menninger K.: The Vital Balance. New York, Penquin Books, 1977.

Perris C.: A study of bipolar (manic-depressive) and unipolar recurrent depressive psychoses. Acta Psychiatr. Scand. Suppl. 194, 1966.

Winokur G., Clayton P., Reich T.: Manic-Depressive Illness, St. Louis, C.V. Mosby Co., 1969.

References for Chapter 18

The Bipolar Spectrum: New Concepts in Classification and Diagnosis

Abrams R., Taylor M.A.: Catatonia: a progressive clinical study. Arch. Gen. Psychiatry 33:579–581, 1976.

Abrams R., Taylor M.A., Gaztanaga P.: Manic-depressive illness and paranoid schizophrenia. Arch. Gen. Psychiatry 31:640–642, 1974.

Adebimpe V.R.: Overview: white norms and psychiatric diagnosis of black patients. Am. J. Psychiatry 138: 279–285, 1981.

Akiskal H.S.: Affective disorders, in Merck Manual of Diagnosis and Therapy, 14th ed. Philadelphia, Merck Sharp & Dohme Research Laboratories, 1982a.

Akiskal H.S.: Age and manner of onset of bipolar spectrum disorders in the offspring and younger sibs of manic-depressives. Paper presented at Psychiatric Research Society Meeting, Salt Lake City, March 1982b.

Akiskal H.S.: Clinical overview of depressive disorders and their pharmacological management, in Neuropharmacology of Central and Behavioral Disorders. Edited by Palmer G.O. New York, Academic Press, 1981a.

Akiskal H.S.: Dysthymic and cyclothymic disorders: a paradigm for high-risk research in psychiatry, in The Affective Disorders. Edited by Maas J., Davis J.M. Washington, D.C., American Psychiatric Press Inc., 1982c.

Akiskal H.S.: External validating criteria for psychiatric diagnosis: their application in affective disorders. J. Clin. Psychiatry 41 (Sec 2):6–14, 1980.

Akiskal H.S.: Hypomanic personality: clinical and sleep EEG study. New research paper presented at Annual Meeting of the American Psychiatric Association, Toronto, Canada, May 1982d.

Akiskal H.S.: Subaffective disorders: dysthymic, cyclothymic and bipolar II disorders in the "borderline" realm. Psychiatr. Clin. North Am. 4:25–46, 1981b.

Akiskal H.S., McKinney W.T. Jr.: Overview of recent research in depression: integration of ten conceptual models into a comprehensive clinical frame. Arch. Gen. Psychiatry 32:285–305, 1975.

Akiskal H.S., Puzantian V.R.: Psychotic forms of depression and mania. Psychiatr. Clin. North Am. 2:419–439, 1979.

Akiskal H.S., Bitar A.H., Puzantian V.R., et al.: The nosological status of neurotic depression: a prospective three-to-four-year examination in light of the primary-secondary and unipolar-bipolar dichotomies. Arch. Gen. Psychiatry 35:756–766, 1978.

Akiskal H.S., Djenderedjian A.H., Rosenthal R.H., et al.: Cyclothymic disorder: validating criteria for inclusion in the bipolar affective group. Am. J. Psychiatry 134: 1227–1233, 1977.

Akiskal H.S., Khani M.K., Scott-Strauss A.: Cyclothymic temperamental disorders. Psychiatr. Clin. North. Am. 2:527–554, 1979a.

Akiskal H.S., King D., Rosenthal T.L., et al.: Chronic depressions: Part I. Clinical and familial characteristics in 137 probands. J. Affective Disord. 3:297–315, 1981.

Akiskal H.S., Lemmi H., Yerevanian B., et al.: The utility of the REM latency test in psychiatric diagnosis: a study of 81 depressed outpatients. Psychiatry Res. 7:101–110, 1982a.

Akiskal H.S., Rosenthal T.L., Haykal R.F., et al.: Characterological depressions: clinical and sleep findings separating "subaffective dysthymias" from "character-spectrum disorders." Arch. Gen. Psychiatry 37:777–783, 1980.

Akiskal H.S., Rosenthal R.H., Rosenthal T.L., et al.: Differentiation of primary affective illness from situational, symptomatic and secondary depressions. Arch. Gen. Psychiatry 36:635–643, 1979b.

Akiskal H.S., Walker P., Puzantian V.R., et al.: Bipolar outcome in the course of depressive illness: phenomenologic, familial, and pharmacologic predictors. J. Affective Disord., 1982b.

Ambelas A.: Psychologically stressful events in the precipitation of manic episodes. Br. J. Psychiatry 135:15–21, 1979.

American Psychiatric Association: Diagnostic and Statistical Manual of Mental Disorders, 2nd ed. Washington, D.C., American Psychiatric Association, 1968.

American Psychiatric Association: Diagnostic and Statistical Manual of Mental Disorders, 3rd ed. Washington, D.C., American Psychiatric Association, 1980.

Andreasen N.C.: Affective flattening and the criteria for schizophrenia. Am. J. Psychiatry 136:944–947, 1979a.

Andreasen N.C.: Thought, language, and communication disorders: II. Diagnostic significance. Arch. Gen. Psychiatry 36:1325–1330, 1979b.

Andreasen N.C., Canter A.: The creative writer: psychiatric symptoms and family history. Compr. Psychiatry 15: 123–131, 1974.

Angst J.: Zur Atiologie und Nosologie endogener depressiver Psychosen. Berlin, Springer Verlag, 1966.

Angst J., Baastrup P., Grof P.: The course of monopolar depression and bipolar psychoses. Psychiatr. Neurol. Neurochir. (Amsterdam) 76:489–500, 1973.

Baldessarini R.J.: Frequency of diagnoses of schizophrenia versus affective disorders from 1944–1968. Am. J. Psychiatry 127:759–763, 1970.

Baldessarini R.J., Cole J.O., Davis J.M.: Tardive Dyskinesia, Task Force Report 18. Washington, D.C., American Psychiatric Association, 1980.

Batchelor I.R.C.: Henderson and Gillespie's Textbook of Psychiatry, 10th ed. London, Oxford University Press, 1969.

Bazzoui W.: Affective disorders in Iraq. Br. J. Psychiatry 117:195–203, 1970.

Berner P.: Modification in the psychopathologic definition of schizophrenia. Alterations during the last two decades: expectations for the future. Compr. Psychiatry 21:475–482, 1980.

Blackburn I.M.: The pattern of hostility in affective illness. Br. J. Psychiatry 125:141–145, 1974.

Bowden C.: Lithium-responsive depression. Compr. Psychiatry 19:227–231, 1978.

Braden W., Bannasch M.A.T., Fink E.: Diagnosing mania: the use of family informants. J. Clin. Psychiatry 41:226–228, 1980.

Braftos O., Haug J.O.: The course of manic-depressive psychosis. Acta Psychiatr. Scand. 44:89–112, 1968.

Brodie H.K.H., Leff M.J.: Bipolar depression: a comparative study of patient characteristics. Am. J. Psychiatry 127:1086–1090, 1971.

Bunney W.E.: Psychopharmacology of the switch process in affective illness, in Psychopharmacology: A Generation of Progress. Edited by Lipton M.A., DiMascio A., Killam K.F. New York, Raven Press, 1978.

Campbell J.D.: Manic-Depressive Disease: Clinical and Psychiatric Significance. Philadelphia, J.B. Lippincott Co., 1953.

Carlson G.A., Goodwin F.K.: The stages of mania. Arch. Gen. Psychiatry 28:221–228, 1973.

Carlson G.A., Strober M.: Manic-depressive illness in early adolescence. J. Am. Acad. Child Psychiatry 17:138–153, 1978.

Carpenter W.T., Strauss J.S., Muleh S.: Are there pathognomonic symptoms in schizophrenia? An empiric investigation of Schneider's first-rank symptoms. Arch. Gen. Psychiatry 28:847–852, 1973.

Carroll B.J.: Clinical applications of the dexamethasone suppression test for endogenous depression. Pharmacopsychiatria 15:19–24, 1982.

Carroll B.J., Feinberg M., Greden J.F., et al.: A specific laboratory test for the diagnosis of melancholia: standardization, validation and clinical utility. Arch. Gen. Psychiatry 38:15–22, 1981.

Clayton P.J.: The epidemiology of bipolar affective disorder. Compr. Psychiatry 22:31–43, 1981.

Clayton P.J., Endicott J., Croughan J., et al.: Schizoaffective disorders divided by polarity. Paper presented at the III World Congress of Biological Psychiatry. Stockholm, Sweden, June/July 1981.

Clayton P.J., Pitts F.N. Jr., Winokur G.: Affective disorder, IV. Mania. Compr. Psychiatry 6:313–322, 1965.

Cole J.O.: Drug therapy of adult minimal brain dysfunction (MBD), in Psychopharmacology Update. Edited by Cole J.O. Lexington, MA., Collamore Press, 1980.

Coryell W., Winokur G.: Diagnosis, family and follow-up studies, in Mania: An Evolving Concept. Edited by Belmaker R.H., Van Praag H.M. New York, Spectrum Publications, 1980.

Cowdry R.W., Goodwin F.K.: Dementia of bipolar illness: diagnosis and response to lithium. Am. J. Psychiatry 138:1118–1119, 1981.

Davis R.E.: Manic-depressive variant syndrome of childhood: a preliminary report. Am. J. Psychiatry 136:702–705, 1979.

Depue R.A., Monroe S.M.: The unipolar-bipolar distinction in the depressive disorders. Psychol. Bull. 85:1001–1029, 1978.

Depue R.A., Slater J.F., Welfstetter-Kausch H., et al.: A behavioral paradigm for identifying persons at risk for bipolar depressive disorders: a conceptual framework and five validation studies. J. Abnorm. Psychol., Suppl. 90:381–438, 1981.

Detre T., Himmelhoch J., Swartzburg M., et al.: Hypersomnia and manic-depressive disease. Am. J. Psychiatry 128:1303–1305, 1972.

Donlon P.T., Rada R.T., Arora K.K.: Depression and the reintegration phase of acute schizophrenia. Am. J. Psychiatry 131:1265–1268, 1976.

Dunner D.L.: Unipolar and bipolar depression—recent findings from clinical and biologic studies, in The Psychobiology of Affective Disorders. Edited by Mendels J., Amsterdam J.D. Basel, S. Karger, 1980.

Dunner D.L., Fieve R.R.: The lithium ion: its impact on diagnostic practice, in Psychiatric Diagnosis: Exploration of Biological Predictors. Edited by Akiskal H.S., Webb W.L. New York, Spectrum Publications, 1978.

Dunner D.L., Fleiss J.L., Fieve R.R.: The course of development of mania in patients with recurrent depression. Am. J. Psychiatry 133:905–908, 1976.

Dunner D.L., Russek F.K., Russek B., et al.: Classification of bipolar affective disorder subtypes. Compr. Psychiatry 23:186–189, 1982.

Egeland J.A.: Bipolarity: the iceberg of affective disorders? New research paper presented at Annual Meeting of the American Psychiatric Association. Toronto, Canada, May 1982.

Extein I., Pottash A.L.C., Gold M.S., et al.: Differentiating mania from schizophrenia by the TRH test. Am. J. Psychiatry 137:981–982, 1980.

Extein I., Pottash A.L.C., Gold M.S., et al.: Using the protirelin test to distinguish mania from schizophrenia. Arch. Gen. Psychiatry 39:77–81, 1982.

Feighner J.P., Robins E., Guze S.B., et al.: Diagnostic criteria for use in psychiatric research. Arch. Gen. Psychiatry 26:57–63, 1972.

Fieve R.R., Dunner D.L.: Unipolar and bipolar affective states, in The Nature and Treatment of Depression. Edited by Flach F., Draghi S. New York, John Wiley & Sons, 1975.

Fischer M., Gottesman I.I.: A study of offspring of parents both hospitalized for psychiatric disorders, in The Social Consequences of Psychiatric Illness. Edited by Robins L.N., Clayton P.J., Wing J.K. New York, Brunner/Mazel, 1980.

Gagrat D.D., Spiro H.R.: Social, cultural, and epidemiologic aspects of mania, in Mania: An Evolving Concept. Edited by Belmaker R.H., Van Praag H.M. New York, Spectrum Publications, 1980.

Ganz V.H., Gurland B.J., Deming W.E., et al.: The study of the psychiatric symptoms of systemic lupus erythematosus. Psychosom. Med. 34:207–220, 1972.

German G.A.: Aspects of clinical psychiatry in sub-Saharan Africa. Br. J. Psychiatry 121:461–479, 1972.

Gershon E.S.: The search for genetic markers in affective disorders, in Psychopharmacology: A Generation of Progress. Edited by Lipton M.A., DiMascio A., Killam K.F. New York, Raven Press, 1978.

Gershon E.S., Liebowitz J.H.: Sociocultural and demographic correlates of affective disorders in Jerusalem. J. Psychiatr. Res. 12:37–50, 1975.

Gershon E.S., Dunner D.L., Sfert L.: Assortative mating in the affective disorders. Biol. Psychiatry 7:63–74, 1973.

Gershon E.S., Goldin L.R., Weissman M.M., et al.: Family and genetic studies of affective disorders in the eastern United States: a provisional summary. Paper presented at the III World Congress of Biological Psychiatry. Stockholm, Sweden, June/July 1981.

Gershon E.S., Hamovit J., Guroff J.J., et al.: A family study of schizoaffectives; bipolar I, bipolar II, unipolar and normal control probands. Arch. Gen. Psychiatry 39:1157–1167, 1982.

Gershon E.S., Mark A., Cohen N., et al.: Transmitted factors in the morbid risk of affective disorders: a controlled study. J. Psychiatr. Res. 12:283–299, 1975.

Goodwin E., Bunney W.E. Jr.: A psychobiological approach to affective illness. Psychiatr. Ann. 3:19–53, 1973.

Greden J.F., Kronfol Z., Gardner R., et al.: Neuroendocrine evaluation of schizoaffectives with the dexamethasone suppression test, in Biological Psychiatry 1981. Edited by Perris C., Struwe G., Janssen B. Amsterdam, Elsevier/North Holland Biomedical Press, 1981.

Grof P., Angst J., Haines T.: The clinical course of depression: practical issues, in Classification and Prediction of Outcome of Depressions. Edited by Angst J. New York, F.K. Schattaves Verlag, 1974.

Guze S.B.: The occurrence of psychiatric illness in systemic lupus erythematosus. Am. J. Psychiatry 123:1562–1570, 1967.

Helzer J.E., Clayton P.J., Pambakian R., et al.: Reliability of psychiatric diagnosis: II. The test/retest reliability of diagnostic classification. Arch. Gen. Psychiatry 34:136–141, 1977.

Himmelhoch J.M., Mulla D., Neil J.F., et al.: Incidence and significance of mixed affective states in a bipolar population. Arch. Gen. Psychiatry 33:1062–1066, 1976.

Jamison K.R., Gerner R.H., Hammen C., et al.: Clouds and silver linings: positive experiences associated with primary affective disorders. Am. J. Psychiatry 137:198–202, 1980.

Johnson D.A.W.: Studies of depressive symptoms in schizophrenia: I. The prevalence of depression and its possible causes. Br. J. Psychiatry 139:89–101, 1981.

Keller M.D., Shapiro R.W.: "Double depression:" superimposition of acute depressive episodes on chronic depressive disorders. Am. J. Psychiatry 139:438–442, 1982.

Kestenbaum C.J.: Children at risk for manic-depressive illness: possible predictors. Am. J. Psychiatry 136:1205–1208, 1979.

Klerman G.L.: The spectrum of mania. Compr. Psychiatry 22:11–20, 1981.

Knights A., Hirsch S.T.: "Revealed" depression and drug treatment for schizophrenia. Arch. Gen. Psychiatry 38:806–811, 1981.

Kotin J., Goodwin F.K.: Depression during mania: clinical observations and theoretical implications. Am. J. Psychiatry 129:679–686, 1972.

Kraepelin E.: Manic-Depressive Insanity and Paranoia. Edinburgh, E. & S. Livingstone, 1921.

Kraines S.H.: Mental Depressions and Their Treatment. New York, MacMillan Co., 1957.

Krauthammer C., Klerman G.L.: Secondary mania. Arch. Gen. Psychiatry 35:1333–1339, 1978.

Kupfer D.J., Broudy D., Spiker D.G., et al.: EEG sleep and affective psychoses: I. Schizoaffective disorders. Psychiatr. Res. 1:173–178, 1979.

Kupfer D.J., Foster F.G., Coble P., et al.: The application of EEG sleep for the differential diagnosis of affective disorders. Am. J. Psychiatry 135:69–74, 1978.

Kupfer D.J., Pickar D., Himmelhoch J.M., et al.: Are there two types of unipolar depression? Arch. Gen. Psychiatry 32:866–871, 1975.

Lehmann H.: The impact of the therapeutic revolution on nosology, in The Schizophrenic Syndrome, vol. 1. Edited by Cancro R. New York, Brunner/Mazel, 1970.

Leonhard K.: Aufteilung der endogenen Psychosen. Berlin, Akademie-Verlag, 1957.

Lewis J.L., Winokur G.: The induction of mania—a natural history study with controls. Arch. Gen. Psychiatry 39:303–306, 1982.

Liebowitz M.R., Klein D.F.: Hysteroid dysphoria. Psychiatr. Clin. North Am. 2:555–575, 1979.

London W.P., Taylor B.M.: Bipolar disorders in a forensic setting. Compr. Psychiatry 23:33–37, 1982.

Loranger A.W., Levine T.M.: Age at onset of bipolar affective illness. Arch. Gen. Psychiatry 35:1345–1348, 1978.

McKnew D.H., Cytryn L., Buchsbaum M.S., et al.: Lithium in children of lithium responding parents. Psychiatry Res. 4:171–180, 1981.

Mellor C.S.: First rank symptoms of schizophrenia. Br. J. Psychiatry 117:15–23, 1970.

Mellor C.S., Sims A.C.P., Cope R.V.: Change of diagnosis in schizophrenia and first-rank symptoms: an eight-year follow-up. Compr. Psychiatry 22:184–188, 1981.

Mendlewicz J., Rainer J.D.: Adoption study supporting genetic transmission in manic-depressive illness. Nature 268:327–329, 1977.

Miles C.P.: Conditions predisposing to suicide: a review. J. Nerv. Ment. Dis. 164:231–246, 1977.

Morrison J.R.: Bipolar affective disorder and alcoholism. Am. J. Psychiatry 131:1130–1133, 1974.

Neil J.F., Himmelhoch J.M., Mallinger A.G., et al.: Caffeinism complicating hypersomnic depressive episodes. Compr. Psychiatry 19:377–385, 1978.

Orvaschel H., Weissman M.M., Padian N., et al.: Assessing psychopathology in children of psychiatrically disturbed parents: a pilot study. J. Am. Acad. Child Psychiatry 20:112–122, 1981.

Ostow M.: The hypomanic personality in history, in Mania: An Evolving Concept. Edited by Belmaker R.H., Van Praag H.M. New York, Spectrum Publications, 1980.

Perris C.: A study of bipolar (manic depressive) and unipolar recurrent depressive psychoses. Acta Psychiatr. Scand., Suppl. 194, 1966.

Perris C.: A study of cycloid psychoses. Acta Psychiatr. Scand., Suppl. 253, 1974.

Petterson U.: Manic-depressive illness: a clinical, social and genetic study. Acta Psychiatr. Scand., Suppl. 269, 1977.

Pope H.G. Jr., Lipinski J.F. Jr.: Diagnosis in schizophrenia and manic depressive illness. Arch. Gen. Psychiatry 35:811–828, 1978.

Post F.: Affective disorders in old age, in Handbook of Affective Disorders. Edited by Paykel E.S. New York, Guilford Press, 1982.

Post F.: The Significance of Affective Symptoms in Old Age. London, Oxford University Press, 1962.

Procci W.R.: Schizoaffective psychosis: fact or fiction? A survey of the literature. Arch. Gen. Psychiatry 33:1167–1178, 1976.

Racamier P.C., Blanchard M.: De l'angoisse à la manie. L'Evolution Psychiatrique III:558–587, 1957.

Rao A.V., Nammalvar N.: The course and outcome in depressive illness. A follow-up study of 122 cases in Mandurai, India. Br. J. Psychiatry 130:392–396, 1977.

Reich L.H., Davies R.K., Himmelhoch J.M.: Excessive alcohol use in manic-depressive illness. Am. J. Psychiatry 131:83–86, 1974.

Rifkin A., Levitan S.J., Galenski, et al.: Emotionally unstable character disorder—a follow-up study: description of patients and outcome. Biol. Psychiatry 4:65–79, 1972.

Rosenthal T.L., Akiskal H.S., Scott-Strauss A., et al.: Familial and developmental factors in characterological depressions. J. Affective Disord. 3:183–192, 1981.

Roth M.: The natural history of mental disorders in old age. Br. J. Psychiatry 101:281–301, 1955.

Roth M.: The psychiatric disorders of later life. Psychiatr. Ann. 6:57–101, 1976.

Roth M., Barnes T.R.E.: The classification of affective disorders: a synthesis of old and new concepts. Compr. Psychiatry 22:54–77, 1981.

Schlesser M.A., Winokur G., Rush A.J.: Dexamethasone suppression test in schizoaffective psychosis. Paper presented at the III World Congress of Biological Psychiatry. Stockholm, Sweden, June/July 1981.

Shopsin B.: Mania: II. Differential diagnostic issues with schizoaffective illness: a critical assessment and implications for future research and treatment, in Manic Illness. Edited by Shopsin B. New York, Raven Press, 1979.

Shulman K., Post F.: Bipolar affective disorder in old age. Br. J. Psychiatry 136:26–32, 1980.

Siris S.G., Harmon G.K., Endicott J.: Postpsychotic depressive symptoms in hospitalized schizophrenic patients. Arch. Gen. Psychiatry 38:1122–1130, 1981.

Smeraldi E., Negri E., Melica M.: A genetic study of affective disorders. Acta Psychiatr. Scand. 56:382–398, 1977.

Sovner R.D., McHugh P.R.: Bipolar course in schizoaffective illness. Biol. Psychiatry 11:195–203, 1976.

Spicer C.C., Hare E.H., Slater E.: Neurotic and psychotic forms of depressive illness—evidence from age-incidence in a national sample. Br. J. Psychiatry 123:535–541, 1973.

Spitzer R.L., Endicott J., Robins E., et al.: Preliminary report of the reliability of research diagnostic criteria (RDC) applied to psychiatric case records, in Psychopharmacology. Edited by Gershon E.S., Baer R. New York, Raven Press, 1975.

Spitzer R.L., Endicott J., Robins E.: Research diagnostic criteria for a selected group of functional disorders, 3rd ed. New York, N.Y. Psychiatric Institute Biometrics Research Division, 1978.

Strober M., Carlson G.: Bipolar illness in adolescents with major depression: clinical, genetic and psychopharmacologic predictors in a three- to four-year prospective follow-up investigation. Arch. Gen. Psychiatry 39:549–555, 1982.

Taylor M.A., Abrams R.: Reassessing the bipolar-unipolar dichotomy. J. Affective Disord. 2:195–217, 1980.

Taylor M.A., Gaztanaga P., Abrams R.: Manic-depressive illness and acute schizophrenia: a clinical, family history and treatment-response study. Am. J. Psychiatry 131:678–682, 1974.

Tsuang M.T.: Schizoaffective disorder: dead or alive? Arch. Gen. Psychiatry 36:633–634, 1979.

Turner W.J., King S.: Two genetically distinct forms of bipolar affective disorder? Biol. Psychiatry 16:417–439, 1981.

Van Praag H.M.: The significance of biological factors in the diagnosis of depressions: II. Hormonal variables. Compr. Psychiatry 23:216–226, 1982.

Weeke A.: Causes of death in manic-depressives, in Origin, Prevention and Treatment of Affective Disorders. Edited by Schou M., Strömgren E. New York, Academic Press, 1979.

Weissman M.M., Myers J.K.: Affective disorders in a U.S. urban community. Arch. Gen. Psychiatry 35:1304–1311, 1978.

Welner A., Liss J.L., Robins E.: Psychiatric symptoms in white and black inpatients. II. Follow-up study. Compr. Psychiatry 14:483–488, 1973.

Wertham F.I.: A group of benign chronic psychoses—prolonged manic excitements. Am. J. Psychiatry 9:17–78, 1928.

Winokur G: Depression—The Facts. London, Oxford University Press, 1981.

Winokur G.: Is there a common genetic factor in bipolar and unipolar affective disorder? Compr. Psychiatry 21:460–468, 1980.

Winokur G., Clayton P.: Family history studies: I. Two types of affective disorders separated according to genetic and clinical factors, in Recent Advances in Biological Psychiatry. Edited by Wortis J. New York, Plenum Publishing Corp., 1967.

Winokur G., Clayton P., Reich T.: Manic-Depressive Illness. St. Louis, C.V. Mosby Co., 1969.

Winokur G., Tsuang M.T., Crowe R.R.: The Iowa 500: affective disorder in relatives of manic and depressed patients. Am. J. Psychiatry 139:209–212, 1982.

Wold P.N., Dwight R.: Subtypes of depression identified by the KDS-3A: a pilot study. Am. J. Psychiatry 136:1415–1419, 1979.

Youngerman J., Canino I.A.: Lithium carbonate use in children and adolescents. Arch. Gen. Psychiatry 35:216–224, 1978.

References for Chapter 19

Drug Treatment of the Acute Manic Episode

American Psychiatric Association: Diagnostic and Statistical Manual of Mental Disorders, 3rd ed. Washington, D.C., American Psychiatric Association, 1980.

Ballenger J.C., Post R.M.: Carbamazepine in manic-depressive illness: a new treatment. Am. J. Psychiatry 137:782–790, 1980.

Bunney W.E. Jr., Goodwin F.K., Davis F.M., et al.: A behavioral-biochemical study of lithium treatment. Am. J. Psychiatry 125:499–512, 1968.

Cade J.F.J.: Lithium salts in the treatment of psychotic excitement. Med. J. Aust. 36:349–352, 1949.

Carlson G.A., Goodwin F.K.: The stages of mania: a longitudinal analysis of the manic episode. Arch. Gen. Psychiatry 28:221–228, 1973.

Chang S.S., Pandey G.N., Casper R.C., et al.: Pharmacokinetics of lithium: predicting optimal dosage, in Lithium: Controversies and Unresolved Issues. Edited by Cooper T.B., Gershon E.S., Kline N.S., Schou M. Amsterdam, Excerpta Medica, 1979.

Cho J.T., Bone S., Dunner D.L., et. al.: The effect of lithium treatment on thyroid function in patients with primary affective disorder. Am. J. Psychiatry 136:115–116, 1979.

Cohen W.J., Cohen N.H.: Lithium carbonate, haloperidol, and irreversible brain damage. JAMA 230:1283–1288, 1974.

Cooper T.B., Bergner P.E., Simpson G.E.: The 24-hour serum lithium level as a prognosticator of dosage requirements. Am. J. Psychiatry 130:601–603, 1973.

Cooper J.E., Kendell R.E., Gurland B.J., et al.: Psychiatric Diagnosis in New York and London. London, Oxford University Press, 1972.

Dunner D.L.: Affective disorders, in Current Therapy. Edited by Conn H.F. Philadelphia, W.B. Saunders Co., 1981.

Dunner D.L.: Rapid cycling bipolar manic depressive illness. Psychiatr. Clin. North Am. 2:461–462, 1979.

Dunner D.L., Fleiss J.L., Fieve R.R.: The course of development of mania in patients with recurrent depression. Am. J. Psychiatry 133:905–908, 1976a.

Dunner D.L., Gershon E.S., Goodwin F.K.: Heritable factors in the severity of affective illness. Biol. Psychiatry II:31–42, 1976b.

Dunner D.L., Murphy D., Stallone F., et al.: Episode frequency prior to lithium treatment in bipolar manic-depressive patients. Compr. Psychiatry 20:511–515, 1979a.

Dunner D.L., Patrick V., Fieve R.R.: Rapid cycling manic depressive patients. Compr. Psychiatry 18:561–566, 1977.

Dunner D.L., Roose S.P., Bone S.: Complications of lithium treatment in older patients, in Lithium: Controversies and Unresolved Issues. Edited by Cooper T.B., Gershon E.S., Kline N.S., Schou M. Amsterdam, Excerpta Medica, 1979b.

Dunner D.L., Russek F.D., Russek B., et al.: Classification of affective disorder subtypes. Compr. Psychiatry 23: 186–189, 1982.

Feighner J.P., Robins E., Guze S.B., et al.: Diagnostic criteria for use in psychiatric research. Arch. Gen. Psychiatry 26:57–63, 1972.

Goodwin F.K., Murphy D.L., Bunney W.E. Jr.: Lithium carbonate treatment of depression and mania. Arch. Gen. Psychiatry 21:486–496, 1969.

Janowsky D.S., Leff M., Epstein R.S.: Playing the manic game. Arch. Gen. Psychiatry 22:252–261, 1976.

Johnson G., Gershon E.S., Burdock E., et al.: Comparative effects of lithium and chlorpromazine in the treatment of acute manic states. Br. J. Psychiatry 109:56–65, 1971.

Johnson G., Gershon E.S., Hekiman L.: Controlled evaluation of lithium and chlorpromazine in the treatment of manic states: an interim report. Compr. Psychiatry 9: 563–573, 1968.

Kocsis J.R.: Treatment of mania. Compr. Psychiatry 22: 596–602, 1981.

Krauthammer C., Klerman G.L.: Secondary mania. Arch. Gen. Psychiatry 35:1333–1339, 1978.

Maggs, R.: Treatment of manic illness with lithium carbonate. Br. J. Psychiatry 109:56–65, 1963.

McCabe M., Norris B.: ECT versus chlorpromazine in mania. Biol. Psychiatry 12:245–254, 1977.

McCabe M.S., Strömgren E.: Reactive psychoses: a family study. Arch. Gen. Psychiatry 32:447–454, 1975.

Murphy D.L., Beigel A.: Depression, elation and lithium carbonate responses in manic patient subgroups. Arch. Gen. Psychiatry 31:643–648, 1974.

Platman S.B.: A comparison of lithium carbonate and chlorpromazine in mania. Am. J. Psychiatry 127:351–353, 1970.

Pollock H.M.: Recurrence of attacks in manic-depressive psychoses. Am. J. Psychiatry 11:562–573, 1931.

Prien R.F.: Clinical uses of lithium—Part I: Introduction, in Lithium: Controversies and Unresolved Issues. Edited by Cooper T.B., Gershon E.S., Kline N.S., Schou M. Amsterdam, Excerpta Medica, 1979.

Prien R.F., Caffey E.M., Klett C.J.: A comparison of lithium carbonate and chlorpromazine in the treatment of excited schizoaffectives. Arch. Gen. Psychiatry 27:182–189, 1972a.

Prien R.F., Klett C.J., Caffey E.M.: Comparison of lithium carbonate in the treatment of mania. Arch. Gen. Psychiatry 26:146–153, 1972b.

Rosenthal N.E., Rosenthal L.N., Stallone F., et al.: Toward the validation of RDC schizoaffective disorder. Arch. Gen. Psychiatry 37:804–810, 1980.

Schou M., Juel-Nielson N., Strömgren E., et al.: The treatment of manic psychoses by the administration of lithium salts. J. Neurol. Neurosurg. Psychiat. 17:250–260, 1954.

Shopsin B., Gershon E.S., Thompson H., et al.: Psychoactive drugs in mania. Arch. Gen. Psychiatry 32:34–42, 1975.

Spring G., Schweid D., Gray G., et al.: A double-blind comparison of lithium and chlorpromazine in the treatment of manic states. Am. J. Psychiatry 126:1306–1309, 1970.

Stallone F., Shelly E., Mendlewicz J., et al.: The use of lithium in affective disorders: III. A double-blind study of prophylaxis in bipolar illness. Am. J. Psychiatry 130: 1006–1010, 1973.

Stancer H.C., Persad E.: Treatment of intractable rapid cycling manic-depressive disorder with levothyroxine. Arch. Gen. Psychiatry 39:311–312, 1982.

Stokes P.E., Shamoian C.A., Stoll P.M., et al.: Efficacy of lithium as acute treatment of manic depressive illness. Lancet 1:1319–1325, 1971.

Takahashi R., Sakuma A., Itoh K., et al.: Comparison of efficacy of lithium carbonate and chlorpromazine in mania. Arch. Gen. Psychiatry 32:1310–1318, 1975.

Thomas C., Tatham A., Jakubowski S.: Lithium/haloperidol combinations and brain damage. Lancet 1:626, 1982.

Winokur G., Clayton P., Reich T.: Manic Depressive Illness. St. Louis, C.V. Mosby Co., 1969.

References for Chapter 20

Long-Term Prophylactic Pharmacologic Treatment of Bipolar Illness

Ahlfors U.G., Baastrup P.C., Dencker S.J., et al.: Flupenthixol decanoate in recurrent manic-depressive illness: a comparison with lithium. Acta Psychiatr. Scand. 63:226–237, 1981.

Angst J., Baastrup P., Hippius W., et al.: The course of monopolar depression and bipolar psychoses. Psychiatr. Neurol. Neurochir. (Amsterdam) 76:489–500, 1973.

Angst J., Grof P.: Selection of patients with recurrent affective illness for a long-term study: testing research criteria on prospective follow-up data, in Lithium: Controversies and Unresolved Issues. Edited by Cooper T.B., Gershon, E.S., Kline N.S., Schou M. Amsterdam, Excerpta Medica, 1979.

Angst J., Grof P.: The course of monopolar depressions and bipolar psychosis, in Lithium in Psychiatry: A Synopsis. Edited by Villeneuve A. Quebec, Les Presses de L'University Laval, 1976.

Baastrup P.C.: The use of lithium in manic-depressive psychosis. Compr. Psychiatry 5:396–408, 1964.

Baastrup P.C., Poulson J.C., Schou M., et al: Prophylactic lithium: double-blind discontinuation in manic-depressive and recurrent depressive disorders. Lancet 2:326–330, 1970.

Baastrup P.C., Schou M.: Lithium as a prophylactic agent. Its effects against recurrent depressions and manic-depressive psychosis. Arch. Gen. Psychiatry 16:162–172, 1967.

Ballenger J.C., Post R.M.: Therapeutic effects of carbamazepine in affective illness: a preliminary report. Commun. Psychopharmacol. 2:159–175, 1978.

Ban T.A.: Adverse effects in maintenance treatment: practical and theoretical considerations. Prog. Neuropsychopharmacol. 3:231–255, 1979.

Ban T.A., Hollender M.H.: Psychopharmacology for Everyday Practice. Basel, Switzerland, S. Karger, 1981.

Bialos D., Giller E., Jatlow P., et al.: Recurrence of depression after discontinuation of long-term amitriptyline treatment. Am. J. Psychiatry 139:325–330, 1982.

Blackwell B., Shepherd M.: Prophylactic lithium: another therapeutic myth? Lancet 1:968–971, 1969.

Braden G., Amsterdam J., Gehab M.: A prospective study of lithium-induced neuropathy: preliminary results, in Abstracts of the 14th Annual Meeting of the American Society of Nephrology. Thorofare, N.J., 1981.

Brown W.T.: The use of lithium carbonate in the treatment of mood disorders. Can. Med. Assoc. J. 108:742–744, 1973.

Brown W.T.: The pattern of lithium side-effects and toxic reactions in the course of lithium therapy, in Handbook of Lithium Therapy. Edited by Johnson F.N. Lancaster, England, MTP Press Limited, 1980.

Bucht G., Wahlin A.: Renal concentrating capacity on long-term lithium treatment and after withdrawal of lithium. Acta Med. Scand. 207:309–314, 1980.

Bunney W.E.: Psychopharmacology of the switch process in affective illness, in Psychopharmacology: A Generation of Progress. Edited by Lipton M.A., DiMascio A., Killam K.F. New York, Raven Press, 1978.

Carroll B.J.: Prediction of treatment outcome with lithium. Arch. Gen. Psychiatry 36:870–878, 1979.

Coppen A., Bishop M.E., Bailey J.E., et al.: Renal function in lithium and non-lithium treated patients with affective disorders. Acta Psychiatr. Scand. 62:343–355, 1980.

Coppen A., Metcalfe, Wood K.: Lithium, in Handbook of Affective Disorders. Edited by Paykel E.S. Edinburgh, Scotland, Churchill Livingstone, 1982.

Coppen A., Noguera R., Baily J., et al.: Prophylactic lithium in affective disorders. Lancet 2:275–279, 1971.

Coppen A., Peet M.: The long-term management of patients with affective disorders, in Psychopharmacology of Affective Disorders. Edited by Paykel E.S., Coppen A. Oxford, Oxford University Press, 1979.

Cundall R.L., Brooks P.W., Murray L.G.: Controlled evaluation of lithium prophylaxis in affective disorders. Psychol. Med. 3:308–311, 1972.

Davenport Y.B., Ebert M.H., Adland M.L., et al.: Couples group therapy as an adjunct to lithium maintenance of the manic patient. Am. J. Orthopsychiatry 47:495–502, 1977.

Davies B., Kincaid-Smith P.: Renal biopsy studies of lithium and prelithium patients and comparison with cadaver transplant kidneys. Neuropharmacology 18:1001–1002, 1979.

Department of Health and Human Services: Medical Practice Information Demonstration Project: A State-of-the-Science Report, Contract 282-17-0068; Office of the Assistant Secretary for Health. Baltimore, Policy Research Inc., 1979.

DePaulo R.J., Correa E.I., Folstein M.F.: Does lithium stabilize mood or affective illness? Presented at the 135th Annual Meeting of the American Psychiatric Association, Toronto, May 1982.

DePaulo J.R., Correa E.I., Sapir D.G.: Renal toxicity of lithium and its implications. Johns Hopkins Med. J. 149:15–21, 1981.

Dunner D.L., Fieve R.R.: Clinical factors in lithium carbonate prophylaxis failure. Arch. Gen. Psychiatry 30:229–233, 1974.

Dunner D.L., Fleiss J.L., Fieve R.R.: Lithium carbonate prophylaxis failure. Br. J. Psychiatry 129:40–44, 1976a.

Dunner D.L., Stallone F., Fieve R.R.: Lithium carbonate and affective disorders: A double-blind study of prophylaxis of depression in bipolar illness. Arch. Gen. Psychiatry 33:117–121, 1976b.

Galenberg A.J.: Lithium and the kidney: ongoing issues. Biological Therapies in Psychology 4:25–26, 1981.

Ghose K.: Lithium salts: therapeutic and unwanted effects. Br. J. Hosp. Med. 18:578–583, 1977.

Giller E.L., Bialos D.S., Docherty J.P.: Chronic amitriptyline toxicity. Am. J. Psychiatry 136:458–459, 1979.

Grof P., Angst J., Karasek M., et al.: Selection of an individual patient for long-term lithium treatment in clinical practice, in Lithium: Controversies and Unresolved Issues. Edited by Cooper T.B., Gershon E.S., Kline N.S., Schou M. Amsterdam, Excerpta Medica, 1979.

Hartigan C.: The use of lithium salts in affective disorders. Br. J. Psychiatry 109:810–813, 1963.

Hestbech J., Hansen H.E., Amdisen A., et al.: Chronic renal lesions following long-term treatment with lithium. Kidney Int. 12:205–213, 1977.

Hullin R.P.: Minimum serum lithium levels for effective prophylaxis, in Handbook of Lithium Therapy. Edited by Johnson F.N., Lancaster, England, MTP Press Limited, 1980.

Jamison K.R.: Psychological issues in bipolar affective illness. Presented at 135th Annual Meeting of the American Psychiatric Association, Toronto, May 1982.

Jamison K.R., Gerner R.H., Goodwin F.K.: Patient and physician attitudes toward lithium. Relationship to compliance. Arch. Gen. Psychiatry 36:866–869, 1979.

Jerram T.C., McDonald R.: Plasma lithium control with particular reference to minimum effective levels, in Lithium in Medical Practice. Edited by Johnson F.N., Johnson S. Baltimore, University Park Press, 1978.

Kane J.M., Quitkin F.M., Rifkin A., et al.: Prophylactic lithium with and without imipramine for bipolar I patients: a double-blind study. Psychopharmacol. Bull. 17:144–145, 1981.

Kielholz T., Terzani S., Pöldinger W.: The long-term treatment of periodical and cyclic depressions with flupenthixol decanoate. Int. Pharmacopsychiatry 14:305–307, 1979.

Kjellman B.F., Karlberg B.E., Thorell L.H.: Cognitive and affective functions in patients with affective disorders treated with lithium. Acta Psychiatr. Scand. 62:32–46, 1980.

Klerman G.L.: Long-term treatment of affective disorders, in Psychopharmacology: A Generation of Progress. Edited by Lipton M.A., DiMascio A., Killam K.F. New York, Raven Press, 1978.

Kukopulos A., Reginaldi D., Giraldi P.: Course of manic-depressive recurrences under lithium. Compr. Psychiatry 16:517–524, 1975.

Lewis J.L., Winokur G.: The induction of mania. Arch. Gen. Psychiatry 39:303–306, 1982.

Loo H., Benyacoub A.K., Rovei V.: Long-term monitoring of tricyclic antidepressant plasma concentrations. Br. J. Psychiatry 137:444–451, 1980.

Nystrom S.: Depressions: factors related to 10-year prognosis. Acta Psychiatr. Scand. 60:225–238, 1979.

Okuma T., Inanaga K., Osuki S., et al.: Comparison of the anti-manic efficacy of carbamazepine and chlorpromazine: double-blind controlled study. Psychopharmacology 56:211–217, 1979.

Okuma T., Kazutoyo I., Saburo O., et al.: A preliminary double-blind study on the efficacy of carbamazepine in prophylaxis of manic-depressive illness. Psychopharmacology 73:95–96, 1981.

Okuma T., Kisimoto A.: Antimanic efficacy of carbamazepine. Paper presented at the VI World Congress of Psychiatry, Honolulu, 1977.

Post R.M.: Cyclic affective illness: alternatives to lithium. Paper presented at the 135th Annual Meeting of the American Psychiatric Association, Toronto, May 1982.

Prien R.F.: Predicting lithium responders and non-responders: illness indicators, in Handbook of Lithium Therapy. Edited by Johnson F.N. Lancaster, England, MTP Press Limited, 1980.

Prien R.F., Caffey E.M.: Long-term maintenance drug therapy in recurrent affective illness: current status and issues. Dis. Nerv. Syst. 38:981–992, 1977.

Prien R.F., Caffey E.M.: The relationship between dosage and response to prophylaxis. Am. J. Psychiatry 133:567–570, 1976.

Prien R.F., Caffey E.M., Klett C.J.: Factors associated with treatment success in lithium carbonate prophylaxis. Arch. Gen. Psychiatry 31:189–192, 1974.

Prien R.F., Caffey E.M., Klett C.J.: Prophylactic efficacy of lithium carbonate in manic-depressive illness. Arch. Gen. Psychiatry 28:337–341, 1973a.

Prien R.F., Klett C.J., Caffey E.M.: Lithium carbonate and imipramine in prevention of affective episodes. Arch. Gen. Psychiatry 29:420–425, 1973b.

Quitkin F., Rifkin A., Klein D.F.: Prophylaxis of affective disorders. Arch. Gen. Psychiatry 33:337–346, 1976.

Rabin E.Z., Garston R.G., Weir R.V.: Persistent nephrogenic diabetes insipidus associated with long-term lithium carbonate treatment. Can. Med. Assoc. J. 121:194–198, 1979.

Rafaelson O., Bolwig T., Bran C.: Lithium and the kidney. Presented at the 132nd Annual Meeting of the American Psychiatric Association, Chicago, May 1979.

Ramsey A.T., Cox M.: Lithium and the kidney. Am. J. Psychiatry 139:443–449, 1982.

Schou M.: Lithium Treatment of Manic-Depressive Illness. London, S. Karger, 1980.

Schou M.: Normothymics, "mood normalizers:" are lithium and imipramine drugs specific for affective disorders? Br. J. Psychiatry 109:803–809, 1963.

Schou M.: Social and psychological implications of lithium therapy, in Handbook of Lithium Therapy. Edited by Johnson F.N. Lancaster, England. MTP Press Limited, 1980.

Schou M., Baastrup P.C., Grof P., et al.; Pharmacological and clinical problems of lithium prophylaxis. Br. J. Psychiatry 116:615–619, 1970.

Schou M., Thomsen K.: Prophylaxis of recurrent endogenous affective disorders, in Lithium Research and Therapy. Edited by Johnson F.N. London, Academic Press, 1975.

Shakir S.A., Volkmar F.R., Bacon S., et al.: Group psychotherapy as an adjunct to lithium maintenance. Am. J. Psychiatry 136:455–456, 1979.

Stallone F., Shelley E., Mendlewicz J.: The use of lithium in affective disorders. III: A double-blind study of prophylaxis in bipolar illness. Am. J. Psychiatry 130:1006–1010, 1973.

Van Putten T.: Why do patients with manic-depressive illness stop lithium? Compr. Psychiatry 16:179–183, 1975.

Vestergaard P.: Renal side effects of lithium, in Handbook of Lithium Therapy. Edited by Johnson F.N. Lancaster, England, MTP Press Limited, 1980.

Vestergaard P., Amdisen A., Schou M.: Clinically significant side effects of lithium treatment: a survey of 237 patients in long-term treatment. Acta Psychiatr. Scand. 62:193–200, 1980.

Vestergaard P., Schou M., Thomsen K.: Monitoring of patients in prophylactic lithium treatment. Br. J. Psychiatry 140:185–187, 1982.

Weinstein M.R.: Lithium treatment of women during pregnancy and in the post-delivery period, in Handbook of Lithium Therapy. Edited by Johnson F.N. Lancaster, England, MTP Press Limited, 1980.

Winokur G., Clayton P., Reich T.: Manic-Depressive Illness. St. Louis, C.V. Mosby Co., 1969.

Zis A.P., Goodwin F.K.: Major affective disorder as a recurrent illness: a critical review. Arch. Gen. Psychiatry 36:835–839, 1979.

References for Chapter 21

Psychotherapeutic Issues in Bipolar Illness

Abraham K.: Notes on the psychoanalytic investigation and treatment of manic-depressive insanity and allied conditions (1927), in Selected Papers of Karl Abraham. London, Hogarth Press, 1968.

Benson R.: The forgotten treatment modality in bipolar illness: psychotherapy. Dis. Nerv. Syst. 36:634–638, 1975.

Benson R.: Psychotherapy and bipolar illness. Unpublished manuscript, 1976.

Bunney W.E. Jr., Hartman E.L., Mason J.W.: Study of a patient with 48-hour manic-depressive cycles. II. Strong positive correlation between endocrine factors and manic defense patterns. Arch. Gen. Psychiatry 12:619–625, 1965.

Cade F.J.F.: Lithium salts in the treatment of psychotic excitement. Med. J. Aust. 2:349–352, 1949.

Cochran S.D.: Strategies for preventing lithium noncompliance in bipolar affective illness. Doctoral dissertation, University of California, Los Angeles, 1983.

Davenport Y.B., Ebert M.H., Adland M.L., et al.: Couples group therapy as an adjunct to lithium maintenance of the manic patient. Am. J. Orthopsychiatry 47:495–502, 1977.

English O.S.: Observation of trends in manic-depressive psychosis. Psychiatry 12:125–134, 1949.

Fitzgerald R.G.: Mania as a message: treatment with family therapy and lithium carbonate. Am. J. Psychother. 26:547–555, 1972.

Fromm-Reichmann F.: Intensive psychotherapy of manic-depressives. Confina. Neurologica 9:158–165, 1949.

Goodwin F.K., Jamison K.R.: Manic-Depressive Illness. New York, Oxford University Press, 1983.

Greenson R.R.: The Technique and Practice of Psychoanalysis. New York, International Universities Press, 1967.

Jamison K.R., Gerner R.H., Goodwin F.K.: Patient and physician attitudes towards lithium. Relationship to compliance. Arch. Gen. Psychiatry 36:866–869, 1979.

Jamison K.R., Gerner R.H., Hammen C., et al.: Clouds and silver linings: positive experiences associated with the primary affective disorders. Am. J. Psychiatry 137:198–202, 1980.

Janowsky D.S., Leff M., Epstein R.S.: Playing the manic game: interpersonal maneuvers of the acutely manic patient. Arch. Gen. Psychiatry 22:252–261, 1970.

Jenner F.A., Eastwood P.R.: Renal effects of lithium, in Lithium in Medical Practice. Edited by Johnson F.N., Johnson S. Baltimore, University Park Press, 1978.

Johnson F.N.: Social and psychological supportive measures during lithium therapy, in Handbook of Lithium Therapy. Edited by Johnson F.N. Lancaster, MTP Press Limited, 1980.

Kerry R.J.: Recent developments in patient management, in Lithium in Medical Practice. Edited by Johnson F.N., Johnson S. Baltimore, University Park Press, 1978.

Klerman G.L.: Combining drugs and psychotherapy in the treatment of depression, in Drugs in Combination with other Therapies. Edited by Greenblatt M. New York, Grune & Stratton, 1975.

Kraepelin E: Lectures on Clinical Psychiatry. London, Balliere, Tindall & Cox, 1904.

Logan J.: Up and Down, In and Out Life. New York, Delacorte Press, 1976.

Lowell R.: Day by Day. New York, Farrar, Strauss & Giroux, 1977.

Mayo J.A., O'Connell R.A., O'Brien J.D.: Families of manic-depressive patients: effect of treatment. Am. J. Psychiatry 136:1535−1539, 1979.

Polatin P., Fieve R.R.: Patient rejection of lithium carbonate prophylaxis. JAMA 218:864−866, 1971.

Rado S.: The problem of melancholia. Int. J. Psychoanal 9:420−438, 1928.

Rosen A.M.: Group management of lithium prophylaxis. Presented at the Annual Meeting of the American Psychiatric Association, San Francisco, 1980.

Rosenfeld H.: Notes on the psychological and psychoanalytic treatment of depressive and manic depressive patients, in Psychiatric Research Report 17. Edited by Azima H., Glueck B.C., Washington, D.C., American Psychiatric Association, 1963.

Rounsaville, B.J., Klerman G.L., Weissman M.M.: Do psychotherapy and pharmacotherapy for depression conflict? Empirical evidence from a clinical trial. Arch. Gen. Psychiatry 38:24−29, 1981.

Schou M.: Social and psychological implications of lithium therapy, in Handbook of Lithium Therapy. Edited by Johnson F.N. Lancaster, MTP Press Limited, 1980.

Schou M., Baastrup P.C.: Personal and social implications of lithium maintenance treatment, in Psychopharmacology, Sexual Disorders and Drug Abuse. Edited by Ban T.A., Boissier J.R., Gessa G.J. Amsterdam & London, North Holland Publishing Co., 1973.

Schou M., Baastrup P.C., Grof P., et al.: Pharmacological and clinical problems of lithium prophylaxis. Br. J. Psychiatry 116:615−619, 1970.

Shakir S.A., Volkmar F.R., Bacon S., et al.: Group psychotherapy as an adjunct to lithium maintenance. Am. J. Psychiatry 136:455−456, 1979.

Van Putten T.: Why do patients with manic-depressive illness stop their lithium? Compr. Psychiatry 16:179−182, 1975.

Volkmar F.R., Shakir S.A., Bacon S., et al.: Group therapy as an adjunct to lithium maintenance. Paper presented at Annual Meeting of the American Psychiatric Association, San Francisco, 1980.

Weissman M.M.: Psychotherapy and its relevance to the pharmacotherapy of affective disorders: from ideology to evidence, in Psychopharmacology: A Generation of Progress. Edited by Lipton M.A., DiMascio A., Killam K.F. New York, Raven Press, 1978.

V

Depressive Disorders

Part V

Depressive Disorders

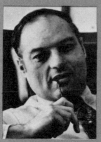

Gerald L. Klerman, M.D., Preceptor

Harrington Professor of Psychiatry
Harvard Medical School
Director of Research
Psychiatry Service
Massachusetts General Hospital

Authors for Part V

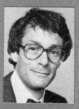

Robert M.A. Hirschfeld, M.D.
Chief, Center for Studies of
  Affective Disorders
Clinical Research Branch
National Institute of Mental Health

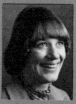

Christine K. Cross, M.A.
Research Assistant
Group Operations, Incorporated
Rockville, Maryland

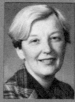

Paula J. Clayton, M.D.
Professor and Head
Department of Psychiatry
University of Minnesota
  Medical School

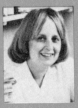

Myrna M. Weissman, Ph.D.

Professor of Psychiatry
  and Epidemiology
Yale University School of Medicine
Director
Depression Research Unit
Connecticut Mental Health Center

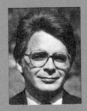

Jeffrey H. Boyd, M.D., M.P.H.

Epidemiology Fellow
Center for Epidemiologic Studies
Division of Biometry and
  Epidemiology
National Institute of Mental Health

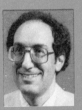

Elliot S. Gershon, M.D.

Section on Psychogenetics
Biological Psychiatry Branch
National Institute of Mental Health

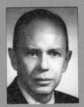

Joseph J. Schildkraut, M.D.

Professor of Psychiatry
Harvard Medical School
Director
Neuropsychopharmacology Laboratory
Massachusetts Mental Health Center
Director
Psychiatric Chemistry Laboratory
New England Deaconess Hospital

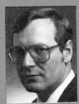

John J. Mooney, M.D.

Instructor in Psychiatry
Harvard Medical School
Massachusetts Mental Health Center

Paul J. Orsulak, Ph.D.

Assistant Professor of Psychiatry
Harvard Medical School

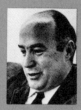

Jonathan O. Cole, M.D.

Chief
Psychopharmacology Program
McLean Hospital

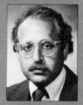

Alan F. Schatzberg, M.D.

Associate Professor
Harvard Medical School
McLean Hospital

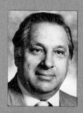

James M. Perel, Ph.D.

Professor of Psychiatry
  and Pharmacology
University of Pittsburgh
  School of Medicine
Director
Clinical Pharmacology Program
Western Psychiatric
  Institute and Clinic

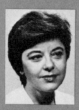

Maria Kovacs, Ph.D.

Associate Professor of Psychiatry
University of Pittsburgh
  School of Medicine and
Western Psychiatric
  Institute and Clinic

V

Depressive Disorders

Introduction

by Gerald L. Klerman, M.D.

Clinical descriptions of depression are found in the writings of many ancient peoples, including the Greeks, the biblical Hebrews, and the Egyptians. Many descriptions of melancholia appear in the later works of medieval writers and in eighteenth and nineteenth century literature. In recent decades, attention to clinical depressions has increased markedly, and with this attention the research and scientific writings on psychopathology, genetics, treatment, and epidemiology have grown in both quality and quantity.

DSM-III crystallizes a number of the significant findings from this recent research. Among the major achievements of DSM-III with regard to depressive disorders are the following five. First, DSM-III groups the Affective Disorders into a separate category. Previously, some forms of depression were considered psychotic disorders (as in major depressive insanity) and others were considered neurotic disorders (psychoneurotic depressive reaction). Second, DSM-III emphasizes syndromal descriptions based on clinical history and manifest symptomatology without presumptions as to etiology. Thus, terms like endogenous or reactive depression are not included in DSM-III. In a third advance, DSM-III includes in the range of Affective Disorders a number of affective conditions previously regarded as personality disorders. The inclusion of Cyclothymic Disorder is a particularly noteworthy example. Fourth, DSM-III separates Bipolar Disorder from other forms of Affective Disorder and clarifies the criteria for what was previously called manic-depressive illness by requiring a current or previous history of mania. This reflects the recent genetic, treatment-response, and neurophysiological data that indicate the value of separating bipolar illness from other forms of Affective Disorder. Fifth and finally, DSM-III includes a new diagnostic category, Dysthymic Disorder. This newly created category brings together a heterogeneous group of conditions with chronic course, fluctuating levels of symptoms and distress, and long-standing personality and interpersonal dysfunctions.

The chapters in this Part review the recent research developments in the diagnosis, epidemiology, genetics, and treatment of depressive disorders within the DSM-III framework. The contents of this Part, however, must be viewed within the context of the literature in the field and in light of the other Parts of this volume and some Parts of *Psychiatry 1982 (Psychiatry Update: Volume I)*. While the emphasis in this Part is on the relevance of recently established research findings for clinical practice, clinicians will find that some important topics are not covered here. In some cases, this is because of limitations of space or because the available research evidence is inadequate. For example, clinicians experienced in psychoanalytic theory and in the use of dynamic psychotherapy may find the discussion of these topics meager, in part reflecting the lack of new research findings in this area. In part this reflects the fact that these topics have been covered elsewhere, and some additional topics are not reviewed here because they have been so systematically reviewed in recent journals. Thus, for instance, no chapter deals in depth with recent neuroendocrine research, particularly with the dexamethasone suppression test developed by Carroll and associates (see Carroll, 1982) or with the important findings that Kupfer and associates have made in the area of sleep neurophysiology (see Kupfer et al., 1976).

Similarly, depression in childhood and adolescence is not covered in this Part, since the topic was reviewed extensively in *Psychiatry 1982* (*Psychiatry Update: Volume I*, Part III). Nor does the Part contain a chapter on depressions occurring in the elderly, although several of the chapters do discuss particular aspects of treating depression in older persons. The special problems of neurological dysfunction and clinical psychopharmacology required that depressive disorders in the elderly be dealt with separately (see Part II of this volume and especially chapter 9). Finally, some of the chapters in this Part apply equally to Part IV of this volume, Bipolar Illness. The review of epidemiologic data by Drs. Weissman and Boyd and the review of genetic and familial data by Dr. Gershon both deal with the broad spectrum of affective disorders and thus are not limited in their applicability to the depressive disorders.

Given the foregoing contextual parameters, the chapters included in this Part attempt a broad if not comprehensive update concerning the current status of research on depressive disorders. The chapters are particularly focused on the clinical and epidemiologic aspects of depression and the important issues most frequently encountered in the drug and psychotherapeutic treatment of depressive disorders.

In the first chapter, the Preceptor reviews the nosology and diagnosis of depressive disorders, beginning with a discussion of the distinctions between depression as a normal emotion or symptom and depression as a clinical syndrome. The chapter discusses each of the DSM-III diagnostic categories and also considers the evidence for refining the nosology and incorporating several additional classificatory dimensions.

Dr. Robert M.A. Hirschfeld and Ms. Christine K. Cross discuss the role of personality factors, life events, and social factors in the development of depressive disorders. Their chapter covers the current methodologically sound research on these factors and organizes the findings according to a fourfold hypothetical schema concerning the relationships between psychosocial factors and depressive disorders. According to their schema, psychosocial factors may be predispositional for depression, they may be subclinical manifestations of depression, and/or they may influence the character of depression; finally, depression may influence the psychosocial factors themselves.

In the next chapter, Drs. Myrna M. Weissman and Jeffrey H. Boyd consider the epidemiologic and risk factors involved in depressive symptoms, in nonbipolar depression, and in bipolar disorder. Their review of the literature and introductory remarks highlight the progress in epidemiologic research made possible by the increased standardization and reliability of diagnostic and classification schemes used in the United States and abroad.

Dr. Paula J. Clayton next presents a concise review of the epidemiologic and risk factors that are involved in completed and attempted suicides. Prefacing her discussion of the scientific literature with a revealing paraphrase from a suicidal literary figure, she illustrates graphically the complex of psychological risk factors and later places them in the context of a wider range of epidemiologic and risk factors.

Dr. Elliot S. Gershon discusses comprehensively the genetic hypotheses regarding affective disorders, drawing evidence from the family, adoption, and twin studies conducted in the United States and abroad. His chapter also details the possible mode of genetic transmission, linkage markers, and etiologic markers, and he concludes that while the evidence for genetic factors in the affective disorders is strong, preventive applications must still generally be limited to secondary and tertiary interventions.

Drs. Joseph J. Schildkraut, Alan F. Schatzberg, John J. Mooney, and Paul J. Orsulak explore the history, status, and possibilities of the emerging field of psychiatric chemistry and review the recent research findings on the neuropsychopharmacology and neuropsychoendocrinology of depressive disorders. Their chapter shows how these findings, with the help of multivariate statistics, are pointing both to a more refined classification of depressive disorders and to the possibility of more precise predictions regarding individual responses to pharmacologic treatments.

In the next chapter, Drs. Jonathan O. Cole and Alan F. Schatzberg review the state of the art in the drug treatment of depressive disorders. Their discussion covers the chemical structures, efficacy, and side effects of the well-known tricyclic antidepressants, as well as the monoamine oxidase inhibitors, and it also presents knowledge to date about a number of promising newer drugs which are in clinical trial or have only recently been released for use in the United States.

Dr. James M. Perel discusses the pharmacokinetics of the tricyclic antidepressants and the use of plasma levels in clinical management. With its practical discussions of single-dose kinetics and assay methods, his chapter is of special interest to the clinician who seeks more precise knowledge and guidance about the dynamics of the tricyclics and the indications and techniques for plasma-level monitoring.

In the last chapter of this Part, Dr. Maria Kovacs reviews several types of psychotherapies for depression. In her discussion of cognitive therapy, behavior therapy, interpersonal psychotherapy, and psychodynamic psychotherapy, she systematically examines the theoretical assumptions, the concept of depression, and the salient tactics within each therapy. Mindful of the theoretical problems associated with psychotherapy research, she then offers some basic guidelines for selecting a psychotherapy for a given depressed patient.

The emphasis in this Part is on empiricism, and theoretical speculation is kept to a minimum. The field of affective disorders in general, and depressive disorders in particular, is changing rapidly. Not only are new empirical data becoming available, but theoretical points of view are themselves becoming more pluralistic and empirical, as more complex views of the interaction of genetics and of metabolic, developmental, and social factors emerge.

Chapter 22

The Nosology and Diagnosis of Depressive Disorders

by Gerald L. Klerman, M.D.

INTRODUCTION

The *affective disorders* include a number of clinical conditions whose common and essential feature is a disturbance of mood, usually depressions and elations, accompanied by cognitive, psychomotor, psycho-physiological, and interpersonal difficulties. *Mood* usually refers to sustained emotional states that color the whole personality and psychic life; thus; mood refers to a pervasive or prevailing emotion. *Affect*, on the other hand, refers to the fluctuating subjective aspect of emotion. In the clinical disorders under consideration, the emotional changes are pervasive and sustained, and some authorities have therefore suggested that *mood disorders* would be a more precise designation than affective disorders. However, historical continuity and clinical usage have preferred the term affective disorders, and that term is used both in DSM-III (American Psychiatric Association, 1980) and in this chapter.

Although human experience includes a variety of emotions, such as fear, anger, pleasure, and surprise, the clinical conditions considered under the affective disorders involve depression and mania. Grouping the affective disorders according to the patient's predominant symptoms does not represent the ideal basis for a nosology. An ideal nosology would base classification on the genetic, psychodynamic, and biological causes of the disorders. These and other causal factors have in fact been proposed as etiologic in the affective disorders, and investigations are underway to establish their precise roles. The conditions grouped together as affective disorders are heterogeneous as to causation, and some or most of them are probably multifactorial in causation, involving complex interactions of genetic, biochemical, developmental, and environmental factors.

In view of our limited current knowledge, however, classification by type of psychological impairment has had great heuristic value. Since the late nineteenth century, mental disorders have been classified according to the psychological faculty that is manifestly the most impaired: intelligence (mental retardation), thinking and cognition (the dementias, the deliriums, the schizophrenias), social behavior (character and personality disorders), and mood (affective disorders). Such an approach to classification parallels the classification of internal physical disorders according to the organ affected (heart, kidney, and so forth). The faculties of the mind assume the role of mental structures and are equivalent to body organs in that they provide a basis for classification when a causal classification has not yet been sufficiently substantiated by research or clinical experience.

Historical Perspectives

Literary and clinical descriptions of mania and of depression, the mental, bodily, and spiritual state that in previous eras was called melancholia, date back to antiquity, as do speculations about the relationships of those emotional states to health and illness and to the human condition. Scientific investigations of affective disorders, however, are only a century or two old. During the nineteenth century, clinicians and especially the French clinicians Falret and Ballenger observed the alternation of depressed and elated states in the same patient. However, it was for Kraepelin to bring together the diverse states into his concept of "manic-depressive insanity."

The classification of manic-depressive insanity was described initially by Kraepelin (1921) and was modified by Bleuler (1951). Over the decades since then, various researchers have further elaborated on the concept. After Kraepelin (1921) first delineated manic-depressive insanity as a diagnostic entity, debates arose over the breadth of the concept, and additional diagnostic labels, such as psychoneurotic-depressive reaction and involutional melancholia, were included in textbooks, governmental classifications, and professional nosologies. The debates were partially resolved by Bleuler's (1951) creation of the general grouping called affective disorders. That particular grouping has had many advantages. It has allowed for multiple subcategories, with possibly differing causes; it has offered more theoretical flexibility than the manic-depressive entity; and it has emphasized affect as a normal human faculty, thus not restricting psychiatrists' attention to insanity and other psychotic phenomena. However, many issues remain unresolved concerning the scope of the affective disorders and the principles on which subcategories are to be delineated and validated.

Kraepelin's textbooks provided a causal basis for the classification of mental disorders. Based on the nineteenth century medical model of illness, disease entities were delineated by syndromal description and were then correlated according to pathology, histology, bacteriology, and natural history. Applied to mental illnesses, this approach proved highly successful, especially for the infectious disorders like general paresis caused by central nervous system syphilis and for nutritional diseases like pellagra. Early in the twentieth century, however, doubts arose about whether this approach was adequate for the functional disorders, those psychiatric syndromes for which no structural CNS pathology could be demonstrated by the methods then available. Among the functional disorders, the affective disorders in particular generated continuing controversy. Kraepelin's concept of manic-depressive illness had brought together a large number of clinical states, including mania, melancholia, and cyclic psychoses, and his concept had clarified many issues, creating a brief period of unity. During the middle decades of the twentieth century, however, the apparent unity achieved by Kraepelin's concept gave way to the proliferation of many new categories.

The endogenous-reactive and neurotic-psychotic distinctions were proposed. Debates arose over the validity of the vaguely defined psychotic-depressive reaction. Adding to the controversy, Kasanin's (1933) description of the schizoaffective psychoses created a nosological overlap between schizophrenia and the manic-depressive disorders. Then, in the 1940s and 1950s, borderline states and pseudoneurotic schizophrenia were described in patients in whom depression and other mood swings were prominent, and this created yet another bridge between psychotic states and neurotic reactions, in this case between schizophrenia and depression. In retrospect, this confusion was a consequence of multiple factors. As psychiatric services expanded outside the mental institutions and into general hospitals, outpatient clinics, social agencies, and private practice, increasing numbers of nonpsychotic and noninstitutionalized patients came to the attention of psychiatrists. Today, most patients with affective disorders are neither hospitalized nor psychotic, and they manifest behaviors and symptom patterns differing in many respects from the classic syndromes formulated in the late nineteenth century. The confusion continued during the period between World War I and World War II and into the early 1950s.

The turning point came in 1952 to 1954 with the development of the new psychopharmacologic agents. The pattern of response to classes of therapeutic drugs proved consistent with Kraepelin's divisions. In particular, the response patterns separated the so-called functional psychosis into schizophrenia, paranoia, and other disorders of thinking which respond to neuroleptics and the disorders of affect which respond either to lithium, in the case of manic states, or to tricyclics, in the case of depressions. While there is overlap among classes of drugs, the general pattern of response follows the separation of the major disorders proposed by the generation of Kraepelin and Bleuler.

The therapeutic efficacy of these drugs has stimulated a search for diagnostic classes that will predict response. The endogenous pattern of depression has been found to predict response to tricyclics. Attempts are underway to develop criteria for "atypical depressions" that may respond specifically to monoamine oxidase inhibitors (MAOIs). These efforts involve rating-scale techniques which were originally designed for the assessment of change under the influence of drugs, but they have also extended to the nosological descriptions of samples to be included in drug studies. In addition to the search for the psychopathological factors that are related to drug response, considerable effort is underway to develop biological laboratory tests. These tests have three purposes: (1) to serve as diagnostic measures in connection with or as replacement for clinical psychopathological criteria; (2) to predict response to treatment; and (3) to guide clinical decision making.

DEPRESSION AS NORMAL MOOD, SYMPTOM, AND CLINICAL SYNDROME

Depression covers a wide range of human emotional and clinical states. As a normal mood, depression is ubiquitous in human existence; not to grieve after losing a loved one is to be "less than human." As a symptom, depression occurs in a wide variety of reactions to stress and to medical and psychiatric conditions. As clinical states, the various depressive syndromes are usually considered to belong to the affective disorders along with mania.

Depression as a Normal Human Emotion

Although the major focus of this chapter is on depression and affective disorders as clinical conditions, understanding their psychopathology and treatment is greatly enhanced by understanding them within the broader context of human experience and behavior. The normalcy of depressed states poses problems for clinical practice and for theory. For clinical practice, criteria are needed to specify the boundaries between the normal mood state and those abnormal states that merit clinical intervention. For theory, it is necessary to understand the nature and function of depression as a normal emotion and to elucidate which features of depression are common to both normal and pathological states and which features are unique to the abnormal states.

Important insights concerning the adaptive value of normal depressive affect derive from Darwin. According to the strictest criterion of evolutionary theory, a trait or behavior is adaptive from the phylogenetic viewpoint if it promotes the survival of the species. Moreover, from the ontogenetic view, a trait is adaptive if it promotes the growth and survival of the individual members of the species. Darwin himself first applied the evolutionary approach to behavior and especially to emotional responses. Darwin postulated the evolution not only of morphological structures but also of "mental and expressive capacities." He also collected material to document the phylogenetic continuity of emotional expressions in animals, particularly in primates and human beings. However, his observations and theory lay dormant for many decades until an interest in the comparative biology of emotional states grew up following World War II. From studies of mammalian behavior, specifically of mother-child development in primates, a significant convergence of findings from neurobiology, ethology, and comparative psychology has emerged.

Psychodynamic studies of human infant development have paralleled these animal researches. Bowlby and others have demonstrated that the genesis of the child's emotion is related to vicissitudes in the child's bond of attachment to mothering figures. Due to their prolonged state of dependency, human infants are highly vulnerable to the effects of separation and attendant feelings of helplessness. The infant's depressive behaviors serve to alert the social group, usually the family, to his or her need for nurturing, assistance, and succor. This generalization is true for the child, but what of the adult living in a modern industrial society? Is a civilized man's or woman's depression merely the automatic perpetuation of previously developed evolutionary responses? If so, is the clinical depression of adults an adaptive response, or is it a maladaptive recurrence of behaviors that were adaptive in an earlier developmental state? The investigations into these questions involve clinical and biological research and theoretical analysis.

The approach of Bowlby and of others who study attachment behavior is in keeping with the psychobiological approach to mental illness first enunciated by Adolf Meyer. In his efforts to apply Darwin's ideas about evolution and adaptation to psychiatric illness, Meyer viewed psychiatric illness in the context of an individual's attempt to adapt to his or her environment. In the history of thought about affective disorders, a tension has existed between the Meyerian approach and the Kraepelinian approach. While the Meyerian approach has tended to view the range of depression, both normal and clinical, within the context of human experience and to emphasize the continuity between normal and clinical states, the Kraepelinian approach has focused upon the pathological aspects and the discontinuity between clinical disorders and normal experience.

The adaptational approach examines the multiple functions of depression. It inquires into the neuroanatomical structures and neurochemical mechanisms by which natural selection, genetic mutation, environmental conditioning, and social learning occur, and it examines how they serve both to mediate the impact of environmental change and to initiate, organize, integrate, and terminate the emotional, metabolic, and goal-directed activities of the organism, in its normal depressive moods as well as in clinical depressive states. The four adaptive functions of affects that are relevant to clinical psychiatry include social communication, physiological arousal, subjective awareness, and psychodynamic defense.

Depression as a Symptom

Depression and mania can occur as symptoms of stress and of medical and psychiatric disorders. Depressive symptoms are seen more commonly than manic symptoms. They seldom occur alone but are usually associated with bodily complaints or with psychological and social impairment. Depressive symptoms may occur as reactions to stressful personal experience, as in grief and bereavement, or they may occur in response to adverse social and economic circumstances, as in poverty or racial or ethnic discrimination. They may also occur as part of a reaction to medical and surgical illnesses. While psychiatric intervention may be useful in these contexts, systematic clinical trials have not been undertaken. The concept is that some patients have depressive symptoms that warrant clinical attention but do not have psychopathological features that meet the diagnostic criteria for the full clinical syndromes.

GRIEF, MOURNING, AND BEREAVEMENT   The prototype for adult depression is grief, the almost universal depressive response to losing a loved one through death. The clinical symptomatology of grief has been widely recognized, and efforts are under way to explore the natural history of grief and to determine which grieving patients may be at risk for clinical depression. Relatively few psychobiological studies of grief have been conducted, and until we know more about neuroendocrine and other changes, important questions about the continuity or discontinuity between normal grief and clinical depression will remain unanswered. No systematic controlled trials have been done except to examine the possible value of imipramine or other tricyclic antidepressants or MAOIs in grieving states. In most clinical circles, the conventional wisdom is that the grieving process is normal and should not be interfered with lest adverse consequences occur. On the other hand, the intensity of affects generated in the grieving reaction may predispose the bereaved individual to a higher risk for cardiovascular and other medical complications. A clinical trial of tricyclic antidepressants against placebo or against counseling would be of both theoretical and practical value.

ADJUSTMENT REACTIONS   A variety of emotional reactions occur in response to stressful or traumatic circumstances. Depressive and other mood symptoms often appear in this context, with mixtures of anxiety, disappointment, frustration, insomnia, and bodily complaints. The concept of adjustment reaction has appeared in many nomenclatures to encompass these responses. Studies of life events such as unemployment, migration, and natural disasters indicate that depressive symptoms occur quite frequently in these transitional adjustment states. Whether they are in continuity with clinical disorders has been the subject of ongoing controversy.

Depression as a Clinical Syndrome

Feelings of sadness, disappointment, and frustration are normal accompaniments of the human condition. Because clinicians and investigators do not fully agree about the complete range of affective phenomena that should be diagnosed as psychopathological, the boundary between normal mood and abnormal depressions is undefined. This has many consequences for practice and theory. In clinical practice, inconsistencies often arise in referrals, and marked variations occur in decisions about psychotherapeutic or psychopharmacologic treatment. Without validated diagnostic criteria, case finding is highly variable, and epidemiologic surveys are inconclusive or ungeneralizable. It is difficult, if not impossible, to calculate accurate estimates of incidence, prevalence, and other basic rates.

DECISION-MAKING CRITERIA   The presence or absence of an overt life stress or precipitating life event poses some diagnostic dilemmas. Psychiatrists tend to think that they can understand emotional fluctuations in relation to the precipitating event, but they often minimize the severity of depressive reactions when a life stress is apparent. It is therefore desirable for clinical states to be classified independently of environmental circumstances. Moreover, regardless of the duration, intensity, or presence of precipitating events, features such as hallucinations, delusions, marked weight loss, and suicidal trends indicate, according to almost all observers, that the boundary between normal and pathological has been passed.

The desirability of operational criteria is increasingly recognized. The diagnostic summaries that appear in textbooks and in official nomenclatures give only general guides. The most common clinical practice has been to list the number of symptoms in various categories, one or more of which may be necessary for the diagnosis. This form of clinical thinking implies a necessary-but-not-sufficient model of diagnosis, in which the emphasis is on salient symptoms derived from clinicians' experience with ideal cases. This model has been successfully translated into operational criteria in the past decade. To meet the diagnosis, the patient must display symptoms that have been operationally defined and categorized and must also not evidence the exclusion criteria that have been elaborated.

Although it is appealing because of its logical simplicity, this approach has been criticized for its lack of quantitative sophistication and its emphasis on pure forms that may be relatively infrequent. An alternative approach uses multivariate statistical methods and generates rating scales to be used in diagnosis. In recent years, much psychometric research has been conducted to develop and validate rating scales for diagnosing depression, and normative data have been collected for a number of scales, particularly the Beck, Zung, and Hamilton scales. It is now possible to identify cutoff points where normal moods are distinguished from clinical states. Recent data from epidemiologic studies that have used such scales indicate that while many persons in the community are distressed by depressive symptoms, only a minority meet the criteria for depressive conditions as defined by DSM-III.

A related approach derives from naturalistic studies of normal states. Prominent in this area are the excellent studies of normal mourning among widows. These studies offer the promise of delineating the duration and intensity of normal grief. In concert with the grief studies, systematic population surveys indicate that although mood complaints are common among normal subjects, clinical states are characterized not only by mood disturbance, but also by associated vegetative and bodily dysfunctions and by persistent and pervasive impairments in usual social performance.

ASSESSMENT AND DIAGNOSIS   Having established that a patient's affective disturbance represents a clinical state, rather than being within the range of normal mood, the clinician then faces the issues of nosology and classification. Since affective symptoms can occur in association with many other psychiatric and medical illnesses, some confusion exists concerning the status of these clinical conditions. The complexity of decisions required of the clinician is a tribute to the recent progress in understanding and treating the affective disorders. Better understanding of the complexity of psychopathology makes assessment and diagnosis both more important and more difficult. Similarly, the availability of many effective treatments, both biological and psychological, presents the clinician with a range of treatment choices but also complicates the decision-making process.

This discussion distinguishes between assessment and diagnosis. *Assessment* is the collection of information relevant to the patient's clinical condition, information which is pertinent to diagnosis, management, and treatment. *Diagnosis* is the clinical process of using the pertinent information to assign the patient to a specific nosological class or disorder.

Assessment involves careful history taking and a review of the current signs and symptoms and suicidal potential, as well as a complete physical examination. Where secondary depression or mania is suspected, assessment also includes laboratory studies. Comprehensive personal, social, and family histories should be obtained, along with a history of previous psychiatric symptoms, treatment, and medication. As Freedman (1978) has summarized it, patients have histories, personalities, skills, defects, and biases, and all of this is part of the total assessment.

Table 1 outlines the components of a comprehensive assessment strategy for patients with depressive syndromes. Assessment should entail history, current status, laboratory tests, and, if possible, interviews with significant others, usually a spouse or other family member. Prior to initiating treatment, it is important to assess the patient's current family and social resources and environmental supports. In practice, most treatment decisions are determined not only by the nature of the patient's psychopathology or severity of illness, but also

Table 1. Assessment of Patients with Depressive Syndromes

History
Family history: psychiatric illness, drug use, response to medication, suicide
Social history: family background, education, occupation
Previous psychiatric history: hospitalization, suicidal ideation, mood changes, response to medication, ECT

Current psychopathology
Preferably along the lines of some standardized format such as the Present State Exam or the Schedule for Affective Disorders and Schizophrenia

Assessment of current social situation
Stresses, social supports, social performance

Physical examination
For differential diagnosis and for ascertainment of conditions that may contraindicate or influence treatment

Laboratory tests
Liver battery, EKG, DST

Interview with significant other
Usually the spouse or another family member or both

Other data
Information from hospital records and social agencies, employment information

by the extent and availability of social support systems, especially the family. Families can give the depressed patient encouragement to counter self-depreciation and to enhance self-esteem. Even with a severely ill patient, hospitalization may be avoided when the patient has a family that is loving, consistently supportive, and encouraging. Such families are in effect willing and able to serve as auxiliary nursing personnel, feeding the patient and maintaining adequate levels of activity. For some suicidal patients, the family may monitor suicidal intent and prevent attempts.

This practical approach is supported by research which shows that the impact of adverse life events is partially offset by the presence of personal, familial, and interpersonal resources. The presence of a spouse and the availability of friends and confidants have been found to be especially significant factors. People who live alone or in poor housing and people who are involved in hostile marital relationships are more likely to require hospitalization since they lack the support of face-to-face primary social supports. Since these persons are also more likely to become depressed in the first place, the negative consequences of their environments are multiplied.

Diagnostic judgments provide a guide to management. In the case of depression, diagnosis involves a sequence of decisions, first the decision that the syndrome is present, and second, an assignment to subgroups. Recent research in psychopathology has clarified many issues in the nosology of affective disorders. As used here, nosology refers to the scientific study of groupings of illnesses and disorders, their reliability, validity, and appropriateness. Research has also indicated the importance of the distinctions between primary and secondary disorders and between unipolar and bipolar disorders.

CAUSES, COURSE, AND PROGNOSIS

Causes

The theories and hypotheses proposed regarding the causation of depressive disorders follow those for affective disorders in general.

The fact that so many patients experience the onset of depression in the late teens and young adulthood suggests an etiologic role for psychodynamic features, particularly those that are related to faulty personality and ego development and that culminate in a difficulty adapting to adolescence and young adulthood. The role of personality in depression has been given considerable attention by the psychiatric community. In a review of psychoanalytic theories of depression and personality, Chodoff (1972) concluded that undue interpersonal dependency and obsessionality often predispose to depression. Several newer approaches from cognitive and behavioral theories have also been applied to depression. Most notable have been the ideas of Beck (1972), Seligman (1974), and Lewinsohn (1974).

In contrast to the theoretical approaches that emphasize predisposition, two alternate formulations about the relationship of personality and depression should be considered. First, certain personality features and certain psychiatric disorders, whether genetic, developmental, or familial, may be manifestations of the same underlying process. That is, a personality trait may represent a subclinical expression of a psychiatric disorder, such as bipolar disorder. If that trait has a familial or genetic basis, one expects to find an increased frequency of the trait in both affected and unaffected relatives, as well as in patients. A second formulation is that personality qualities may be altered by the experience of the chronic and recurrent affective disorder. Chronic diseases, both medical and psychiatric, often lead to changes in individual personality patterns. The precise extent to which such changes may occur in patients with chronic depressions is at present unknown. Weissman and Paykel (1974) found that personality features such as dependency, guilt, and passivity did not return to normal levels after the depressive symptoms had relapsed and the illness was in remission. Kahn (1975) described several pervasive personality traits, especially low self-esteem, that are strongly associated with what he called "the depressive character."

Differences of opinion exist concerning the role of psychosocial stressors as precipitants of chronic episodes. One hypothesis is that the chronic disorder represents the poorly treated or partially resolved residual of acute depressions that occurred earlier in adult life and that themselves had psychosocial precipitants (Weissman and Klerman, 1977). On the other hand, in their Kansas City community survey, Hornstra and Klassen (1977) found no relationship between life stress and depressive symptoms of an enduring nature.*

Many chronic depressive conditions may represent the residual effects of secondary depressions due to the chronic use of alcohol, amphetamines, or barbiturates. Or they may be related to a long-standing medical illness, such as a gastrointestinal disorder or arthritis or a thyroid or other endocrine disorder.

Course and Prognosis

AGE OF ONSET Many patients report that their depressive symptoms began in late adolescence or in young adulthood and that the symptoms have been chronic for so long that they have become ingrained as part of their characters. A distinction should be drawn between the personality features that predispose to depression (Chodoff, 1972) and the clinical personality disorder with guilt, dependency, irritability, and passivity. Patients can have both depressive disorder and personality constellations that predispose them to affective disorders (Chodoff, 1972). In a patient with onset early in life, it is important to reconstruct the patient's history carefully, seeking episodes of acute onset, especially in the transition from adolescence to young adulthood. Obtaining the family history to detect a history of affective disorders is also valuable, since the dysthymic patient may have a mild form of depression whose severity has not been sufficient to reach the criteria for classification as Major Depression.

Onset is most commonly in maturity and middle age. The history is likely to show relatively good social adjustment and normal mood through adolescence and young adulthood, with a gradual or insidious onset of depressive symptoms, or with poorly remembered episodes of acute depression or residual symptoms following a grief reaction to the death of a parent, sibling, or child. A careful history may reveal that there has in fact been an impairment of marital functioning, with

*Preceptor's note: Hirschfeld and Cross review these issues in greater detail, and they consider several ways in which psychosocial factors and depression may be interrelated.

disputes, irritability, and poor sexual functioning, and impairment of parental functioning, particularly with teenage children (Weissman and Paykel, 1974), or an impairment in occupational functioning.

Onset in old age often leads to a difficult diagnostic problem because of the need to differentiate depressive pseudodementia from dementia. Many elderly patients present with an impairment of cognitive functions, complaints of decreased memory, inability to concentrate, poor attention, and slowing of functioning. The differential diagnosis of dementia due to central nervous system disorders such as Huntington's chorea or, more often, senile brain disease may be difficult. Moreover, since the disorders may coexist, the issue is not so much dementia versus depression as the coexistence of the two disorders.*

RISK AND IMPAIRMENTS In all affective disorders, the risk of suicide is increased. One should probe for potential suicide, reconstructing the history of previous suicide attempts, eliciting suicidal ideation, and exploring suicidal fantasies. If these signs exist, attention should be given to the patient's history of medication use, particularly since suicide-prone patients are often heavy users of the health care system and have a tendency to accumulate partially used bottles of medication. Attention should also be given to the patient's proneness to accidents, particularly in automobile driving.

Patients with chronic and intermittent depressions are probably at greater risk for serious medical illnesses than are other persons. Studies indicate that the death rate is higher than average, often because of cardiovascular disease (Avery and Winokur, 1976). Some suggestions have been made that depressive patients may be more prone than average to cancer. The apparent increase may, however, be attributable to the fact that depressed persons delay seeking medical attention or are misdiagnosed because of their previous history of chronic complaints.

Mental hospitalization for depressive disorders has become uncommon since the development of modern somatic treatments in the 1940s (electroconvulsive therapy) and the 1950s (psychopharmacology). Before the availability of these therapies, psychiatric hospitals often had a moderate number of patients with long-standing hospitalizations because of chronic depressive conditions.

The most common impairments are in the areas of social functioning, manifested by a reduced ability to sustain emotional intimacy, a reduction of sexual interest, lowered sexual performance (often manifested by impotence), and a decreased frequency of intercourse. Dysthymic patients may also have difficulty maintaining their usual levels of social activity and show reduced interest and participation in hobbies, games, sports, or social activities (Paykel and Weissman, 1973). Divorce, unemployment, and business or professional failure are often consequences.

The most important determinant of the course and outcome of depressive disorder is whether or not the disorder is recognized. Left to themselves, patients often have continuing episodes of chronic or intermittent symptoms, with gradual impairment of social functioning.

*Editor's note: The chapters by Sloane and Friedel in Part II present detailed discussions of the problems in differential diagnosis in the elderly and of some techniques for improving diagnostic reliability.

They may have frequent hospitalizations or emergency room visits because of suicide attempts or aggravated somatic complaints. When the depression is recognized and treated intensively, the prognosis improves greatly in the majority of cases.

THE DSM-III CLASSIFICATIONS

The DSM-III category of Affective Disorders groups all of the affective disorders together, regardless of the presence or absence of psychotic features or precipitating life experiences. Within that group, the subcategory Bipolar Disorder includes Mixed, Manic, or Depressed forms, and the subcategory Major Depression includes Single Episode or Recurrent forms. Affective Disorders also include two additional subcategories, Other Specific Affective Disorders, including Cyclothymic Disorder and Dysthymic Disorder, and Atypical Affective Disorders, including Atypical Bipolar Disorder and Atypical Depression. Table 2 shows the DSM-III categories for Affective Disorders.

The classification system in DSM-III is a result of modifications and refinements in previous classifications, and some terms used previously for a variety of affective disorders have been changed. For example, involutional melancholia is now classified as Major Depression, Single Episode, with Melancholia or with Mood-congruent Psychotic Features. Manic-depressive illness, manic type, is now classified as Bipolar Disorder, Manic type; manic-depressive illness, depressed type, as Major Depression, Single Episode or Recurrent; and manic-depressive illness, circular type, as Bipolar Disorder, Manic, Depressed, or Mixed type. Depressive neurosis is now classified as either Major Depression, Single Episode or Recurrent, without Melancholia, as

Table 2. DSM-III Classification of Affective Disorders

MAJOR AFFECTIVE DISORDERS

Code major depressive episode in fifth digit: 6 = in remission, 4 = with psychotic features (the unofficial non-ICD-9-CM fifth digit 7 may be used instead to indicate that the psychotic features are mood-incongruent), 3 = with melancholia, 2 = without melancholia, 0 = unspecified.
Code manic episode in fifth digit: 6 = in remission, 4 = with psychotic features (the unofficial non-ICD-9-CM fifth digit 7 may be used instead to indicate that the psychotic features are mood-incongruent), 2 = without psychotic features, 0 = unspecified.

	Bipolar disorder
296.6x	mixed, _____
296.4x	manic, _____
296.5x	depressed, _____

	Major depression
296.2x	single episode, _____
296.3x	recurrent, _____

OTHER SPECIFIC AFFECTIVE DISORDERS
301.13   Cyclothymic disorder
300.40   Dysthymic disorder (or Depressive neurosis)

ATYPICAL AFFECTIVE DISORDERS
296.70   Atypical bipolar disorder
296.82   Atypical depression

Source: American Psychiatric Association (1980).

Dysthymic Disorder, or as Adjustment Disorder with Depressed Mood. DSM-III accepts the evidence that points to the importance of distinguishing between unipolar and bipolar forms of affective disorders.

Leonhard (1957) originally proposed separating depressed patients with a history of manic episodes (the bipolar group) from those depressed patients whose history included only recurrent episodes of depression (the unipolar group). More recently, the bipolar-unipolar distinction has achieved rapid acceptance. Considerable evidence now exists concerning genetic, familial, personal, biochemical, physiological, and pharmacologic differences between bipolar and unipolar affective disorders. When the possible genetic factors were studied carefully, patients with bipolar disorder showed a far higher frequency of positive family history than did patients with only depression (Gershon, 1978; Winokur et al., 1978). Psychopharmacologic studies have also indicated differences in bipolar and depressed patients' responses to psychoactive drugs, especially lithium. Patients with bipolar disorder are more likely to develop hypomanic responses to levodopa or to imipramine and other tricyclics than are patients with depression.

Although the concept of bipolar disorder is well defined and amply substantiated by research and clinical experience, the status of unipolar disorder (depression) is still uncertain. The criterion for bipolar disorder is clear: evidence of a current or a past manic episode. In some studies, a depressive psychosis has been a necessary criterion for bipolar disorder. In other reports, all depressions, psychotic or not, have been included. Some investigators require not only evidence of psychotic forms of depression but also evidence of frequent recurrences. Perris (1966) specified three recurrences, and Schou (1968) specified two recurrences within a one- or two-year period. Since virtually all individuals with manic episodes eventually develop depressive episodes, most investigators now consider that manic episodes are evidence of bipolar disorder. Therefore, in DSM-III the diagnosis of Bipolar Disorder is made when there is a manic episode, whether or not there has been a depressive episode. All other types of depression are now regarded as unipolar.

The Major Depressive Syndrome

Most patients with one or more episodes of depression will not fit the criteria for Bipolar Disorder, since bipolar patients make up only about 10 percent of patients with depression. The previous classifications have included such distinctions as agitated-retarded, endogenous-reactive, and psychotic-neurotic, but since many of these terms embodied etiologic presumptions, DSM-III created the broader category of Major Depression. The criteria shown in Table 3 are purely descriptive and are independent of any presumed etiology, whether biological, psychological, or situational. It must be emphasized that there is no one depressive syndrome. The DSM-III classification outlined in Table 3 provides the reference point for a clinical subclassification, a subject to which the chapter will return. As shown in the table, the symptoms of depression are broad, and to further aid the clinician, two important qualifiers are designated in DSM-III, Melancholia and Psychotic Features.

Table 3.   DSM-III Diagnostic Criteria for Major Depressive Episode

A.   Dysphoric mood or loss of interest or pleasure in all or almost all usual activities and pastimes. The dysphoric mood is characterized by symptoms such as the following: depressed, sad, blue, hopeless, low, down in the dumps, irritable. The mood disturbance must be prominent and relatively persistent, but not necessarily the most dominant symptom, and does not include momentary shifts from one dysphoric mood to another dysphoric mood, e.g., anxiety to depression to anger, such as are seen in states of acute psychotic turmoil. (For children under six, dysphoric mood may have to be inferred from a persistently sad facial expression.)

B.   At least four of the following symptoms have each been present nearly every day for a period of at least two weeks (in children under six, at least three of the first four):
   (1)   poor appetite or significant weight loss (when not dieting) or increased appetite or significant weight gain (in children under six consider failure to make expected weight gains)
   (2)   insomnia or hypersomnia
   (3)   psychomotor agitation or retardation (but not merely subjective feelings of restlessness or being slowed down) (in children under six, hypoactivity)
   (4)   loss of interest or pleasure in usual activities, or decrease in sexual drive not limited to a period when delusional or hallucinating (in children under six, signs of apathy)
   (5)   loss of energy; fatigue
   (6)   feelings of worthlessness, self-reproach, or excessive or inappropriate guilt (either may be delusional)
   (7)   complaints or evidence of diminished ability to think or concentrate, such as slowed thinking, or indecisiveness not associated with marked loosening of associations or incoherence
   (8)   recurrent thoughts of death, suicidal ideation, wishes to be dead, or suicide attempt

C.   Neither of the following dominate the clinical picture when an affective syndrome is [absent (i.e., symptoms in criteria A and B above)] . . . :
   (1)   preoccupation with a mood-incongruent delusion or hallucination . . .
   (2)   bizarre behavior

D.   Not superimposed on either Schizophrenia, Schizophreniform Disorder, or a Paranoid Disorder.

E.   Not due to any Organic Mental Disorder or Uncomplicated Bereavement.

Source: American Psychiatric Association (1980).

MAJOR DEPRESSION WITH MELANCHOLIA   Recent clinical research has led to reevaluation of the classic concept of endogenous depression. DSM-III substitutes the term melancholia for the older term endogenous depression, as shown in Table 4. DSM-III thus avoids the implication that the syndrome is etiologically based on internal or endogenous biological or constitutional features. Recent research indicates no correlation between the presence of the melancholic syndrome and the presence or absence of life events. Diagnosis of a situational or reactive stimulus is therefore not precluded by the presence of the syndrome summarized in Table 4. The endogenous or melancholic syndrome can occur with both primary and secondary forms of depression, including those that are secondary to drugs such as the rauwolfias or the steroids or to viral disorders.

One clinically important consequence of this descriptive diagnosis is the increasing evidence that the endogenous or melancholic pattern predicts a positive response to both tricyclic antidepressants

Table 4.   DSM-III Criteria for Melancholia

Loss of pleasure in all or almost all activities, lack of reactivity to usually pleasurable stimuli (dosen't feel much better, even temporarily, when something good happens), and at least three of the following:

(a) distinct quality of depressed mood, i.e., the depressed mood is perceived as distinctly different from the kind of feeling experienced following the death of a loved one

(b) the depression is regularly worse in the morning

(c) early morning awakening (at least two hours before usual time of awakening)

(d) marked psychomotor retardation or agitation

(e) significant anorexia or weight loss

(f) excessive or inappropriate guilt

Source: American Psychiatric Association (1980).

and ECT and a negative response to psychotherapy. Among inpatients, 40 to 60 percent of patients who meet the DSM-III criteria for Major Depressive Episode will have significant endogenous or melancholic symptom features. It is not clear how to classify the remaining group. They are variously labeled as having atypical depression, neurotic depression, or reactive depression.

MAJOR DEPRESSION WITH PSYCHOTIC FEATURES   By the late nineteenth century, *psychotic* had come to indicate conditions in which the patient manifested a disturbance in higher-level mental functions, including language, orientation, perception, and thinking. These disturbances would appear as delusions, hallucinations, confusion, and impaired memory. Freud and other psychoanalysts concluded that psychoses involved the "loss of reality testing," one of the functions of the ego. Another use of the term psychotic is also derived from psychoanalytic theory. This usage is based on Fenichel's influential work, *The Psychoanalytic Theory of Neurosis* (1945), and it employs the degree of ego regression as the criterion for illness. Other meanings or criteria have evolved during the decades since. In the most common usage, the term psychotic has become synonymous with severe impairment of social and personal functioning, manifested by social withdrawal and the inability to perform the usual tasks of household and occupation.

The diagnosis of psychotic depression correlates with severe impairment, higher suicidal risk, and possibly the need for hospitalization. Patients with psychotic depressions do not respond to tricyclic and phenothiazine treatment or to ECT. Pending further research, the psychotic-nonpsychotic distinction should be regarded as a continuum descriptive of clinical judgments, rather than as a means for distinguishing clear-cut nosological groupings which have established etiologic differences.

Psychotic depressions are relatively infrequent in current clinical practice. Only 10 percent of patients show delusions, hallucinations, confusion, or impaired reality testing. With better diagnostic criteria, more mental health facilities, greater willingness of patients to seek psychiatric help, and new psychopharmacologic agents, treatment is being initiated earlier in the clinical course, before psychotic stages develop.

OTHER FORMS OF MAJOR DEPRESSION Ambiguities have surrounded the term *neurotic*. Sometimes neurotic depressions have referred to nonpsychotic forms of depression. At other times neurotic has been used synonymously with reactive, although little evidence exists that precipitating events are highly correlated with nonpsychotic symptom states. At still other times clinicians have used the term neurotic to refer to those depressions that arise in patients with long-standing character problems or chronic maladaptive personality patterns. Furthermore, attempts to separate psychotic and neurotic patients into distinct, statistically verifiable nosological groups have been unsuccessful. Current evidence indicates that psychotic-neurotic distinctions, like those within the endogenous-reactive dichotomy, occur on a continuum that would be better called psychotic-nonpsychotic than psychotic-neurotic.

Etiologic assumptions have also confused the psychotic-neurotic dichotomy. Biological causes and disturbances in brain function are presumed to account for psychotic forms of depression. Neurotic forms, on the other hand, have been ascribed to social and psychosocial causes that lead to impairments in personality function. Evidence for these presumed etiologic correlations is minimal at best. In clinical practice, moreover, the endogenous-reactive dichotomy has unfortunately been used interchangeably with the psychotic-neurotic distinction. This usage is not valid, since psychotic states often follow reactions to stressful life events such as losses. Similarly, individuals with endogenous features, particularly sleep disturbance and weight loss, may not have psychotic symptoms such as delusions or hallucinations.

Most older classifications and textbooks separate neurotic depressions from other forms of affective disorders, particularly from the affective psychoses and manic-depressive illness. While the latter were treated as psychoses and often grouped together with schizophrenia, neurotic depressions were grouped in the same category as other neuroses. The newer classifications like DSM-III combine all forms of affective disturbance, independent of whether or not they have previously been categorized as neurotic or psychotic with regard to symptoms, degree of severity, or impairment of social functioning.

Recent evidence indicates that neurotic depressives respond well to tricyclics. The efficacy of tricyclics, particularly imipramine and amitriptyline, was established for psychotic forms of depression in the 1950s and 1960s, even though the samples included admixtures of patients that today would be diagnosed as bipolar. The Veterans Administration-National Institute of Mental Health studies (Prien et al., 1973) have since indicated that bipolar depressives treated with tricyclics do less well than those treated with placebo.

Dysthymic Disorder

Clinical experience and numerous studies have shown that most depressions are episodic. Although a large proportion of adults experience acute depressions and usually do not come to the attention of physicians, let alone psychiatrists, a significant percentage experience their condition as chronic.

For example, Barrett et al. (1978) surveyed 293 nonpatient air-traffic controllers and found that almost 30 percent reported some degree of depression during at least one month of the year. The vast majority had symptoms that were nonpsychotic and of relatively short duration. Only a small percentage sought medical attention. However, about 9 percent had been bothered by an enduring depressed mood, with only intermittent periods of normal feeling state during the year of observation. Similarly, in a follow-up study of 150 patients treated for acute depression, Weissman and the author found that about 12 percent had a chronic course that although distressing was not sufficiently disabling to require hospitalization (Weissman and Klerman, 1977). Most chronic depressions probably represent the inadequately recognized and poorly treated residual of unresolved or partially remitted acute depressions. As the studies summarized in Table 5 indicate, about 15 to 20 percent of patients experiencing acute depressions do not make a complete recovery but show some intermittent, fluctuating, and chronic symptoms, often persisting for years.

The creation of a separate category in DSM-III for patients with Dysthymic Disorder represents an important step forward. This advance in diagnosis is particularly important in the era of community psychiatric treatment, since most of these patients are not institutionalized and are able to continue in the community. They have moderate to severe fluctuating symptom levels but can maintain some degree of occupational, family, and community roles. Families, co-workers, and friends are affected by the patients' emotional stress, however, since impairments in social functioning are often severe. Many are heavy users of the health care system and complain predominantly of hypochondriacal and bodily ailments, posing major diagnostic and therapeutic problems.

The essential feature of Dysthymic Disorder is a chronic nonpsychotic disturbance involving depressed mood or a loss of interest or pleasure in all or almost all usual activities and pastimes. Usually, associated symptoms are not of sufficient severity to meet the criteria for Major Depression. Dysthymic Disorder is a long-standing illness of at least two years in duration with either sustained or intermittent disturbances in depressed mood and associated symptoms. The disorder may begin in early adult life, often without a clear onset.

Table 5. Summary of Studies Reporting Depressed Patients with a Chronic Course

Year of Publication	Investigator	N	Duration of Follow-Up (Years)	Percent Chronic
1921	Kraepelin	899	10 to 40	4 to 5
1945	Lundquist	638	20	9
1948b	Huston and Locher	80	6.8	9
1948a	Huston and Locher	93	6.5	18
1952	Stenstedt	216	2 to 20	1 to 14
1956	Watts	387	Up to 8	14
1959	Astrup, Fossum, and Holmboe	278	7 to 19	8
1968	Bratfos and Haug	207	1 to 12	28
1973	Morrison, Winokur, and Crowe	202	4.3	20
1974	Murphy, Woodruff, Herjanic, and Super	43	2.8 to 6.5	16
1974	Paykel, Klerman, and Prusoff	190	0.8	21

The category includes those who would in the past have been diagnosed as having depressive neurosis. Subgroups of patients with Dysthymic Disorder include those with masked depression or depressive equivalents.

The depressed mood may be determined by the patient's reports of feeling sad, blue, down in the dumps, or low. Life may be described as dark, black, or bleak. The depressed mood and associated features may be either relatively persistent, in which case the disorder is considered chronic, or the mood may be intermittent, in which case the periods of symptoms are separated by intervals of normal mood. The relatively normal periods may last from a few days to a few weeks and are characterized by the capacity to enjoy pleasure and to function at some normal level of social activity.

The patient may have manifestations of the nonpsychotic features of the depressive syndrome, such as impaired self-esteem, sleep difficulty (particularly early morning awakening), loss of energy, slowing of speech and thinking, loss of appetite, decreased sexual drive and performance, and thoughts of suicide. The patient usually experiences these as discontinuous and ego-alien changes from his or her usual or former self. The presence of delusions and hallucinations is by definition inconsistent with the diagnosis of Dysthymic Disorder. In distinguishing the dysthymic disorder from cyclothymia (see below), one must ascertain whether the patient experiences the return to normal as a relief from depression or whether the patient shows positive signs of euphoria, increased activity, and poor judgment. In the latter case, the patient should be considered cyclothymic.

VARIANTS OF DYSTHYMIC DISORDER   Although the clinical presentation with predominant depressive mood, as described above, is most common, it is important to recognize a number of major variants. The variants include masked depression, hypochondriacal and somatic complaints, pessimism and hopelessness, alcohol abuse, and drug ingestion.

In patients with masked depressions (Kielholz, 1973; Lesse, 1977), the mood disturbance may not be readily apparent, but the patient may present with chronic pain, insomnia, weight loss, or other bodily complaints. That mode of presentation is most often seen by psychiatrists working in general hospitals and as consultants to medical practitioners.

A number of studies by psychiatrists working in general hospitals and outpatient medical clinics (Jacobs et al., 1968; Lipsitt, 1970) have documented that a large number of patients with recurrent undiagnosed medical complaints, often called hypochondriacs or crocks, are unrecognized, intermittent or chronic depressives whose ticket of admission to the health care system is through their bodily complaints. They are usually middle-aged and elderly patients, most often women. They are often referred from one specialty clinic or specialist to another, especially for complaints related to gynecology, thyroid and other endocrine disorders, gastrointestinal functioning, and arthritis and rheumatism.

Patients with helplessness, pessimism, and discouragement represent another mode of presentation. Their difficulties may be directed against the self, as with feelings of self-reproach, low self-esteem, and feelings of failure in life, or their problems may be manifested by inadequate functioning in their work or marriages. Such patients may be labeled masochistic personalities. On the other hand, their pessimism may be directed outward, with tirades against the world and feelings of having been treated poorly by relatives, children, parents, work colleagues, or the system. It is important to distinguish these pessimistic depressed patients from paranoid patients, and the main difference is that the depressives do not have the paranoid persons' sense that malicious intent is directed at them.

Clinicians must recognize that a high percentage of chronic alcoholics develop secondary depressions. The rates range from 25 to 50 percent (Pottenger et al., 1978). Whether the depression is psychogenic or caused by pharmacologic toxicity is not certain. Weissman and Myers (1980) have suggested that the chronic depression of alcoholism, associated with as many as 50 percent of a large series of alcoholics, was due to the alcohol's toxic effect on the central nervous system. The depressive features come after long periods of heavy drinking and often occur during the rehabilitation following acute withdrawal reactions.

Selected drugs, particularly the steroids, amphetamines, barbiturates, and other central nervous system depressants are known to produce depression after periods of heavy use. A chronic depression secondary to heroin use or long-term methadone use has also been described.

Cyclothymic Disorder

The term *cyclothymia* was first coined by Kahlbaum in the middle of the nineteenth century for what was then called circular insanity. Following Kraepelin (1921), the common usage is to regard cyclothymia as a personality condition which is manifest in a chronic nonpsychotic disturbance with numerous periods marked by symptoms characteristic of either the manic or the depressive syndrome or both. Usually the symptomatic periods are not of sufficient intensity to meet the full criteria for Bipolar Disorder. Furthermore, patients generally experience them as ego-syntonic and do not present themselves for psychiatric treatment. Family members, relatives, and co-workers, however, may be disturbed by the mood swings and behavior fluctuations and recommend treatment.

With the recent success of lithium in treating full-blown manic episodes and in preventing the recurrence of episodes in patients with bipolar disorder, more patients with cyclothymic disorder are coming to psychiatric attention, and a new focus on the disorder is developing (Akiskal et al., 1977; Tellenbach, 1977). There are still only a few systematic studies, however, and the most important of these was done by Akiskal et al. (1977). Pending further quantitative research, the conclusions described below must be regarded as tentative.

A general consensus exists, following Kraepelin, that cyclothymia is a mild or attenuated form of bipolar disorder. That consensus is based on several sources of evidence. First is the symptomatic and phenomenological similarity between symptoms and the behavior of persons with cyclothymic disorder and the full-blown bipolar disorder. The second source of evidence is the distribution of affectively disordered biological relatives among the family members of patients with cyclothymic disorders (Akiskal et al., 1977). Third are the observations based on follow-ups that a significant proportion of cyclothymic disorders evolve into the clinical picture of bipolar disorder and that they show similar responses to pharmacologic treatment, including the tendencies for hypomanic response to tricyclic therapy and for favorable response to lithium. Finally, Gershon and his associates have demonstrated an increased frequency of cyclothymic personality disorders in the biological relatives of probands with bipolar disorders (Gershon, 1978). Similar findings were also reported by Akiskal et al. (1977).

Although the genetic hypothesis as to cause is the most favored, there are also some important psychodynamic and cultural hypotheses. These hypotheses derive in large part from observations of patients in long-term psychotherapy, particularly by Jacobson (1971) and by Mabel Blake Cohen et al. (1954). The psychodynamic theories place the emphasis on early childhood experience, often postulating trauma and fixation during the early oral stages of infant development. Although attempts have been made to describe a specific family constellation, the differentiation of cyclothymic disorder from other forms of bipolar disorder is not clear.

Uncomplicated Bereavement

DSM-III contains a category for Uncomplicated Bereavement, reflecting the fact that a full depressive syndrome frequently occurs as part of the normal reaction to losing a loved one. Symptoms such as weight loss, insomnia, and poor appetite may occur. In the author's opinion, this category should be used only in those instances where there has been a recent death of a significant family member, a close friend, or a spouse.

In the various complicated forms of grief, suicide may occur, the reaction may be prolonged, or the person may show excess morbid preoccupation with feelings of worthlessness and prolonged functional impairment beyond usual social convention. In such cases, consideration should be given to a diagnosis of Adjustment Reaction or Major Depression.

Adjustment Reaction

Depressive symptoms often occur as part of a maladaptive response to an identifiable psychosocial stressor. For an Adjustment Disorder diagnosis, DSM-III requires that the psychosocial stressor be identifiable and that the symptoms occur within three months after the onset of the stressor. Stressors such as divorce, unemployment, failure to be promoted, chronic illness in a loved one, moving, and so forth have been shown to increase the risk of various kinds of emotional difficulties, particularly depression, but also anxiety and insomnia. In such instances, the individual may often increase the use of alcohol or sedatives and other psychotropic drugs. If the level of symptoms reaches that of the criteria for major depressive disorder or other depressive disorder, then that diagnosis should take precedence.

CLASSIFICATIONS SUPPLEMENTAL TO DSM-III

Although DSM-III represents a major advance, a number of current research efforts suggest the need to extend the DSM-III classification for depressive disorders. The major needs are to subclassify Major Depression further and to develop some system for handling depressive reactions associated with or secondary to other psychiatric or medical disorders.

Depressive Disorders Secondary to Other Psychiatric Illnesses

Robins and Guze (1972) proposed making a distinction between primary and secondary affective disorders. The initial distinction was based on two criteria, the chronology of onset in relation to the patient's psychiatric history and the evidence of associated psychiatric illnesses. Within this classification, primary affective disorders occur in those patients who have previously been well or whose only previous psychiatric disease was mania or depression, while secondary affective disorders occur in persons who have had another previous psychiatric illness. Since this distinction makes no reference to immediately apparent life stress or specific symptom patterns, the knotty etiologic questions posed by the endogenous-reactive distinction can be postponed. The distinction is also independent of severity, so that the etiologic biases implicit in the older psychotic-neurotic diagnostic classification are again circumvented.

On the other hand, the fact that the criteria for primary and secondary affective disorders do not refer to precipitating life events or to psychotic features does not mean that these features are unimportant in assessment, treatment decisions, or prognosis. Rather, the Washington University group simply proposes that the diagnostic criteria for primary-secondary affective disorders not include these features as necessary or sufficient for assignment to the primary or secondary subclassification.

Since the depressive states can occur secondarily in the temporal sense but be associated with other psychiatric disorders, diagnostic criteria for the nonaffective psychiatric disorders must be specified. Toward this end and to their credit, Robins and his associates have published their criteria for a number of nonaffective disorders, including schizophrenia, hysteria, and alcoholism (Feighner et al., 1972). The association of depression with alcoholism and schizophrenia, for example, has been well documented.

Exact prevalence rates for primary and secondary affective disorders are not available. Clinical experience shows that the majority of affective disorders do not occur in clear association with other medical or psychiatric disorders, and the primary affective disorders receive the greatest attention in both research and clinical practice. In a large sample of patients with depression seen in emergency rooms of general hospitals, 55 percent were found to have primary affective disorders, and 33 percent had secondary affective disorders. For approximately 10 percent of the patients, the diagnostic assignment could not be made (Robins and Guze, 1972).

Secondary manic states also occur. Elated mood and overactive behavior may be secondary to organic states or to the effects of drugs. In patients with schizophrenic symptoms or with histories of a previous schizophrenic episode, an elated or manic episode would be considered a part of the schizophrenic syndrome according to the Robins criteria. Some psychiatric investigators, however, would label such an episode schizoaffective.

The primary-secondary distinction is not a final diagnostic subclassification. Rather, it is a valuable initial separation toward classifying multiple diagnostic groups. The decision-tree approach which the distinction makes possible is shown in Figure 1.

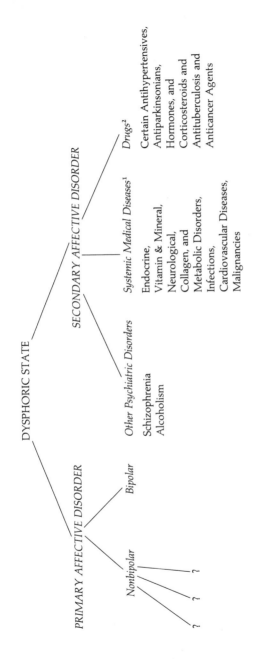

Figure 1. Nosology of depression

[Image content:]

DYSPHORIC STATE

PRIMARY AFFECTIVE DISORDER

Nonbipolar
? ? ?

Bipolar

SECONDARY AFFECTIVE DISORDER

Other Psychiatric Disorders
Schizophrenia
Alcoholism

Systemic Medical Diseases[1]
Endocrine,
Vitamin & Mineral,
Neurological,
Collagen, and
Metabolic Disorders,
Infections,
Cardiovascular Diseases,
Malignancies

Drugs[2]
Certain Antihypertensives,
Antiparkinsonians,
Hormones, and
Corticosteroids and
Antituberculosis and
Anticancer Agents

[1]See Table 6.
[2]See Table 7.

Table 6.   Medical Conditions Frequently Associated
with Higher Risk for Affective Disorder

Endocrine Disorders
  Acromegaly
  Hyperadrenalism
  Hypoadrenalism
  Hyperinsulinism secondary to insulinoma
  Hyperparathyroidism
  Hypoparathyroidism
  Hypopituitarism
  Hyperthyroidism
  Hypothyroidism
  Inappropriate antidiuretic hormone (ADH) secretion

Vitamin and Mineral Disorders
  Beriberi (vitamin B_1 deficiency)
  Hypervitaminosis A
  Hypomagnesimia
  Pellagra (nicotinic acid deficiency)
  Pernicious anemia (vitamin B_{12} deficiency)
  Wernicke's encephalopathy

Infections
  Encephalitis
  Hepatitis
  Influenza
  Malaria
  Mononucleosis
  Pneumonia
  Syphilis
  Tuberculosis

Neurological Disorders
  Multiple sclerosis
  Tuberous sclerosis
  Wilson's disease

Collagen Disorders
  Systemic lupus erythematosus
  Polyarteritis nodosa

Cardiovascular Diseases
  Cardiomyopathy
  Cerebral ischemia
    Hypotension of cardiac origin
    Cerebral arteriosclerosis
    Cerebral embolization
  Congestive heart failure
  Myocardial infarction

Malignancies
  Carcinoid
  Pancreatic carcinoma
  Pheochromocytoma

Metabolic Disorder
  Porphyria

Source: Griest and Griest (1979).

Depressive Disorders Secondary to Medical Illnesses

Robins and Guze (1972) originally applied the concept of secondary affective disorder only to affective disorders secondary to psychiatric disorders such as schizophrenia and alcoholism. The author and others have proposed extending the concept to affective disorders associated with and following general medical conditions or drug reactions (Klerman and Barrett, 1973). These investigators have noted that affective disorders are also often associated with general medical illnesses or drug reactions. Affective states, particularly depressions, often occur in patients with pneumonia, infectious hepatitis, or mononucleosis. Endocrine disorders, especially those of the thyroid, adrenal, and pituitary glands, are often associated with mood dysfunction (see Table 6). Another important group of affective disorders results from the effects of drugs such as the rauwolfias, amphetamines, and steroids (see Table 7). The concept of secondary affective disorders therefore should be expanded to include affective states not only secondary in time to other well-defined psychiatric syndromes, but also secondary to or associated with concomitant systemic medical diseases or drug reactions.

This usage is similar to the distinction in hypertension between essential hypertension and symptomatic hypertension. Similar distinctions are often used for anemias where the anemia may be secondary to infection, tumor, or chronic ingestion of toxic substances such as benzene. Applied to psychiatric practice, the usage requires recognizing the many medical illnesses and drugs which can render the patient at greater risk for affective illness, both depression and mania.

Attention should be given to the particular aspects of depression manifest in association with the various medical disorders. In many instances, the symptomatology has been sufficiently studied to allow specific statements as to diagnostic and treatment aspects. In many

Table 7.   Drugs Frequently Associated with Depressive Reactions as Adverse Effects

Class Name	Generic Name	Trade Name
Antihypertensives	Reserpine	Serpasil, Sandril
	Methyldopa	Aldomet
	Propranolol hydrochloride	Inderal
	Guanethidine sulfate	Ismelin sulfate
	Hydralazine hydrochloride	Apresoline hydrochloride
	Clonidine hydrochloride	Catapres
Antiparkinsonian agents	Levodopa	Dopar, Larodopa
	Levodopa, carbidopa	Sinemet
	Amantadine hydrochloride	Symmetrel
Hormones	Estrogen	Evex, Menrium
	Progesterone	
Corticosteroids	Cortisone acetate	
Antituberculosis	Cycloserine	Seromycin
Anticancer	Vincristine sulfate	Oncovin
	Vinblastine sulfate	Velban

Source: Klerman and Hirschfeld (1979).

other instances, however, a new research agenda arises: to study, disorder by disorder, the circumstances leading to and the characteristics of the depressive reactions associated with the various medical illnesses. Such research would not only be important in clinical diagnosis and management, but would also help to identify possible clues to etiology and pathogenesis. For example, knowledge of the role of viral disease in depressive reactions may give clues to those parts of the central nervous system which are vulnerable to viral infection and which may also be involved in regulating affect and mood expression. Similarly, studies of depression associated with thyroid and adrenal disease have provided insights into the interaction between steroid metabolism and thyroid metabolism and into the role of catecholamines as neurotransmitters, particularly in the hypothalamic and pituitary centers which regulate peripheral-adrenal organ responses.

Winokur's Subclassification of Primary Depressive Disorders

Winokur and his colleagues (1978) presented a system of diagnosis in unipolar depression that is based on specific familial backgrounds. In their system, patients with primary depression are assigned to one of several distinctive subgroups that may be identified by different familial constellations of illness. Some patients are classified as having depression spectrum disease, in which a first-degree family member has alcoholism or an antisocial personality or both. Others are classified as having pure depressive disease, in which the family history shows depression and includes a depressed first-degree family member.

Although Winokur and his colleagues have found few differences between the two groups in either their presenting clinical pictures or the precipitating factors, the evidence did indicate differences in the areas of personal problems and personality, as well as in the course of illness (Van Valkenburg et al., 1977; Winokur, 1979). The depression spectrum patients were less likely to have experienced the symptom of losing interest in usual activities than were the pure depressive disease patients. They were more likely, however, to have had a history of sexual problems, to have been divorced or separated, to have been described as irritable, and to report prior episodes of depression. Depression spectrum patients were also found to be more likely to recover completely than were the pure depressive disease patients (Van Valkenburg et al., 1977).

SUMMARY AND CONCLUSIONS

DSM-II and ICD-9 did not have composite categories for the affective disorders but separated them into psychotic and neurotic disorders. The recent trend in the United States has been to group the affective disorders together as a diagnostic class. This grouping has blurred, but not eliminated completely, the distinction between the psychotic and neurotic forms. This trend is seen clearly in the research employing the RDC and in the creation of a separate DSM-III category for affective disorders. The creation of this category for affective disorders in DSM-III crystallized a large body of research on the psychopathological, biological, and therapeutic aspects of depression and mania.

The bipolar concept has been widely accepted for its clinical utility in predicting positive response to lithium and adverse response to tricyclics. The bipolar diagnosis has also proven a strong spur to research on genetic and biochemical correlates. The unipolar concept is less well accepted. There is increasing awareness that all that is not bipolar is not unipolar, and DSM-III has no separate unipolar category.

The concept of neurotic depression has been radically revised. The DSM-II diagnosis of psychoneurotic depressive reaction was one of the most common diagnoses in clinical practice. Research and clinical experience have increasingly challenged the utility and validity of this concept. Neurotic depression has multiple definitions. Among other definitions, neurotic depression has been defined by (1) long-term personality difficulty, (2) precipitation by acute stress, and (3) underlying unconscious conflicts. Criticisms of the concept and its definitions (Klerman et al., 1979) resulted in the omission of neurotic depression as a separate category in DSM-III.

Considerable research on the possible role of life events in precipitating various forms of affective disorder has led to questioning about whether a separate category of reactive or situational depression is warranted. Life events may increase the risk for a wide variety of disorders, not only for affective disorders, but also for schizophrenic and medical conditions. The specificity of life events for any clinical form of affective disorders is therefore increasingly in question.

Attention to endogenous depression has increased. Kuhn (1957) observed that patients with endogenous depressions responded to tricyclics. Factor-analytic studies were initially undertaken by Kiloh and Garside (1963) and the Newcastle group. Numerous replications of the factor-analytic studies in the United States (Mendels and Cochrane, 1968) identified a cluster of symptoms including early morning awakening, loss of interest in activities and pleasure, loss of appetite, loss of weight, and psychomotor change in the form of either retardation or agitation. Evidence has accrued that this symptom cluster is independent of precipitating life events, while it is highly predictive of response to ECT and to tricyclic antidepressants.

Another major advance in the understanding of affective disorders was the Robins and Guze (1972) proposal to separate primary and secondary depressions based upon the criterion of temporal preexistence of other psychiatric conditions, particularly schizophrenia and alcoholism. The author and others have proposed that the diagnosis of secondary depression be extended to include conditions associated with preexisting medical disorder or drug reactions (Klerman and Barrett, 1973). The occurrence of mania secondary to medical conditions has led to a proposal for the category of secondary mania (Krauthammer and Klerman, 1978).

The large number of ambulatory patients with symptoms of both anxiety and depression causes nosological uncertainty. In clinical practice these patients tend to be diagnosed as having anxiety disorders and are most often treated with antianxiety drugs of the chlordiazepoxide series. A number of studies have cast doubt on the therapeutic efficacy of this class of drugs for depressions. Whether a separate category for anxiety-depression will appear in future nomenclatures is still in question.

Although the classic psychotic-neurotic separation of depression has diminished, the presence of delusions and other manifestations of psychoses, narrowly defined, is of clinical and therapeutic importance. Patients with delusions and hallucinations seem to respond poorly to tricyclic antidepressants. While the nosological significance of this finding for the classification of affective disorders is still undefined, the practical significance for treatment decisions has gained increasing attention. Uncertainty remains about whether depressed patients with delusions are best treated with a combination of tricyclics and neuroleptics or with ECT.

Chapter 23 **Personality, Life Events, and Social Factors in Depression**
by Robert M.A. Hirschfeld, M.D. and
Christine K. Cross, M.A.

INTRODUCTION

Today we believe that depression results from a combination of biological and psychosocial factors, including biochemical, genetic, general health, neuroendocrine, familial, personality, and social factors, as well as life events. At times the search for biological concomitants of depression seems to have eclipsed the interest in other variables, as evidenced by the number of biologically oriented articles in the major psychiatric journals. Historically, however, psychosocial factors have predominated in theories and treatments of depression, and particular emphasis has been given to early loss, "weak" personality, stress, and social deprivation. This chapter focuses on the extent to which the research findings support a role for these and other psychosocial factors in the development, nature, and course of depressive disorders.

The authors begin by reviewing conceptually the nature of the relationship between psychosocial factors and depression. Following this is a critical review of the research literature as it pertains to this relationship. As much as possible, the discussion focuses on the major subclasses of affective disorders (i.e., bipolar disorder, primary [nonbipolar] major depression, with or without melancholia, and secondary depressive disorder). Major findings from the literature are summarized and discussed, and recommendations are made for future research.

Psychosocial factors encompass a wide variety of conditions, and the chapter concentrates on three major types—personality, life events, and social factors. *Personality* refers to relatively enduring traits, the response sets or characteristic modes of behavior which an individual exhibits and which may be constitutional in origin (temperament) or acquired during development (character). *Life events* refer to changes which occur in an individual's social matrix and which may be considered social stressors inasmuch as they cause disruptions in the person's customary life pattern and necessitate adaptation. Life events may be recent (6 to 12 months prior to onset of the depressive episode) and include such events as marriage, change in residence, death of a significant other, and so forth. Or they may be remote, such as the death of or separation from a parent during childhood. Finally, *social factors* refer to the interpersonal resources such as family ties and social relationships and to the life circumstances which may influence an individual's vulnerability to stress.

APPROACHES TO PSYCHOSOCIAL FACTORS AND DEPRESSION

The nature of the relationship between psychosocial factors and depressive disorders can be conceptualized using several alternative, but not necessarily mutually exclusive, hypothetical approaches. Four approaches are reviewed here and serve as the organizational scheme for the literature review which follows.

The *predisposition approach* proposes that certain personality characteristics, certain types of life events, and the lack of supportive social conditions are antecedent to depressive disorders and render an individual especially vulnerable to depression. The importance of personality characteristics in the etiology of depression has been emphasized in various theories of depression (Chodoff, 1972; Lewinsohn, 1976; Seligman, 1975), although disagreement exists with regard to the terminology and the etiology of the characteristics themselves. Psychoanalytic theorists have described qualities such as undue interpersonal dependency, orality, and obsessionality as keys to the pathogenesis of depression. Social learning theorists have emphasized poor social skills and limited behavioral repertoires in depressed patients. Similarly, stressful life events, particularly those involving real or threatened interpersonal loss, have been considered of etiologic significance in depression.

The *subclinical approach* proposes that psychosocial factors represent subclinical manifestations of depressive disorders. As such, psychosocial factors and depressive disorders are expressions of the same underlying genetic or constitutional endowment. Thus, certain enduring behavior patterns or personality characteristics are considered to be part of a continuum, with depressive disorders defining one clinically observable endpoint.

The *pathoplasty approach* proposes that psychosocial factors act to influence the character of the depressive disorder. So instead of exerting a pathogenic influence in depression, psychosocial factors may affect the symptomatic expression or the course of the depressive episode or both. In this regard, psychosocial factors may be associated with specific symptom profiles or may serve as predictors of outcome and course.

The *deterioration approach* proposes that depression may act as an influence on psychosocial factors. That is, changes in psychosocial factors may result from the experience of the depressive episode itself, particularly if it is severe and protracted. These changes may include changes in personality characteristics such as an individual's attitude toward him- or herself, an individual's style of interacting with others, or an individual's perception of the environment. Changes may also occur in an individual's vulnerability to stressful life events and in the structure of his or her social support system.

The relationships among the psychosocial factors, as well as the relationships between these factors and depression as described in the four approaches, may be independent and direct, or they may be interactive. For example, life events have been viewed both as direct causal factors in depression and as precipitating factors in a person predisposed or vulnerable to depression. According to the latter interactive view, certain personality characteristics may act to predispose the individual to depressive episodes by making him or her more sensitive to the impact of life stress.

METHODOLOGICAL ISSUES

Several substantive methodological problems have hampered investigations of the relationship between psychosocial factors and depression. Since these problems affect both the feasibility of conducting research and the quality of the published reports, a brief review of four particular problems precedes the discussion of findings.

(1) *The heterogeneity of depressive disorders.* Since depressive disorders encompass several distinct subclasses which are considered to be heterogeneous with respect to etiology, clinical picture, and course (Klerman and Barrett, 1973), the nature of the relationship between the various psychosocial factors and specific depressive subtypes may differ. Failure to differentiate among depressive subtypes may therefore lead to considerable heterogeneity within study populations, and this in turn may either produce inconsistent results or obscure potentially important findings or both.

(2) *Operational criteria for defining depressive disorders and psychosocial factors.* In addition to more homogeneous samples of depressed subjects within a study, operational criteria are needed to define and specify the class rules by which persons are assigned a diagnosis. Similarly, psychosocial constructs such as dependency needs, obsessionality, loss events, major difficulties, and the like are ambiguous and open to idiosyncratic interpretation, and they also require operational definitions. Without diagnostic rigor in identifying patient populations and specificity in defining psychosocial variables, findings may be misleading and may not be comparable across studies.

(3) *Reliable measures of depressive disorders and psychosocial factors.* Reliable and standardized instruments or ratings to assess psychosocial variables and to diagnose and subtype depressive disorders are critical to sound methodology. Such methods help to ensure the replicability of research findings and facilitate the interpretation of results by providing objective and reliable reflections of operationally defined variables.

(4) *Influences on assessments.* Two major sources of bias may influence investigations of psychosocial factors and depression. The first of these arises from clinical state influences on assessments of psychosocial factors if measurements are obtained during the morbid state. That depressed patients do not provide valid reports of their premorbid functioning, but rather tend to distort their views of themselves and their life circumstances, has been well documented. For example, one of the authors and his colleagues (Hirschfeld et al., 1982) compared self-report personality inventories of patients obtained while patients were depressed with self-reports obtained at one-year follow-up when their symptoms had completely remitted. They found that clinical state strongly influenced personality scales related to emotional strength, interpersonal dependency, and extraversion. During the morbid period, patients appeared significantly more neurotic, more dependent, and more introverted than they did in remission. Similarly, Liebowitz et al. (1979) reported that even mild levels of depressive symptoms influenced measures of neuroticism in their study of personality traits in unipolar and bipolar depressives. This occurred despite test instructions that expressly directed patients to respond as to their "usual" functioning.

With regard to life events research, investigators in the area have warned against potentially misleading reports of the occurrence or dating of events when reports are obtained from patients during the depressive episode (Hudgens et al., 1970; Brown et al., 1973). They recommend using corroborative reports from relatives or obtaining information from patients after symptoms have abated. Barring premorbid assessments, which would of course be ideal, reliable information concerning premorbid psychosocial functioning must be obtained from patients during an intermorbid, symptom-free period.

A second possible source of influence on assessments of psychosocial factors is experimenter bias. The formulation of research hypotheses, the design of the study, the selection of dependent measures, and the interpretation of results are experimental factors. These are appropriately guided by the investigator's theories concerning depression, theories which are based largely on repeated observations of patients during depressive episodes. What is not appropriate, however, is the intrusion of theoretical views on the ratings of dependent measures. In order to minimize the introduction of such experimenter bias, independent blind ratings and standardized procedures are essential. Accordingly, psychosocial assessments must either be performed by individuals unaware of the research hypothesis and the subject's diagnostic status or be obtained via patient self-report.

Largely in light of these methodological problems, the authors have imposed several restrictions on the selection of studies for the review. Also, since several reviews of psychosocial factors and depression have recently appeared in the literature (e.g., Hirschfeld and Cross, 1982; Lloyd, 1980a; 1980b), the more recent research is emphasized. These studies are, however, placed in the context of previous theory and research. Among the recent studies, only those which provide operational or well-specified criteria for depression are included. Furthermore, the review includes only studies that employed objective and reliable assessments of psychosocial factors and obtained them during an intermorbid, symptom-free period. With these restrictions in mind, the authors aim to present only the most valid data concerning psychosocial factors in depression and to increase thereby the critical quality of the review.

REVIEW OF THE LITERATURE

Personality

THE PREDISPOSITION APPROACH Of the four approaches concerning the nature of the relationship between personality and depression, the predisposition hypothesis has enjoyed the greatest interest among clinicians and researchers. Much of the research in this area is an outgrowth of the psychoanalytic viewpoint. Psychoanalytic theorists since Abraham have described several personality characteristics associated with depression. Although Abraham (1948) stressed obsessional characteristics, most psychoanalytic writers since then have focused more on the area of interpersonal dependency. In his review of this literature, Chodoff (1972) concluded that a liberal mixture of "anal" and "oral" traits were the theorized hallmarks of depression-prone personalities. He described depressed individuals as "inordinately and almost exclusively dependent on narcissistic supplies derived directly or indirectly from other people for maintenance of their self-esteem. Their frustration tolerance is low and they may employ various techniques— submissive, manipulative, coercive, piteous, demanding or placating—to maintain their desperately needed but essentially ambivalent relationships with the external or internalized objects of their demands" (Chodoff, 1972, 670).

Although most psychoanalytic theorists do not specify the diagnosis beyond "depression," a study by Mabel Blake Cohen and her colleagues (1954) provides a significant exception. In their investigation of a group of patients who would be termed bipolars today, the authors described the patients as ambitious, driven, relatively extraverted, and concealing strong dependency needs while appearing superficially well adjusted.

Several recent studies have examined personality traits in euthymic depressed patients using standardized procedures for both diagnosis and personality assessment (see Table 1). Benjaminsen (1981a) investigated the Eysenck Personality Inventory (EPI) neuroticism and introversion scores of three groups of depressed patients: primary melancholics, primary nonmelancholics, and secondary depressives with a primary diagnosis of neurotic disorder. In his analyses, Benjaminsen found that nonmelancholic patients were significantly more neurotic and more introverted than melancholic patients. Secondary depressives were intermediate in introversion, differing significantly from no group, but they were significantly more neurotic than either of the primary depressed groups. A comparison of the EPI scores for these patient groups against the published norm reveals that the secondary depressives to some extent and the nonmelancholic depressives to a much greater extent were more introverted than the norm. The melancholic depressives, on the other hand, had scores very close to the norm for introversion. On neuroticism, melancholics again scored at the norm, while both the nonmelancholic and secondary depressives scored within the neurotic range. Further analyses conducted with the melancholic patient group, categorized by polarity, revealed that the unipolar and bipolar melancholic patients did not differ in their levels of neuroticism and introversion. Comparisons of the unipolar and bipolar melancholic groups with nonmelancholics and secondary depressives showed the nonmelancholic patients to be significantly more introverted than the bipolars but not the unipolars. Secondary depressives were more neurotic than either the bipolar or the unipolar melancholic group, but they did not differ from them in introversion. With regard to the published norms, bipolar melancholics scored within the normal range on both neuroticism and introversion, whereas nonbipolar melancholics were normal in neuroticism level but scored in the slightly introverted range.

Bech et al. (1980) compared personality scale scores in bipolar and nonbipolar melancholic patients using three inventories in addition to the EPI: the Marke-Nyman Temperament Scale (MNTS), which measures Sjobring's three personality dimensions; the von Zerssen Personality Scale, which consists of two scales measuring melancholia and cyclothymia; and the Cesarec-Marke Personality Scale, which consists of 11 subscales based on Murray's theory of psychogenic needs (1938). Consistent with Benjaminsen's results, Bech et al. found no difference in neuroticism and introversion levels between bipolar and nonbipolar patients. Furthermore, a pattern similar to that described by Benjaminsen emerged in normative comparisons. Both groups evidenced normal levels of neuroticism, and whereas normal levels of introversion were found in bipolars, nonbipolars were more introverted than the norm.

On the MNTS, bipolars and nonbipolars differed significantly, with nonbipolars scoring higher than bipolars on the solidity scale. In addition, nonbipolars scored significantly lower than bipolars on the guilt, succorance, and autonomy subscales of the Cesarec-Marke scale. The groups showed no differences on the von Zerssen subscales.

Liebowitz et al. (1979) also assessed personality characteristics in bipolar and nonbipolar melancholic patients using the MNTS and Eysenck's Maudsley Personality Inventory (MPI). As in the Benjaminsen and Bech et al. studies, these investigators found no differences between patient groups on either neuroticism or introversion, and in normative comparisons they obtained patterns consistent with those described above. Unlike the Bech et al. findings, no significant differences in MNTS subscales emerged between the nonbipolar and bipolar groups.

In a two-year follow-up assessment of primary major depressive patients, Hirschfeld and Klerman (1979) reported findings much in agreement with those described above for depressives compared with the norms. Whereas several personality scales showed significant departures from published norms when assessments were made during the depressive episode, only the extraversion scale of the MPI differed in these patients when assessed during remission, and it was significantly lower than the norm. No differences were observed in comparisons with norms on the MPI-Neuroticism (MPI-N) scale, the three MNTS scales, or the Lazare-Klerman-Armor Personality Inventory measures of orality, obsessionality, and hysterical pattern.

With regard to the above-described findings of marked similarity between euthymic unipolar and bipolar melancholic patients, Donnelly et al. (1976) compared Minnesota Multiphasic Personality Inventory (MMPI) profiles of unipolar and bipolar primary depressives in remission. No significant differences emerged on any of the ten clinical subscales between these groups, nor did the scores of any of the scales show a significant elevation (i.e., greater than 70).

One relatively recent study compared the scoring patterns of different depressive subtypes on the 16 Personality Factor Questionnaire and reported significant differences between recurrent unipolar and bipolar patients upon recovery. Murray and Blackburn (1974) found that the scores of unipolar patients differed significantly from those of bipolar patients. Unipolar patients showed lower levels of emotional stability, surgency, adventurousness, and extraversion, and they showed higher levels of anxiety. On all differing scales, the scores of bipolar patients approximated the norm.

Finally, two factor analytic studies by Wittenborn and his associates have investigated in women those personality characteristics associated with depression in general (Altman and Wittenborn, 1980; Cofer and Wittenborn, 1980). They obtained the responses of groups of formerly depressed women to self-descriptive questionnaires and compared these responses with those of matched groups of normal controls. They then factor analyzed items which they found discriminated between the two groups in each study. Several similar factors were characteristic of depressives in both studies: (1) an unhappy outlook, (2) narcissistic vulnerability, and (3) low self-esteem, a sense of helplessness, and a lack of confidence or sense of competence. In addition, Cofer and Wittenborn found that two factors representing perception of

Table 1. Summary of Studies on Personality Characteristics and Depression

Source	Sample[1]	Methods[1]		Results
		Diagnostic	Personality	
		PREDISPOSITION HYPOTHESIS		
1. Benjaminsen (1981a)	146 Dep inpts: 46 Pr Mel (23 BP, 23 NBP) 41 Pr Nmel 59 Neur with Sec Dep	Feighner Criteria	Eysenck Personality Inventory (EPI)	Nmel UP had sig lower extraversion scores than BP; Sec Dep had sig higher neuroticism scores than all other grps; Nmel UP had sig higher neuroticism scores than Mel UP and BP. Mel UP and BP did not differ on either scale.
2. Bech et al. (1980)	36 Manic-Mel outpts: 13 UP 23 BP	Multiclad System	EPI Marke-Nyman Temperament Scale (MNTS) von Zerssen Personality Scale (ZPS) Cesarec-Marke Personality Scale (CMPS)	No sig differences emerged between UP and BP on either the neuroticism or extraversion scales of the EPI, nor did the two grps differ sig on the ZPS. UP scored sig higher on the solidity scale of the MNTS and sig lower on the guilt, succorance, and autonomy subscales of the CMPS.
3. Liebowitz et al. (1979)	110 outpts with Pr Aff Dis: 71 BP I and II 21 UP (18 BP-Other)	Feighner Criteria	Maudsley Personality Inventory (MPI) MNTS	No sig differences were obtained on any of the pers measures when comparisons of euthymic pts were made.
4. Hirschfeld and Klerman (1979)	15 inpts with Aff Dis at follow-up	SADS/RDC	MPI Lazare-Klerman-Armor Personality Inventory (LKA) MNTS	Of all pers measures, only the MPI extraversion scale differed from the norm in recovered Dep.

5.	Donnelly et al. (1976)	34 Dep inpts in Remission: 17 Pr UP 17 Pr BP	Feighner Criteria	MMPI	No sig differences were found in MMPI subscale scores between UP and BP pts in remission.
6.	Murray and Blackburn (1974)	36 Recovered Dep: 18 UP Mel pts with at least 3 previous episodes 18 BP pts	Psych Dx	16 Personality Factor Questionnaire (16 PF)	Recovered UP pts differed sig from recovered BP pts in showing lower scores on Emotional Instability, Surgency, Adventurousness, and the secondary factor Extraversion, while showing sig higher scores on the secondary factor Anxiety. On all scales, the scores of BP pts approximated the norms.
7.	Altman and Wittenborn (1980)	88 Dep female inpts (in remission) 88 Matched community C females	Psych Dx	134-item self-report inventory	Correlational and subsequent factor analyses of the discriminating items yielded 5 factors which differentiated formerly Dep pts from never-ill C: (1) low self-esteem; (2) preoccupation with failure; (3) unhappy outlook; (4) narcissistic vulnerability; and (5) lack of self-confidence and a lack of sense of competence. A general factor of Dep-prone pers did not emerge.
8.	Cofer and Wittenborn (1980)	48 Previously hospitalized Dep females 90 Matched community C females	Psych Dx	50-item self-report inventory with each presented to reflect the pts' (1) self-perception; (2) perception of mother; and (3) perception of father	43 of the 150 items were found to discriminate the formerly Dep from Cs. Factor analysis of these items yielded 5 factors: (1) unhappy outlook; (2) narcissistic vulnerability; (3) low self-esteem; (4) critical dissatisfied mother; and (5) overprotective, dependency-fostering father.

Table 1. Continued

Source	Sample[1]	Methods[1]		Results
		Diagnostic	Personality	
		SUBCLINICAL HYPOTHESIS		
1. Gershon et al. (1975)	70 Pr UP & BP inpts 524 1st-degree relatives of Dep 75 Medical C pts 619 1st-degree relatives of C	Feighner Criteria	Diagnostic interview to ascertain presence of various psych disorders	The overall prevalence of Aff Dis, dep spectrum dis, moderate dep, and cyclothymic pers did not differ in comparisons of the relatives of UP and BP probands. Relatives of both Dep grps had sig higher rates of moderate dep and cyclothymic pers than C relatives.
2. Wetzel et al. (1980)	65 Pr UP Dep inpts 215 1st-degree relatives of Dep 16 "Normal" C subjects 62 1st-degree relatives of C	Feighner Criteria	16 PF	Age- and sex-corrected scores were compared in both proband grps and both relative grps to assess traits related to Dep which appeared to be both familial and related to Dep included Reserved, Emotional Instability, Shyness, Apprehensiveness, and Tense. All of these factors, with the exception of Reserved, load highly on the secondary factor Anxiety, found previously to have considerable genetic loading.
		PATHOPLASTY HYPOTHESIS		
1. Paykel et al. (1976)	185 Dep inpts, outpts, and day pts	Psych Dx	MPI LKA LKA-Relative Version	MPI neuroticism scores, obtained after substantial clinical improvement had occurred, were sig correlated with several symptoms considered to be characteristic of Neur as opposed to Mel Dep. These included guilt, obsessionality, helplessness, anxiety, irritability, and initial insomnia

#	Study	Sample	Measures	Results
2.	Snaith et al. (1971)	50 Pr UP Dep	Psych Dx MPI Sandler-Hazari Scale	(all positive correlations), and loss of insight and severity (both negative correlations). Pts displaying a more Neur symptom pattern also tended to have more oral dependent and less obsessional pers, as assessed by the LKA, whereas pts with hysterical pers tended to be less severely Dep and to show more irritability and less anxiety. Clinical assessments of suicidal propensities, phobic symptoms, obsessional symptoms, guilt, hypochondriasis, irritability, and agitation/retardation showed no sig relationship to any of the pers variables.
3.	Weissman et al. (1978)	150 female UP, nonpsychotic Dep pts (predominantly Nmel) placed on amitriptyline	Psych Dx MPI (at 1, 8, 20, and 48 mo after initiation of treatment)	MPI neuroticism scores at initial testing (1 mo) were the best predictor of long-term outcome. Pts who had a complete remission at 8 mo which was maintained during the course of the study had the lowest neuroticism scores at 1 mo (these approximated normal scores), whereas chronic pts who maintained a moderate level of Dep symptoms had the highest neuroticism scores (greater than 30 at all testings) initially and at each follow-up testing. The "fluctuating" grp showed intermediate neuroticism scores on initial assessment and at subsequent testing, at each time showing scores above the norm. MPI extraversion scores did not relate to outcome. NOTE: Initial severity ratings did not predict outcome (i.e., pers and severity appear to be separate dimensions).

[1]Key

Dep = Depressed/Depressives; Neur = Neurotic; Nmel = Nonmelancholic; Aff Dis = Affective Disorder; BP = Bipolar; UP = Unipolar; C = Controls; Pr = Primary; Sec = Secondary; Sig = Significant; Pers = Personality; SR = Self-reports.

parents differentiated the depressed group, a view of mother as critical and dissatisfied and a view of father as overprotective and dependency fostering. (Altman and Wittenborn did not asssess this aspect of personality.) Neither study identified a general factor of depression-prone personality which could account for the difference between the depressed and nondepressed groups.

From this body of research, several conclusions may be drawn on the predispositional role of personality in depression. First, some evidence suggests that nonmelancholic and secondary depressives may be predisposed to depressive episodes by the increased levels of neuroticism which characterize their premorbid personalities. In addition, major depressives generally appear to be both more introverted and more anxious compared with the norm and with bipolar depressives, and they have been found to differ from control subjects on several self-esteem-related measures. In contrast, however, neither melancholic major depressives nor bipolar depressives have been found consistently to be more neurotic and dependent than the norm. The similarities between these two groups and their lack of deviation from the norm are in fact more striking than their differences in these areas. The studies which have subdivided depressives most consistently report no personality differences between melancholic major depressives and bipolar patients; the differences that other authors report in introversion, anxiety, and self-esteem are therefore likely due primarily to their having included nonmelancholic major depressives in their heterogeneous samples.

THE SUBCLINICAL APPROACH The hypothesis that both personality characteristics and depressive disorders represent a trait-state continuum which is genetically determined was first postulated by Kraepelin (1921). On the basis of clinical observation, Kraepelin described depressive, manic, irritable or mixed, and cyclothymic affective temperaments which he considered to be milder versions of affective illnesses. Schneider's (1958) writings on the depressive and hypomanic personality types and Kretschmer's (1936) on the cycloid and schizoid types extended Kraepelin's original views.

Investigations of personality characteristics as subclinical manifestations of depressive disorders have generally been directed at differentiating unipolar and bipolar patients from normal controls on the basis of temperamental differences in their relatives. Data bearing on this hypothesis are available from two recent studies (see Table 1). Gershon et al. (1975) examined the rates of cyclothymic personality, moderate depression, and cyclic depressive personality in the first-degree relatives of unipolar depressives, bipolar depressives, and normal controls. These investigators found cyclothymia and moderate depression to be significantly more prevalent in the relatives of both depressed groups as compared with control relatives, lending support to the subclinical view of personality.

In a second study of the subclinical hypothesis, Wetzel et al. (1980) used the 16 Personality Factor Questionnaire and compared the scores of unipolar depressed probands, their first-degree relatives, control probands with no history of psychiatric illness, and the controls' relatives. With this design they aimed to ascertain those personality factors which are both familial and related to depression. A factor was judged to be both familial and depression related if depressed probands and their relatives scored in a similar manner and if the score differed from that of control probands and their relatives, who would also have to score in a fashion similar to each other. According to these criteria, several factors appeared to be both familial and depression related. Nearly all of these factors were contained in a higher-order factor related to anxiety, which had previously been demonstrated to have considerable genetic loading. The depressives and their relatives scored higher on this factor as compared with controls. Although Wetzel et al. had hypothesized that the unipolar patients and their relatives would show higher scores on a factor considered indicative of cyclothymia, they instead found the reverse, that unipolars and their relatives scored lower than controls on cyclothymia.

Obviously, the data concerning the view of personality as a sub-clinical manifestation of depressive disorders are insufficient at present to evaluate the validity of this hypothesis. The contradictory nature of the available reports is undoubtedly due to differences in the timing and methods of assessment.

THE PATHOPLASTY APPROACH   The hypothesis that person-ality characteristics may affect the symptom picture or the course of the depressive episode or both has been tested in three relatively recent studies (see Table 1). In a large group of depressed patients, Paykel et al. (1976) compared symptom ratings and scores on three personality scales, the MPI, Lazare-Klerman-Armor Personality Inventory (LKA), and a relative version of the LKA. They aimed to determine whether certain features of premorbid personality were associated with specific symptom patterns. The most reliable findings to emerge from these analyses were that patients with high premorbid neuroticism scores on the MPI tended to show a more neurotic, rather than an endogenous/melancholic symptom picture. These patients were also found to be more "oral" and less "obsessional" on the LKA. Patients with hysterical premorbid personality features tended to be rated as less severely de-pressed and to show more irritability and less anxiety than patients without such characteristics.

In contrast to the findings of Paykel et al., Snaith et al. (1971), in an earlier and similarly designed study, had found no significant asso-ciations between symptom measures and personality characteristics in their group of unipolar depressives.

Finally, in a study designed to investigate personality attributes as predictors of outcome of depressive disorders, Weissman et al. (1978) obtained symptom ratings and MPI scores in a group of female neu-rotic depressives at 1, 8, 20, and 48 months following initiation of treatment. These investigators found one-month MPI-N scores to be the best predictors of outcome, as measured by symptom levels at each follow-up assessment period. Those patients who remained chronically symptomatic at follow-up had the highest initial MPI-N scores, and those who were considered asymptomatic for the entire follow-up period had the lowest initial MPI-N scores, these being in the normal range.

Although personality as an influence on the symptom picture and course of the depressive episode has yet to be convincingly demon-strated, some evidence suggests a relationship between a nonneurotic premorbid personality and the development of melancholic symptomatology. This finding is reinforced by reports of nonneurotic premorbid personalities in melancholic depressives. The evidence also suggests a relationship between high levels of neuroticism and a more chronic, unremitting depression.

THE DETERIORATION APPROACH To date, studies have not been carried out to test the proposition that depression influences personality.

Life Events and Social Factors

Life events and social factors may render an individual vulnerable to depression. As in the case of personality factors, however, they may "color" the episode (pathoplasty) rather than predispose a person to it. And, of course, the depression may lead to changes in the whole social situation (deterioration). Since the overwhelming majority of research has been directed toward the predisposition approach, the following review focuses on that hypothesis in some detail and briefly reviews the two studies that have examined the pathoplasty hypothesis with regard to life events. Finally in this section, six studies of the possible predispositional effect of social factors are reviewed.

Life events research is characterized by two different methodologies. The first follows from the work of Holmes and Rahe, who defined stress as a weighted sum of recent life events (Holmes and Rahe, 1967; Rahe et al., 1964). These weights may reflect distress on the basis of ratings by a general population sample; they may reflect the proportion of desirable and undesirable events; or they may reflect the number of events categorized according to controllability. Comparisons of depressed and control subjects are generally based on total numbers, weighted totals of life events experienced, or totals within a category. This approach typifies the research conducted by Paykel and his associates (1969) and the National Institute of Mental Health Collaborative Study on the Psychobiology of Depression (Hirschfeld, 1981).

The second methodology is employed by George Brown and his associates (1973), who argue that standard weights cannot be applied to events. Instead, these investigators consider each event experienced within its objective content and rate events according to the degree of threat they pose to the individual. Analyses of depressed and control populations generally consist of comparisons of the percentage of each group experiencing at least one threatening life event.

LIFE EVENTS AND PREDISPOSITION (OR PRECIPITATION)
In the case of life events, as compared with personality factors, the predisposition approach might more properly be called the precipitation approach, but the interrelationship with depressive disorders is nonetheless analogous. Life events research related to the predisposition approach stems in part from observations that under conditions of severe, life-threatening environmental stress, the incidence of psychiatric disorder rises sharply. Following this lead, several investigators have demonstrated an association between everyday stressful events and psychiatric impairment in general (e.g., Myers et al., 1971;

1972) and depression more specifically (e.g., Brown et al., 1973; Paykel et al., 1969; Thomson and Hendrie, 1972).

Moreover, certain types of life events, rather than life change in general, have been linked to the onset of depressive disorders. Depressives have been found to experience significantly more exit events (i.e., loss of a significant other through death or separation), more undesirable events, more severely threatening events, and more uncontrollable events in the six months prior to onset than general population controls (Brown et al., 1973; 1975; Paykel et al., 1969) or schizophrenic controls (Jacobs et al., 1974). Attempts to differentiate subtypes of depressive disorders on the basis of the occurrence of life events, however, have found no difference in the rates for bipolar compared with nonbipolar depressives (Patrick et al., 1978) or between endogenous and reactive depressives (Thomson and Hendrie, 1972).

Recent research efforts have confirmed and extended these earlier findings (see Table 2). Fava et al. (1981) replicated the original Paykel et al. study (1969) which formed the basis for much of our current knowledge concerning life events. Comparing the rate of specific types of life events in the six months prior to onset, Fava et al. found that depressives reported significantly more life events than a matched group of normal controls. Furthermore, these investigators showed that the excess of events reported by depressives was attributable to the types previously found to relate to the onset of depression: events with a negative impact, events out of the control of the individual, undesirable events, and events involving loss. No differences in rates of controllable, desirable, or entrance events were found between the two groups.

Finlay-Jones and Brown (1981) compared rates of events, evaluated in terms of the severity of loss or danger they posed, in the 12 months prior to onset in groups of depressed, anxious, mixed depressed-anxious, and community control women. A significantly higher proportion of "cases" than controls reported at least one severe event in the 3-, 6-, 9-, and 12-month periods prior to onset, and some specificity of events was noted among patient groups. Whereas no difference was found in rates of severe loss between controls and anxiety cases, significantly more cases of depression and mixed depression-anxiety had experienced a severe loss in the three months prior to onset than either controls or anxiety cases. With regard to events involving severe danger, significantly more anxiety cases had experienced these events in the three months prior to onset than either depressed cases or noncases. Such events did not know the same degree of specificity that characterized loss events, however, in that significantly more depressed and mixed depressed-anxious cases than noncases also experienced dangerous events in the three months prior to onset. No difference in rates of either loss or dangerous events were found between mixed depressed-anxious and depressed cases.

Few differences among depressive subtypes have been reported in the frequency and types of events preceding onset. Benjaminsen (1981b) compared event rates in the six months prior to onset in a group of depressed inpatients assigned to five alternative dichotomies representing various definitions of neurotic/nonneurotic depression: melancholic/nonmelancholic, psychotic/nonpsychotic, mild/severe, primary/secondary (with neurosis as primary diagnosis), and self-pitying/non-self-pitying. No differences between the various dichotomies were

Table 2. Summary of Studies on Life Events in Relation to Depression

Source	Sample[1]	Methods[1] Diagnostic	Methods[1] Life Events	Results[1]
1. Fava et al. (1981)	40 1st episode Pr Major Dep 40 matched normal C	RDC	Paykel's Recent LE Scale (6 mo)	Dep reported sig more total and independent E; E with moderate, marked or severe impact; and uncontrollable, undesirable, and exit E than C. No differences in controllable, desirable, or entrance E were found between the two grps.
2. Finlay-Jones and Brown (1981)	164 females attending London G.P. Clinic: 17 Rated as "Case Dep" 13 Rated as "Case Anx" 15 Rated as "Mixed Case" 80 With No Psych Dis	PSE/Consensus Dx by 2 Psychiatrists and 2 Sociologists	Brown's Semistructured LE Interview (12 mo). E evaluated for severity of loss and severity of danger	A sig higher proportion of cases than noncases reported at least 1 severe E in the 3, 6, 9, and 12 mo periods before onset. In addition, sig more cases of Dep and mixed cases than either C or Anx cases experienced a severe loss in the 3 mo prior to onset. No differences were found in severe loss between Dep and mixed cases, or between Anx and noncases. With regard to severe danger, sig more Anx cases than Dep or noncases experienced such E in the 3 mo prior to onset. However, sig more Dep. and mixed cases than noncases also experienced dangerous E.
3. Benjaminsen (1981b)	89 Pr and Sec Dep inpts assigned to 5 alternative dichotomies: Mel/Nmel Psychotic/Nonpsychotic Pr/Sec Self-pitying/Non-self-pitying	Feighner Criteria	Paykel's Recent LE Scale (6 mo)	The percentage of pts in each of the 5 Neur/Nneur comparison grps experiencing at least 1 LE in the 6 mo prior to onset did not differ. Sig more Neur than Nneur Dep experienced multiple E's, regardless of how the grps were defined. However, these differences did not emerge when comparisons of multiple unrelated E's and severe personal losses were made.

Study	Sample	Diagnosis	LE Measure	Findings
4. Benjaminsen (1981a)	145 Dep inpts: 45 Pr Mel (23 BP, 23 NBP) 41 Pr Nmel 59 Neur with Sec Dep	Feighner Criteria	Paykel's Recent LE Scale (6 mo)	No sig differences in type or frequency of LE were found in comparisons of the three grps.
5. Hirschfeld (1981)	38 Situational Dep 68 Nonsituational Dep	SADS/RDC	Psychiatric Epidemiology Research Inventory—Modified (3 and 6 mo)	In comparisons of 3 and 6 mo total LE scores and LE scores by content area (e.g., school, work, health, etc.), the only difference to emerge between the two grps was a higher number of love-related E's at 6 mo in Situational Dep.
6. Matussek and Neuner (1981)	90 Mel Dep 38 Neur Dep 41 Normal C	Psych Dx from Medical Records/RDC in unclear cases	Loss of 1st-degree relatives, including spouse (in adulthood), through death or separation	An equal percentage of Mel and Neur Dep and C had experienced adulthood loss, including when losses were categorized by close person concerned (e.g., sib, parent, etc.). Sig more Neur Dep than Mel Dep became Dep in the yr following loss of any close person, with the difference attributable solely to loss through separation, particularly from a partner.
7. Brown et al. (1979)	62 Psychotic Dep 49 Neur Dep	Psych Dx	Brown's Interview of LE and Major Difficulties	No differences between the two grps were found in the proportion of pts reporting severe LE or long-term difficulties prior to onset. Incidence of "past" loss was higher in Psychotics and, whereas Psychotics had experienced sig more past losses through death, Neur had experienced sig more past losses through separation.

Table 2. Continued

		Methods[1]		
Source	Sample[1]	Diagnostic	Life Events	Results[1]
8. Lloyd et al. (1981)	50 Pr UP Major Dep undergoing antidepressant treatment: Good responders Bad responders	Psych Dx	Paykel's Recent LE Scale for 1 yr prior to onset (antecedent E's) and for 1 mo treatment period (concurrent E's)	Good and poor responders did not differ in total number, content area, or number of desirable antecedent E's for either the 12 mo or 2 mo prior to onset. Poor responders reported sig more concurrent E's than did good responders. When these were broken down into categories, poor responders were found to have experienced more undesirable, health-related, and uncontrollable E's. No differences were seen in exit, independent, controllable, desirable, or entrance E's.
9. Weissman et al. (1978)	150 F UP Nonpsychotic Dep Pts (predominantly Nmel) placed on amitriptyline	Psych Dx	Paykel's Recent LE Scale (6 mo)	Pts were categorized as asymptomatic, moderately symptomatic, or chronically symptomatic at 8, 12, 20 and 48 mo after onset. At none of these assessment periods were antecedent LE's found to differentiate the chronic pts from either of the other two grps.

[1]Key
E = Event(s); LE = Life Event; Dep = Depressives/Depressed; Nmel = Non melancholic; UP = Unipolar; C = Controls; Pr = Primary; Sec = Secondary; Sig = Significant; Anx = Anxiety.

found in the percentage of patients in each group experiencing at least one life event in the six-month period prior to onset. Nor were differences in loss events, undesirable events, or severely upsetting events found among these pairs. Significantly more neurotic than non-neurotic depressives did experience multiple events, regardless of how the groups were defined. These differences held only for related or possibly related events, however. When comparisons of multiple un-related events were made, no differences between groups emerged.

In a second study, Benjaminsen (1981a) compared melancholic, nonmelancholic, and secondary depressives with regard to frequency and types of events occurring in the six months prior to onset. He found no differences among these groups on any of the life events measures.

Similarly, Hirschfeld (1981) compared life events rates in total and within area of life affected (e.g., school, work, love, and so forth) in situational and nonsituational depressives in the three- and six-month periods prior to onset. Only a single difference emerged between the two groups. Situational depressives had a higher rate of love-related events at six months than nonsituational depressives.

Matussek and Neuner (1981) examined the rates of loss in adulthood, restricting their definition of loss to death or separation from a first-degree relative or partner, in groups of melancholic depressives, neurotic depressives, and normal controls. These investigators found that although the incidence of adulthood loss was equal in all three groups, a significantly higher percentage of neurotic depressives be-came depressed in the year following such a loss than did melancholic depressives. When they separated losses as to whether they were due to death or separation, they found an equal proportion of melancholic and neurotic depressives became depressed in the year following the death of a close person, but significantly more neurotic depressives than melancholics became depressed following separation from a close person, particularly a partner.

Finally, Brown et al. (1979) investigated the rates of severe life events and long-term difficulties prior to onset in groups of psychotic and neurotic depressives. While they found no difference in the proportion of patients reporting such events or difficulties, they noted that the incidence of past loss through death was significantly higher in psychotics, whereas the incidence of past loss through separation was higher in neurotics.

Added to studies conducted previously, these studies suggest that life events, particularly those involving losses and those having a negative impact or representing a severe threat, play a precipitating role in depression in general. From the findings presented, however, the contributory role of life events is clearly not associated differ-entially with any specific subtype of depression. Moreover, many depressions of a melancholic, neurotic, or psychotic type develop without an apparent stressful precipitant, and conversely many stress-ful life events are not followed by depression. Life events are there-fore neither a necessary nor a sufficient cause of depression.

LIFE EVENTS AND PATHOPLASTY   Lloyd et al. (1981) examined the relationship between life events and response to tricyclic antide-pressant therapy in a group of unipolar depressives. They assessed events for the one year prior to admission (antecedent events) and for the one-month treatment period (concurrent events), categorized patients as good or poor responders as reflected by improvement in Hamilton scores, and then compared the response groups with regard to occurrence of life events. Good and poor responders did not differ in the total number of antecedent life events they experienced, the content areas that were affected, or the number of undesirable antecedent life events they had experienced. Poor responders, however, reported significantly more undesirable, health-related, and uncontrollable concurrent life events than did good responders. No differences between the two response groups were found for exit, independent, controllable, desirable, or entrance events.

The finding that antecedent life events were unrelated to drug therapy outcome is consistent with a report by Weissman et al. (1978). Weissman and her colleagues categorized female depressed patients on the basis of their response to antidepressant therapy at 8, 12, 20, and 48 months after onset and found no difference in the rates of antecedent life events.

Together, the results of these two studies on the course of the depressive episode suggest that while antecedent life events have little impact on the outcome of the depressive episode, events occurring during the treatment period may have a detrimental effect on the outcome of treatment. Lloyd et al. do make a good case for explaining the effects of concurrent events with the pathoplasty hypothesis: concurrent life events may interfere with the therapeutic effects of antidepressant drugs. An alternative explanation more in line with the deterioration hypothesis could be offered, however: nonresponders, who by definition remain depressed, could be contributing to the occurrence of negative events via their depression-related behavior.

SOCIAL FACTORS   In a 1975 investigation of the relationship between life events and depression in a community sample of women, Brown et al. identified four social factors which appeared to mediate the effects of life events. Brown et al. called these factors vulnerability factors since their presence increased the likelihood of a depressive episode in the face of a provoking agent (i.e., a stressful life event). Three of the four factors represent current life circumstances: unemployment, three or more children at home under the age of 14, and lack of a confiding relationship with a partner. The fourth represents a remote life event: childhood loss of a parent through death or separation. All four of these factors are presumed to contribute to depression by rendering an individual less able to cope with stress.

Three recent studies have been designed to test Brown's vulnerability model (see Table 3). In a replication of the original findings of Brown et al. (1975) in a sample of urban-dwelling women, Brown and Prudo (1981) examined whether threatening life events and long-term difficulties and social factors played an etiologic role in depression among a sample of rural women. As in their urban sample, significantly more women with an onset of depression in the one year before the interview had experienced at least one severely threatening event or difficulty prior to onset, as compared

Table 3. Summary of Studies on Social Factors in Relation to Depression

| Source | Sample[1] | Methods[1] | | Results[1] |
		Diagnostic	Social Factors	
1. Brown and Prudo (1981)	355 rural Community females 39 with case Dep	Present State Exam (PSE)/ Consensus Dx	Brown's Interview Schedule for LE and Major Difficulties	Sig more women with case Dep had experienced at least 1 severely threatening LE or major difficulty than noncase women. Three or more children at home under age 14 was the only vulnerability factor which sig increased the likelihood of Dep in the presence of a provoking agent (LE).
2. Costello (1982)	449 Community females 38 with case Dep	PSE/ID-Catego Method	Brown's Interview Schedule for LE and Major Difficulties (12 mo) Sociodemographic and Marital Interviews	A sig association was found between the occurrence of severe E's and the onset of Dep which held for both independent and possibly independent E's. Similarly, a sig association was found between the occurrence of severe difficulties and the onset of Dep, but only for possibly independent difficulties, not for independent difficulties. Of Brown's vulnerability factors, only lack of a confiding relationship was sig related to Dep. No interaction between social factors and life stress was obtained.
3. Solomon and Bromet (1982)	2 samples of Community females: 311 high-risk females living within 10 mi of Three Mile Island nuclear plant (TMI) 124 C females living within 10 mi of Beaver Valley nuclear plant (BV)	SADS-L/RDC (either Dep or Anx)	LE Scale Sociodemographic Interview	One-yr prevalence rate of Aff Dis was sig higher in the TMI sample, with the onset of the majority of these subsequent to the TMI accident. Of Brown's vulnerability factors, only failure to name husband as confidant was associated with Dep, but this held only in the high-stress grp. Similarly, when high- and low-stress grps were identified by the occurrence of a major stressor (other than the TMI accident), failure to identify husband as confidant was sig associated with Dep, but only in the TMI sample; no support for the vulnerability model was provided in the BV sample.

Table 3. Continued

| Source | Sample[1] | Methods[1] | | Results[1] |
		Diagnostic	Social Factors	
4. Roy (1981a)	88 Pr UP, Nonpsychotic females 88 Matched Normal C females	Psych Dx	Sociodemographic and Marital Interviews	Parental loss before age 17, poor marital relationship, and unemployment were reported sig more frequently in Dep women.
5. Roy (1981b)	71 Pr UP, Nonpsychotic Dep males 71 Matched Normal C males	Psych Dx	Sociodemographic and Marital Interviews	Parental loss before age 17 and unemployment were reported sig more frequently in Dep men.
6. Roy (1981c)	94 Pr UP, Nonpsychotic Dep inpts 94 Matched Psychotic pts with Pers Dis	Psych Dx (Dep)/DSM-III Criteria (Pers Dis)	Sociodemographic and Marital Interviews	Parental loss before age 17 and unemployment were found to differentiate Dep from Pers Dis women, whereas only parental loss was associated with Dep in men. Poor marital relationship did not discriminate between the grps.

[1]Key

E = Events; LE = Life Events; Dep = Depression/Depressives/Depressed; Aff Dis = Affective Disorders; UP = Unipolar; Pr = Primary; Sig = Significant; Anx = Anxiety.

with nondepressed women. With regard to vulnerability factors, having three or more children under the age of 14 at home was the only factor that increased the likelihood of depression in the presence of a provoking agent (life event or long-term difficulty).

In the second study, Solomon and Bromet (1982) investigated stressful life events and social factors in two samples of community women, a high-stress group of women living within ten miles of the Three Mile Island nuclear plant (TMI) and a matched control group of women living within ten miles of the Beaver Valley nuclear plant (BV). The prevalence rate of affective disorder in the one year following the TMI accident was significantly higher in the TMI sample than in the BV sample, and the onset of most of the disorders followed the accident. Of Brown's four vulnerability factors, the failure to name a partner as confidant was the only one associated with depression, and this held only in the TMI (high-stress) group. Similarly, when high- and low-stress groups were further defined by the occurrence of a major life event, the failure to name a partner as confidant was again the only vulnerability factor found to be associated with depression, and this again held only in the TMI sample. None of the vulnerability factors was associated with depression in the BV sample.

In the third study, Costello (1982) assessed the independent and interactive effects of threatening life events, major difficulties, and social factors in a community sample of women. He found a significant association between the onset of depression and the occurrence of severely threatening life events when such events were classified as either independent or possibly independent of the disorder. He also found a significant association between the onset of depression and the occurrence of major difficulties, but only when the difficulties were possibly independent difficulties. As in the study reported by Solomon and Bromet, among Brown's vulnerability factors only the lack of a confiding relationship was found to be significantly related to depression. Furthermore, Costello found no interaction between social factors and life stress.

Roy (1981a; 1981b; 1981c) has reported the results of three investigations of the independent contribution of social factors to depression. One compared female unipolar depressives with matched normal controls, one compared male unipolar depressives with matched normal controls, and the third compared unipolar depressives with matched psychiatric controls who had personality disorder as a diagnosis. In female depressives, Roy found three of Brown's four vulnerability factors to be associated with depression, parental loss before age 17, a poor marital relationship, and unemployment. In male depressives, only two of Brown's vulnerability factors were associated with depression, parental loss before age 17 and unemployment. Finally, in his investigation of the specificity of these factors to depression, Roy found that parental loss before age 17 and unemployment differentiated female depressives from personality-disordered women, while only parental loss differentiated depressed from personality-disordered men.

As a whole, these studies do not support Brown's vulnerability model across populations. Aspects of it, especially the presence of a heterosexual confidant among women (but not men), have been associated with depression. However, the factors do not form a constellation that precedes depression any more often than other conditions. Therefore, Brown's earlier findings may be somewhat specific to his sample or possibly specific to women living in an urban area. The later three studies were based on either nonurban areas (Brown and Prudo; Solomon and Bromet) or an area less urbanized than London (Costello).

With regard to the independent contribution of social factors to depression, the findings are mixed. One of Brown's vulnerability factors, three or more children under the age of 14 at home, was not associated with depression in any study following Brown and his colleagues'. Both unemployment and lack of a confiding relationship with a partner appear to be significant only in some depressed populations compared with normal control populations. Since neither of these two factors can be viewed as independent of depression, however, their role cannot be assumed to be causal, but rather may be considered interactive. Evidence concerning the role of the fourth vulnerability factor, parental loss in childhood, is inconsistent. Although this factor has long and widely been viewed as a predisposing factor in depression (Freud, 1917; Bowlby, 1969), several recent reviews of the literature have concluded that parental death during childhood has yet to be established as an etiologic factor in adult depression (Crook and Eliot, 1980; Lloyd, 1980a; Orvaschel et al., 1980; Tennant et al., 1980). These conclusions are further supported by the mixed results of the studies discussed here.

DISCUSSION

The following conclusions may be drawn concerning the four approaches to the nature of the relationship between psychosocial factors and depression.

The *predisposition approach* proposes that psychosocial factors are antecedent to and etiologic in depression and, on the basis of the current literature, certain psychosocial factors do appear to precede clinical depression. Predisposing personality characteristics include poor sociability (introversion) and modest emotional instability (general neuroticism). Precipitating or predisposing life events include interpersonal losses, severely threatening events, and long-term difficulties. The social background factors of childhood bereavement and lack of a confiding heterosexual relationship also appear influential.

Psychosocial factors also differentiate among affective subtypes. Bipolar patients have relatively normal intermorbid personalities. Nonbipolar melancholic patients are somewhat introverted, but are otherwise normal. Other primary major depressive disorder patients (nonmelancholic nonbipolar) are introverted as well, but they also show modest emotional instability, and secondary major depressives (with premorbid characterological conditions) show even more emotional instability. Life events, however, do not appear to differentiate between bipolars and major depressives or between melancholic or psychotic and nonmelancholic subtypes. To date, the role of social factors within depressive subtypes has not been investigated.

Regarding the *subclinical approach*, the evidence suggests that subclinical manifestations of depression do run in families, supporting the theory of a genetic spectrum of affective disorders. To test this issue definitively, however, substantially more research is needed. Life events and social factors can be fit into the subclinical framework only by invoking personality as a mediating factor. That is, an individual's response to adverse life events and circumstances and the nature of his or her social environment would be hypothesized to represent factors which are constitutionally determined. No research has been conducted to test this hypothesis.

Pathoplasty, the symptom picture and outcome of a depressive episode, appears to be influenced by personality characteristics, in particular by premorbid level of neuroticism. In addition, some evidence has been offered to suggest that treatment response may be influenced by concurrent life events. No researchers have investigated the role of social factors in the course or symptom picture of depression.

To date, the prospective research necessary to test the hypotheses of the *deterioration approach* has not been carried out.

CLOSING REMARKS

At first glance, it is surprising how many questions remain on the relationship between psychosocial factors and depression. A careful review of the research literature nonetheless does reveal remarkable consistency in many areas, as well as the significant methodological problems which hamper further progress. The authors believe that the time is now propitious to undertake more definitive studies to resolve the most salient questions in this area. Findings to date must be replicated in carefully controlled studies, and tools now exist to overcome methodological obstacles.

The first type of study to launch is the family study that will test the subclinical approach. Families of carefully diagnosed patients with several types of affective disorders, along with appropriate control groups, should be evaluated independently and blindly in terms of psychopathology, personality, and other psychosocial factors. Biological trait variables should also be included. Such an approach, in concert with adoption studies, can resolve the spectrum question as it relates to affective disorders and subsequently lead to a better understanding of the etiology of at least some types of affective disorders.

The second type of study needed is a longitudinal and prospective follow-up of psychosocial factors in populations at high risk for affective disorders. Only this approach will allow truly premorbid assessments of psychosocial factors, which is essential to definitive resolution. Such an approach will also allow an examination of the interaction of psychosocial variables and depression. As with so many other areas of research, we will probably find that aspects of all of the hypothetical approaches to psychosocial factors and depression have some validity, especially if viewed from a dynamic perspective. Personality and social factors, for example, may well predispose a person to a depression. But the depression itself may lead to changes in the family unit, employment, and social networks, and this in turn may increase the likelihood of a recurrence. A longitudinal and prospective study would enable us to separate the individual effects and the interactive effects of these factors over time.

Chapter 24

The Epidemiology of Affective Disorders: Rates and Risk Factors[†]
by Myrna M. Weissman, Ph.D. and
Jeffrey H. Boyd, M.D., M.P.H.

INTRODUCTION

Epidemiology is the study of variations in the distribution of specific disorders in populations and the factors that influence that distribution. Epidemiologic studies can generate three types of information about a disorder: (1) rates (prevalence and incidence); (2) variations in these rates by person, time, and place; and (3) identification of risk factors which increase the probability of developing the disorder. Such information can potentially generate new ideas about etiology, pathogenesis, treatment, and prevention and can also yield insights that will improve practice and planning for care. In recent decades the scope of epidemiology expanded markedly from its origins in the study of infectious disease to include studies of chronic conditions such as heart disease, stroke, and cancer (MacMahon and Pugh, 1970). More recently, the scope of chronic disease epidemiology also has expanded to include psychiatric disorders, particularly the affective disorders (Silverman, 1968; Weissman and Klerman, 1978).

Because of the high prevalence and morbidity of affective disorders, as well as the increase in effective treatments, there has been considerable interest in their epidemiology. Reviews of the epidemiology of depression are nearly as common as the studies on which they are based (Bebbington, 1978; Boyd and Weissman, 1981; Hirschfeld and Cross, 1982; Klerman and Barrett, 1973; Krauthammer and Klerman, 1979; Perris, 1966; Silverman, 1968; Turns, 1978). All reviews acknowledge and reflect the problem of case definition. Many variations in rates and findings between studies may be accounted for by diagnostic differences.

In this chapter, the authors describe the current state of information on the epidemiology of affective disorders, focusing on rates and risk factors. The discussion is confined to available data, primarily from population surveys published in the English language, and the authors have divided the affective disorders into three groups—depressive symptoms, bipolar disorder, and nonbipolar (major) depression.

Historical Trends in Diagnoses

The study of the epidemiology of depression has been hindered by major differences in diagnostic classification over time, between coun-

[†]The research reported in this chapter was supported in part by Alcohol, Drug Abuse, and Mental Health Administration Grant No. MH 34224, "Epidemiologic Catchment Area Program," from the NIMH Center for Epidemiologic Studies and by the Yale Mental Health Clinical Research Center NIMH Grant No. MH 30929.

Permission has been granted to reproduce portions of the chapter from:

Boyd J.H., Weissman M.M.: The epidemiology of affective disorders: a reexamination and future directions. Arch. Gen. Psychiatry 38:1039–1046, 1981.

Boyd J.H., Weissman M.M.: Epidemiology, in Handbook of Affective Disorders. Edited by Paykel E.S. Edinburgh, Churchill-Livingstone, 1982.

Weissman M.M., Boyd J.H.: Epidemiology of affective illness, in The Neurobiology of Mood Disorders. Edited by Post R.M., Ballenger J.C. Baltimore, Williams & Wilkins, in press.

tries, and among investigators and clinicians within countries. The same terms have different meanings in different diagnostic schemes, and different terms have similar meanings in different diagnostic schemes (Klerman, 1980).

The cross-cultural conceptual differences in psychiatric diagnoses were highlighted by the United States-United Kingdom Collaborative Study in the late 1960s. The purpose of this study was to understand why the prevalence of schizophrenia was greater in the United States than in England, while the reverse was true for manic-depressive disorder (Chodoff, 1972; Klerman and Barrett, 1973; Kramer, 1969; Zubin, 1969). In their studies of patients in treatment, the investigators found that patients with similar symptoms were given different diagnoses in the two countries.

In addition to the conceptual and theoretical differences between diagnostic systems, there has been unreliability within the diagnostic systems. This unreliability stemmed from imprecise definitions of the diagnostic terms and nonstandardized methods of collecting data on signs and symptoms (Spitzer et al., 1975). In order to avoid diagnostic unreliability, United States psychiatric epidemiologists avoided diagnoses following World War II (Weissman and Klerman, 1978). Community surveys in the United States during this period were based on a unitary view of mental disorders that did not differentiate specific psychiatric disorders from overall psychological malaise. Mental illness was seen as a continuum, and diagnostic groups were considered to be quantitatively different manifestations of the same causes of mental malfunctioning. It was presumed that social factors such as migration, poverty, stress, and urbanization underlay the malfunctioning.

United States investigators during this era used overall impairment scales which were independent of diagnoses, and this made surveys easier to administer. Furthermore, the scales did not require highly trained personnel to administer them. Above all, the problem of the unreliability in psychiatric diagnoses was avoided. Unfortunately, the data from these United States studies could not be related to clinical psychiatry and the emerging developments in psychiatric genetics, neurobiology, and psychopharmacology. Quite simply, it was unclear what the relationship was between a high impairment score and clinical depression, schizophrenia, phobias, and so forth.

The European and Scandinavian tradition, by contrast, has been heavily influenced by Kraepelin (1921). Epidemiologic studies in this tradition made the underlying assumption that there were distinct psychiatric entities. However, the Kraepelinian taxonomic system gave rise to difficulties in classifying the depressive disorders. Following Kraepelin's delineation of manic-depressive insanity as a diagnostic entity, debate arose over the breadth of the concept and the definition of additional diagnostic labels such as neurotic depressive reaction, psychogenic depression, endogenous depression, psychotic depression, and involutional melancholia. The Kraepelinian classification of manic-depressive psychosis was particularly difficult to apply in outpatient or community settings, where most of the people suffering from depressions were not psychotic. The discrepancy between American and European concepts of a case and the unreliability of diagnoses made it difficult to interpret or to compare the findings of different epidemiologic surveys.

Standardized Diagnostic Procedures

In order to obtain reliable data that can be used comparatively among studies, cross-culturally, and over time, rules of case definition must be laid down, and a standardized examination procedure must be undertaken. Such advances in psychiatric diagnosis have taken place and are being applied in epidemiologic studies.

THE UNITED STATES EXPERIENCE In 1972 the Washington University Department of Psychiatry in Saint Louis, Missouri, published precise criteria for diagnosing 15 major disorders (Feighner et al., 1972) and developed a structured interview, the Renard Diagnostic Interview, for obtaining information sufficient for applying the criteria (Robins et al., 1977). Spitzer et al. modified and elaborated these criteria and published specific criteria for making 25 psychiatric diagnoses, and they called them the Research Diagnostic Criteria (RDC) (Spitzer et al., 1978a; 1978b; Endicott and Spitzer, 1979). The RDC focuses on episodes of illness, past or present, and provides inclusion and exclusion criteria which facilitate diagnosing and studying homogeneous groups of patients. The RDC is supplemented by a structured interview called the Schedule for Affective Disorders and Schizophrenia (SADS), which elicits information on signs and symptoms and their duration (Spitzer et al., 1978c). It has since been shown that using the SADS and the RDC greatly improves diagnostic reliability. DSM-III was based on this approach (American Psychiatric Association, 1980). The SADS-RDC has been applied to a community sample in New Haven, Connecticut, to obtain rates of specific psychiatric disorders which include both treated and untreated cases (Weissman and Myers, 1978a; 1978b).

Robins et al. (1981) recently refined the Renard Diagnostic Interview and the SADS interview to be used specifically by lay interviewers in large-scale epidemiologic surveys in the United States. This interview, the National Institute of Mental Health (NIMH) Diagnostic Interview Schedule (DIS), is highly structured, thus reducing the need for judgments by clinically trained interviewers. Computer diagnoses based on the RDC, the Feighner criteria, and some of the DSM-III diagnoses can be generated from the results. The DIS is now being used in major epidemiologic studies of the Epidemiologic Catchment Area (ECA) Program in five centers located in Connecticut, Missouri, Maryland, North Carolina, and California (Eaton et al., 1981). The first ECA study went into the field in 1981, and over the next five years the five centers will generate data on more than 15,000 subjects.

THE UNITED KINGDOM EXPERIENCE A parallel development in psychiatric diagnosis has occurred in England. Wing and his collaborators developed the Present State Exam (PSE), which applies standardized techniques of defining, eliciting, and recording symptoms with a reasonably high degree of reliability (Wing et al., 1978; Orley et al., 1979). The PSE includes 140 items which are either observations made by the interviewer during the interview or symptoms reported by the patient for the preceding four-week period. A computer diagnosis (CATEGO Class) can be generated from the results. According to Wing, when classificatory rules embodying the hierarchical principles commonly used in clinical diagnosis are specified precisely enough to be incorporated in a computer program (CATEGO) and applied to the symptom ratings, the resulting broad categories agree very well with the diagnoses made by clinicians (Wing et al., 1978).

Wing et al. (1978) point out that in outpatient psychiatric work and in community surveys one constantly faces the problem of where to establish the threshold for a diagnosis. Above this threshold, one has some assurance that one has a "case" and can legitimately make a diagnosis; below it, one has no such assurance. The threshold is defined by an Index of Definition (ID), which is a scale (0 to 8) measuring the degree of likelihood that there are sufficient components of key syndromes present to allow classification (Wing et al., 1978). Any person with an ID score of 5 or more is considered with reasonable assurance to be a "case" for whom a diagnostic classification is appropriate.

The CATEGO system of diagnosis is related to the official nomenclature of the ICD-9 (the International Classification of Diseases, ninth edition). It has been used to make diagnoses in four epidemiologic community surveys, in the Camberwell section of London, in the Outer Hebrides, in two African villages, and in Canberra, Australia (Brown et al., 1977; Duncan-Jones and Henderson, 1978; Orley et al., 1979).

There have been almost no studies comparing the American and British systems of diagnosis. One study suggests that the two approaches might lead to quite different findings when applied in an epidemiologic survey. In a survey of the general population, Wing et al. (1978) identified 22 persons with depressive disorder by PSE-ID-CATEGO criteria. When the Feighner criteria were applied to these 22 persons, however, only one person was found to have definite depressive disorder, and two had probable depression. The Feighner criteria appear to define either a much smaller group of depressives in the general population than the PSE-ID-CATEGO or a different group of depressives. The Alcohol, Drug Abuse, and Mental Health Administration in the United States, in collaboration with the World Health Organization, is now launching an effort to understand and to test empirically the differences between European and American diagnostic schemes.

Depressive Symptoms, Nonbipolar Depression, and Bipolar Disorder: Rationale

Most diagnostic systems agree that the affective disorders refer to a group of psychiatric conditions in which disturbances of mood predominate and that depression and elation are the major affective disorders. But they do not agree on what affects should be included and how much weight should be given to symptom patterns, precipitants, severity, or chronology. In order to avoid the debates about how to subclassify, for the purposes of this discussion the authors have divided the epidemiologic data on affective disorders into three parts: depressive symptoms, nonbipolar depression, and bipolar disorder.* This division is admittedly unorthodox, but it reflects areas

*Preceptor's note: In several of the chapters in this Part, approaches to subclassification are reviewed. In the last section of his chapter, the Preceptor discusses Winokur's schema, as well as the evidence for distinguishing primary and secondary depressions. Gershon presents some of the genetic evidence, and Schildkraut and his colleagues demonstrate the contributions of neuropsychopharmacological and neuropsychoendocrinological data in the identification of depressive subtypes. In Part IV, Akiskal describes the concept of a spectrum of affective disorders with a wide variety of subtypes within both the depressive and the bipolar disorders.

of international agreement in diagnostic systems. Most agree that some people have depressive symptoms that are not of sufficient intensity to warrant a clinical diagnosis or that appear in a variety of disorders. There is also some agreement that bipolar disorder (defined by one or more episodes of mania) is a distinct diagnostic entity. However, those with clinical depression who are not bipolar constitute a heterogeneous group. There is considerable international disagreement about how to define or subdivide this latter group, who are the majority of depressives. Therefore, the authors have aggregated these depressives into the category of nonbipolar depression.

Any attempt to translate these diagnostic distinctions directly into the terms of DSM-III will be imprecise. Roughly, though, bipolar disorder would most closely conform to the DSM-III classification Bipolar Disorder (Mixed, Manic, or Depressed type) or to Atypical Bipolar Disorder. Nonbipolar depression would include DSM-III Major Depression (Single Episode or Recurrent), Cyclothymic Disorder, Dysthymic Disorder, Atypical Depression, or Adjustment Disorder with Depressed Mood. The depressive symptoms category could include any of those symptoms common to the DSM-III Affective Disorders or other psychiatric and physical disorders which have symptoms that overlap with depression, as well as states of dysphoria and demoralization not sufficiently persistent or severe to meet any diagnostic criteria.

All of the epidemiologic studies discussed here except the NIMH ECA study were completed prior to the publication of DSM-III. The preliminary results of the ECA study will be described, but most of the data discussed are based on a variety of diagnostic schemes, usually DSM-II, ICD versions 7 through 9, and in a few cases the RDC. In order to compare more recent United States data based on the RDC and DSM-III with both the older United States data based on DSM-II and the European data based on the ICD, the authors have recalculated the data from the older and the European studies where possible. As much as possible, persons with bipolar disorder are assigned to that category, and the remaining persons are aggregated into the nonbipolar category; as noted, the nonbipolar category ignores the heterogeneity of nonbipolar depressions and the debate about how to subdivide them.

Definitions of Epidemiologic Terms

Before reviewing the epidemiologic findings in the three categories chosen for discussion, some definitions of basic epidemiologic terms are in order. *Point prevalence* is defined as that proportion of the population which has the disorder being studied at a given point in time. *Morbid risk* is the individual's lifetime risk of having a first episode of illness. For nonbipolar depression, the period of risk lasts as long as a person is alive, so some difficulty arises in using the term morbid risk for nonbipolar depression. For bipolar disorders the period of risk for a first attack probably ends by age 60, so the term morbid risk is meaningful there. *Incidence* is the number of new cases of a disorder occurring in the population per year. A *risk factor* is an epidemiologic concept for a condition which increases the likelihood of a person developing the disorder under study.

Definition

Feelings of sadness and disappointment are part of the human condition. All people experience them at some point in their lives, whether or not they are clinically depressed. The boundary between normal mood and abnormal symptoms remains undefined. Usually symptoms that are intense, pervasive, and persistent and that interfere with a person's ordinary functioning are considered pathological. But an incompletely defined gradient exists between normal mood and the clinical state.

In recent years considerable psychometric research has focused on developing rating scales for measuring depressive symptoms. Self-report scales are attractive because they are economical and easy to administer in community surveys. Normative data have been collected for several standard self-report scales which measure depressive symptoms, and cutoff points have been identified to distinguish normal mood from clinical states.

It is unclear what may be the clinical significance of depressive symptoms (i.e., whether they are prodromal of a depressive syndrome) and what therapeutic interventions they may warrant. Recent epidemiologic studies indicate that although many persons in the community are sad and have depressive symptoms, scoring high on a depressive symptom scale does not correlate strongly with meeting the criteria for a major depression according to the RDC or DSM-III (Myers and Weissman, 1980). One recent study found that many clinically depressed persons were missed by the self-report scale (a false-negative rate of 36 percent) and that some persons who were not clinically depressed scored high on depressive symptoms (a false-positive rate of 6 percent). Many of the misclassified subjects were persons with no psychiatric disorders or persons with psychiatric disorders other than depression.

Point Prevalence

Table 1 shows the point prevalence of depressive symptoms as determined by self-report questionnaires in nine community studies conducted between 1957 and 1979 in the United States and England. These findings show some consistency in that the point prevalence of depressive symptoms ranges from 13 to 20 percent of the total population.

Risk Factors

SEX In a comprehensive review of studies of depression, covering more than thirty countries and a period of forty years, one of the authors and Klerman found that almost all studies showed depression and depressive symptoms to be more common in women than in men (Weissman and Klerman, 1977). Although the authors reached no conclusions, they offered several categories of reasons for the difference. Women may be more vocal about their depressions (artifactual reasons). Hormones and childbirth may influence depression (biological reasons). Contemporary women's lives may subject them to circumstances that cause depression (social reasons). Finally, women's

Table 1. Point Prevalence Rates for Depressive Symptoms

Source	Location	Rates per 100		
		Men	Women	Total[1]
Husaini et al. (1979)	Tennessee, USA	—	—	13
Weissman and Myers (1978b[2])	New Haven, CT, USA	12	20	16
Weissman and Myers (1978b[3])	New Haven, CT, USA	16	20	18
Comstock and Helsing (1976)	Missouri, USA	16	22	20
Comstock and Helsing (1976)	Maryland, USA	12	21	17
Blumenthal (1975)	Pennsylvania, Indiana, Kentucky, and Michigan, USA	12	32	—
Mellinger et al. (1974)	USA	19	34	—
Warheit et al. (1973)	Florida, USA	13	24	—
Martin et al. (1957)	London, England	10	24	17

[1]Totals do not represent sums but overall rates. Sample sizes for men and women varied within studies, and three studies reported no overall rate. One study did not report separate rates for men and women.
[2]1969 survey
[3]1967 survey

early training may teach them to be helpless, and they may thus be less able to master stress (psychological reasons).

AGE Findings on the relationship between age and depressive symptoms have been inconsistent and have been different for the two sexes. Weissman and Myers (1978b) found that the rates of moderate depression were higher in younger women and tended to decrease with age. The opposite pattern was found for men, where the prevalence of depressive symptoms was lower in young men and increased with age. These findings are consistent with those of Mellinger et al. (1974). On the other hand, Martin et al. (1957) found that women had an increase of depressive symptoms up to the age of 65 and a decrease thereafter and found no age trend for men. Leighton et al. (1963) noted an increase with age up to 70 and then a decrease in both sexes. Blumenthal (1975) found no variation with age, and Comstock and Helsing (1976) found a decrease with age after adjustments for other variables were made.

There is no increase in depressive symptoms during the involutional period in women (Hällström, 1973). This finding in several studies has led researchers to discard involutional depression as a real entity (Weissman and Klerman, 1977; Weissman, 1979; Winokur, 1973a).

SOCIAL CLASS A number of studies have found that social class is inversely related to depressive symptoms (Blumenthal, 1975; Comstock and Helsing, 1976; Mellinger et al., 1974; Weissman and Myers, 1978b). Hällström (1973), however, in his study of Swedish women aged 38 to 54, did not find an association between depressive symptoms and social group, income, or education. The lack of association in the Swedish study may be related to the greater homogeneity of social class and income levels in that country.

RACE Several studies have found an increased risk for depressive symptoms in nonwhite subjects (Mellinger et al., 1974; Warheit et al., 1973; Weissman and Myers, 1978b). However, when sex and social class have been controlled, the differences in rates between the races have disappeared (Comstock and Helsing, 1976).

MARITAL STATUS Many studies have found an increased rate of depressive symptoms in people who are divorced and separated (Blumenthal, 1975; Comstock and Helsing, 1976; Mellinger et al., 1974; Weissman and Myers, 1978b). Hällström (1973), however, found that single women had lower rates than single men. Similarly, Radloff (1975) noted that the prevalence of depressive symptoms and marital status should be considered separately by sex, since she found that increased risk for depressive symptoms was largely accounted for by married women and single men.

URBAN VS. RURAL RESIDENCE According to the review by Hirschfeld and Cross (1982), limited data are available to assess rural-urban differences in depressive symptoms, since few epidemiologic surveys have included both rural and urban samples in their study designs. While levels of psychiatric impairment in general have been found to be substantially higher in urban settings, such differences tend to hold only for neurosis and personality disorders. Comstock and Helsing (1976) compared rural and urban populations and found no significant difference in the rates.

LIFE EVENTS The relationship between life events (defined as changes in a person's social milieu) and depressive symptoms has been well reviewed by Hirschfeld and Cross (1982). They note a positive relationship between life events and the development of depressive symptoms based on two large-scale community surveys. In a study of depressive symptoms in the community, Warheit et al. (1973) found a positive relationship between the level of depressive symptoms and the number of life events experienced in the months prior to the interview.

Ilfeld (1977) investigated the relationship between depressive symptoms and current social stressors (defined as problematic or undesirable stressors in marriage, parenting, work, or neighborhood). In a sample of more than 2,000 Chicago-area residents, he found that the level of depressive symptoms was strongly related to the number and level of current social stressors experienced. Marital stressors had the highest correlation with symptoms, followed by parental stressors for women and job stressors for men. Taken together, the five categories of stressors accounted for more than 25 percent of the variance in the level of depressive symptoms, while demographic characteristics (i.e., sex, age, marital status, and income) accounted for only 8 percent.

PERSONAL RESOURCES AND SOCIAL SUPPORT Hirschfeld and Cross (1982) have also examined the role of personal resources, the current interpersonal and extrinsic factors such as family ties and relationships with significant others that can serve as support systems in times of crisis. They cite the Brown et al. (1977) study which found that a confiding relationship was a significant mediator in the impact of life events for a sample of women in the community. Women who enjoyed a close relationship with a significant other were less likely to report high levels of depressive symptoms in the face of high numbers of life events than were women with many life events without such a relationship. Similarly, Paykel et al. (1980) studied factors contributing to clinical depression in community women attending postnatal clinics within six to eight weeks postpartum. They found that poor marital support contributed to the onset of depression, but only in the presence of stressful life events.

The finding that marriage per se serves a protective role in moderating the influence of life events is reinforced in studies of the sociodemographic characteristics of depressives as well. These studies report higher rates of depression among the unmarried.

An independent contribution of personal resources to depressive symptoms also has been demonstrated. Warheit et al. (1973) reported that low socioeconomic status, absence of a spouse, and the absence of friends correlated with high loss scores and high depression scores.

Summary: Epidemiology of Depressive Symptoms

Depressive symptoms have been found to have a point prevalence which ranges between 13 percent and 20 percent of the population. The factors which increase the risk of depressive symptoms are being a young woman or an older man, being of lower socioeconomic class, being divorced or separated, experiencing an increase in life events, particularly marital stress, and having fewer personal resources and social supports.

NONBIPOLAR DEPRESSION

Definition

Patients with depression are often given diagnoses such as neurotic depression, reactive depression, endogenous depression, involutional depression, psychogenic depression, psychotic depression, unipolar depression, the depressed type of manic-depressive illness, and depression not otherwise specified. As noted, however, no international agreement currently exists about which of these subclassifications of depression are meaningful. Many of these terms mean different things to different researchers or clinicians within countries, and many have different meanings in one country versus another. For example, the term *unipolar depression* is sometimes assumed to mean any depression (including neurotic depression) that is not bipolar disorder. At other times, unipolar depression is assumed to mean only psychotic depression or recurrent depression. The authors have collected all these subdivisions of depression into one group called nonbipolar depression.

Point Prevalence

Table 2 gives the point prevalence rates of nonbipolar depression from 25 studies, most of which are community surveys. Studies based on hospitalization have been omitted since only a small fraction of nonbipolar depressives are hospitalized. Studies of period prevalence were also omitted unless point prevalence could be estimated from them.

The first 15 studies in Table 2 present data on the full range of nonbipolar depression based on various diagnostic methods. These studies show that the point prevalence of nonbipolar depression in industralized countries is between 1.8 and 3.2 cases per 100 for men and between 2.0 and 9.3 cases per 100 for women. The highest rates are reported in Africa: 14.3 for men and 22.6 for women.

The next two studies in Table 2 are limited to the study of psychotic depression. Pederson et al. (1972) defined psychotic depression loosely as severe depression and found prevalence rates of 2.6 per 100 for men and 5.0 per 100 for women. The study by Mayer-Gross (1948), conducted in 1943, found considerably lower rates for psychotic depression, but since the study obtained information from records and key informants, underreporting may have occurred.

The remaining eight studies in Table 2 were limited to the study of manic-depressive illness and included patients who are bipolar along with those who were nonbipolar. However, this classification probably included only the more severe depressives, and the prevalence rates were usually less than 1 percent.

As can be seen, only the first six studies used the newer research diagnostic techniques. If the analysis is limited to studies in industrialized nations that used the new diagnostic techniques, the findings among different studies are somewhat convergent. The point prevalence is 2.3 to 3.2 per 100 for males and 4.5 to 9.3 per 100 for females.

Incidence

Since incidence is the number of new cases of a disorder over a period of time (usually one year), its measurement requires a longitudinal study design. Table 3 gives incidence data from 17 studies.

The first two studies were longitudinal and were based on interviews of a sample of persons who had not had a depression at the outset of the study. The goal was to determine how many new depressions would develop over time. These studies yield an incidence of nonbipolar depression between 247 and 598 per 100,000 per year for women and between 82 and 201 for men. There are difficulties in interpreting these data. The first study, by Essen-Möller and Hagnell (1961), consisted of interviews of a cohort of people who were then interviewed again ten years later. People tend to forget depressions that they have had in the past, and over such a long time span considerable amnesia is probable. Essen-Möller and Hagnell (1961) may have therefore underestimated the incidence of depression.

The next nine studies in Table 3 were based on case registries and included persons with depression who entered some form of treatment for the first time. Between 130 and 201 per 100,000 men per year were found to enter treatment for depression for the first time. For women the figure was between 320 and 500 per 100,000 per year. However, these studies probably underreported incidence since only 20 to 25 percent of people with nonbipolar depression ever get treated for

Table 2. Point Prevalence Rates for Nonbipolar Depression

Source	Location	Diagnostic Criteria[1]	Rates per 100		
			Men	Women	Total[2]
Full Range of Nonbipolar Depression:					
Weissman et al. (1982)	New Haven, CT, USA	DSM-III (DIS)	2.3	5.1	3.9
Weissman and Myers (1978a)	New Haven, CT, USA	RDC (SADS)	3.2	5.2	4.3
Wing et al. (1978)	Camberwell Section, London, England	ICD-9 (PSE)	—	9.3	—
Duncan-Jones and Henderson (1978)	Canberra, Australia	ICD-9 (PSE)	—	—	10.8
Brown et al. (1977)	Outer Hebrides, Scotland	ICD-9 (PSE)	—	4.5	4.5
Orley et al. (1979)	Ugandan Villages, Africa	ICD-9 (PSE)	14.3	22.6	—
Nielsen and Nielsen (1969)	Samsø Island, Denmark	Unspecified	—	—	0.95
Thacore et al. (1975)	Northern India	DSM-II	—	—	1.16
Bash and Bash-Liechti (1974)	Shiraz, Iran	ICD-8	—	—	1.07
Bash and Bash-Liechti (1969)	Khuzestran, Iran	Unspecified	1.0	1.0	—
Hällström (1973)	Gothenburg, Sweden	Unspecified	—	7.8[3]	—
Sørensen and Strömgren (1961)	Samsø Island, Denmark	Unspecified	1.8	6.3	3.9
Helgason (1961)	Iceland	Unspecified	2.7	4.9	3.8
Essen-Möller and Hagnell (1961)	Two Swedish Parishes	Unspecified	1.8	2.0	—
Roth and Luton (1943)	Tennessee, USA	Unspecified	—	—	4.7

Psychotic Depression only:

Study	Location	Method			
Pederson et al. (1972)	Monroe County, NY, USA	DSM-I	2.6	5.0	3.7
Mayer-Gross (1948)	Dumfries, Scotland	Unspecified	—	—	0.35

Manic-Depressive Illness only:

Study	Location	Method			
Nielsen (1976)	Samsø Island, Denmark	ICD-7	1.04	1.60	1.31
Katsrup et al. (1976)	Aarhus, Denmark	ICD-8	0.05	0.08	—
Katsrup et al. (1976)	Randers, Denmark	ICD-8	0.04	0.15	—
Dube and Kumar (1973)	Uttar Pradesh, India	Unspecified	0.1	0.15	—
Crocetti et al. (1971)	Croatia, Yugoslavia	ICD-7	—	—	0.42
Kulcar et al. (1971)	Croatia, Yugoslavia	ICD-7	—	—	0.06–0.24
Watts et al. (1964)	England and Wales	Unspecified	—	—	0.19
Watts et al. (1964)	Scotland	Unspecified	—	—	0.18

[1]Interview method shown in parentheses where applicable

[2]Totals do not represent sums but overall rates. Sample sizes for men and women varied within studies, and some studies reported no overall rate. In many other studies, the authors did not report separate rates for men and women.

[3]Hällström's "disability grades" 2–4

Table 3. Incidence Rates for Nonbipolar Depression[1]

Source	Location	Rates per 100,000 per Year		
		Men	Women	Total[2]
Longitudinal Studies:				
Essen-Möller and Hagnell (1961)	Southern Sweden	82	247	162
Hällström (1973)	Gothenburg, Sweden	—	598[3]	—
Case Registries:				
Nielsen and Nielsen (1979)	Samsø Island, Denmark	—	—	519
Helgason (1977)	Iceland	—	—	110[4]
Bebbington (1978)	Camberwell, England	201	381	295
Bebbington (1978)	Salford, England	156	320	240
grad de Alarcón et al. (1975)	Chichester, England	—	—	350
grad de Alarcón et al. (1975)	Salisbury, England	—	—	246
Nielsen and Nielsen (1979)	Aarhus County, Denmark	—	—	204
Weeke et al. (1975)	Aarhus County, Denmark	130	330	—
Juel-Nielsen et al. (1961)	Aarhus County, Denmark	200	500	350

Psychotic Depression:				
Pederson et al. (1972)	Monroe County, NY, USA	27	37	—
Adelstein et al. (1968)	Salford, England	65	123	97
Manic-Depressive Illness:				
Krauthammer and Klerman (1979)	Review of 8 studies from USA, UK, and Scandinavia	—	—	10–150
Nonbipolar Depressives among those with Manic Depression:				
Johannes Nielsen, (personal communication, 1979)	Samsø Island, Denmark	127	209	169
Tomas Helgason, (personal communication, 1979)[5]	Iceland	55	152	—
Anita Weeke, (personal communication, 1979)	Aarhus County, Denmark	59	82	—

[1]Studies limited to hospitalized cases are not included.
[2]Totals do not represent sums but overall rates. Sample sizes for men and women varied, and some studies reported no overall rate. In a number of other studies, the authors did not report separate rates for men and women.
[3]Data for disability grade 3, meaning unable to work
[4]Data include affective and reactive depressive psychoses.
[5]Data from Larus Helgason

their depressions (Juel-Nielsen et al., 1961; Klerman and Barrett, 1973; Lehmann, 1971; Weissman et al., 1982).

The last three sections of Table 3 show the results of six studies on the incidence of selected subclassifications of nonbipolar depression, including psychotic depression, manic-depressive illness, and the depressed subtype of manic-depressive illness. The incidence rates here are somewhat lower, with rates ranging from 27 to 209 per 100,000 per year.

Risk Factors

SEX In almost all studies of depression in industrialized countries, roughly twice as many women as men are found to become depressed (see Tables 2 and 3). Weissman and Klerman (1977) reviewed the literature on the preponderance of women in studies of depression and arrived at the conclusion that the sex difference is real and is not an artifact of help-seeking behavior or reporting bias. Although women do seek treatment more readily than men, women also predominate in community studies where help-seeking behavior is not a source of bias.

AGE A number of studies are in agreement that the incidence and prevalence rates of depression in women reach a peak at the age range of 35 to 45 years (Essen-Möller and Hagnell, 1961; grad de Alarcón et al., 1975; Weissman and Myers, 1978a). There may also be an increase for women over the age of 55. The pattern for men is less evident, but it appears that the rates for men increase with age.

MENOPAUSE Although the incidence and prevalence of nonbipolar depression are high for women aged 35 to 45 years, they show no tendency to rise in the menopausal years. In fact, the rates tend to fall during those years. Recent research has suggested that menopause does not predispose to depression and that depression occurring in the menopausal period is not a distinct entity in terms of symptom patterns, severity, or absence of precipitants (Weissman, 1979; Weissman and Klerman, 1977; Winokur, 1973a). Hällström (1973) reported a very careful study which demonstrated that the incidence of depression does not increase in the menopausal years.

SOCIAL CLASS There is no particular pattern to the distribution of nonbipolar depression across various socioeconomic classes (Weissman and Myers, 1978a). This lack of association between the rates of nonbipolar depression and social class contrasts with the findings for depressive symptoms, which are found more often in the lower social classes. It also contrasts with the findings for bipolar disorder, which apparently occurs slightly more often in the higher social classes.

RACE Silverman (1968) reported on seven studies which showed that treatment for depression is less common among blacks than whites. However, prevalence rates should not be based solely on treated cases. These findings were biased by the fact that treatment facilities were less accessible to blacks than to whites. In fact, one study showed that when hospitals became integrated in the United States, the rates of treatment for depression rose substantially among blacks.

FAMILY HISTORY A family history of depression or alcoholism increases the risk for depression. For example, in a follow-up of the

"Iowa 500" study, interviewers who were blind to the probands' diagnosis contacted the first-degree relatives of unipolar depressives and relatives of controls. A 9.4 percent rate of depression was found among the relatives of depressed patients, compared with a 4.5 percent rate of depression among the relatives of controls (p < .05) (Winokur, 1979; Winokur and Morrison, 1973).

Whether this familial concentration of depression should be attributed to genetic, cultural, or environmental transmission of the disorder is in question. The evidence for genetic transmission is less clear for nonbipolar depression than for bipolar disorder (Kidd and Weissman, 1978). At the present time, we cannot say what sort of interaction takes place between genotype and environment in the etiology of nonbipolar depression.

CHILDHOOD EXPERIENCES   The relationship of early parental death to subsequent depression is controversial. A review by Orvaschel et al. (1980) concluded that when studies are carefully controlled no relationship is found. On the other hand, Brown and Harris (1978) found that parental loss before age 11 is a risk factor for subsequent depression. There is evidence that a disruptive, hostile, and generally negative environment in a child's home constitutes a risk factor for depression. Case-control studies have found such a home environment more frequently in the backgrounds of depressed adults than in the backgrounds of the control group (Orvaschel et al., 1980).

PERSONALITY ATTRIBUTES   Personality as a risk factor for depression has been a subject of considerable interest to clinicians and psychotherapists. Hirschfeld and Klerman (1979) reported a study of the personality profiles of 73 depressed patients. Diagnoses were based on SADS-RDC criteria, and the patients were studied after recovery from their depression. The results suggested that persons who develop depression have the following personality characteristics: likelihood to break down under stress, lack of energy, insecurity, introversion and sensitivity, tendency to worry, lack of social adroitness, unassertiveness, dependency, and obsessionality. While such a profile is generally consistent with the literature from psychoanalytic, cognitive, and behavioral schools about the personality attributes of depressives (Chodoff, 1972; Hirschfeld and Klerman, 1979), this work requires replication before it can be accepted. Moreover, future research in this area must separate the cause from the consequence of depression by studying persons prior to their first episode of the disorder.

RECENT LIFE EVENTS   In general, studies have shown that many (but not all) depressed patients, as compared with a normal control sample, tend to have an excess of negative life events prior to the onset of a depressive episode. However, the precise magnitude of the effect of life events is unclear (Bebbington, 1978; Brown and Harris, 1978).

ABSENCE OF AN INTIMATE CONFIDING RELATIONSHIP
The absence of a satisfying intimate heterosexual relationship has been shown to be a risk factor for depression. In a study of women in the Camberwell section of London, Brown and Harris (1978) examined social factors predisposing women to depression, as defined by the PSE. They found that if a woman does not have an intimate tie, someone

she can trust and confide in, particularly a husband or boyfriend, she is four times as likely to break down in the presence of a severe event or major difficulty (Brown and Harris, 1978). Brown and his colleagues also found that a lack of employment and the presence of young children in the home are risk factors for depression.*

POSTPARTUM PERIOD In the postpartum period, significant hormonal changes occur, and depressive mood changes are commonly reported. Transient emotional disturbances in the first weeks following delivery, the "new-baby blues," occur with such frequency as to be considered normal, and they generally resolve without treatment. However, there is overwhelming evidence that the period up to six months postpartum also carries an excess risk for more serious psychiatric disorders (Paffenbarger and McCabe, 1966; Pugh et al., 1963; Weissman and Klerman, 1977).

Most authors agree that endocrine changes may be involved in postpartum psychiatric illness. In a previous era, many of the acute psychotic states that occurred postpartum, including delirium, were probably related to infections, fever, dehydration, and hemorrhage following childbirth. With better medical care, these symptoms are rare in industrialized countries, and today the severe postpartum psychiatric reactions are almost entirely of a depressive nature. It must be concluded that women are at greater risk for psychiatric disorders, particularly depression, in the postpartum period. But if any specific endocrine abnormality is involved, the mechanism is not understood (Weissman and Klerman, 1977). The role. changes and psychosocial events of the postpartum period may also contribute to the increased risk of depression.

Summary: Epidemiology of Nonbipolar Depression

When the new diagnostic techniques are used, the point prevalence of nonbipolar depression in industrialized nations is found to be 2.3 percent to 3.2 percent of the adult male population and from 4.5 percent to 9.3 percent of the adult female population. In longitudinal and case registry studies in industrialized countries, the incidence of nonbipolar depression is 82 to 201 new cases per 100,000 men per year (or 0.08 to 0.2 percent) and 247 to 598 new cases per 100,000 women per year (or 0.2 to 0.6 percent).

Risk factors for nonbipolar depression include being female, particularly aged 35 to 45 years, having a family history of depression or alcoholism, having lived as a child in a disruptive, hostile, and generally negative home environment, having had recent negative life events, particularly exits, lacking an intimate confiding relationship, and having had a baby in the preceding six months.

BIPOLAR DISORDER

Definition

Bipolar disorder today refers to patients who experience both mania and depression and those who experience only mania. In this regard, bipolar disorder could be considered a subclass of the older classification of manic-depressive illness. The latter consisted of patients who had

---

*Preceptor's note: As the authors note above, Hirschfeld and Cross have reviewed the relationships between psychosocial factors and depression. Their chapter in this volume is a succinct evaluation of the current research in this area.

episodes of mania (who would be considered bipolar in this discussion) and patients who had only depression (who would be considered as nonbipolar depressives in this discussion). Leonhard (1957) made the original proposal for classifying depressed patients with a history of manic episodes (the bipolar group) separately from those who had only depression. The proposal was subsequently developed by Perris (1966; 1976) in Scandinavia, by Winokur (1973b) in the United States, and by Angst (1966) in Switzerland. The separation of the bipolar group has achieved rapid acceptance because of accumulating evidence for its possible genetic, biochemical, and pharmacologic validity.

The criterion for bipolar disorder is relatively clear—evidence of a current or past manic episode. A manic episode is usually defined as a period of euphoric mood associated with other symptoms: irritability, hyperactivity of a motor, social, and/or sexual nature, pressure of speech, flight of ideas, grandiosity, loss of sleep, distractibility, buying sprees, poor judgment, and social intrusiveness.

There is evidence that a small percentage of persons experience only manic episodes. In a longitudinal study Helgason (1977) followed a cohort of 5,395 persons and found that by age 61, 32 (0.5 percent) persons had experienced an episode of mania. Of these, seven (0.1 percent) had never experienced a known depression. Helgason therefore makes a distinction between the term *bipolar* (by which he means mania and depression) and *mania*. Most investigators, however, do not separate unipolar manics from bipolars (Krauthammer and Klerman, 1979). Bipolar disorder has been further divided into bipolar I and II. In bipolar I patients have a full-blown manic episode, and in bipolar II they have mild hypomania only. More recently, several additional divisions of bipolar disorder have been suggested.*

The relationship between bipolar disorder and manic-depressive illness has been uncertain. Data gathered on patients with manic-depressive illness were rarely broken down to show who had episodes of mania and who did not. Krauthammer and Klerman (1979) reviewed seven studies of consecutive hospital admissions where the distinction was made between bipolar and manic-depressive illness. Between 15 percent and 31.7 percent of all those with Kraepelinian manic-depressive illness had bipolar affective disorder, with an average of approximately 20 percent. Since mania is more likely than depression to result in hospitalization, the percentage of bipolars in studies of nonhospitalized persons is lower, in the range of 10 to 12 percent.

Morbid Risk

The morbid risk of bipolar affective disorder is of interest because it focuses on the number of people who are vulnerable to a recurrence of their disorder. Table 4 includes data from six studies which have examined the morbid risk of bipolar disorder. The morbid risk for both sexes ranges from 0.6 percent to 0.9 percent in industrialized nations and is estimated at 0.24 percent in New Zealand.

Incidence

Table 5 includes data from the nine studies which have reported the incidence of bipolar disorder. Studies of the incidence of manic-depressive illness are omitted, unless data for bipolar disorder were also

*Editor's note: For a summary of these proposals, see the chapter by Akiskal in Part IV.

Table 4. Morbid Risk of Bipolar Disorder[1]

| Source | Location | Risk as Percent of Patient Population | | |
		Men	Women	Total[2]
Helgason (1977)	Iceland	0.67	0.91	0.79
Weissman and Myers (1978a)	New Haven, CT, USA	—	—	0.6[3]
Weissman et al. (1982)	New Haven, CT, USA	0.6	1.0	0.9
James and Chapman (1975)	New Zealand	—	—	0.24
Parsons (1965)	England	—	—	0.88
Krauthammer and Klerman (1979)	Denmark	—	—	0.61

[1]Studies of manic-depressive illness are omitted if persons with bipolar disorder are not separated from nonbipolars.
[2]Totals do not represent sums but overall rates. Some studies reported no separate rates for men and women.
[3]Lifetime prevalence rates for bipolar with mania only (bipolar I). If bipolars with hypomania (bipolar II) are included, the total lifetime prevalence is 1.2 percent

reported. The best estimates of incidence are from the first three studies in the table. The incidence of bipolar disorder ranges from 9 to 15.2 new cases per 100,000 men per year and from 7.4 to 32 new cases per 100,000 women per year.

The rate of first hospitalization for bipolar disorder for both sexes ranges from 2.8 to 22.2 per 100,000 per year. In general, the hospitalization studies would be expected to underestimate the incidence of bipolar disorder, since the hypomanics and bipolar II patients who are treated as outpatients would not be counted. The Faris and Dunham (1939) data are particularly difficult to interpret. Their use of the word rates leaves one uncertain whether they were referring to first admissions or to all admissions, and unclear whether they were referring to annual rates or to rates for a 12-year period (from 1922 to 1934). Faris and Dunham (1939) also present data on two series of manic-depressives, and the rates for bipolar disorder are ten times as high in the first series as in the second. Both sets of data are given in the table.

Risk Factors

SEX While all affective disorders are more prevalent in women than in men, the sex differences in rates of bipolar disorders are not as great. Different studies report a ratio of women to men for bipolar disorder in the range of 1.3:1 to 2:1 (Krauthammer and Klerman, 1979; Pope and Lipinski, 1978).

AGE Published reports which include age-specific figures are in disagreement on age differences in the incidence of bipolar disorder. Faris and Dunham (1939) found a rising incidence until age 35 and then a decline, although more than 20 percent of the new cases occurred after

Table 5. Incidence Rates for Bipolar Disorder for Persons 15 Years or Older[1]

| Source | Location | Rates per 100,000 | | |
		Men	Women	Total[2]
Incidence Studies				
Anita Weeke (personal communication, 1979)	Aarhus County, Denmark[3]	15.2	17.4	—
Johannes Nielsen (personal communication, 1979)	Samsø Island, Denmark[4]	14.1	7.4	10.8
Tomas Helgason (personal communication, 1979)[5]	Iceland	9.0	32.0	—
Studies of First Hospitalization for Bipolar Disorder				
Anita Weeke (personal communication, 1979)	Central Danish Registry[6]	4.8	4.7	—
Anita Weeke (personal communication, 1979)	Central Danish Registry[7]	2.4	3.2	—
Johannes Nielsen (personal communication, 1979)	Samsø Island, Denmark[4]	—	—	6.1
Spicer et al. (1973)	England and Wales	3.0	3.9	3.5
Faris and Dunham (1939)	Chicago, IL, USA[8]	—	—	22.2
Faris and Dunham (1939)	Chicago, IL, USA[9]	—	—	2.8

[1]Studies of manic-depressive illness are omitted if persons with bipolar disorder are not separated from nonbipolars.
[2]Totals do not represent sums but overall rates. Sample sizes for men and women varied within studies, and some studies reported no overall rate. Three of the studies did not report separate rates for men and women.
[3]Data for 1960 to 1964
[4]Data for 1957 to 1974, with population size estimated in 1964
[5]Data from Larus Helgason
[6]Data for 1978
[7]Data for 1965 and 1966
[8]Series 1, consisting of 734 patients with manic-depressive psychosis, 440 of whom were bipolar
[9]Series 2, consisting of 2,311 patients with manic-depressive psychosis

the age of 50. Spicer et al. (1973) found that the incidence of mania increased with age, without any decline in the incidence rates, and that half of the new cases occurred in those over the age of 50. These observations on the age of onset were gathered from longitudinal studies and contradict the findings of a number of retrospective studies in which the age of onset ranges from 24 to 31 years, with a modal age of onset of 30 years (Krauthammer and Klerman, 1979).

The age distribution of bipolar disorder is also affected by the pattern in the recurrence of episodes. Episodes recur every 2.7 to 9 years. With increasing age, the interval between episodes becomes shorter, and the length of each episode increases (Klerman and Barrett, 1973). Thus, a person with bipolar disorder will have an increasing risk of experiencing a manic or depressive episode as he or she grows older.

SOCIAL CLASS Bipolar disorder may occur more frequently in the upper socioeconomic classes (Krauthammer and Klerman, 1979;

Weissman and Myers, 1978a). This finding is inconstant, however. In a review of the subject, Bagley (1969) offered three possible explanations for the excess of manic-depressive illness in the upper socioeconomic classes. (1) A diagnostic bias may cause patients from lower socioeconomic classes to be inaccurately diagnosed. (2) A particular type of personality may dispose certain individuals both to the disorder and to a rise in the social scale. (3) The stresses of life in the upper socioeconomic classes, or the stress of having moved up into such classes, may predispose certain individuals to the disorder. Bagley (1969) found some evidence in the literature to support the first two hypotheses and indirect evidence to support the third.

In a classic study, Faris and Dunham (1939) showed that the distribution of bipolar disorder and manic-depressive disorder was strikingly different from that of schizophrenia. Areas of the city of Chicago marked by poverty and social disintegration showed a higher concentration of schizophrenia, but they did not show a similar concentration of affective disorders. More affluent areas of the city had slight concentrations of people with manic-depressive illness and bipolar disorder.

In clinical studies, Cohen et al. (1954) and Gibson (1958) found that manic-depressive patients, when compared with schizophrenics, came from family backgrounds with low prestige. The chief interest of the manic-depressive's family was the child's potential usefulness in improving the family's position or in meeting the parents' prestige needs.

More recently, a retrospective study which paid careful attention to methodology demonstrated that bipolar subjects achieved higher levels of education and somewhat higher occupational status than did a control group of patients with nonbipolar depression (Monnelly et al., 1974; Woodruff et al., 1971).

RACE Faris and Dunham (1939) found no relationship between race and bipolar disorder. As noted by Silverman (1968), however, Wagner reported that blacks had a higher admission rate for manic-depressive illness than whites.

MARITAL STATUS Many studies suggest that bipolar disorder may be slightly more common among single and divorced persons. However, marital status may change as a result of the disorder rather than leading to the onset of the disorder (Krauthammer and Klerman, 1979).

For example, Faris and Dunham (1939) found a slight increase in the percentage of divorced people among those with manic-depressive illness when compared with the general population, but found no greater frequency of being single, married, or widowed. Similarly, in the Iowa 500 study, 51 percent of manics were currently married, compared with 58 percent of the general population (Krauthammer and Klerman, 1979). In the Scandinavian literature, Weeke et al. (1975) found that manic-depressives were less likely to be married than the general population and more likely to be separated or divorced. They cautioned, however, that in many cases the illness preceded and probably contributed to the divorce. Therefore, we cannot say that being single or divorced is a risk factor for bipolar disorder.

Stevens (1969) showed that the marital status and fertility of women with affective disorders in the London area were similar to the general population, as contrasted with schizophrenics who have a lower likelihood of marriage or reproduction.

FAMILY HISTORY The evidence is reasonably good for a genetic component in the familial transmission of bipolar disorder. Bipolar probands have both bipolar and unipolar first-degree relatives in roughly equal frequencies (about 7 percent and 8 percent, respectively), and these rates are higher than might be expected in the general population (Kidd and Weissman, 1978).

Summary: Epidemiology of Bipolar Disorder

The morbid risk of bipolar disorder for both sexes ranges from 0.6 percent to 0.9 percent in industrialized nations. The incidence of bipolar disorder is 9 to 15.2 new cases per 100,000 per year for men (or 0.009 percent to 0.015 percent) and for women 7.4 to 32 new cases per 100,000 per year (or 0.007 percent to 0.03 percent).

The major risk factor for bipolar disorder is having a family history of bipolar disorder. The data suggest that people under the age of 50 are at higher risk of a first attack of bipolar disorder, whereas those who already have the disorder face an increasing risk of a recurrent manic or depressive episode as they grow older. Bipolar disorder seems to be associated with the upper socioeconomic classes.

CONCLUSION

Epidemiologic studies of psychiatric disorders have been difficult to interpret because of differing case definitions. The emergence of new methods for making reliable and well-defined diagnoses (SADS-RDC; DSM-III; PSE-ID-CATEGO) offers the promise of conducting comparable and reproducible studies in the field of epidemiology. Six studies using these new diagnostic techniques have been reported earlier in this chapter (Table 2).

In order to review the literature on the epidemiology of affective disorders, the authors had to decide what diagnostic classifications make sense at the. present time. Since there is now international agreement on how to measure depressive symptoms independent of diagnosis and on how to define bipolar disorder, the authors used these classifications in their review. However, because the classification and subtyping of the large remaining group suffering from depression is still an area of disagreement, the authors chose to aggregate them all into the category of nonbipolar depression.

Despite the diversity of methodologies employed in epidemiologic studies, some findings are consistent. The point prevalence of depressive symptoms seems to be in the range of 13 to 20 percent of the population. The point prevalence of nonbipolar depression in industrialized nations, using the new diagnostic techniques, is 2 to 3 percent for men and 5 to 9 percent for women. The annual incidence of nonbipolar depression is 0.08 to 0.2 percent for men, and 0.2 to 0.6 percent for women. The morbid risk of bipolar disorder in industrialized nations is less than 1 percent for both sexes. The annual incidence of bipolar disorders is 0.009 to 0.015 percent for men and 0.007 to 0.03 percent for women.

When we compare risk factors, certain trends emerge. For all three categories (depressive symptoms, nonbipolar depression, and bipolar disorder), women have higher rates than men, although the sex difference is less pronounced for bipolar disorder. Depressive symptoms are higher in the lower social classes; nonbipolar depression shows no particular social class distribution; and bipolar disorder tends to be higher in the upper socioeconomic classes.

Improved diagnostic techniques are already in use. Efforts are being made to clarify existing international differences in diagnosis. The United States has recently launched the Epidemiologic Catchment Area Program. In light of these advances, more precise data on the incidence, prevalence, and risk factors for affective disorders are sure to come forth.

Chapter 25 Epidemiologic and Risk Factors in Suicide[†]
by Paula J. Clayton, M.D.

INTRODUCTION

Every student who wants to develop an in-depth understanding of the clinical picture of a depressive disorder should be required to read *The Bell Jar*, Sylvia Plath's autobiographical novel (Plath, 1963). In it she not only beautifully describes the development and course of a major depression, but also clearly emphasizes the suicidal preoccupation that the depressed patient may develop.

In her book Plath describes how, as a college student, she competed for and won a summer job with a women's magazine in New York City. She experiences depressive symptoms. Untreated, she returns home. Then because of insomnia and her use of sleeping pills, she is referred to a psychiatrist. He gives her one outpatient electroconvulsive treatment. She decides not to return. After this her hopelessness becomes evident, and she becomes totally engrossed with the idea of committing suicide. Not only does she have detailed thoughts about suicide, but most of these thoughts are accompanied by some attempt to carry them out. At one point when she has not slept for 21 nights, she locks herself in the bathroom, runs a tub of hot water, and plans to cut herself with a razor blade. She succeeds only in cutting her calf with a guillotine-like stroke which necessitates the use of a band-aid.

Next she takes a complicated train and bus ride to a remote island made into a peninsula. There she sits on the beach with 19 Gillette blades in her pocket, considering whether she should rent a seaside room in which to commit suicide. As she sits, the tide comes in, the water begins to come up around her feet, and she is warned by a little boy that this is happening. She considers death by drowning.

The book continues in a humorous yet melancholic way, as she goes on to detail her attempt to hang herself, which also fails. She is later cajoled into taking a blind date. During the course of this date she engages her male friend in a discussion of suicide.

[†]The preparation of this chapter was supported in part by a United States Public Health Service Grant No. MH 25430.

She asks him how he might do it, and he replies, "I'd blow my brains out." This causes her to muse about how she would find a gun and what she would shoot, and she concludes that she would probably end up maiming herself without dying. She nonetheless continues to question her friend about the kind of gun he would use and where he would get one. When he replies that he would get one from his father, she asks him where his father lives and is disappointed to learn that he lives in England. She and her friend then swim out to sea. He becomes tired and turns back, and she tries to drown herself by diving but finds that she keeps popping back up.

Last she decides that when the money from her prize-winning summer job runs out, she will commit suicide. The day that this occurs she writes her mother a note saying that she is going out for a long walk, unlocks her mother's strongbox, gets out a new bottle of sleeping pills, dresses, takes her new black raincoat, and goes to the basement. There she hides herself in the crawl space, laying over it the fireplace logs that had covered the opening before she crawled in. Once inside, she takes all of the sleeping pills. Apparently she remains missing for several days and is found accidentally by her mother as she is in the cellar doing the laundry. She is admitted to a psychiatric hospital and slowly recovers with psychotherapy and five electroconvulsive treatments. In the hospital she meets a college friend who is depressed and whimsically suicidal and who does commit suicide by hanging. The book ends on the more optimistic note of her impending discharge from the hospital.

The book was published in 1963. Sylvia Plath committed sucide on 11 February 1963 by carbon monoxide poisoning from the kitchen stove, one of the few ways she hadn't contemplated in the book.

COMPLETED SUICIDE

Risk Factors

On the basis of psychological autopsies (systematic interviews shortly after the death with close friends, relatives, physicians, and so forth), we have long known that the majority of people who commit suicide are psychiatrically ill. In 1959, Robins et al. showed that of 134 consecutive suicides, 98 percent were chronically ill, 94 percent being psychiatrically ill and 4 percent being medically ill. More important, 68 percent of the suicides were found to be suffering from one of two disorders, manic-depressive disease (45 percent) or chronic alcoholism (23 percent). In 1960, Dorpat and Ripley reported that all of 108 consecutive completed suicides had psychiatric illnesses. The diagnoses were depression in 30 percent, alcoholism in 27 percent, schizophrenia in 12 percent, personality disorder in 9 percent, chronic brain syndrome in 4 percent, and miscellaneous and nonspecific psychiatric illness in 19 percent. Finally, Baraclough et al. (1974) found that 93 percent of 100 suicides were diagnosed as mentally ill. The diagnoses were depressive illness in 70 percent, alcoholism in 15 percent, schizophrenia in 3 percent, phobic anxiety state in 3 percent, barbiturate dependence in 1 percent, and schizoaffective psychosis in 1 percent.

Thus, as Sylvia Plath exemplifies, between 30 and 70 percent of people who commit suicide are suffering from a potentially treatable illness, major depression. Guze and Robins (1970) have also emphasized this. When they reviewed 17 studies of the outcomes of affective disorder patients, they found that 15 percent of all deaths were by suicide. A more recent follow-up study by Tsuang (1978) indicated that the suicide rate among depressives had not changed much. This study also pointed out for the first time that the rate was similar in bipolars, unipolars, and schizophrenics. Tsuang reported that 10 percent of the schizophrenics, 11 percent of the bipolars, and 9 percent of the unipolar depressive patients died by suicide. These rates contrasted strikingly with those of a matched control group who had a suicide rate of 2 percent. As shown in other studies, the suicides in the unipolar depressives occurred early in the course of the illness. In a similarly designed study of schizoaffective patients, Tsuang et al. (1979) showed that their suicide rate was 16 percent. Thus, all the major "functional" psychoses carry a high risk for death by suicide.

Because base prevalence rates for depressive disorders and alcoholism are much higher than for schizophrenia or schizoaffective illness, depression and alcoholism stand out in the psychological studies after completed suicides. Still, when thinking about risk factors, the first and most important factor to consider is diagnosis, and the diagnoses associated with suicidal risk include bipolar or unipolar depressive disorder, schizophrenia, and the schizoaffective disorders, as well as alcoholism and other depressive disorders (Clayton, 1982). Most recent studies on secondary depression (a major depression that occurs during the course of another psychiatric disorder such as drug or alcohol abuse, panic disorder, and so forth) indicate that patients with two disorders also have a high suicidal risk (Clayton, 1983). But data on the percent of patients with such diagnoses who die by suicide are not yet available. The high suicide rate in alcoholism and schizophrenia may be an example of this, as is the recently reported excess in panic disorder patients (Coryell et al., 1982).

Before going on to discuss other risk factors associated with the individual, several points need to be made about other sources of risk. Numerous studies have shown that a large number of patients are under a physician's care at the time they commit suicide (Barraclough et al., 1974; Dorpat and Ripley, 1960; Murphy, 1975b; Robins et al., 1959). The most recent study (Murphy, 1975b) indicated that 82 percent of sixty subjects who had committed suicide saw their physicians within six months of their deaths and 53 percent of them within one month or less. These and other studies have also indicated that at least two thirds of the patients who complete suicide communicate their suicidal ideas to those around them, families, friends, or physicians (Barraclough et al., 1974; Dorpat and Boswell, 1963; Murphy, 1975b; Robins et al., 1959; Sainsbury, 1973). The most frequent manner of communicating the suicide intent was a direct and specific statement of the intent to commit suicide. And these studies emphasize that a large number of those who died by barbiturate poisoning used barbiturates recently prescribed by their physicians (Barraclough et al., 1974; Murphy, 1975a; Sainsbury, 1973). The conclusion reached repeatedly is that physicians are treating these patients for symptoms of depression (e.g., low mood or insomnia) without asking enough questions to make a definitive diagnosis of depressive disorder. Or if they do diagnose depression, they conclude that the depression is understandable (social or economic stresses explain the affect), and they fail to ascertain the seriousness of the illness. Death wishes, suicidal thoughts, and/or suicide attempts are not inquired about, and if they are and are found to be present, they are not correctly evaluated (Murphy, 1977). There is some indication that ECT may decrease premature death by suicide (Avery and Winokur, 1976; Tsuang et al., 1979). Based on these findings, thoughtful researchers question the soundness of the "rational suicide" concept (Brown, 1981; Murphy, 1973).

Murphy (1972) has reviewed the literature on clinical suicidal risk factors. In addition to psychiatric diagnosis, which was already emphasized, several demographic factors seem to be well correlated with increased risk: being older (over 45), being male, being white, being separated, widowed, or divorced, living alone, and being unemployed or retired. Thus, a *depressed* white man who has recently retired, is widowed, and lives alone would be a high suicidal risk. Based on studies of professional women and additional reports, the author and her colleagues (Clayton et al., 1980) have suggested that high intelligence may correlate with suicide, especially in those younger than 45. In addition, certain stresses have been identified as possible precipitants in those who have the depressive diathesis or who are already mildly depressed. One is a recent change in dwelling (Sainsbury, 1973). Another is a recent loss from separation, divorce, estrangement, or death (Murphy et al., 1979). In the latter instance, the stress is particularly significant in patients who have a diagnosis of alcoholism.

The symptomatic correlates of patients who go on to complete suicide are difficult to tease out. Certainly the person who has made a suicide attempt is more likely to commit suicide than someone from the general population. However, most of those who attempt do not eventually commit suicide. If it is possible to classify suicide attempts as nonserious and serious (and some would argue that it is not), then there is some correlation between a serious suicide attempt and completed suicide (Pallis and Barraclough, 1977; Pallis and Birtchnell, 1977). Beck (1963) and Minkoff et al. (1973) found that completed suicide was related to hopelessness and negative expectations about the future. Other symptoms, however, such as extreme guilt or psychotic symptoms, do not predict an outcome of suicide.

Traskman et al. (1981) reported that depressed and nondepressed patients who had attempted suicide had lower levels of spinal 5-hydroxyindoleacetic acid (5-HIAA), a serotonin metabolite, than healthy volunteers. A one-year follow-up of these patients, plus 89 additional depressives, revealed a 20 percent mortality by suicide in those with below-median CSF 5-HIAA.

Although these correlates are all of interest, predicting a rare event like suicide is difficult (Murphy, 1972). For instance, marital status may be a significant distinguishing factor between those who commit suicide and nonsuicidal individuals who are appropriately matched on other variables. More widowed people, for example, commit suicide than their nonwidowed counterparts. Nonetheless, the majority of people who commit suicide are married. The relative weight of each correlate has yet to be tested on a large group of individuals who commit suicide, and many questions remain unanswered.

Genetic and Epidemiologic Data

The familial aspects of suicide are controversial. Juel-Nielsen and Videbech (1970) looked at concordance for suicide in monozygotic and dizygotic twins from the twin registry in Denmark. They found four concordant pairs in 19 monozygotic twins and no concordant pairs in 58 dizygotic twins. Their review of the cases led them to believe that there was a high frequency of affective disorder in the suicides and that this would explain some of the genetic influence. The cases also showed that there were other suicides in the families of the concordant (monozygotic) twins. Blath et al. (1973) reported on a pair of monozygotic twins who were depressed and made serious suicide attempts, and there are several other reports of suicide in families (Dabbagh, 1977; Khin-Maung-Zaw, 1981). Kety (1979) reported a higher incidence of suicide in the biological relatives of adoptees who suffered from depression than in their adoptive relatives or in the biological or adoptive relatives of nondepressed adoptee controls.

Finally, without regard to depression, Schulsinger et al. (1979) reported that 57 of 5,483 adoptees in a Copenhagen sample committed suicide. A comparable group of controls from the community had only 34 suicides, and the difference was significant. When the 57 adoptees who committed suicide were internally matched to other adoptees who had not, Schulsinger et al. found significantly more suicides in the biological relatives of the adoptees who had committed suicide than in the biological relatives of the other adoptees. There were no suicides in the adoptive families of either group of adoptees. Even in the community control group who were raised by their biological families, Schulsinger et al. found significantly more suicides in the families of the individuals who committed suicide than in the families of the internally matched adopted controls whose lives did not end in suicide. The suicides in the adoptees and the relatives were equally distributed between those who had been in a psychiatric hospital and those who had not. Because the authors found suicides in both adoptees and biological relatives who had not been in psychiatric hospitals, they concluded that genetic factors do play a role in transmitting suicidal behavior and that this role might be somewhat independent of the role played by the mental disorders frequently associated with suicide (alcoholism and depression).

This latter conclusion, however, seems premature in light of other data. All the studies that have linked depression and alcoholism to completed suicides show clearly that although many of these people were physicians, they were not seeing psychiatrists and had not been in psychiatric hospitals. The fact that the adopted probands and their biological families had not been in a psychiatric hospital does not mean that they were free of the two major mental disorders linked to suicide.

The strongest conclusion from this study would have to be that there is a genetic component to suicide, but how this component operates is not yet clear. Actually, Schulsinger et al. (1979) dealt with this quite nicely in their introduction. They questioned whether some psychological reactions or personality traits might be genetically transmitted and predispose certain people to suicide under given circumstances. They then speculated that these traits could be such things as a combination of decisiveness and impulsivity, or an inability to cope with and resist adverse conditions, or a tendency toward hoplessness and giving up, or a tendency toward feelings of inadequacy. Thus, certain personality traits, under the circumstances of depression or excessive drinking, could lead certain individuals to commit suicide. This is an interesting speculation. Evoking some personality trait as a vulnerability factor might help to explain the very puzzling findings that although two thirds of depressives are women, men have significantly higher suicide rates, and far more people with depression do not end their illness by suicide than do. It would be helpful to have a personality assessment, ascertained during the depression or a well state or both, that might predict an outcome of suicide.

Suicide rates vary slightly from country to country, and rates also fluctuate over time. These variations can sometimes be traced to environmental factors. For instance, the fluctuation of suicide rates in Australia may be partially explained by the availability of sedative drugs (Oliver and Hetzel, 1972). When sedative drugs were more available, suicide rates were higher. Similarly, suicide rates in the United Kingdom have decreased, and this may be because the methods most commonly used have become less lethal (a reduction in the carbon monoxide content of domestic gas), and perhaps because methods of resuscitation have improved (Brown, 1979). In the North American continent, overall suicide rates have been rising, particularly the rates among people between the ages of 15 and 29 (Hellon and Solomon, 1980; Murphy and Wetzel, 1980). In an interesting study of birth cohorts, Murphy and Wetzel (1980) showed that the number of young suicides is steadily increasing. Based on cohort trends, it seems likely that as these young people get older, their suicide rates will continue to rise. From this standpoint, the number of suicides in the United States will increase substantially in the near future.

ATTEMPTED SUICIDE

In the early 1950s investigators in two countries simultaneously conducted pioneering research on attempted and completed suicides. Stengel in England (reported in 1965) and Robins in the United States (Schmidt et al., 1954; Robins et al., 1957) proposed that those who attempt suicide and those who complete suicide come from two separate but overlapping populations. This concept is important because it may shed some light on why suicide prevention centers have for the most part been unable to alter the suicide rates (Murphy et al., 1969). Most people who attempt suicide do not go on to complete suicide. On the whole, however, the person who attempts suicide is at greater risk of committing suicide than the person who does not (Resnik, 1968). Using emergency room visits as an index of the number of persons who attempt suicide, approximately eight people attempt suicide for every one who completes it. Two percent of those who attempt suicide do kill themselves within one year after the first attempt, and about 10 percent are shown, if they are followed long enough, to kill themselves eventually. This rate is 35 to 100 times the rate of completed suicide in the general population.

People who attempt suicide are usually women, are under 30 years old, do not have specific psychiatric diagnoses or carry such diagnoses as sociopathic personality or Briquet's syndrome, make their attempts impulsively, are relatively public about their attempts, and may use relatively less serious means than those who complete suicide. In contrast, as already noted, those who complete suicide are more likely to be men, are over 45 years old, have specific diagnoses such as depression and alcoholism, give previous warnings of their intention to commit suicide, make their suicide attempts in private ways, and use highly efficient means. An example of efficiency (and high risk) came from a study of women physicians. A woman physician who was subject to severe depressive episodes confided that she had decided that the only way to commit suicide was to do it in two ways simultaneously. If one way failed, the other would succeed. She also reasoned that people initiating the suicide rescue would be distracted by one means so that the other way would then have time to work.

As indicated, much controversy surrounds the matter of judging the seriousness of a suicide attempt. When a person uses a highly efficient method such as firearms, hanging, drowning, or jumping, one can easily feel that the attempt was serious. However, many men and women also make "serious" attempts with drugs, as evidenced by the fact that the number of men and women who complete suicide by overdose is increasing. This is also reflected in physicians' suicides (Rich and Pitts, 1979). Here, the author and others have concluded that those who are knowledgeable about the means they use are more likely to complete the act (Carlson and Miller, 1981; Clayton et al., 1980). Finally, since some people make trivial first attempts, the degree of danger to life in a first attempt is not a reliable index of future suicidal risk. Sylvia Plath is a good example of this.

It does seem reasonable to conclude that people who attempt suicide are asking for help. Every person who makes a suicide attempt should be evaluated, and most should be referred for treatment. Treatments are varied and depend on the diagnosis of the patient, as well as on the number of attempts (Liberman and Eckman, 1981; Montgomery and Montgomery, 1983). Studies from all countries have indicated that suicide attempts are increasing (Brown, 1979; Grove and Lynge, 1979; Kreitman, 1977; Liberman and Eckman, 1981). Preventative intervention is difficult, but it seems likely that intervention should begin with the first suicide attempt.

Chapter 26 # The Genetics of Affective Disorders[†]
by Elliot S. Gershon, M.D.

INTRODUCTION

Within many of our professional lifetimes, any belief in the inheritance of psychiatric illness was considered uninformed, and a patient who feared that a psychiatric illness might be hereditary was assured that this was not the case. More recently, mental health professionals have

[†]This chapter includes materials originally published in:

Gershon E.S.: Genetic factors from a clinical perspective, in The Psychobiology of Affective Disorders. Edited by Mendels J., Amsterdam J.D. Basel, S. Karger, 1980.

Gershon E.S.: Genetics of the affective disorders. Hospital Practice 14:117–122, 1979.

Gershon E.S.: Genetic perspectives, in Manic-Depressive Illness. Edited by Goodwin F.K., Jamison K.R. New York and Oxford, Oxford University Press, 1983.

Gershon E.S.: New approaches in clinical studies, in Genetic Strategies in Psychobiology and Psychiatry. Edited by Matthysse S., Ciaranello R.D., Breakefield X.O. Pacific Grove, CA., Boxwood Press, 1981.

accepted with reluctance the idea of genetic differences in people's emotional vulnerabilities and intellectual capacities. One reason for resisting the idea of genetic factors in psychiatric illnesses is the fear of inducing therapeutic nihilism and stigmatizing the victims of illness. However, the evidence for genetic factors in bipolar illness is strong, and it is increasingly well known to the public. In light of this, mental health professionals should begin to assimilate this knowledge into their clinical practices and to focus on the implications this new genetic knowledge has for the characterization, treatment, and secondary prevention of affective disorders.

The clinical evidence for genetic factors playing a major role in manic-depressive illness is persuasive and generally accepted. A century ago Galton suggested that twins be studied to explore the role of nature versus nurture in human traits. Identical (monozygotic) twin pairs share the same environment, and all their genes are identical by descent. Fraternal (dizygotic) twin pairs share their environment to the same degree, but only half their genes are identical by descent. Therefore, differences in concordance on a trait between identical and fraternal twin pairs suggest hereditary predominance in determining the trait, while similarity in concordance suggests environmental predominance. In the case of affective disorders, twin concordance studies consistently show very much greater concordance in monozygotic twins than in dizygotic twins, strongly supporting a predominantly genetic contribution to vulnerability.

A second type of clinical design separates genetic from postnatal environmental factors by studying the biological relatives of people who have been separated from their natural parents by adoption. A tendency for illness to be concordant in biological relatives separated in this way implies genetic transmission of illness. Although this design does not rule out prenatal environmental factors, adoption studies of affective illness have supported the hypothesis of prenatal genetic transmission.

A third clinical prediction that can be made for a genetic disease is that the illness will be concentrated in a relatively limited number of families in the population. This is a necessary but not sufficient condition of genetic transmission, since there are numerous familial characteristics that are not genetic. Bipolar illness is clearly familial in this epidemiologic sense. Perhaps the best-developed epidemiologic-genetic studies in psychiatry have been done on the affective disorders. Studies have yielded a wealth of data on diagnostic prevalence in the population and in relatives of patients, as well as data on the role of factors such as diagnostic criteria and differential mortality in the observed familial prevalences.

Three major areas are unsettled and to some extent controversial. First, what is the genetic relationship of unipolar to bipolar illness?

Gershon E.S., Hamovit J.R.: Genetic methods and preventive psychiatry. Prog Neuro-Psychopharmacol 3:565–573, 1979.

Gershon E.S., Goldin L.R., Weissman M.M., Nurnberger J.I. Jr.: Family and genetic studies of affective disorders in the Eastern United States: a provisional summary. Presented at the Third World Congress on Biological Psychiatry, Stockholm, Sweden, July 1981.

Gershon E.S., Hamovit J.R., Guroff J.J., et al.: A family study of schizoaffective, bipolar I, bipolar II, unipolar and normal control probands. Arch. Gen. Psychiatry 39:1157–1167, 1982.

Nurnberger J.I. Jr., Gershon E.S.: Genetics of affective disorders, in Neurobiology of Mood Disorders. Edited by Post R., Ballenger J. Baltimore, Williams & Wilkins, 1983.

This is part of the general question of whether there is a spectrum of disorders genetically transmitted with bipolar illness or whether there are discrete and independent genetic entities defined by clinical diagnosis.* Second, what is the mode of genetic transmission? In particular, does any X-chromosome or autosomal single-major-gene inheritance exist in bipolar affective disorders, and are there subgroups with genetic linkage to the human leukocyte antigen (HLA) region on chromosome 6 and/or to the color blindness-glucose-6-phosphate dehydrogenase (G6PD) region of the X chromosome? And third, are there biological markers of genetic vulnerability? Is there biological or genetic heterogeneity in these disorders? This chapter goes into each of these issues in some depth, with the goal of enabling the reader to appreciate and perhaps to anticipate future developments.

The clinician dealing with bipolar illness will encounter genetic issues in two general ways. As an increasingly sophisticated population of patients, relatives, spouses, and prospective spouses are recognizing the role of genetics, requests for genetic counseling are increasing. The informed mental health professional can deal with these requests as a specialized problem of psychotherapeutic importance to the patient and the family, as discussed later in this chapter. In a second clinical use, genetic knowledge can serve as an aid in decisions on diagnosis and psychotropic drug management.

Finally, recent advances in genetics offer new opportunities in biological research in manic-depressive illness. One can confidently predict that the question of whether there is single-gene transmission and linkage to chromosomal markers in some or all bipolar pedigrees will be resolved within a generation. Recently it has become technically feasible to isolate single chromosomes using cell-sorting technology, and the DNA in these chromosomes can be mapped using existing recombinant DNA technology (Ruddle, 1981). Geneticists have repeatedly predicted that within a decade or two it will be possible to map the entire human genome. With this map and with the several-orders-of-magnitude increase in linkage markers provided by the DNA probes, single-locus transmission in pedigrees can be confidently identified or ruled out. Based on the studies which the author and his colleagues are conducting (see below), it would not be surprising to find that single-locus transmission in bipolar illness is either rare or nonexistent.

Resolving the question of the genetic transmission of bipolar illness may require identifying the inherited pathophysiological vulnerability or vulnerabilities, and this in turn may require a major shift in clinical research strategies. The classical model of psychiatric illness is that it results from stress in an otherwise normal person, and the model has an underlying but unstated concept that there is a homogeneous population substrate upon which stress acts to induce a pathophysiology of illness. This model leads to clinical research strategies which compare the ill versus the well states in patients with episodic disorders, since the model implies that in the well state patients are essentially equivalent to normal controls. The clinical and biological effects of psychotropic drugs are extrapolated from their universal effects on

*Editor's note: In his chapter in Part IV, Akiskal presents the clinical evidence and some of the genetic evidence for the concept of a spectrum of affective disorders that would include bipolar and unipolar illness and a number of subtypes.

brain metabolism in experimental animals ("the pharmacologic bridge") rather than from their differential effects on genetic variants.

A new model is implied by genetic vulnerability. Persons who become ill are presumed to have a continuous and chronic constitutional vulnerability which is present even when they are well. A second important implication is that the etiologic importance of any specific biological factor can be tested by observing whether it is genetically transmitted along with the illness or whether it is transmitted independently of the illness. The concept of genetic vulnerability therefore dictates new research strategies. One becomes enormously interested in the euthymic bipolar patient. This patient is interesting not simply as a control for observations made while he or she is ill. The patient is interesting as a person who has a vulnerability for an illness which is not manifest but which should still be detectable in a properly chosen comparison with normal control individuals. Unmasking this vulnerability becomes the major goal of clinical, biological, and pharmacologic research. For example, one might use provocative pharmacologic challenges to unmask biological or behavioral variants in these patients and later conduct pharmacogenetic studies of their relatives. Pedigree studies of biological variants and illness would also become most valuable. In the author's opinion, this sort of biological-genetic study will gradually supplant the epidemiologic-diagnostic-genetic studies which have so far dominated the research literature.

FAMILY STUDIES

Unipolar and Bipolar Disorder

Family studies here mean case-controlled studies of illness in the relatives of patients or in normal controls. The key questions that can be answered by family studies are whether bipolar disorder is genetically independent of unipolar disorder (and other forms of affective disorder), whether specific genetic models fit the illness, and what is the familial concentration of bipolar disorder and other affective disorders in the population.

Table 1 shows a great inconsistency in reported prevalences in relatives, and this necessitates a methodological digression on family studies. The inconsistency is present even though the table is restricted to studies with explicit diagnostic criteria and direct examination of relatives. Some of the discrepancies are undoubtedly due to differences in procedures and criteria and to population differences. But could the inconsistencies reflect a basically unreliable methodology? Using recently developed family study procedures and criteria, good reliability of diagnosis is routinely attained. In collaborative studies, good reliability between centers can be established, and very similar prevalences in relatives can be found, as evidenced by the similarity of findings in the collaborating studies by the author and his colleagues (Gershon et al., 1981) and Weissman et al. (1981). But within studies which had good reliability and which used quite similar procedures, cognitive or cultural factors have been shown to lead to differences in diagnostic rates in family studies (Gershon et al., 1982). These include urban-rural differences, generational differences, and differences between American and Israeli Jews (who are genetically similar). Urban setting, younger generation, and American nationality are associated with higher diagnostic rates, principally for unipolar disorder.

Table 1. Lifetime Prevalence of Affective Illness in First-Degree Relatives of Patients and Controls

	Number at Risk	Morbid Risk (%)	
Bipolar Probands		Bipolar	Unipolar
Perris, 1966	627	10.2	0.5
Winokur and Clayton, 1967	167	10.2	20.4
Goetzl et al., 1974	212	2.8	13.7
Helzer and Winokur, 1974	151	4.6	10.6
Mendlewicz and Rainer, 1974	606	17.7	22.4
James and Chapman, 1975	239	6.4	13.2
Gershon et al., 1975b	341	3.8	8.7
Smeraldi et al., 1977	172	5.8	7.1
Johnson and Leeman, 1977	126	15.5	19.8
Pettersen, 1977	472	3.6	7.2
Angst et al., 1979; 1980	401	2.5	7.0
Taylor et al., 1980	601	4.8	4.2
Gershon et al., 1981; 1982	598 (572)[1]	8.0	14.9
Unipolar Probands			
Perris, 1966	684	0.3	6.4
Gershon et al., 1975b	96	2.1	14.2
Smeraldi et al., 1977	185	0.6	8.0
Angst et al., 1979; 1980	766	0.1	5.9
Taylor et al., 1980	96	4.1	8.3
Weissman et al., 1981 (Severe)[2]	242 (234)	2.1	17.5
Weissman et al., 1981 (Mild)[3]	414 (396)	3.4	16.7
Gershon et al., 1981; 1982	138 (133)	2.9	16.6
Normal Probands			
Gershon et al., 1975b	518 (411)	0.2	0.7
Weissman et al., 1981	442 (427)	1.8	5.6
Gershon et al., 1981; 1982	217 (208)	0.5	5.8

[1]Number at risk (corrected for age) for bipolar illness appears first in at-risk column; in parentheses is number at risk for unipolar illness when this is available separately.
[2]Hospitalized for depression
[3]Never hospitalized for depression

The fact that cognitive or cultural factors appear to be a general aspect of morbid risk estimates has several implications. First, there is not a "true" rate of diagnosable affective illness in the population (see the chapter by Weissman and Boyd) or in relatives of patients. The rates may be a function of procedures and criteria (Coryell et al., 1981; Weissman et al., 1981; in preparation), the culture of the population in which they are observed, and genetic factors. Second, clinical anamnestic criteria now available do not, across populations, consistently define a phenotype for affective illness, even though these procedures can be reliably applied.

Despite these methodological difficulties, it is still possible to observe consistencies in within-study comparisons. First, the rate of affective illness is consistently several times higher in relatives of patients than in relatives of controls. This is evidence for a strong familial contribution to diagnostic variance within the population. Second, in nearly all studies a great deal of unipolar illness is found in relatives of bipolar patients, although the reverse is generally not found. This implies at least partial genetic overlap between bipolar and unipolar illness, as do the twin data to be reviewed in a later section. As described below, in much of the family study data, the hypothesis cannot be rejected that bipolar and unipolar disorders generally represent more (bipolar) and less (unipolar) severe states of the same underlying genetic vulnerability.

Are there genetic differences between clinically defined subdivisions of bipolar disorder? Angst et al. (1980) subdivided their bipolar probands into three groups: (1) the Dm group, those who were hospitalized for depression and slight manic or hypomanic episodes, probably comparable to bipolar II (N = 43); (2) the MD group, those who were hospitalized for both mania and depression (N = 36); and (3) the Md group, those who were hospitalized with mania with slight depressive episodes (N = 16).* They found that the risk for affective disorder in first-degree relatives was 18.2 percent in the Dm group, 10.8 percent in the MD group, and 4.0 percent in the Md group. The difference between Dm and Md risks was significant (p = .005). However, Angst's study of a second sample did not replicate this difference (Angst, 1981). More recently, the author and his colleagues in Bethesda found that morbid risks of affective illness in relatives of bipolar I and bipolar II probands were similar (Gershon et al., 1981; 1982). Thus, it does not appear that a genetic distinction can be made between these subgroups.

The clinical genetic spectrum of bipolar disorders can be constructed by comparing the prevalence of illness in relatives of patients with the prevalence in relatives of controls. Based on such data, schizoaffective disorder and cyclothymic personality, in addition to unipolar illness, may be considered part of the spectrum of bipolar illness. The existence of a clinical spectrum with shared genetic factors has implications for etiology and for treatment, particularly with regard to lithium responsiveness in schizoaffective, unipolar, and cyclothymic relatives of bipolar patients (for example, see Kupfer et al., 1975).

Schizoaffective Disorder

From the viewpoint of familial transmission of affective illness, is there a separate entity of schizoaffective disorder? This question arises from the repeated observations of patients with episodic (as opposed to chronic) periods of schizophreniform psychosis along with affective symptoms and patients with some episodes which appear schizophrenic and some which appear affective in nature, again episodic over the lifetime. Most studies of first-degree relatives of patients with schizoaffective illness have shown more affective illness (particularly bipolar illness) and (to a lesser extent) schizophrenia in the relatives than schizoaffective illness. The 1979 work of Angst et al. reviewed most studies done to that time (see Table 2). Among the studies, only that of Perris (1974) showed increased homotypically ill relatives as opposed to relatives with affective illness and schizophrenia. Angst et al. (1979), however, criticized this study for having too inclusive a definition of schizoaffective illness. Referring to schizoaffective illness as cycloid

*Editor's note: The bipolar I and bipolar II distinction has been used to differentiate patients who have a history of one or more full-blown manic episodes (bipolar I) from those whose history shows hypomania and depression but no full-blown manic episode (bipolar II). The chapters by Akiskal, Dunner, and Prien in Part IV elaborate further on these subgroups, their clinical characteristics, and their responses to treatment.

Table 2. Genetic Studies on Schizoaffective and Related Psychoses

| AUTHOR | YEAR | PROBANDS (N) | DIAGNOSIS | FIRST-DEGREE RELATIVES | | | | | |
| | | | | Number at Risk | | Secondary Cases | | | |
				Schizophrenic	Affective Disorder	Schizophrenic (%)	Schizoaffective (%)	Affective Disorder (%)	Other Depressive (%)
Angst	1966	73	schizoaffective	372.7	321.3	5.9	3.8	3.4	5.3
Clayton et al.	1968	39	—	58[1]	58[1]	3		14	
Perris	1974	60	cycloid psychoses	262.5	182.5	0.8[2]	9.1[2]	1.6[2]	4.9
Abrams and Taylor	1976	7	schizoaffective	36[1]	36[1]	—		14	
McCabe and Cadoret	1976	45	atypical psychoses	45	38	4.4	2.2	5.3	2.6
Mendlewicz et al.	1976	45	schizoaffective	118.2	118.2	11.0	0.8	35.5	
Shopsin et al.	1976	12	schizoaffective	24	24	8.0⁻		12.5	
Suslak et al.	1976	10	schizoaffective	23[2]	23[2]	4.0[2]	—	6.5[2]	
Tsuang et al.	1976	85	atypical schizo.	?	?	1.3		7.6	
Felder[3]	1977	85	—	520.5	520.5	4.6	3.1	4.6	1.0
Tsuang et al.	1977	53	schizoaffective	228[1]	228[1]	0.9		11.8	

[1] N-Number of relatives
[2] Figures calculated by the author
[3] Study of Angst (N = 73) with follow-up and 12 new probands

Source: Angst et al. (1979); used with permission.

psychosis, Perris included Leonhard's categories of "motility psychoses" and "confusion psychoses" in his diagnostic definition. Even in the study of Perris, though, there is a considerable frequency of bipolar affective illness and some schizophrenia in the relatives of the schizoaffective patients.

Similarly, McCabe (1975) found a high frequency of reactive psychosis in relatives of patients with bipolar illness, but his reactive psychosis category included schizoaffective and some other diagnoses. Asano (1967) distinguished between typical and atypical manic-depressive patients and classified 81.5 percent of his probands as atypical. He also classified many of their relatives as atypical, but it should be noted that this classification is not the same as schizoaffective disorder. For example, Asano would have included depression with compulsive or depersonalization symptoms under atypical manic-depressive psychosis. In a study of sibling pairs, Tsuang (1979) also found a relative lack of schizoaffective-schizoaffective pairs as compared with schizoaffective-schizophrenic and schizoaffective-affective-disorder pairs. Mendlewicz et al. (1980b) reported a morbid risk of 34.6 percent for affective illness and 10.8 percent for schizophrenia in the relatives of 55 schizoaffective probands, while the risk for schizoaffective illness was "too low to be tabulated." The author and his colleagues have found that among 84 first-degree relatives of schizoaffective probands the morbid risk is 6.1 percent for schizoaffective disorder, 10.7 percent for bipolar I disorder, 6.1 percent for bipolar II, 14.5 percent for unipolar, and 3.6 percent for schizophrenia.

Though schizoaffective probands tend to have a high frequency of affective illness in relatives (and a low incidence of schizoaffective illness), the twin studies present a very different picture. McCabe (1975) reviewed and combined the twin data of Kringlen (1967), Essen-Möller (1963), Tienari (1963), Fischer et al. (1969), and Cohen et al. (1972). Thirteen out of 44 monozygotic twins versus one out of 45 same-sex dizygotic twins were concordant for type of illness. As noted above, McCabe's definition included as concordant those persons who were ill with reactive schizophreniform psychosis, as well as schizoaffective psychosis. While the twin studies thus show that the same form of psychosis appears to be genetically transmitted, this does not appear true in the family studies.

Where the monozygotic twin concordance appears so much greater than the concordance among first-degree relatives, the data may be reflecting a peculiar form of inheritance. The phenomenon may be produced by interaction among several loci, such that there is greatly increased concordance in monozygotic twins, as compared with concordance in dizygotic twins and other first-degree relatives. This is produced by the fact that monozygotic twins will be identical by descent at all loci, but the chances of two siblings (for example) being identical by descent at a given locus is one half. The probability of being identical by descent at n loci is therefore 0.5^n, which becomes a vanishingly small number as the number of loci involved increases. An example of this type of inheritance appears to be found in the visual evoked response (Dustman and Beck, 1965).

The author speculates that there are peculiar genetic factors which cause the psychosis to have a schizoaffective expression, since there is a high twin concordance. But these factors in turn are superimposed on the genetic diathesis for bipolar affective illness, since this is consistently the most frequent disorder in relatives of schizoaffective patients. The literature does presently suggest factors that predispose to the schizoaffective expression of psychosis.*

Alcoholism

Helzer and Winokur (1974) found an increase in alcoholism in the relatives of male bipolar probands. Elsewhere in the United States Dunner et al. (1976) found no increased alcoholism in the families of bipolar or unipolar patients as compared with control families, although they did find an increase in the families of bipolar II patients. Morrison (1975) found no increase in alcoholism in the families of bipolar patients unless the bipolar patient was him- or herself alcoholic. The author and Liebowitz reported no increase in alcoholism in families of either unipolar or bipolar patients in Israel (Gershon and Liebowitz, 1975).

Similarly, current United States data of the author and his colleagues (Gershon et al., 1982) show no increase in alcoholism in the relatives of affectively ill probands compared with the relatives of controls. Although bipolar illness and alcoholism are not uncommonly found in the same individual, alcoholism by itself (without affective disorder) does not appear to belong in the genetic spectrum of bipolar manic-depressive illness.

Anorexia Nervosa

Cantwell et al. (1977) reported in a family history of anorectics that an excess of affective disorder was present in relatives. In a family study, Winokur, March, and Mendels (1980) investigated 25 anorectic women and 192 of their first- and second-degree relatives. A group of 25 age-matched women with no history of anorexia or depression were used as controls. Of the relatives of the anorectics, 17.7 percent had unipolar illness, and 4.7 percent had bipolar illness (not age corrected). The corresponding figures for controls' relatives were 9.2 percent and 0.6 percent. The difference in total incidence of affective illness was significant (p < .005), suggesting a genetic relationship between the two disorders.

The author and his colleagues (Gershon et al., 1983) have had similar findings, a modest amount of anorexia in relatives of anorectics (2 percent) and as much affective disorder as in relatives of bipolars (8.3 percent bipolar and 13.3 percent unipolar). In relatives of bipolars, however, there is very little anorexia (0.6 percent). It appears that anorexia has a unique familial vulnerability factor, possibly genetic, which is superimposed on a genetic tendency to bipolar and unipolar affective disorder. This appears to be even less common than the similar tendency to schizoaffective disorder.

Other Diagnoses

Cyclothymic personality has been reviewed as a separate entity by Akiskal, Djenderedjian, and Rosenthal (1977) and Akiskal, Khan, and Scott-Strauss (1979). Evidence from family studies of the author and his colleagues (Gershon et al., 1975b; 1981; 1982) suggests that it

*Editor's note: Akiskal, in his chapter in Part IV, discusses several hypotheses regarding the nosological status of the schizoaffective states. (See the section of his chapter titled "The Question of Schizoaffective Psychosis.")

may be related to bipolar affective disorder. Hyperactive syndrome of childhood or attention deficit disorder (Dyson and Barcai, 1970) and agoraphobia and anxiety disorder (Gardos, 1980) have also been hypothesized to be related to affective illness.

Suicide was frequent in the biological relatives of Danish adoptees with affective disorder. In the new family study data of the author and his colleagues, the suicides in the proband's own and later generations occur largely in persons with symptoms of antecedent affective disorder (determined by history from relatives and medical records). But in the earlier generations (proband's parents, aunts and uncles, grandparents) there were 15 suicides (among about 1,000 individuals), and 13 were in people who had no known antecedent psychiatric disorder. The intergenerational difference seems to be a cognitive difference in "psychological mindedness" between the generations, not a finding that nonpsychiatric suicide is a separate entity in the affective spectrum.

Risk Implications of Family Studies

RISK TO OFFSPRING   For the clinician, family studies are an important source for estimating the risk of recurrence in patients' relatives. In estimating this risk, the clinician must rely on family studies that are contemporaneous, that are conducted in a population comparable to the person seeking counsel, and that use diagnostic criteria and procedures with which the clinician is familiar.

The risk to offspring is of most interest in genetic counseling. Where one parent is ill, the age-corrected risk to 614 adult children of patients with major affective illness was 27 percent in a recent study (Gershon et al., 1982). In 300 children who each had one bipolar parent and one not ill, the risk was 29.5 percent (1 percent schizoaffective, 13 percent bipolar I or II, 15 percent unipolar). With two parents ill, the risk of major affective disorder was 74 percent in 28 offspring. Winokur, Clayton, and Reich (1969) reported 50 percent risk in 31 offspring of bipolar patients. It should be borne in mind that assortative mating, the tendency for persons with the same disorder to mate at greater-than-chance rates, has been reported in several but not all studies of affective disorder, as reviewed elsewhere (Negri et al., 1979). Therefore, in estimating risk to offspring, the putatively well parent should be carefully evaluated.

EARLY- AND LATE-ONSET BIPOLAR ILLNESS   Most studies have shown increased morbid risk of affective disorder in the relatives of probands whose illness had an early onset (see review in Gershon et al., 1976). Taylor and Abrams (1981) divided 134 bipolar probands into 80 who had early onset (under age 29) and 54 who had late onset (age 30 or older), with onset defined as the beginning of the first "definite" episode. Relatives of early-onset probands had a morbid risk of 9.6 percent for bipolar illness and 4.6 percent for unipolar illness. Relatives of late-onset probands had 0.8 percent risk of bipolar illness and 3.0 percent risk of unipolar illness. Recent data on 96 bipolar I probands, however, do not confirm this finding (Gershon et al., 1982).

TWIN STUDIES

As noted elsewhere (Gershon et al., 1976), the clear difference between monozygotic and dizygotic concordance in numerous twin studies of affective illness over a fifty-year period argues strongly for heritability of affective illness. Price (1968) has reviewed 12 cases of monozygotic twins raised apart in which at least one twin had affective disorder. In that series eight pairs (67 percent) were concordant. While this is quite similar to findings for monozygotic twins raised together, one must note the study's lack of systematic sampling for twins raised apart.

Bertelsen et al. (1977; Bertelsen, 1979) reported on a study using the Danish Twin Register (Hauger et al., 1968). This register includes all same-sex twins born from 1870 to 1920. Bertelsen et al. sent questionnaires to twins or, if the twins were deceased, to their relatives and followed this with a personal interview if necessary, thus establishing a high degree of completeness in their information. Zygosity was checked either serologically or, if both twins were not living, anthropometrically. They ascertained that there were 110 twin pairs in which one or both had manic-depressive illness (using Kraepelinian criteria). The concordance for monozygotes (55 pairs) was 0.67 and for dizygotes (52 pairs) was 0.20. This is in close agreement with the data previously summarized. Concordance was higher for bipolar monozygotic probands (0.79) than for unipolar monozygotic probands (0.54). Dizygotic rates were similar (0.24 for bipolar and 0.19 for unipolar). Concordance was also related to severity of illness. Bipolar I probands showed 80 percent concordance in monozygotes, and bipolar II probands showed 78 percent concordance. Unipolar probands with three or more episodes of depression showed 59 percent concordance, and unipolars with fewer than three episodes showed 33 percent concordance. The unipolar data may reflect the fact that the population with fewer episodes had not yet passed through the age of risk.

Further analysis of concordant pairs for polarity revealed 11 unipolar-unipolar, 14 bipolar-bipolar, and 7 unipolar-bipolar. This suggests some genetic specificity for polarity, but it also suggests that unipolar and bipolar illness can be associated with the same genetic makeup. These data clearly demonstrate the inherent ambiguity in biological comparisons of bipolar versus unipolar patients. At the very least, a substantial proportion of unipolar patients have the same genetic and biological vulnerability as bipolar patients. Family study data and mathematical models of the observed distribution of diagnoses in families support the same conclusion.

The question of what causes some patients to display mania or hypomania at some point in their careers of mood disorders, while others never do, is crucial. But the question cannot be approached by assuming that unipolars generally lack this capacity and should therefore be clearly distinguished, even on this key characteristic, from bipolars.

ADOPTION STUDIES

Adoption studies are critical to any demonstration that prenatal and perinatal events are sufficient to predispose a person to an illness. Unfortunately, only one study deals specifically with bipolar disorder.

Mendlewicz and Rainer (1977) reported on a study of bipolar adoptees. They found affective disorder (including spectrum disorder) in 31 percent of the biological parents of these probands compared with 12 percent in the adoptive parents. The morbid risk in biological parents was comparable to the risk these investigators found in the parents of nonadopted bipolars (26 percent) and higher than it was in the biological or adoptive parents of normal adoptees (2 percent and 9 percent, respectively).

Schulsinger et al. (1979) and Kety (1979) reported preliminary data on an adoption study of suicide. The biological relatives of 71 adoptees with affective disorder had a disproportionate number of suicides (3.9 percent), in comparison with the adoptive relatives of the probands (0.6 percent) or with the biological or adoptive relatives of control adoptees (0.3 percent and 0.6 percent respectively). The difference between biological relatives of affective patients and the biological relatives of controls is statistically significant at the .01 level. Non-psychiatric suicide, defined as suicide with no preceding psychiatric hospitalization, also appeared to be genetically transmitted in this Danish adoption study. Whether this entity is independent of affective disorders is not clear from the published data.*

MODE OF GENETIC TRANSMISSION

Specific genetic hypotheses can be tested on clinical diagnostic data in patients and relatives. Or they can be tested by combining diagnostic data with chromosomal linkage markers or pathophysiological vulnerability markers in the members of a pedigree. A set of genetic hypotheses can constitute a testable genetic model. Two major classes of models have been proposed for affective illness, and they are called unitary and heterogeneous in this discussion. In the *unitary* models, all patients with a given diagnosisis are hypothesized to be part of a genetic liability distribution. The assumption is that the only way to subdivide a particular class of patients into heterogeneous groups is by clinical diagnosis in the patient or the relatives. Unitary models can be quite complex. For example, they can include hypotheses that a certain proportion of patients has no genetic liability to illness (that is, are phenocopies), or they may hypothesize that bipolar illness and its several associated clinical diagnoses are more and less severe manifestations of the same type of genetic liability. *Heterogeneous* models, on the other hand, can hypothesize that within a diagnostic entity some cases are caused by one genetic disorder and others by a second and distinct disorder. The well-known hypothesis that some proportion of bipolar pedigrees show X-linkage and others do not have X-linked transmission represents a model of genetic heterogeneity, as does a similar hypothesis on HLA linkage.

So far it has not been possible to detect genetic heterogeneity of this kind, although there have been demonstrations that a linkage marker or vulnerability trait can distinguish patients and ill relatives from well relatives in some but not other pedigrees. In the discussion which follows, when there are no markers, the mathematical analyses of clinical pedigree data are based on unitary models.

Pedigree and Segregation Analyses of Clinical Diagnosis
SINGLE-AUTOSOMAL-LOCUS MODELS   In the past few years, computational procedures have become available to test specific genetic models. Elston and Stewart (1971) developed a general model for single-locus inheritance that allows estimation of the maximum likelihood that

*Preceptor's note: In her chapter on epidemiologic and risk factors in suicide, Clayton also discusses the Schulsinger et al. (1979) study, and she evaluates the concept of "nonpsychiatric suicide."

a particular (set of) pedigree(s) would be found under each of the different types of transmission subsumed in the model. The likelihoods of each transmission mode can be compared with each other and with the most general case, which is a powerful way of ruling out possible transmission modes or specific parameter values. This model is applicable to multigenerational families, variable age of onset, and different conditions of pedigree ascertainment (Elston, 1973; Elston and Yelverton, 1975; Elston and Sobel, 1979).

Bucher and Elston (1981) and Bucher et al. (1981) have used this method to test hypotheses of single-locus transmission of affective illness in several sets of bipolar family study data collected from 1919 to 1971 in Europe and the United States. Even though the original investigators each came up with different conclusions with regard to the mode of genetic transmission, the results of segregation analyses indicated that there was some form of vertical transmission of illness in families but that it was not consistent with a single Mendelian locus. Using a different method of segregation analysis with data from an Italian study, Smeraldi et al. (1981) could not distinguish a single-major-locus hypothesis from a polygenetic hypothesis.

Goldin et al. (1982; 1983) tested hypotheses of single-major-locus transmission (autosomal and X-chromosome) of major affective disorder (bipolar, unipolar, and schizoaffective). They used the Elston-Stewart likelihood method of pedigree segregation analysis on a sample of families of varying size ascertained through patients treated at the National Institute of Mental Health (NIMH) in Bethesda. Hypotheses were tested on subsamples of families according to: (1) diagnosis of proband (75 bipolar I, 22 bipolar II, 18 unipolar, and 6 schizoaffective); (2) extreme value of a biological trait in the proband ("low" monoamine oxidase or "low" CSF 5-hydroxyindoleacetic acid [5-HIAA, the serotonin metabolite]); and (3) positive response to lithium in the proband. They did not find evidence for single-major-locus transmission of major affective disorder from segregation analysis in any subsample of families, even when they widened the diagnostic classification of ill phenotypes to include possible affective "spectrum" diagnoses.

Crowe et al. (1981) report on a unipolar pedigree with 98 subjects. A dominant model of genetic transmission provided a better fit than the environmental model, but not significantly better. They tested thirty genetic markers for linkage in 86 family members and found no linkage or association.

X-CHROMOSOME MODELS   The hypothesis that bipolar illness is transmitted by a dominant gene at a single locus on the X chromosome was suggested by Winokur and his associates (Winokur and Clayton, 1967; Winokur et al., 1969). They based their proposition on the finding that in families of bipolar patients, rates of mother-son transmission were high and father-son transmission was virtually absent (Helzer and Winokur, 1974; Winokur and Clayton, 1967). Other family studies have not found an absence of father-son transmission (Gershon et al., 1975b; 1981; Goetzl et al., 1974; James and Chapman, 1975; Mendlewicz and Rainer, 1974; Stenstedt, 1952). A more comprehensive test of the X-chromosome-transmission hypothesis in family data is to test the prevalences in all types of relatives, taking into account incomplete penetrance and possible differences in penetrance between males and females. Threshold models of genetic-environmental liability can provide one means to test this hypothesis (Van Eerdewegh et al., 1980).

Several hypotheses on the relationship of bipolar to unipolar illness can be subsumed under X-chromosome transmission. Perhaps the most interesting is the hypothesis that in families of bipolar patients, bipolar illness and unipolar illness are genotypically identical manifestations of a single dominant X-chromosome allele. This hypothesis is an underlying assumption of all the X-chromosome-linkage marker studies reported to date. As a general hypothesis for the populations studied, it can be rejected in the family study data of Mendlewicz and Rainer (1974) and of the author and his colleagues (Gershon et al., 1975b), but not in the family study data of Winokur and his associates (Winokur et al., 1969, their Table 2.5), as discussed elsewhere (Van Eerdewegh et al., 1980).

MULTIFACTORIAL TRANSMISSION The multiple-threshold model of Reich et al. (1972) has been applied to prevalences of affective illness in first-degree relatives (Gershon et al., 1976; 1981; 1982). This model postulates an underlying quantitative liability to affective disorders, with bipolar illness representing higher liability than unipolar illness. The model used an isocorrelational form in the studies reported, and no specific modifications were introduced for environmental factors, sex effects, assortative mating, or inbreeding. In this form, the model tests whether the transmission of the different diagnostic entities fit a single dimension of underlying vulnerability. Greater vulnerability is associated with more transmission of illness and more transmission of the higher-liability forms of illness. The key question this model tests is whether there is shared or independent transmission of several disease entities under multifactorial inheritance. The parameters of the model are liability thresholds for each form of illness and the correlations between relatives. The liability to illness must fit the normal (Gaussian) distribution, so that the frequency of each form of illness in relatives of each type of patient is predicted from the parameters.

Several data sets can be fit to this model (Angst, 1966; Gershon et al., 1975a; 1975b; 1981; 1982), and one other (Perris, 1966) might fit if the definition of unipolar illness were altered to include "other depressions and suicide." Baron et al. (1981a) concluded that this model also fit their data, but their computational procedure can be criticized. Schizoaffective disorders can be placed on the same continuum as bipolar and unipolar disorders as an extreme form of affective disorder in the data of the author and his colleagues (Gershon et al., 1981; 1982), but apparently not in the data of Angst (Angst et al., 1980; Angst, 1981).

The biological implications of this multifactorial model are that the bipolar vulnerability includes all of the unipolar genetic vulnerability, plus added factors which may be genetic or environmental. A similar statement can be made for schizoaffective compared with bipolar vulnerability in the data of the author and his colleagues (Gershon et al., 1981; 1982). In other words, the model predicts that there are more biological abnormalities to be found in bipolar or schizoaffective than in unipolar patients. This corresponds with the shared intuition of many clinical investigators who have focused their biological studies on bipolar and schizoaffective patients, even though unipolar illness is the more common form of affective illness.

LINKAGE MARKERS

X-Linkage

Based on their earlier family studies which were compatible with X-chromosome transmission of bipolar illness, Winokur and his colleagues were the first to present evidence using genetic linkage markers to support this hypothesis (Reich et al., 1969; Winokur and Tanna, 1969). Later a larger series of informative families were reported by Mendlewicz and his co-workers (Mendlewicz and Fleiss, 1974; Mendlewicz et al., 1972; 1975). Combining their data and Winokur's data, they concluded that in families of bipolar patients, affective illness is closely linked to protan and deutan color blindness, and that linkage to the Xg blood group is also present. Since families were excluded from analysis if there was apparent father-son transmission, these authors qualified their conclusion as being applicable to a subgroup of patients with bipolar illness.

These reported data are problematic, and the presence of linkage may be seriously questioned, as the author and Bunney have reviewed elsewhere (Gershon and Bunney, 1976). The chief problem is that the reported close linkage of bipolar illness to both the Xg locus and the protan-deutan region of the X chromosome is not compatible with the known large chromosomal map distance between the Xg locus and the protan-deutan region. The author and his co-workers have not been able to replicate either of these linkages in their data. For both Xg and protan-deutan color blindness, which are far removed from each other, as noted above, close linkage to affective illness could be ruled out (Leckman et al., 1979; Gershon et al., 1979c). The pedigrees were not heterogeneous with each other, and there were no instances of single pedigrees strongly suggesting linkage to either marker. In studying large pedigrees among the Amish, with affective disorder and color blindness present, Egeland also did not report linkage between the two conditions (Egeland, 1980). On the other hand, Mendlewicz et al. (1979) reported eight new Belgian families in which linkage to color blindness was suggested in at least one.

The studies from the author's group and the original study from Mendlewicz and co-workers (Mendlewicz and Fleiss, 1974; Mendlewicz et al., 1972; 1975) were done at comparable research settings two hundred miles apart in the northeastern United States in clinics with predominantly white patients. Population differences therefore probably do not account for the discrepancy. Findings from the two color blindness linkage series are the most opposite. Each of the two studies is statistically significant by the lod-score test, but in support of opposite conclusions. Both are statistically homogeneous. Baron et al. (1981b) and Mendlewicz (1981) have proposed that genetic heterogeneity accounts for these differences, but the author's group finds this difficult to accept. Since one group of investigators is responsible for the bulk of the positive findings in the literature and another group produced the bulk of the negative findings, it is simply possible that the finding cannot be replicated. Methodological errors in diagnostic or ascertainment procedures could have produced the unique homogeneity of the initial 1972 to 1974 pedigree series of Mendlewicz and his group. This would explain why the initial strikingly positive results were not replicated either in the series of the author's group or in the later series of Mendlewicz et al. (1979).

This is not to say that linked pedigrees do not exist. The pedigree series that the author's group has developed on red-green color blindness and bipolar illness contains six pedigrees. This is small enough that in reality a proportion of all pedigrees might be linked but none would show up in this series. Strongly positive, multigenerational, individual pedigrees for the red-green color blindness region have been reported by Winokur et al. (1969), Mendlewicz and Linkowski (1978), and Baron (1977). But since these reports were not based on large pedigree-series studies, they do not have the assurance of independent, systematic, and unbiased ascertainment and diagnostic procedures. Several large-scale studies are now being conducted by multicenter collaborators who have enough personnel and exchange of records and procedures to give the needed assurances.

Mendlewicz, Linkowski, and Wilmette (1980a) recently reported a family with linkage between manic-depressive illness and glucose-6-phosphate dehydrogenase (G6PD) deficiency, a marker on the X chromosome very close to the red-green color blindness loci. The new DNA probe for this region of the X chromosome (Persico et al., 1981) may serve to make virtually all pedigrees informative for linkage and lead to a resolution of the controversy.

Autosomal

HLA (human leukocyte antigen) associations with bipolar affective illness have been reported (Bennahum et al., 1975; Bennahum, unpublished data; Shapiro et al., 1976; Stember and Fieve, 1977). Statistical significance has been lacking, however, and the reports are not compatible with each other (Gershon et al., 1977b). Moreover, recent reports have not supported the presence of any association (Temple et al., 1979; Smeraldi et al., 1978b; Beckman et al., 1978; Targum et al., 1979). Within pedigrees, genetic heterogeneity of illness can be expected to be minimal or absent. The author's group therefore performed a pedigree study of linkage of HLA antigens to bipolar affective illness, using the multigenerational methods described above and starting with 130 bipolar pedigrees. Linkage (with 15 percent or less recombination) could be ruled out definitively (Targum et al., 1979). Association with specific HLA antigens also could be ruled out, even after matching controls for ethnic origin.

Smeraldi et al. (1978a) applied the identical-by-descent method to HLA types in sibling pairs where both had affective illness, and they noted increased concordance, suggesting a possible linkage. Turner and King (1981) analyzed five pedigrees with no father-son transmission and two pedigrees with such transmission. The families with father-son transmission showed suggestive linkage to HLA (lod score = 2.61), whereas the other families showed no such linkage. They proposed that bipolar illness is a heterogeneous condition with 10 to 30 percent not HLA linked and most of the rest linked to HLA on chromosome 6. Their assignment of phenotypes is confusing: from their description of the "inclusion-in-the-taxon" procedure, the assignment might have been based on other than diagnostic factors.

In a recent publication, Weitkamp et al. (1981) concluded that a major susceptibility gene for depression is located in the HLA region, based on the increased sharing of common HLA types in ill pairs of siblings (identical-by-descent method) in twenty families. However, the increased sharing was not found in the entire sample of sibling pairs, but only in families where *two* siblings were ill and not in families where *three* or more were ill. These researchers argued that the group of families with two ill siblings were more informative for this test since parents were likely to have relatively few susceptibility genes, whereas in the families with three or more affected offspring the parents were likely to have relatively more susceptibility genes. Goldin et al. (1982) have argued that this criterion for dividing a sample is not theoretically sound: families with two out of two children affected and families with two out of ten children affected clearly cannot be considered genetically equivalent. In addition, their new data on 18 families, combined with data on 9 families previously studied by Targum et al. (1979), did not support the hypothesis of a relationship of the HLA locus to depression.

In linkage studies of 21 autosomal markers to affective illness, Goldin et al. (1982; 1983) found no suggestive linkages. Rinieris et al. (1979) report a positive association between bipolar and unipolar disorders and blood type O in 190 affective patients in Greece. Other investigators have not found this (Tanna et al., 1976; Crowe et al., 1981; Goldin et al., unpublished data).

POTENTIAL ETIOLOGIC MARKERS

A central goal of genetic studies of affective disorders is to identify distinct entities that are genetically transmitted (Rieder and Gershon, 1978). Although the biological and pharmacologic characteristics of the affective illnesses could be an excellent means of identifying genetic entities, relatively few studies have attempted to identify the biological factors that are inherited in these disorders.

What is needed is a genetic marker which can be applied to each individual in a pedigree and which successfully predicts who is at risk and who is not. Ideally we would seek a biological variant (such as an altered protein) that could be assigned a specific locus on an identifiable chromosome. But since stable biochemical differences can also suggest genetic differences (Childs, 1976; Stewart and Elston, 1973), virtually any biological finding that was clearly associated with the tendency to affective illness in a subgroup of patients might be studied as a possible genetic marker. The converse is also valid: genetic strategies may be used to demonstrate the validity of a particular biological component of the affective disorders, even in the absence of an established mechanism of genetic transmission.

A characteristic can be investigated as a possible genetic marker of vulnerability to an illness if it meets certain prior qualifications. (1) The characteristic must be associated with an increased likelihood of the psychiatric illness. (On the other hand, the proposition that persons who have the illness should generally show the characteristic need not be true since there may be biological heterogeneity in the illness.) (2) The characteristic must be heritable and must not be a secondary effect of the illness. (3) The characteristic must be observable (or evocable) in the well state, so that we can determine its presence independently of the illness and evaluate well relatives. Meeting these three criteria is still not enough to demonstrate that a biological characteristic is a necessary or contributing genetic factor in an illness. We must also demonstrate the characteristic's nonindependent assortment with the illness within pedigrees. That is, the transmission of the illness and the transmission of the characteristic must be related within pedigrees. Since the twin and family data strongly suggest that some persons with the genetic tendency to mood disorder will be phenotypically well, some relatives who are well may also show the putative marker. The critical prediction would be that frank illness should not be transmitted without the marker. If some ill persons in a pedigree show the marker and others do not, the illness can clearly be transmitted without the marker.

Much of the clinical investigation of affective disorder has centered on state-dependent phenomena, changes that occur within an individual while the individual is ill compared with when the individual is well or that occur when pharmacologic manipulations result in an improvement or worsening of the disorder. Phenomena that are demonstrable only in the presence of active illness have limited usefulness in the genetic investigation of an illness with incomplete penetrance. For example, if a urinary metabolite is decreased only during episodes of illness, it is theoretically impossible to determine whether well relatives or controls would have the same marker. To increase genetic understanding based on comparisons of ill and well relatives, the most valuable two findings will be those abnormalities that do not change from the ill to the well state or those abnormalities that can be unmasked in the well state, such as by pharmacologic challenge.

Stable characteristics that have been examined in the hope of identifying a marker include measures of monoamine metabolism (enzyme and metabolites), measures of cation transport, neuroendocrine variables, responses to pharmacologic stimuli, and the brain protein Pc 1 Duarte.

Monoamine Enzymes and Metabolites

The data on dopamine-β-hydroxylase (DBH) have been summarized by the author and his colleagues (Gershon et al., 1977b) and more recently by Weinshilboum (1979). DBH has been shown to have high heritability (Ross et al., 1973; Levitt and Mendlewicz, 1975; Winter et al., 1978). Segregation analysis has confirmed single-gene transmission (Elston et al., 1979). Data from the author's group suggest codominant inheritance, in which a heterozygote is phenotypically distinguishable from either homozygote (Gershon et al., 1980; Goldin et al., 1982; 1983). Summaries of data in patients and controls do not suggest that there is a difference in DBH levels, except in the study by Meltzer et al. (1976) in which DBH was decreased in psychotic unipolar patients. Unpublished data from the author's group do not confirm this. Levitt (Levitt and Mendlewicz, 1975; Levitt et al., 1976) and the author's group (Gershon et al., 1980) tested for segregation of DBH with affective illness and did not find it.

Red blood cell catechol-O-methyltransferase (COMT) has high heritability (Winter et al., 1978). Data of the author's group on thirty families shows single-gene inheritance of COMT with codominant transmission most likely (Gershon et al., 1982). COMT was found to be different in patients and controls in several studies, but unchanged in others. The author and Jonas reported that COMT segregates with affective illness (Gershon and Jonas, 1975), but more recently the author and his colleagues found no differences between patients and controls (Gershon et al., 1979a). Using a more powerful test of segregation with illness in this study, it was clear that COMT and illness segregated independently.

Two forms of monoamine oxidase (MAO) have been found. MAO-A is predominant in fibroblasts (Groshong et al., 1977; 1978). MAO-B is found in platelets (Collins and Sandler, 1971; Edwards and Chang, 1975; Donnelly and Murphy, 1976) and in primate brain (Murphy et al., 1979). MAO activity in platelets is heritable (Nies et al., 1974; Winter et al., 1978). The data of the author's group show it to be familial (Gershon et al., 1980), but it does not fit any single-gene hypothesis. Platelet MAO has been reported decreased in bipolar patients by some but not all investigators (see review in Gershon et al., 1977b; Edwards et al., 1978; Takahashi, 1977; Gershon et al., 1977a). Pandey et al. (1979b) report that low MAO sorts with illness in bipolar and alcoholic relatives of bipolar probands. The author and his colleagues have reported data which indicate that in their sample low MAO does not sort with affective illness in relatives of low-MAO probands (Gershon et al., 1979b). The differences between these studies remain to be explained.

CNS metabolites of serotonin and dopamine are measurable in CSF without interference from the peripheral sources of these metabolites. 5-Hydroxyindoleacetic acid (5-HIAA), the principal metabolite of serotonin in CSF, was bimodally distributed in two series of depressed patients (Asberg et al., 1976; Van Praag and Korff, 1971). A substantial proportion of depressed patients studied have reduced 5-HIAA in CSF, although not all studies show significant patient-control differences, as reviewed elsewhere (Gershon et al., 1977a). Sedvall et al. (1980) have demonstrated a significant correlation in CSF 5-HIAA between twins, suggesting genetic control. Van Praag and de Haan (1979) reported that in the majority of patients with reduced 5-HIAA, the reduced level persists after recovery. When they compared family history of patients with persistent reduced 5-HIAA with the family histories of patients with normal 5-HIAA, they found higher depressive admissions in relatives of the reduced 5-HIAA group. These data are compatible with a genetically distinct subgroup of affective patients defined by reduced central serotonin turnover. But the evidence is incomplete, since there are no data on segregation of 5-HIAA and illness in relatives. Moreover, the family study data are presented without diagnostic definitions or estimates of the number of relatives at risk.

Cation Transport Parameters

Alterations in cell membranes have been posited as a source of vulnerability to affective disorder (Mendels and Frazer, 1973; Hokin-Neaverson et al., 1974).

For an individual treated with a constant dose of lithium, the ratio of lithium inside the red cell to that outside is generally a stable characteristic of an individual over time (Carroll and Feinberg, 1977; Dunner et al., 1978). It may be measured *in vivo* or *in vitro*, so that individuals not treated with lithium may have an assessment of their ratio by incubating a sample of red cells in a lithium-containing solution, and there is a high correlation between these measurements (Pandey et al., 1979a).

Dorus et al. (1974; 1975; in press) have demonstrated genetic control of the ratio. Several studies have directly related the ratio to the genetics of affective disorder. Rybakowski (1977) found a higher ratio in bipolar patients with a family history of affective disorders than in those without such a history. This may, however, relate to better compliance in those with a positive family history. Pandey et al. (1977) reported lower phloretin-sensitive lithium-Na counterflow, and thus a high lithium ratio, in a manic patient and in his well father and several well siblings.

Dorus et al. (1979b) reported nonindependent assortment of high lithium ratio and affective disorder within pedigrees. They studied 66 first-degree relatives of 31 bipolar I patients. None of the relatives were taking any medication regularly, and they were free of whatever intermittent medications they may have been taking for one week. Dorus et al. found that the relatives with a history of major affective illness or minor affective illness had higher ratios than relatives with no history. (Means for the three groups were 0.17 ± 0.05, 0.18 ± 0.04, and 0.15 ± 0.03.) Affected relatives had a significantly higher ratio than a group of 291 normal controls without a family history (0.15 ± 0.04), whereas the unaffected relatives were not different from controls. Their category of major affective disorder included unipolar illness, mania, bipolar I illness or alcoholism, bipolar II illness, and schizoaffective illness. Nurnberger et al. (1982) have recently found that the Li^+ ratio is affected by previous treatment with lithium and that it stays elevated for three or more weeks, longer than had previously been thought. This may introduce an artifact into family studies of the lithium ratio.

In another study, Dorus et al. (1979a) used a two-variable strategy to assess the value of lithium ratio and platelet MAO together in predicting illness in relatives. In this study of 61 first-degree relatives, they did not report on psychotropic drug status, and they used the same diagnostic categories noted above. Dividing the group into four subgroups according to whether they were above or below the median value for the two biological variables, they found a nonrandom distribution ($\chi^2 = 9.61$; $p < .02$). Thirteen out of 13 individuals in the low-MAO, high-lithium-ratio subgroup were ill (one family accounted for 4 of these individuals). The ratio of affected to unaffected relatives was nearly 1:1 in the other three subgroups. Use of several independent heritable factors to predict illness is a promising strategy.

Duarte Protein

Comings (1979) reported experiments using a two-dimensional protein electrophoretic technique by which he identified a mutant protein, Pc 1 Duarte (Pc for perchloric acid extract) and found an increased frequency in brain specimens taken at autopsy from individuals with affective disorder, alcoholism, or both. In a group of 152 controls, 31.6 percent carried the abnormal protein, compared with 61.9 percent of a group of 42 depressed and alcoholic individuals and 72.7 percent of a group of 11 bipolar patients. Comings found no increased frequency of Duarte protein in samples from schizophrenic patients. In a group of 40 patients with multiple sclerosis, however, he found a 52.5 percent frequency, all heterozygotes, and he found associations in a small sample of brains from persons who died with subacute sclerosing panencephalitis and amyotrophic lateral sclerosis. All these illnesses are suspected of having a viral etiology. Comings suggested that Pc 1 Duarte may be a product of a single major gene involved in depressive disease, combining etiologically with environmental factors.

Extension of this finding into pedigree studies of living persons might appear to be impossible, since the protein is detectable only in brain, not in peripheral tissues. However, Comings (1981) has suggested that recombinant DNA techniques could be used to identify the gene for Pc 1 Duarte, since they would enable the detection of brain protein polymorphisms in DNA from lymphocytes and fibroblasts. This is one example of the clinical applicability of recombinant DNA technology in neurobiological genetics.

Critique of Current Vulnerability Marker Studies

Some criticisms of the current status of genetics in psychobiological clinical research are warranted. First, we have not yet formulated and tested a specific hypothesis of pathophysiology in the genetic transmission of vulnerability. Two important partial exceptions to this first criticism are the studies of Schuckit and Rayses (1979) on acetaldehyde production in relatives of alcoholics and the studies of Dorus et al. (1979a) on ion transport in manic-depressive illness. In their own work on the enzymes of monoamine metabolism in bipolar illness (Gershon et al., 1980), the author and his colleagues have made a complete test of the transmission in relation to enzyme activities according to this definition. But they have never explicitly formulated a hypothesis of pathophysiology that would be tested by enzyme activities. In any case, the results have been negative. Illness is transmitted independently of activities of each of the enzymes studied: erythrocyte COMT, platelet MAO, and plasma DBH.

A second criticism focuses on the paucity of clinical investigative interest in genetic variation among biological characteristics within a psychobiological framework. For example, genetic variation might exist in neurotransmitter receptors (manifested in affinity or number of receptors or in postreceptor events) or in neurobiological peptides (structural or quantitative variations). Many clinical biological variables, such as monoamine metabolites, could also be studied for genetic variation. Psychopharmacogenetic studies of variations in biological response (as opposed to variations in drug metabolism) could also be pursued. Such studies, however, have been unusual in both psychobiology and clinical genetic studies. Instead, the emphasis has been on extensive clinical epidemiologic-diagnostic studies in patients and relatives and much less on extensive studies of biological variables in patients and relatives or in the population as a whole.

A CLINICAL PERSPECTIVE ON GENETICS AND BIPOLAR ILLNESS

Prevention

In light of current knowledge, the possibilities for prevention are limited. We know that families of patients with bipolar illness have greatly increased risk for affective and related disorders compared with the rest of the population, but we cannot identify individuals at risk before the onset of illness. Nor can we identify any environmental manipulation, including genetic counseling, that would reduce this risk. Primary prevention, in the sense of decreasing the number of new cases of manifest disease, is therefore not within our current capabilities.

One exception to these generalizations is based on an unusual case seen several years ago at NIMH. A 22-year-old woman, the identical twin of a bipolar patient, asked if she should take lithium. After examination revealed no psychopathology, it was decided not to prescribe lithium. However, she and her husband were offered information on signs of incipient mania or depression. Within six months she developed mania, which was promptly treated with inpatient hospitalization. Since that time, the patient has had a very good response to lithium prophylaxis. In retrospect, it would have been well to consider the 65 percent risk (without age correction) to the identical twin of the bipolar patient. Since the risk would be closer to 100 percent with age correction, lithium treatment was perhaps indicated when this patient first sought consultation. In other classes of relatives, however, prophylactic lithium treatment would not seem justifiable, and to date no other primary prevention maneuver appears promising.

Secondary prevention of an illness in a population is the early recognition and treatment of cases as they arise, with the goal of reducing their morbidity. Here the family concentration of severe primary affective disorder offers an important opportunity for prevention. In a systematic study of first-degree relatives (parents, siblings, and offspring) and second-degree relatives (grandparents, aunts and uncles, and half-siblings) of patients with bipolar disorder, the author's group made extensive efforts to locate and examine all relatives. This included relatives at a considerable geographic distance from the patient and those who had little knowledge of or interaction with the patient. In the first-degree relatives, the author's group found the expected high incidence of affective disorders (comparable to their previous studies), which was considerably higher than the population prevalence. As Table 3 shows, one fifth of the relatives with diagnosed treatable affective disorder had never been treated. Since such persons constitute a

Table 3. Treated and Untreated Illness in First-Degree Relatives of 86 Bipolar I Patients

	Ill %	Alive and ill %	Alive and ill, untreated %	No information about treatment %
Affective disorders				
Bipolar I and bipolar II	5.9	6.1	1.2	0.2
Unipolar I	10.4	11.1	2.7	1.0
Minor depression	5.0	5.7	2.0	1.2
Cyclothymic disorder	2.1	2.8	1.0	0.5
Depressive personality	1.8	1.7	1.0	0.5
Behavioral disorders				
Sociopathy, drug abuse, alcoholism, sexual deviation	5.2	4.9	2.0	1.7
Minor emotional disorders				
Obsessive compulsive disorder, generalized anxiety disorder, panic disorder, Briquet's disorder, other psychiatric disorder without hospitalization	1.5	2.0	0.5	2.0
Major disorders				
Schizophrenia, schizoaffective disorder, unspecified functional psychosis, other psychiatric disorder with hospitalization	2.3	1.5	0.2	0.7

Note: There are 405 living and 105 dead first-degree relatives. Percentage ill not corrected for age.

Source: Gershon and Hamovit (1979).

population at very high risk for future episodes, they present an excellent opportunity for intervention.

Genetic Counseling

Generally, the onset of affective illness is in young adulthood. The needs for genetic counseling are therefore different from the needs in cases of disorders that are manifest as birth defects (Targum and Gershon, 1980). Incipient or possible future affective illness in a teenage or young adult relative of a patient is the most frequent concern of persons who seek genetic counseling. The next most frequent concern in relation to affective disorders is whether or not to have children. Patients and their spouses usually do not consider that the empirical risk for the disorder is prohibitively high (either before or after counseling), and they generally decide to reproduce. Except in the case of clinically unmanageable affective disorder, which makes the parental role impossible to assume, the author does not advise patients against having children. Since only 15 percent of the bipolar patients seen by the author and his group at NIMH have a bipolar parent, even from the most hardheaded primary prevention viewpoint such advice is not necessary.

From the practicing psychiatrist's point of view, genetic counseling is best subsumed within the psychotherapy. The first goal is a realistic and appropriate appreciation of the patient's own family history and of the risk to relatives. Second, one must offer the patient a means of coping with the anxiety and narcissistic injury that stem from the knowledge about genetic risk. Third, one must make appropriate plans to respond to the risk, including early treatment for relatives who are beginning to show signs of mood disorder.

How can one estimate the risk to the person? Generally the author and his group use the empirical risk estimates shown in Table 1, assuming that the estimates should be halved for each degree that the known ill relative is removed from the person seeking counseling. It is also most important to take a very careful family history, preferably from sources in addition to the person seeking counseling. Extensive multigeneration pedigrees are uncovered in a distinct minority of patients, as shown in Figure 1. In those cases, the risk should be considered greater than the general risk to siblings or offspring, and in each case the particular pedigree will need to be inspected and interpreted to give an estimate of risk.

A second clinical use of a known family history of a major affective disorder is to take a pharmacologically aggressive approach to a newly discovered illness, particularly a mild form of illness. For example, the author would treat moderate depression in a late adolescent child of a patient with bipolar illness as if it were a major affective disorder rather than treating it as if it were the ubiquitous developmental depressive crisis of late adolescence.

Finally in counseling we must consider the patient's spouse. A tendency for assortative mating or for persons with similar affective disorders to marry has been reported repeatedly (Negri et al., 1979). Whether this increases the genetic risks is not known, but it does give a peculiar quality to many of the marriages (Ablon et al., 1975). Among the NIMH inpatients, a majority of bipolar patients get divorced (Brodie and Leff, 1971). The divorce is often attributed to symptoms of the illness, usually mania. Occasionally the author has

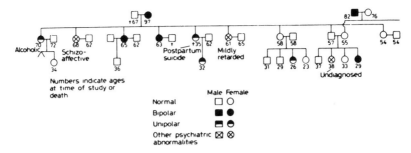

Figure 1. This pedigree of a large family in New England exemplifies several aspects of the affective disorders in addition to their tendency to run in families. Presence of both unipolar and bipolar disorders and a case of schizoaffective disorder suggests that these conditions are etiologically related. Major affective illness is present in each of three generations of this pedigree with both consanguinity and assortative mating. The two ancestral persons are distantly related (not illustrated for space reasons). Two well persons, each having a parent with bipolar manic depressive illness, have married (a form of assortative mating) and have two daughters who have had psychiatric hospitalization, one of them with bipolar illness. Adapted and reprinted by permission from Gershon (1979); artist: Albert Miller.

been confronted with blunt questions. "My fiancé is a manic-depressive. Should I marry him?" "My wife is a manic-depressive. Should we have children?" Answering these questions requires clinical skill and compassion. Recently the author and his colleagues gave a questionnaire to a group of married bipolar patients and their "well" spouses (Targum et al., 1981). The responses are worth recalling. One of the questions asked, "If you had known then what you know now, would you have married?" Nine out of ten of the bipolar patients said yes, but more than half of the spouses said no.

Chapter 27   # Depressive Disorders and the Emerging Field of Psychiatric Chemistry[†]
by Joseph J. Schildkraut, M.D., Alan F. Schatzberg, M.D., John J. Mooney, M.D., Paul J. Orsulak, Ph.D.

INTRODUCTION

The search for possible biological abnormalities in the depressive disorders received a major stimulus in the late 1950s when it was first established that specific pharmacological agents were effective in treating certain types of depressive disorders (Schildkraut, 1970). These drugs became useful tools for research into behavioral and biochemical neuropharmacology, and that research has led to fundamental discoveries concerning the neurobiology of the central nervous system.

[†]This work was supported in part by Grant No. MH 15413 from the National Institute of Mental Health. The authors wish to thank Mrs. Gladys Rege for her assistance in the preparation of this chapter.

The brain consists of billions of neurons that interact with each other through increasingly well-understood electrical and neurochemical processes. We now know that pharmacological agents or environmental stimuli ultimately exert their effects in the brain by altering the processes regulating neurotransmission, i.e., the communication within and between the neurons in the brain. When a neuron is stimulated, the nerve impulse or electrical action potential causes chemical neurotransmitters to be released from specialized regions at the neuronal ending which are in close proximity to another neuron. When neurotransmitters are released into the synaptic cleft (the space between the neurons) from the presynaptic neuron (the neuron leading into the synaptic cleft), they interact briefly with receptors on the postsynaptic neuron (the neuron leading away from the cleft). This interaction results either in electrical stimulation, which increases the likelihood of an action potential, or in electrical inhibition, which decreases the likelihood of an action potential, in the postsynaptic neuron. Neurobiologists have now identified many different neurochemical substances that act as neurotransmitters in the neuronal systems of the brain, and many other chemical substances that serve as neuromodulators and neuroregulators, producing subtle alterations in the processes of neurotransmission.

While it is now generally recognized that genetic disorders are expressed biochemically, it is less often recognized that environmental or psychological factors may also produce long-term neurochemical and neurophysiological changes that can in turn alter an individual's vulnerability to depressive episodes. Because of this, sharp distinctions cannot be drawn between genetically induced depressions and environmentally induced depressions, or between biological depressions and psychological depressions. To a greater or lesser degree, all of these factors are involved in virtually all cases of depressive disorders.

This chapter begins by reviewing briefly the development of neuropsychopharmacological and neuropsychoendocrinological knowledge about the depressive disorders. Following this, the authors describe in detail selected aspects of recent and clinically relevant research on the depressive disorders. Based on this material, the chapter concludes with a brief discussion of the emerging field of psychiatric chemistry.

AN OVERVIEW OF THE NEUROPSYCHOPHARMACOLOGY AND NEUROPSYCHOENDOCRINOLOGY OF THE DEPRESSIVE DISORDERS

Approximately 25 years ago, two major classes of antidepressant drugs, the monoamine oxidase inhibitors and the tricyclic antidepressants, were first introduced into psychiatry. Evidence soon began to suggest that these medications worked at least in part through their effects on brain catecholamines, which make up one of the many groups of chemical substances that function as neurotransmitters within the central nervous system. Of these catecholamines, norepinephrine appeared to be particularly important in the pathophysiology of certain types of depressive disorders. One of the two classes of antidepressants, the monoamine oxidase inhibitors, increased brain concentrations of norepinephrine by blocking its metabolism by the enzyme monoamine oxidase. Shortly thereafter, the tricyclic antidepressant imipramine was found to enhance the physiological effects of norepinephrine. At about the same time, reserpine (a drug which is used in the treatment of hypertension) was found to cause clinical depressions in some patients and to deplete catecholamines in the brain.

These and other data led to the formulation of the catecholamine hypothesis of affective disorders (Schildkraut, 1965). This hypothesis proposed that some depressive disorders may be associated with an absolute or relative deficiency of catecholamines, particularly norepinephrine, at functionally important synapses in the brain, whereas manias might be associated with an excess of such catecholamines. From the outset, the proponents of the hypothesis recognized that this focus on catecholamine metabolism was at best an oversimplification of extremely complex biological states and that abnormalities in many other neurotransmitter or neuromodulator systems, as well as endocrine changes and other biochemical abnormalities, were undoubtedly involved. Nonetheless, the initial formulation focused on the possibility that different subgroups of patients with depressive disorders might be characterized by differences in the metabolism of norepinephrine and in the physiology of noradrenergic (norepinephrine-containing) neuronal systems, including alterations in noradrenergic receptor sensitivity. Studies by many research groups subsequently provided data supporting this possibility.

In addition to studies related to norepinephrine metabolism in depressive disorders, studies of other neurotransmitters or neuroregulators in the brain have yielded major leads concerning the possible underlying pathophysiology of various subtypes of depressive disorders. Such studies have focused, for instance, on dopamine, which is also a catecholamine, and serotonin, which is an indoleamine (Schildkraut, 1970; Garver and Davis, 1979).

During the last decade, another hypothesis that has received considerable attention suggested that depressive disorders could be dichotomized into "noradrenergic" or "serotonergic" depressions on the basis of pretreatment biochemical data and differential responses to various tricyclic antidepressant drugs (Maas, 1975). However, this notion, which was based in part on the differing effects of various tricyclic antidepressant drugs on the inhibition of norepinephrine and serotonin uptake, no longer seems viable. Recent findings from studies of depressed patients (Schatzberg et al., 1982; Maas et al., 1982) and data concerning the complex neuropharmacological effects of antidepressant drugs (Charney et al., 1981) render the hypothesis untenable. In this context, an early review of the catecholamine hypothesis of affective disorders is of some historical interest. The review specifically cautioned against attempts to separate depressions on the basis of simple dichotomies and emphasized the broad clinical and biological heterogeneity of these disorders (Schildkraut, 1965).

Of considerable interest, too, are the recent studies that suggest an important role for acetylcholine in the pathophysiology of at least certain types of depressive disorders (Janowsky et al., 1972; Garver and Davis, 1979). Drugs which stimulate acetylcholinergic activity have been found to induce depressions in control subjects and to exacerbate depressions in depressed patients, as well as to decrease manias in patients during manic episodes. Many of the commonly prescribed antidepressant drugs of course have anticholinergic properties, and their anticholinergic effects have long been known to be responsible for some of their side effects (such as dry mouth and constipation). Only recently, however, has it been recognized that in some depressed patients the anticholinergic effects of antidepressant drugs may also be important in their antidepressant effects (Schildkraut et al., 1981; Kasper et al., 1981).

Neurotransmitters interact with specific receptors in order to exert their effects on neurotransmission. Recent studies have shown that alterations in the biochemical and physiological properties of these receptors may be involved in the mechanisms of action of many antidepressant drugs (Charney et al., 1981), and that abnormalities in these receptors may also be involved in the pathophysiology of depressive disorders. These possibilities are currently under active investigation in a number of laboratories throughout the world.

In recent years it has been well documented that many patients with depressive disorders show abnormalities in various endocrine hormone systems (Rubin and Marder, 1983). A major finding, which has been replicated extensively, is that secretion of the adrenal hormone cortisol is significantly increased in certain depressed patients and that the normal circadian (daily) rhythm of cortisol secretion is abnormal in some depressed patients. In normal subjects, administration of the drug dexamethasone suppresses cortisol secretion. This observation forms the basis of the dexamethasone suppression test, which is increasingly being used by psychiatrists, since certain depressed patients do not show a normal suppression of cortisol secretion after administration of dexamethasone (Carroll et al., 1981). Secretion of cortisol by the adrenal gland is controlled in part by a hormone secreted by the pituitary gland, which is in turn controlled by a releasing factor that derives from the hypothalamus. The neurotransmitters norepinephrine, serotonin, and acetylcholine all appear to be involved in the regulation of this hypothalamic-pituitary-adrenocortical (HPA) endocrine axis.

In addition to the HPA axis abnormalities observed in depressed patients, the hypothalamic-pituitary-thyroid axis has shown functional abnormalities in some depressed patients (Kirkegaard, 1981; Gold et al., 1981; Whybrow and Prange, 1981). Abnormalities in the secretion of growth hormone have also been observed in depressions (Rubin and Marder, 1983).

The pathophysiology of depressive disorders is clearly not restricted to abnormalities in brain function. Rather, the depressive disorders must be conceptualized as complex neuro-endocrinologic-metabolic disorders that involve many different organ systems throughout the body. On this basis, it seems reasonable to predict that during the course of this decade the specialized clinical laboratory tests which are now starting to be used in psychiatry will play an increasingly important role in the diagnostic evaluation and treatment of patients with depressive disorders.

URINARY MHPG LEVELS

Since the late 1960s, it has been acknowledged that urinary 3-methoxy-4-hydroxyphenylglycol (MHPG) is a major metabolite of norepinephrine (NE) originating in the brain (Maas and Landis, 1968; Schanberg et al., 1968a; 1968b). Urinary MHPG may also derive in part from the peripheral sympathetic nervous system, and the fraction of urinary MHPG deriving from NE originating in the brain remains uncertain (Maas et al., 1979; Blombery et al., 1980; Mardh et al., 1981). Nonetheless, many investigators have explored the possibility that measuring urinary MHPG levels might be of value in elucidating the pathophysiology of depressions and in discriminating among biologically meaningful and therapeutically relevant subgroups of depressive disorders.

In longitudinal studies of patients with naturally occurring or amphetamine-induced bipolar manic-depressive episodes, many investigators have found that urinary MHPG levels were lower during periods of depression and higher during periods of mania or hypomania than during periods of remission (Greenspan et al., 1970; Schildkraut et al., 1971; Schildkraut et al., 1972; Watson et al., 1972; Bond et al., 1972; 1975; DeLeon-Jones et al., 1973; Post et al., 1977). All depressed patients, however, do not excrete comparably low levels of MHPG (Maas et al., 1968; 1972). Consequently, a number of investigators have explored the possibility that urinary levels of MHPG, as well as other catecholamine metabolites, might provide a biochemical basis for differentiating among the depressive disorders.

In the initial reports, urinary MHPG levels were significantly lower in patients with bipolar manic-depressive depressions than in patients with unipolar nonendogenous chronic characterological depressions (Schildkraut et al., 1973a; 1973b). The initial finding of reduced urinary MHPG levels in patients with bipolar manic-depressive depressions was subsequently confirmed by a number of studies (Maas et al., 1973; DeLeon-Jones et al., 1975; Goodwin and Post, 1975; Garfinkel et al., 1977; Schildkraut et al., 1978a; 1978c; Goodwin and Potter, 1979; Beckmann and Goodwin, 1980; Edwards et al., 1980). Of particular interest among these studies, Garfinkel et al. (1977) found that when the peripheral contribution to urinary MHPG was reduced with carbidopa, a decarboxylase inhibitor that does not cross the blood-brain barrier, the differences in urinary MHPG levels in depressed bipolar manic-depressives and control subjects became more pronounced and statistically significant.

In contrast, no differences were found in the urinary 3-methoxy-4-hydroxymandelic acid (VMA) levels of patients with unipolar and bipolar depressions (Schildkraut et al., 1978c; Schatzberg et al., 1982). This is an important finding, since some researchers have reported that circulating MHPG may be converted to VMA (Blombery et al., 1980; Mardh et al., 1981). These reports in turn raised questions concerning the specific value of urinary MHPG (e.g., in contrast to VMA) as an index of norepinephrine metabolism in the brain or as a biochemical marker in studies of depressed patients (Linnoila et al., 1982).

In various studies of patients with unipolar depressions, low (DeLeon-Jones et al., 1975; Maas, 1978; Taube et al., 1978; Casper et al., 1977), normal (Goodwin and Post, 1975; Goodwin and Potter, 1979; Beckmann and Goodwin, 1980), or high (Garfinkel et al., 1979) urinary MHPG levels have been reported. Diagnostic heterogeneity may account for these differences. Previously reported findings from the authors' laboratory (Schildkraut et al., 1978c) revealed a wide range of urinary MHPG levels in patients with unipolar depressive disorders, and these findings have been confirmed and extended in the more recent investigations at the laboratory. In the earlier study, a series of 16 patients with unipolar endogenous depressions had a mean urinary MHPG value of 1,950 μg/24 hours (Schildkraut et al., 1978c). In a subsequent study of an enlarged sample of 70 patients (Schatzberg et al., 1982), 50 of the 70 had unipolar depressions. Of the 50, 26 had urinary MHPG levels higher than 1,950 μg/24 hours. Twenty of the 70 patients had bipolar manic-depressive or schizoaffective depressions, identified according to clinical criteria of the authors' group (Schildkraut et al., 1978c). Only 3 of the 20 had MHPG levels higher than 1,950 μg/24 hours ($\chi^2 = 6.6$; $p < .25$). A scatter plot of MHPG levels for the whole series of patients revealed a natural break in MHPG levels around 2,500 μg/24 hours, suggesting the possible existence of a subgroup of unipolar depressions with MHPG levels higher than 2,500 μg/24 hours. For example, in this series, 17 of 50 patients with unipolar depressions had urinary MHPG levels higher than 2,500 μg/24 hours, while only 1 of the 20 patients with bipolar manic-depressive or schizoaffective depressions had an MHPG level higher than 2,500 μg/24 hours ($\chi^2 = 4.9$; $p < .05$).

These data further substantiate the biochemical heterogeneity of unipolar depressions. As the data demonstrate, some patients have low MHPG levels (comparable to values seen in the bipolar manic-depressive or schizoaffective depressions), while others have higher MHPG levels (sometimes higher than control values), and still others have MHPG levels in an intermediate range. However, it should be stressed that urinary MHPG levels in most depressed patients (including unipolar, bipolar, and schizoaffective depressions) fall within the broad range of values observed in normal control subjects (Hollister et al., 1978; Schatzberg et al., 1982). Thus, while urinary MHPG levels may help to differentiate among subtypes of depressive disorders once a clinical diagnosis of depression has been made, urinary MHPG levels cannot be used to make a diagnosis of depression per se.

In support of these findings, data on the distribution of urinary MHPG levels in a series of 102 patients with unipolar major depressive disorders revealed a cluster of patients with urinary MHPG levels above 2,500 μg/24 hours, in addition to clusters with lower MHPG levels (Schildkraut et al., 1982). Moreover, the distribution of pretreatment urinary MHPG levels in a study of an independent series of more than 200 patients with unipolar major depressive disorders revealed a similar pattern. This collaborative multicenter study is examining urinary MHPG levels as predictors of responses to oxaprotiline (BA49802), amitriptyline, or placebo and is being coordinated by Mark Roffman of Ciba-Geigy in conjunction with the authors' laboratory. A cluster of depressed patients has been observed with urinary MHPG levels above 2,500 μg/24 hours. In contrast, a comparable discrete clustering (i.e., peaking) of values above 2,500 μg/24 hours, with relatively few values between 2,300 and 2,500 μg/24 hours, was not observed in the urinary MHPG levels of more than 100 control subjects.

The existence of a biologically meaningful subgroup of unipolar depressions with elevated urinary MHPG levels is also supported by the findings of a study by the authors' research group (Rosenbaum et al., in press). This study of patients with very severe unipolar depressions revealed a subgroup with very high urinary MHPG levels (above 2,500 μg/24 hours) and also very high levels of urinary free cortisol (UFC) (above 200 μg/24 hours). To rule out the possibility that the high UFC and urinary MHPG levels observed in this series of severely depressed patients might be secondary to anxiety, the authors' group also studied urinary MHPG and UFC levels in patients with moderate to severe anxiety states, and they did not observe comparably elevated UFC levels (above 200 μg/24 hours) in these patients. The very high UFC levels observed in the series of severely depressed patients may be related to the severity of the depression, since preliminary data from a study of UFC levels in patients with less severe depressions revealed few patients with markedly elevated UFC levels (Rosenbaum et al., 1981).

Discussion

One explanation for the existence of a subgroup of severely depressed patients with high urinary MHPG levels and markedly elevated UFC levels could be that the high urinary MHPG and UFC levels may occur in these patients secondary to an increase in cholinergic activity. This possibility is consistent with the hypothesis that central cholinergic factors may play a role in the etiology of depressive disorders (Janowsky et al., 1972; Sitaram and Gillin, 1980; Risch et al., 1981a), and it is particularly intriguing in view of four other sets of findings related to physostigmine, an anticholinesterase. (1) Physostigmine and other pharmacological agents which increase brain cholinergic activity have been found to exacerbate depressive symptoms in depressed patients (Janowsky et al., 1972; Garver and Davis, 1979) and to induce depressive symptoms in normal controls (Risch et al., 1980). (2) Physostigmine also produces an increase in plasma cortisol levels in normal controls (Risch et al., 1980). (3) Physostigmine can also overcome suppression of the hypothalamic-pituitary-adrenocortical axis by dexamethasone in normal subjects, thereby mimicking the abnormal escape from dexamethasone suppression seen in some patients who show cortisol hypersecretion (Carroll et al., 1980). (4) Physostigmine also has been found to produce an increase in CSF levels of MHPG in normal subjects (Davis et al., 1977). Thus, the markedly elevated UFC levels observed in some patients with severe unipolar depressive disorders could result from an increase in cholinergic activity, and the elevated urinary MHPG levels in these patients could represent a secondary noradrenergic response to such cholinergic hyperactivity. This formulation suggests that the anticholinergic effects of certain antidepressant drugs may in fact contribute to their antidepressant effects in patients with this subtype of depressive disorder.

The findings of recent studies therefore further substantiate the biochemical heterogeneity of the unipolar depressive disorders, and they suggest that at least three subtypes of unipolar depressions can be discriminated on the basis of differences in urinary MHPG levels. Subtype I, with low pretreatment urinary MHPG levels, may have low NE output because of a decrease in NE synthesis or because of a decrease in the release of NE from noradrenergic neurons. In contrast, Subtype II, with intermediate urinary MHPG levels, may have normal NE output but have abnormalities in other biochemical systems. And Subtype III, with high urinary MHPG levels, may have high NE output in response to alterations in noradrenergic receptors and/or in response to an increase in cholinergic activity, as described above. The further studies necessary to confirm these findings are currently in progress and are exploring the possible pathophysiological abnormalities that may be associated with these subtypes of unipolar depressive disorders.

URINARY CATECHOLAMINES AND METABOLITES: MULTIVARIATE ANALYSES

Construction and Validation of the Model

In the early studies of the authors' laboratory (Schildkraut et al., 1978c), MHPG was the only catecholamine metabolite to show a pronounced difference in values between bipolar, manic-depressive depressions and unipolar nonendogenous depressions of the chronic characterological type. To explore the possibility that NE and other catecholamine metabolites, including VMA, normetanephrine (NMN), and meta-nephrine (MN), might provide further information that would aid in differentiating among subtypes of depressions, the authors' group used a multivariate discriminant function analysis (Schildkraut et al., 1978a). Applied to data on urinary catecholamines and metabolites, the stepwise analysis generated an empirically derived equation that discriminated even more precisely than urinary MHPG alone between bipolar manic-depressive and unipolar nonendogenous (chronic characterological) depressions. In generating this equation, a metric was established so that low scores were related to patients with bipolar manic-depressive depressions, whereas high scores were related to patients with unipolar nonendogenous depressions. The group then obtained preliminary validation of the equation in a sample of patients whose data had not been used in deriving the equation (Schildkraut et al., 1978a). The discrimination equation was designed to compute a Depression-type (D-type) score and had the form:

$$\text{D-type score} = C_1(\text{MHPG}) - C_2(\text{VMA}) + C_3(\text{NE})$$
$$- C_4 \frac{(\text{NMN} + \text{MN})}{\text{VMA}} + C_0$$

The equation was generated mathematically to provide the best least-squares fit of the data, and the terms were not selected by the investigators. Nonetheless, the inclusion of VMA, as well as other urinary catecholamines and metabolites (of peripheral origin), may be correcting for that fraction of urinary MHPG that comes from peripheral sources rather than from the brain (Schildkraut et al., 1978a).

To evaluate the contribution of each of the terms in this four-term discrimination equation, the group then derived separate discrimination equations based on one, two, and three, as well as on four terms, using the biochemical data obtained from the initial series of patients with bipolar manic-depressive and unipolar nonendogenous depressions (Schildkraut et al., 1978a). D-type scores based on these equations were then generated for a series of depressed patients in the validation sample whose biochemical data had not been used to derive the equations.

D-type scores for the patients with bipolar manic-depressive and schizoaffective depressions were then compared with the scores for patients with unipolar nonendogenous depressions, using the one-, two-, three-, and four-term discrimination equations. The one-term equation, based on MHPG alone, tended to separate these groups with some overlap. The two-term equation, based on MHPG and VMA, provided a better discrimination between the groups, but some overlap remained. The three-term equation, based on MHPG, VMA, and NE, removed all overlap between the two groups. And the four-term equation, based on MHPG, VMA, NE, and $\dfrac{NMN + MN}{VMA}$, improved on the discrimination by providing a very wide separation of the D-type scores in these two groups without any overlap. (Recall that the patient groups included only patients from the validation sample, not those whose biochemical data had been used to derive the equations.)

Applications of the Model

Subsequently the authors' laboratory has obtained D-type scores on more than eighty depressed patients whose data were neither used in the original derivation of the equation nor in its preliminary validation. In the light of their finding that patients with unipolar depressive disorders appear to be biochemically heterogeneous with respect to urinary MHPG levels, the authors' group was particularly interested in the distribution of D-type scores in the newly studied patients with "unipolar" depressions. (Patients were diagnosed according to the authors' system of classification on the basis of clinical histories and presenting signs and symptoms [Schildkraut et al., 1978c].) Recent analyses of these data showed that the D-type scores computed with the original D-type equation and with the previously derived coefficients and constant segregated the new patients with unipolar depressions into two widely separated groupings. One group had D-type scores less than 0.5, in the range of values comparable to the range previously observed in bipolar manic-depressive depressions (Schildkraut et al., 1978a). The group of these patients with unipolar depressions had considerably higher D-type scores.

A similar separation of depressed patients with D-type scores less than 0.5 was observed in patients with nonschizotypal unipolar major depressive disorders diagnosed according to the RDC (Spitzer et al., 1978). Analysis of these data showed that this separation was not evident when MHPG levels alone were examined., i.e., when only the scores on the one-term (MHPG) D-type equation were examined. But scores on the four-term D-type equation clearly delineated a cluster of patients with low D-type scores (under 0.5). These analyses also showed that all but one of the patients with urinary MHPG levels above 2,500 $\mu g/24$ hours had D-type scores over 0.9.

On the basis of earlier findings, the authors' group had hypothesized that low D-type scores in patients with so-called unipolar depressions might help identify those patients who had latent bipolar disorders, even before their first clinical episode of mania or hypomania. Pilot follow-up data have focused on patients who had an initial diagnosis of unipolar depression and low D-type scores (in the range usually seen in bipolar manic-depressive depressions) when they were initially studied. Consistent with the hypothesis, a number of these patients went on to develop their first manic, hypomanic, or schizoaffective psychotic episodes several months to several years after their biochemical studies were completed. These findings do suggest that low D-type scores can predict subsequent occurrences of manic or maniclike episodes even in the absence of a history of prior manic episodes.

Relatively few patients with typical bipolar manic-depressive depressions could be included in the recent studies, since most patients with this diagnosis now receive maintenance lithium treatment, and the treatment could not ethically be discontinued in order to conduct the biochemical studies. However, many of the patients in the new group of 80 had depressive disorders that could not be assigned unambiguously to one of the diagnostic categories in the laboratory's classification system. Usually such patients had clinical features that suggested the possibility of a bipolar disorder or a schizophrenia-related disorder with chronic asocial, eccentric, or bizarre behavior. The distribution of D-type scores in 37 patients with diagnostically unclassifiable depressions was significantly different from that observed in patients with unipolar depressions. Moreover, in contrast to the findings in patients with unipolar depressions, the D-type scores in these diagnostically unclassifiable depressions were not separated into discrete clusters.

With regard to these diagnostically unclassifiable depressive disorders, the authors were particularly interested in exploring the hypothesis that patients with low D-type scores would show clinical features suggesting a bipolar disorder, even when the clinical diagnosis of a bipolar disorder could not definitely be made. In support of this hypothesis, they found that of the 8 diagnostically unclassifiable depressed patients with the lowest D-type scores, 7 met the criteria for at least a probable bipolar disorder in the authors' own classification system and would qualify for at least a probable bipolar I or bipolar II diagnosis according to the RDC. In contrast, of the 29 remaining patients with diagnostically unclassifiable depressions, only 7 showed comparable evidence for bipolarity ($\chi^2 = 8.2$; $p < .01$).

To examine the unclassifiable groups further, the authors' laboratory applied the separate equations to the entire group of patients with unclassifiable depressions. They used one term (MHPG), two terms (MHPG and VMA), and three terms (MHPG, VMA, and NE), as well as the four-term discrimination equation. A graphic plot revealed that with the addition of each successive term the D-type scores of patients who did not meet the diagnostic criteria for probable bipolar disorders gradually shifted upward. However, only the four-term D-type equation identified a discrete subgroup of patients with low D-type scores and with probable bipolar disorders.

In regard to its possible pathophysiological implications, several years ago the authors' group suggested that the fourth term $\left(\text{the ratio } \dfrac{NMN + MN}{VMA}\right)$ might be inversely related to monoamine oxidase (MAO) activity, since the O-methylated metabolites NMN and MN could be converted to VMA by deamination (Schildkraut et al., 1978a). Indeed, they recently documented such an inverse correlation between the ratio $\dfrac{NMN + MN}{VMA}$ and platelet MAO activity based on concurrent measurements in a series of ninety patients ($r = -.29$; $p < .005$). This finding confirms that the fourth term of the D-type equation is related to platelet MAO activity. In addition, the correlation, although modest, suggests that measuring platelet MAO activity may provide functionally relevant information with respect to mono-amine metabolism, since it relates logically to a ratio of levels of nondeaminated to deaminated urinary catecholamine metabolites.

PLATELET MAO ACTIVITY

Initial studies of Nies et al. (1971) showed increased MAO activity in a heterogeneous group of depressed patients (most of whom had unipolar depressions), and those of Murphy and Weiss (1972) showed decreased platelet MAO activity in bipolar depressions. Since then, many investigators have examined platelet MAO activity in patients with depressive disorders (Nies et al., 1974; Landowski et al., 1975; Takahashi and Karasawa, 1975; Belmaker et al., 1976; Leckman et al., 1977; Sullivan et al., 1977; Edwards et al., 1978; Schildkraut et al., 1978b; Mann, 1979; Davidson et al., 1980; White et al., 1980; Gottfries et al., 1980; Fieve et al., 1980; Honecker et al., 1981; Reveley et al., 1981). This literature has recently been reviewed by Sandler et al. (1981). In recent studies of unipolar depressions, some investigators (Landowski et al., 1975; Mann, 1979) have reported an increase in platelet MAO activity in unipolar endogenous depressions, whereas other investigators (Davidson et al., 1980; White et al., 1980) have found increased MAO activity in nonendogenous depressions. Since the researchers used different criteria for the diagnosis of endogenous and nonendogenous depressions and used different methods to deter-mine platelet MAO activity, it is not possible to clarify these differences at the present time.

In a recent study, Gudeman et al. (1982) examined platelet MAO activity in relation to clinical signs and symptoms in a series of patients with unipolar depressions. Confirming Mann's (1979) earlier findings, they found a statistically significant and positive correlation between platelet MAO activity and severity of depression as measured by the Hamilton Depression Rating Scale. They also obtained signifi-cant positive correlations between platelet MAO activity and specific clinical signs and symptoms in the spheres of depression, psychic anxiety, and somatic complaints. The clinical items that correlated with platelet MAO activity corresponded to the symptoms that other investigators have found to be associated with favorable responses to treatment with MAO inhibitors (Tyrer, 1976).

Previous studies of patients with depressive disorders reported high platelet MAO activity in many patients with schizophrenia-related depressions characterized by chronic asocial behavior (Orsulak et al., 1978). Adler et al. (1980) recently found a positive correlation between platelet MAO activity and social introversion in a series of male psychiatric patients. A number of research groups have found an association of high platelet MAO activity with social introversion or asociality and low platelet MAO activity with social extraversion or sensation seeking in normal control subjects and psychiatric patients. These findings have been briefly summarized in a recent paper (Gattaz and Beckmann, 1981).

Additional studies are therefore needed and are in progress to determine whether differences in these clinical (psychometric) variables may help to account for the differences in platelet MAO activity that have been observed in these variously defined subgroups of depres-sions. Further research is also required to examine and compare the kinetic parameters (and other properties) of platelet mitochondrial

MAO obtained from patients with various subtypes of depressive disorders and from control subjects.

URINARY MHPG LEVELS AS PREDICTORS OF ANTIDEPRESSANT DRUG RESPONSES

Studies from a number of laboratories have indicated that pretreatment levels of urinary MHPG may aid in predicting responses to certain tricyclic and tetracyclic antidepressant drugs. Specifically, depressed patients with "low" pretreatment urinary MHPG levels have been found to respond more favorably than patients with "high" levels to imipramine (Maas et al., 1972; Beckmann and Goodwin, 1975; Steinbook et al., 1979; Cobbin et al., 1979; Rosenbaum et al., 1980; Schatzberg et al., 1980–1981; Maas et al., 1982), to desipramine (Maas et al., 1972), to nortriptyline (Hollister et al., 1980), or to maprotiline (Rosenbaum et al., 1980; Schatzberg et al., 1981; Gaertner et al., 1982). In contrast, some studies have found that depressed patients with "high" pretreatment levels of urinary MHPG respond more favorably to treatment with amitriptyline than do patients with lower MHPG levels (Schildkraut, 1973; Beckmann and Goodwin, 1975; Cobbin et al., 1979; Modai et al., 1979; Gaertner et al., 1982). But this has not been observed in all studies (Sacchetti et al., 1979; Coppen et al., 1979; Spiker et al., 1980; Maas et al., 1982; Mark Roffman, personal communication). Clearly, further research is required to account for the differences in these findings. Nevertheless, the findings of these studies do point to differences between amitriptyline and imipramine. While many studies have shown that "low" pretreatment urinary MHPG levels predict more favorable responses to imipramine, none of the studies of amitriptyline have had such a finding.

Recently published prospective studies from the authors' group have confirmed that patients with relatively low urinary MHPG levels (at or below 1,950 μg/24 hours) respond more favorably to treatment with imipramine or maprotiline than do patients with higher MHPG levels (Schatzberg et al., 1980–1981; Schatzberg et al., 1981). The findings reported earlier in the chapter suggested that at least three subtypes of unipolar depressive disorders may be discriminated on the basis of differences in pretreatment urinary MHPG levels (Schatzberg et al., 1982). Thus, the authors' group combined the data from the two studies of pretreatment urinary MHPG levels as predictors of responses to imipramine and maprotiline and thereby obtained a large enough series of patients to compare treatment responses in the three subtypes of unipolar depressive disorders. While further studies in a larger series of patients will be required for confirmation and are currently in progress, findings to date suggest that depressed patients with elevated MHPG levels (above 2,500 μg/24 hours) may be more responsive to treatment with imipramine or maprotiline than patients with intermediate MHPG levels (1,951 to 2,500 μg/24 hours). Neither group, however, is as responsive to these drugs as are patients with low pretreatment urinary MHPG levels (at or below 1,950 μg/24 hours). Moreover, as described in a recently published paper (Schatzberg et al., 1981), the authors' group found that although patients with low pretreatment urinary MHPG levels responded rapidly to relatively low doses of maprotiline, the patients with higher MHPG levels who responded to maprotiline required significantly higher doses and longer periods of drug administration.

In contrast to these findings with imipramine and maprotiline, preliminary analysis from a multicenter collaborative study (Roffman et al., 1982) has revealed an unexpected finding. Patients with intermediate urinary MHPG levels responded more favorably to treatment with oxaprotiline than did patients with low or high MHPG levels. Moreover, among all the patients with intermediate urinary MHPG levels, those treated with oxaprotiline responded more favorably than those treated with amitriptyline or placebo. While pretreatment urinary MHPG levels provided a predictor of responses to oxaprotiline, pretreatment urinary MHPG levels did not appear in this study to predict responses to placebo or amitriptyline (maximum dose 150 mg/day).

Complex effects on noradrenergic, dopaminergic, and other neurotransmitter systems, including alterations in various indices of presynaptic and postsynaptic receptor functions, are observed after chronic administration of various antidepressant drugs (Sulser et al., 1978; Charney et al., 1981; Waldmeier 1981). This suggests that empirical trials will be required to assess the value of urinary MHPG levels, or of any other biochemical measure, as clinically useful predictors of responses to a specific antidepressant drug. For example, patients with normal or high urinary MHPG levels who show suppression of cortisol in response to dexamethasone reportedly respond favorably to treatment with mianserin, whereas patients with low urinary MHPG levels whose cortisol secretion is not suppressed by dexamethasone do not respond to mianserin (Cobbin et al., 1981).

MONOAMINERGIC RECEPTORS AND RELATED MEASURES

Several authors have proposed that patients with affective disorders may show alterations in the sensitivity of one or another type of monoaminergic receptor (Schildkraut, 1965; Bunney et al., 1977; Cohen et al., 1980). As noted above, many antidepressant drugs have been found after chronic treatment to alter the sensitivity of various neurotransmitter or neuromodulator receptors in the brain (Sulser et al., 1978; Segawa et al., 1979; Peroutka and Snyder, 1980; Maggi et al., 1980; Enna and Kendall, 1981; Waldmeier, 1981; Charney et al., 1981). These changes in receptor function coincide with the time course of clinical improvement during antidepressant therapy. Pharmacological challenges that produce peripheral effects such as changes in blood pressure and neuroendocrine responses such as release of cortisol or growth hormone, which are under central control mechanisms, have been undertaken to clarify both the central noradrenergic receptor function (Charney et al., 1981; Siever et al., 1981) and the relationships between central cholinergic, noradrenergic, and other neurotransmitter or neuromodulator systems (Risch et al., 1981a; 1981b; 1981c). These results suggest that alterations in receptor sensitivity may play a role both in the pathophysiology of the depressive disorders and in the mechanisms of action of various antidepressant drugs.

Adrenergic receptors on human blood cells have been suggested as a readily available source of material for the study of adrenergic receptors in psychiatric patients (Bunney and Murphy, 1975). β-Adrenergic receptors have been identified on leukocytes (Scott, 1970; Williams et al., 1976). One group of investigators (Extein et al., 1979) found the specific binding of the β-adrenergic antagonist ^{3}H-dihydroalprenolol to lymphocytes was decreased in depressed and manic patients when compared with control subjects and euthymic patients. Moreover, β-adrenergic-receptor-mediated stimulation of the production of cyclic adenosine monophosphate (cAMP) by isoproterenol was reduced in leukocytes (Pandey et al., 1979) and lymphocytes (Extein et al., 1979) from depressed patients. It has been cautioned that the decreased β-adrenergic receptor function in lymphocytes from depressed patients may reflect homeostatic regulation of peripheral β-adrenergic receptors in response to increases in plasma catecholamines (Extein et al., 1979). However, β-adrenergic stimulants (e.g., salbutamol) have been reported to be rapidly effective in the treatment of depressed patients (Lecrubier et al., 1980).

Human platelets possess α_2-adrenergic receptors (Hoffman et al., 1979; Wood et al., 1979) which suppress the activity of platelet adenylate cyclase (Lefkowitz, 1978; Fain and Garcia-Sainz, 1980). Neither basal (Scott et al., 1979) nor α-adrenergic-receptor-mediated suppression of prostaglandin-stimulated cAMP production (Murphy et al., 1973; Wang et al., 1974) has been found to be altered in the platelets of depressed patients. However, depressed patients have been reported to have greater platelet α_2-receptor numbers than control subjects in several recent studies (Kafka et al., 1980; Garcia-Sevilla et al., 1981a; 1981b; 1981c), but not in all (U'Pritchard et al., 1982). This discrepancy could possibly reflect differences in platelet α_2-adrenergic receptors across subgroups of depressed patients.

[3]H-imipramine binds to high-affinity sites in the brain (Langer et al., 1980; Rehavi et al., 1980; Langer et al., 1981) and in platelets (Briley et al., 1979; Talvenheimo et al., 1979; Paul et al., 1980; Langer et al., 1981). And cellular uptake regulation sites for serotonin have been labeled with ^{3}H-imipramine (Talvenheimo et al., 1979; Langer et al., 1980; Paul et al., 1981a). A highly significant decrease in the number of ^{3}H-imipramine binding sites, with no significant change in the apparent affinity constant, has been observed in platelets from depressed patients compared with those from control subjects (Langer et al., 1981; Briley et al., 1980; Paul et al., 1981b). Others have observed decreased platelet serotonin uptake in patients with depressive disorders (Coppen et al., 1978; Tuomisto et al., 1979; Meltzer et al., 1981). One group has proposed that the decreased platelet ^{3}H-imipramine binding observed in depressed patients may reflect a deficiency in the platelet serotonin transport mechanism in these patients (Paul et al., 1981b).

THE EMERGING FIELD OF PSYCHIATRIC CHEMISTRY

Monitoring serum lithium levels during the administration of lithium to patients with bipolar manic-depressive disorders has been routine for many years. More recently it has become possible to measure plasma levels of many of the currently prescribed antidepressant drugs. At similar doses, different individual patients can show marked differences in plasma levels of these drugs, largely because of variability in drug metabolism. Whether the plasma levels of antidepressants should be monitored routinely is as yet an unresolved issue.

Some clinical investigators believe that measuring plasma levels of antidepressant drugs is not necessary in routine treatment, but that it may be useful under certain specific conditions, such as the failure to respond to a standard dose or the occurrence of pronounced side effects on a small dose. Other clinical investigators recommend that plasma levels of antidepressant drugs be monitored routinely whenever possible. Routine monitoring would aim to identify patients who develop very high plasma levels on low doses, to document therapeutic levels at the time of clinical response as a guide to treating future episodes, and to document compliance or possible short-term metabolic changes in patients who respond and then relapse on a given dose.

Measurement of specific plasma levels of MAO inhibitors is not considered to be clinically useful. The degree of MAO inhibition produced by these drugs can be assessed in blood platelets. Since several studies have suggested that clinical response to MAO inhibitors, particularly phenelzine, may be related to the degree of inhibition of platelet MAO activity that occurs during the course of drug administration, this assessment may be clinically useful.

We have clearly now reached the point where the clinical laboratory can be used in psychiatry as it is in other fields of medicine, both to assist the physician in making more specific diagnoses and to aid the physician in prescribing more effectively. Recognizing this fact, in 1977 the authors' group established a psychiatric chemistry laboratory to serve as a model academic laboratory facility for the integration and translation of biochemical research into clinical psychiatric practice and to serve as a resource for education and consultation in the emerging field of psychiatric chemistry.

One may now draw an analogy between the pneumonias and the depressions, in that both disorders are diagnosed on the basis of clinical data. In the case of pneumonias, the physician makes a diagnosis on the basis of a history and a physical examination (including a chest X ray). Having made the diagnosis of pneumonia, the physician can then obtain sputum cultures from the clinical laboratory to aid in determining the specific type of pneumonia and the specific antibiotic or other forms of treatment that may be most effective. Similarly, in the case of depressions, the physician diagnoses depression on the basis of clinical history, coupled with physical and mental status examinations. Having made the diagnosis of depression, the physician can then use specialized clinical laboratory tests to assist in determining the type of depression the patient may have and the forms of treatment most likely to be effective. While the biochemical tests that we have today do not necessarily enable physicians to select a clinically effective treatment on the first trial, they can increase the probability of an effective choice. Considering the time it takes for antidepressant drugs to exert their clinical effects, even a small increase in the percentage of patients who receive an effective drug on the first clinical trial would represent a major advance in the treatment of patients with depressive disorders.

Chapter 28

Antidepressant Drug Therapy
by Jonathan O. Cole, M.D. and Alan F. Schatzberg, M.D.

A steadily growing number and variety of drugs for treating depression are now available in the United States or will soon become available. In addition to the older tricyclic antidepressants and monoamine oxidase inhibitors, there are now available in this country a tetracyclic, maprotiline, a neuroleptic-tricyclic, amoxapine, and a heterocyclic, trazodone. Several other drugs of unusual structure seem to be within a year or two of entering general clinical use.

This chapter reviews the use of the older standard drugs and their assets and liabilities and describes the probable special properties of the newer drugs, drawing both from the available literature and from the authors' clinical experience.

THE TRICYCLIC ANTIDEPRESSANTS

Imipramine, the first tricyclic antidepressant (TCA), was developed as a potential neuroleptic drug. In his initial study, however, Kuhn (1957) found no antipsychotic effect but did note that depressive symptoms improved after one to three weeks on the drug. There are now eight drugs in this class available in the United States (see Table 1). The "newest" of these, trimipramine, was first marketed in this country three years ago but had been available in Europe

Table 1.   Marketed Antidepressants

Generic Name	Trade Name	Approximate Dosage Range[1]
Tricyclics		
Imipramine	(Tofranil, SK-Pramine, others)	150–300 mg
Desipramine	(Norpramin, Pertofrane)	150–300 mg
Amitriptyline	(Elavil, Endep, others)	150–300 mg
Nortriptyline	(Pamelor, Aventyl)	50–150 mg
Protriptyline	(Vivactil)	15–40 mg
Doxepin	(Sinequan)	150–300 mg
Trimipramine	(Surmontil)	150–300 mg
Amoxapine	(Asendin)	150–600 mg
Tetracyclic		
Maprotiline	(Ludiomil)	150–300 mg
MAO Inhibitors		
Phenelzine	(Nardil)	45–75 mg
Tranylcypromine	(Parnate)	20–40 mg
Isocarboxazid	(Marplan)	10–30 mg
Other		
Trazodone	(Desyrel)	150–600 mg
Alprazolam[2]	(Xanax)	1.5–8.0 mg

[1]These dosage ranges will be adequate for many patients. A few will respond to substantially lower doses while others will require and tolerate higher doses (see text).
[2]Marketed only for use in anxiety

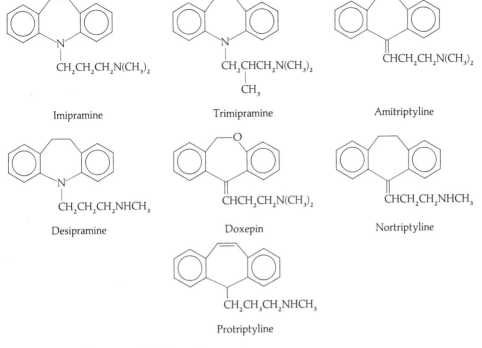

Figure 1. Tricyclic antidepressants

for over a decade. The TCAs are all reasonably similar in structure and pharmacology (see Figure 1). All are more effective than placebo, but no one of them has been convincingly shown to be more effective than any of the others or to be regularly more rapid in its onset of action. While such claims have been made in the past for the desmethyl metabolites of imipramine (desipramine) and of amitriptyline (nortriptyline), no large-scale, convincing studies have documented that their onset of action is reliably more rapid. Occasional depressed patients do respond rapidly, after only a few days, to tricyclics, and in any series of double-blind studies comparing tricyclics, one drug will occasionally turn out by chance to be faster acting than the other.

The other possible reasons for significant differences in efficacy are of scientific interest but are not yet firmly established. Several studies have shown that patients with low levels of 3-methoxy-4-hydroxyphenylglycol (MHPG) in their pretreatment 24-hour urine samples respond better to imipramine, desipramine, nortriptyline, and maprotiline than do patients with high MHPG urine levels (Maas et al., 1972; Beckmann and Goodwin, 1975; Steinbook et al., 1979; Rosenbaum et al., 1980; Hollister et al., 1980; Schatzberg et al., 1980; Schatzberg et al., 1981). The presumed logic behind this lies in the potent effects that such antidepressants exert on the reuptake of noradrenaline. More recent data, growing out of the authors' work with Schildkraut's laboratory, suggests that patients with low MHPG in the urine respond more rapidly and to lower dosages of maprotiline, in contrast to patients with high MHPG levels, who respond more slowly and at higher dosages (Schatzberg et al., 1981). Early studies

Table 2. Reuptake Inhibition of Antidepressants

Drug	Noradrenaline	Serotonin	Dopamine
Tricyclics			
Amitriptyline	+	+ +	0
Nortriptyline	+ +	±	0
Imipramine	+ +	+	0
Desipramine	+ + +	±	0
Protriptyline	+ + +	±	0
Doxepin	+	±	0
Trimipramine	±	0	0
Other Antidepressants			
Amoxapine	+ +	+	
Maprotiline	+ +	0	0
Trazodone	0	+	0
Alprazolam	0	0	0
Nomifensin	+ + +	0	+ +
Fluoxetine	±	+ +	0

on amitriptyline indicated that patients with high MHPG levels responded more favorably to treatment with this drug than did their counterparts with low MHPG levels (Beckmann and Goodwin, 1975; Schildkraut, 1973). Subsequent studies, however, have failed to confirm the earlier findings with any uniformity (Spiker et al., 1980; Modai et al., 1979).

This area is currently in flux for several reasons. First, the reuptake inhibition seen with TCAs occurs after single doses, while relief of depressive symptoms comes on more slowly, sometimes beginning after two or three days, sometimes after one to three weeks. Second, newer data from animal research suggest that desensitization of noradrenaline receptors correlates better with antidepressant drug efficacy than does reuptake inhibition of either noradrenaline or serotonin (Sulser, 1982; Crews and Smith, 1978). It is of course possible that inhibition of reuptake could facilitate such receptor desensitization. Several new and apparently effective unmarketed antidepressants (e.g., buproprion, alprazolam) lack reuptake inhibition completely.

Despite the remaining questions, the TCAs and other antidepressants can be rated by their effects on reuptake, as shown in Table 2 (Maas, 1975). Desipramine is the most purely noradrenergic of the available TCAs, and amitriptyline is the most serotonergic. However, these statements by themselves are a bit deceptive. Since amitriptyline is metabolized to nortriptyline, a relatively noradrenergic TCA, most patients have more nortriptyline than amitriptyline in their plasma when under amitriptyline treatment for one or more weeks. Furthermore, imipramine is metabolized to desipramine, so that most patients on imipramine have about equal amounts of the two TCAs in their blood. Trimipramine was developed and marketed in Europe before the reuptake phenomena became of scientific interest, and work with this drug is now in progress. Doxepin is racemic and has desmethyl metabolites whose reuptake properties have not been studied.

Side Effects

The current tricyclics differ appreciably in their side effects, particularly in the degree to which anticholinergic effects are caused, the extent of sedation or stimulation, orthostatic hypotensive effects, and effects on cardiac conduction. It is tempting, though perhaps simplistic, to relate the frequency and severity of various side effects to the effects which these drugs have on various receptors. Richelson (1981) and Baldessarini (1982) have reviewed this well and have suggested that potency at the histamine (H_1) receptors may be responsible for both the sedation and the weight gain seen with some tricyclics (see Table 3). Whether H_2-receptor effects relate to mental confusion is more speculative, but it is interesting to see that some tricyclics should be good antihistamines, especially amitriptyline and doxepin, and some might be as effective as cimetidine on H_2 receptors. A word of caution is appropriate. The potencies given in Table 3 apply to drug interactions with specific receptor sites in specific animal preparations, and they may not generalize with absolute fidelity to the relative potencies with which these drugs attach to the human brain or autonomic nervous system receptors that are responsible for the side effects seen clinically. Also, the same side effects may be generated by different mechanisms. Trazodone has no anticholinergic properties in animal systems but sometimes does cause dry mouth in patients. The monoamine oxidase inhibitors are also not anticholinergic but cause "anticholinergic" side effects, probably by increasing adrenergic activity.

Table 3.   Anticholinergic and Antihistaminic Potency of Tricyclic Antidepressants

Drug	Relative Anticholinergic Potency	Relative Antihistaminic Potency	
		H_1	H_2
Amitriptyline	+ + +	+ +	+ +
Nortriptyline	+	±	±
Imipramine	+ +	±	+
Desipramine	+	0	0
Protriptyline	+ + +	0	0
Doxepin	+ +	+ + +	+
Trimipramine	+ +	+ +	?

Amitriptyline and protriptyline are the most anticholinergic and desipramine the least so, but even desipramine can cause urinary retention occasionally. Dry mouth is the most common anticholinergic side effect of TCAs, and most patients notice this effect to at least a small degree. Constipation is the next most common. The heart rate may be increased, but the change is usually trivial and not noticed by the patient. Narrowing of the urinary stream can occur, and real urinary retention can occasionally result. Blurred vision can happen, and narrow-angle (but not wide-angle) glaucoma can be aggravated. Fortunately, the latter is rare and is often found to be currently or to have been previously treated by an ophthalmologist. Impotence can also occur. Central anticholinergic side effects can range from a mild, barely noticeable memory difficulty, through speech blocking and clear-memory and orientation difficulties, to frank delirium (Cole and Schatzberg, 1976; Schatzberg et al., 1978; Baldessarini and Willmuth, 1968).

Although TCAs clearly can have a deleterious effect on memory (Branconnier et al., 1982), some depressed patients with prominent complaints about poor memory will have improved memory, at least subjectively, after TCA treatment. Glass et al. (1981) have complicated this area further: they found that imipramine improved memory in depressed outpatients without improving the depression! It is also well documented that patients with senile dementia of the Alzheimer's type have decreased acetylcholinergic activity in their brains. Theoretically, TCAs might well increase dementia in older depressed patients with preexisting or concomitant early senile dementia of the Alzheimer's type. There is no evidence for this, however. Clinically, the TCAs seldom make organically impaired elderly people with depressions any worse. In the absence of more data and in the absence of reliable methods for discriminating pseudodementia from real dementia, the clinician should keep this issue in mind when treating elderly depressed patients. The possibility of improving the patient's "dementia" by raising his or her mood seems more important than the possibility that the dementia might be temporarily aggravated by a TCA.*

All these anticholinergic side effects should be watched for, and patients should probably be informed about the possibility of dry mouth, constipation, and urinary problems. Moreover, TCAs are worth avoiding when the patient is a male with prostate problems. Bethanechol (Urecholine) is a short-acting peripheral cholinergic drug that can be used in a dosage of 25 to 50 mg three or four times a day to counteract bothersome peripheral anticholinergic effects (Everett, 1976). Physostigmine has been used for a temporary reversal of central anticholinergic symptoms (Granacher and Baldessarini, 1975), but its brief duration of action and convulsant properties make its regular use questionable (Preskorn and Irwin, 1982).

Several of the TCAs, particularly amitriptyline, but also imipramine and doxepin, and probably nortriptyline and trimipramine, can be effective hypnotics even in modest dosages (about 50 mg at bedtime). Some patients, however, find that unpleasant sedation and grogginess can persist for hours after arising, particularly with amitriptyline. Desipramine and protriptyline are more commonly a little stimulating. Since tricyclics generally have longish half-lives (twenty to eighty hours), they are equally effective when given all at bedtime and when given three or four times a day. Generally, the more sedative TCAs can be given only at bedtime, and the stimulant ones are best tolerated when given three times a day. It should be noted that *any* TCA can be either sedative or stimulant in a given patient. Since some patients tolerate some TCAs badly, it is sensible to begin TCA therapy with a low dose (25 mg of imipramine or amitriptyline, 10 mg of protriptyline or nortriptyline). Dosage can then be increased by one pill every day or two until the therapeutic dosage is reached, and the patient can be stabilized at that dose level for one or two weeks before going on to higher dosages in the event that clear clinical improvement has not occurred by two weeks.

The dosage required for improvement varies widely from 50 mg to 500 mg a day of a standard drug like imipramine or amitriptyline, though 150 mg is a common dose for outpatients and 250 mg for

*Editor's note: In Part II of this volume Friedel discusses the choice and trial of TCAs with elderly patients and the symptoms which may contraindicate the use of TCAs with such patients.

more seriously depressed inpatients. Data on imipramine plasma levels help to explain this diversity. Glassman and colleagues found that a fixed dose of 3.5 mg/kg yielded steady-state plasma levels ranging from 14 ng/ml to 1,014 ng/ml, summing the plasma levels of desipramine and imipramine (Glassman et al., 1977). From this study it appears that total plasma levels over 225 ng/ml may be optimal unless side effects intervene. For nortriptyline, the other well-studied TCA, there appears to be a "therapeutic window." Levels between 40 ng/ml and 150 ng/ml are associated with improvement, while levels higher or lower are not (Asberg et al., 1971). For other tricyclics, the evidence is limited, or in the case of amitriptyline, present but very confusing.* Even for the other tricyclics, plasma levels are worth using, particularly in patients who fail to respond. Very low levels (e.g., 40 to 60 ng/ml) indicate that a dosage increase is worth trying, while very high levels (e.g., 400 to 800 ng/ml) suggest that a lower dosage might be tried. There is little evidence that high plasma levels alone are any basis for lowering TCA dosage in healthy adults who are experiencing no bothersome side effects. In elderly patients or those with a cardiac disease, however, a high plasma level may pose a problem. In patients who have no limiting side effects or medical complications, low tricyclic plasma levels have been used to justify going above the upper dosage levels specified in the drug labeling approved by the Food and Drug Administration (FDA).

CARDIOVASCULAR EFFECTS   Plasma levels of tricyclics may be relevant to the postural hypotension which sometimes limits the use of TCAs, particularly but not exclusively in the elderly. The work of Glassman and colleagues suggests that this hypotension is characterized by a lack of compensatory tachycardia when the patient first stands up. With this lack, the normal mild orthostatic blood pressure drop is not rectified by increased heart output (Glassman et al., 1979). This effect seems to occur at about 100 ng/ml of imipramine and desipramine but not to be worsened at higher plasma levels, since the effect plateaus at about that point. Glassman's group (Roose et al., 1980) has noted that nortriptyline has the same threshold for orthostatic hypotension. Since improvement on nortriptyline (but not on imipramine) often occurs at plasma levels below 100 ng/ml, nortriptyline may be particularly useful in elderly depressed patients or patients prone to orthostatic hypotension.

Thayssen et al. (1981) carried out a formal study comparing the effects of nortriptyline and imipramine in depressed patients and confirmed Glassman's findings. Nortriptyline did not cause orthostatic hypotension, while imipramine caused major problems. It is not clear that elderly patients are more likely than younger patients to become hypotensive on imipramine, but they are more likely to sustain more serious complications such as fractures after falls. Since adverse cardiovascular effects of TCAs are almost certainly related to plasma levels (Preskorn and Irwin, 1982), monitoring plasma levels regularly to avoid inadvertent escalation to levels well over 300 ng/ml is particularly important in the elderly and in patients with cardiac disease.

*Preceptor's note: In the next chapter, Perel systematically reviews the findings concerning therapeutic plasma levels for imipramine, nortriptyline, and amitriptyline, and he presents some tentative data on doxepin, protriptyline, and desipramine.

In the authors' experience, patients often adapt over time to orthostatic hypotension. Patients barely able to tolerate 50 mg of TCA initially may well be gently inched up to 150 to 250 mg over a few weeks and finally respond well. Temporary measures which can help orthostatic hypotension include advising patients to get up slowly, to use belly binders or corsets, to wear elastic stockings, or if a drug approach is indicated, to add salt tablets or fludrocortisone (Florinef), a salt-retaining corticosteroid, to elevate blood pressure.

Some tachycardia, asymptomatic or symptomatic, can occur in patients on tricyclics. A rise in blood pressure is occasionally seen.

TCAs have other important effects on heart function. They slow impulse conduction, a beneficial quinidinelike effect which can actually suppress premature contractions (Giardana et al., 1981). However, TCAs can also throw a patient with partial heart block into complete heart block, and at toxic doses they can cause a variety of arrhythmias and decreased myocardial contractility, presumably by acting on the membranes as local anesthetics. If patients with cardiac pacemakers are to receive TCAs, it is worth making sure that the stimulating electrode is below the A-V node. A pacemaker stimulating the atrium is of little use if a TCA causes heart block.

The question of whether TCAs are safe in patients with cardiac disease is still unsettled. Early serious complications of TCAs in cardiac patients were reported before plasma levels were generally available. Glassman has informally stated that orthostatic hypotension is even more prevalent in hospitalized cardiac patients on multiple cardiac drugs than it is in healthy adults (Alexander Glassman, personal communication). Veith et al. (1982), on the other hand, have reported a detailed small study comparing imipramine with doxepin and placebo in cardiac patients. They found that both drugs were clinically useful and had minimal adverse effects other than a few instances of symptomatic postural hypotension with each drug. Maprotiline has also been reported to have somewhat fewer cardiac complications (Gelenberg, 1982a). Doxepin's reputation for greater safety in cardiac patients is, in the authors' opinion, not strongly supported by available data.

All this may be helpful to the psychiatrist needing to treat a cardiac patient for depression, and collaboration with an internist and electrocardiographic monitoring would also seem sensible. Many internists, however, are unfamiliar with the recent work on tricyclics and cardiac function and may need access to some of the literature cited here. In particular, in the case of TCA overdose, one should warn the treating physician *not* to treat arrhythmias with quinidine. Preskorn and Irwin (1982) have discussed in some detail the pros, cons, and ignorance surrounding the proper treatment of depressed cardiac patients.

OTHER SIDE EFFECTS   A tremor, usually faster than that seen in pseudoparkinsonism, can occur and may respond to propranolol, as may symptomatic tachycardia due to TCAs. Myoclonic twitches of one muscle group or whole body areas can occur, and grand mal seizures are seen rarely.

Recurrent drenching sweats can occur. The mechanism is unclear. Weight gain, possibly secondary to H_1 blockade, is often a problem. It seems less common, but can still occur, with desipramine.

Although overdoses can be fatal, they are often successfully managed in the intensive care units of general hospitals.

Indications

In the past, it was often claimed that severe endogenous depressions respond best to tricyclics (Kiloh et al., 1962). While this may still be true, it is also increasingly clear that the less severe and less endogenous depressions often respond quite well. A three-clinic collaborative study sponsored by the National Institute of Mental Health (NIMH) has now added to the complexity of this issue. The study compared imipramine (about 125 mg a day), the benzodiazepine chlordiazepoxide (about 40 mg a day), and placebo in primarily anxious outpatients and found imipramine to be superior to both chlordiazepoxide and placebo after four and six weeks, though the benzodiazepine was the most effective treatment at the end of the first week (Kahn et al., 1981). A recent study by Donald Klein's group showed that outpatients with mild depressions, who would not have qualified for most standard antidepressant drug studies because of their low symptomatology, nevertheless did significantly better on desipramine than on placebo (Stewart et al., 1981). The data from the two studies cited suggest that tricyclics can be effective both in anxiety alone and in milder, nonendogenous depressions.

Much has also been said in the literature about the superiority of monoamine oxidase inhibitors (MAOIs) to tricyclics in the so-called atypical depressions, variously defined (Tyrer, 1976). Moreover, most clinicians assume, on the one hand, that tricyclics are superior in patients with endogenous symptoms such as guilt, psychomotor retardation or agitation, anhedonia, anorexia and weight loss, early morning awakening, and lessening in the intensity of the depression toward evening. The MAOIs, they assume on the other hand, are indicated in patients with overeating, hypersomnia, worsening of symptoms toward evening, anxiety, phobias, irritability, and "reactivity" of mood (feeling better if good things happen). This may be true, but two recent large studies, one British (Rowan et al., 1982) and one American (Ravaris et al., 1980) contradict these assumptions. Comparing amitriptyline and phenelzine in large samples of depressed outpatients, both studies failed to find any response differences of the sort outlined above, though they did both find that the MAOI was slightly better in relieving the symptoms of anxiety. The authors' experience has been that patients with severe and chronic endogenous depressions may respond to MAOIs after failing to respond to TCAs (Schatzberg et al., 1981).

This leaves the whole matter a bit up in the air. Certainly patients qualifying for the DSM-III diagnosis of Major Depressive Episode (American Psychiatric Association, 1980) and probably patients qualifying for the DSM-III diagnosis of Dysthymic Disorder (depressive neurosis) are reasonable candidates for tricyclic medication. The criteria specified are broad enough to cover both endogenous and atypical depressions of a good range of intensities from mild to severe.

When should tricyclics *not* be used in patients with symptoms of depression and no physical contraindications? This is harder to define. Certainly some patients with a clear schizophrenic illness are made worse by tricyclics. These are probably mainly schizophrenic patients who have histories of maladjustment since childhood or severe disorganization beginning in adolescence (Pollack et al., 1965), but some depressed schizophrenics are helped by tricyclics, usually added to their antipsychotic medication.

A related problem is the ability of tricyclics to elicit manic or hypomanic reactions in patients with past histories of spontaneous mania (bipolar I affective disorder) and sometimes in patients who have only become manic on medications (bipolar II). Since manic-depressive illness overlaps with schizoaffective illness, some worsenings seen in schizophrenic patients are due to the manic reaction elicited on top of the preexisting schizophrenia. But some nonaffective process schizophrenics also have their psychosis worsened by tricyclics.

Patients with varying degrees of organic dementia and depression can improve on tricyclics, but they may also be at risk for anticholinergic impairment of brain functioning. Hypochondriacal patients and patients with borderline personality or marked mood lability are sometimes helped and sometimes worsened by tricyclics (Cole and Sunderland, 1982).

The best treatment of patients with psychotic and/or paranoid depressions is unclear at present. They may respond to tricyclics, though various authorities have suggested that either electroconvulsive therapy or a combination of antipsychotic and tricyclic medication is superior (Glassman et al., 1975; Nelson and Bowers, 1978; Minter and Mandel, 1979). An ongoing controlled study by Duane Spiker at the University of Pittsburgh is showing the antipsychotic-TCA combination to be superior to either a TCA or a neuroleptic alone. Because of the risk of tardive dyskinesia, an initial trial on tricyclics alone seems sensible unless paranoid psychotic symptoms are far more prominent than depressive symptoms.

Choice of Tricyclic

Since the relationship of plasma level to response is clearest for imipramine, this probably is the drug of choice where plasma levels are available. In patients with insomnia, imipramine or possibly amitriptyline, trimipramine, or doxepin is useful. These drugs improve sleep almost immediately. Amitriptyline's side effects are bothersome to a fair number of depressed outpatients. Desipramine, or possibly protriptyline or amoxapine, may be preferable in patients with hypersomnia and fatigue, because these drugs lack sedation and have occasional energizing properties. Where other tricyclics cause unpleasant anticholinergic side effects, desipramine can be substituted with frequent benefit. There are small studies in the literature suggesting that patients who feel better on D-amphetamine or methylphenidate will do best on imipramine or desipramine (Fawcett et al., 1972). Fawcett et al. (in press) have recently reported that patients who fail to respond to desipramine will often go on to respond to nortriptyline and vice versa. In the authors' experience, this has worked in a few cases. If true, this may be the first clear evidence that patients who fail on one TCA ever regularly benefit from a trial on a second TCA. Studies of this issue are not available in the literature. The one exception, in which patients who failed on desipramine were randomly assigned to clomipramine, was a notable failure. Only five of forty initial patients failed to improve on desipramine, and the three patients who failed and were randomly assigned to clomipramine did not improve (Stewart et al., 1980).

In patients with marked anergia, methylphenidate has been combined with a tricyclic early in treatment and may help either by a direct stimulant effect or by elevating plasma levels of the tricyclic (Wharton et al., 1971). Antipsychotics probably also raise tricyclic plasma levels. A benzodiazepine may help by relieving anxiety in the first week or so of treatment. Limbitrol, a chlordiazepoxide-amitriptyline combination, is clearly superior to amitriptyline alone only in the first week of treatment, but there is abundant evidence that standard benzodiazepines alone are not as effective as tricyclics in depression (Schatzberg and Cole, 1978).

Triiodothyronine has been reported to speed clinical response to imipramine and amitriptyline and to elicit improvement in patients previously unresponsive to these drugs (Gelenberg, 1982b; Goodwin et al., 1982). The authors have found it useful in their practices only occasionally.

Adding lithium is indicated in mania-prone depressions, but its efficacy as an antidepressant alone and its ability to improve response to tricyclics is still unclear. Lithium alone can probably be effective in depressed bipolar patients who are not already on it. A recent Canadian paper has reported obtaining excellent responses by adding lithium to the medications of depressed patients who responded inadequately to TCAs or MAOIs (de Montigny et al., 1981). The authors' limited experience with this adjuvant since reading the paper has not been encouraging. Moreover, the authors have rarely found patients who do well on TCAs plus lithium but do not do well on either drug alone.

Management

Once a patient has improved on a tricyclic, he or she should probably be maintained on it for at least six months, since relapse frequently occurs if the drug is stopped too soon (Klerman et al., 1974). Patients improving on tricyclics after depressive illnesses which have persisted for years may well need indefinite maintenance therapy. To date no clear adverse effects of long-term maintenance with tricyclics have been reported. Long-term treatment could, however, induce receptor changes that might be associated with some untoward effect.

If the tricyclic is to be stopped, it should be gradually tapered. Abrupt cessation often results in a variety of autonomic and flulike symptoms. These can be relieved by a single dose of the tricyclic, and they probably represent true withdrawal symptoms, possibly on the basis of cholinergic rebound. As an example of a possible long-term receptor change, the authors recently described seven patients who became hypomanic after abruptly stopping the tricyclic that they had been taking for several months to several years (Mirin et al., 1981).

One large-scale double-blind study (Prien et al., 1973) has compared the effectiveness of imipramine with that of lithium and placebo in preventing depressive episodes in patients who had histories of at least three affective episodes in the preceding two years. Imipramine and lithium were equally effective and were both superior to placebo in averting depressive episodes. In a review, Davis (1976) found that other smaller studies supported this thesis. Lithium-treated patients were, however, less likely to develop mania while on maintenance therapy. On the other hand, when Quitkin et al. (1976) reviewed the same literature, they concluded that lithium is better at preventing mania and less clearly effective in preventing depression. A preliminary report from a recently completed NIMH collaborative study has suggested that lithium is less effective than imipramine in preventing early depressive relapses in patients who have recurrent depressive episodes unless they have been essentially free of depression for at least twenty weeks (Prien, 1981). All in all, it may make more clinical sense to continue patients who have relatively frequent (e.g., one or two a year) depressive episodes on the tricyclic to which they have responded well than to shift them to lithium, unless the tricyclic gives them bothersome side effects.

MONOAMINE OXIDASE INHIBITORS

The first MAOI, iproniazid, was found to have antidepressant effects by two rather different approaches in the late 1950s. The drug, a chemical congener of isoniazid, was tried in tuberculous patients where it proved to have euphoriant but not antibiotic effects. Crane (1957) followed up on this observation by using it successfully to treat depression. At the same time the drug's ability to inhibit the enzyme monoamine oxidase was known, and Kline reasoned that since this enzyme destroyed noradrenaline and serotonin intracellularly, blocking it might relieve depression. He also carried out a successful trial of the drug in depression (Kline, 1958). Although iproniazid is probably an effective antidepressant, it is no longer used in this country following a flurry of reports that its use was associated with acute hepatic necrosis. It is, however, still on the market in Britain.

Currently three MAOIs are in general use in this country, phenelzine (Nardil), tranylcypromine (Parnate), and isocarboxazid (Marplan). Pargyline (Eutonyl), another MAOI, is marketed only for use in hypertension but has been used in depression. Only phenelzine and, to a lesser extent, tranylcypromine have been well studied in controlled clinical trials with depression (see Figure 2).

Tranylcypromine was briefly withdrawn from clinical use in the 1960s because of its association with hypertensive crises, which may be more frequent with it than with the other MAOIs. Although tranylcypromine is now approved by the FDA for use only in "severe reactive or endogenous depressions," evidence and clinical experience suggest that it may be at least as effective in the milder or more atypical nonendogenous depressions.

Phenelzine has now been most thoroughly studied. Its lack of clear efficacy in earlier studies was presumably a dosage problem. Ravaris et al. (1976) showed that at a dose of 30 mg/day phenelzine is no different from placebo, while at 60 mg/day it is clearly effective. They further showed that clinical response is associated with over 80 percent inhibition of the MAO in platelets. Phenelzine blood levels

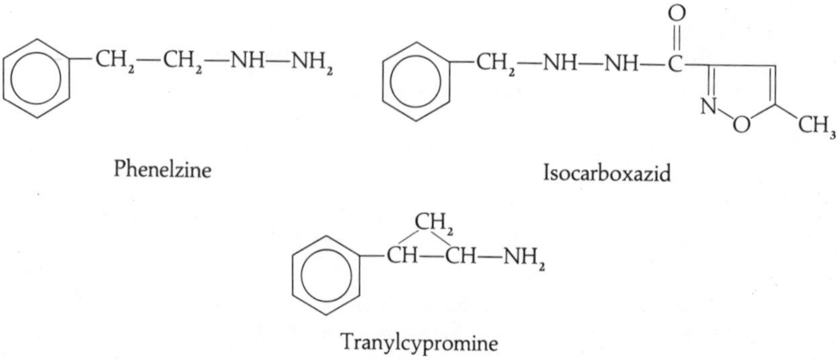

Phenelzine

Isocarboxazid

Tranylcypromine

Figure 2. Monoamine oxidase inhibitors

are probably also correlated with improvement. Earlier suggestions that the differences in improvement could be due to interindividual differences in the rate of acetylation, the chief metabolic route for phenelzine, have not been borne out by subsequent trials. It had been suggested that rapid acetylators responded less well to phenelzine than slow acetylators (Johnston and Marsh, 1973). Clinical experience shows that many patients who fail to respond to even 60 mg of phenelzine after two to four weeks may respond to dosages of 75 or 90 mg a day.

The effective dose of tranylcypromine has been less well studied, but 20 to 40 mg a day is a common dosage range, and the authors have occasionally gone to 60 mg a day or higher in nonresponding patients. Since even low dosages of tranylcypromine will produce significant reduction in MAO activity, serial platelet MAO-activity measures may be less useful in monitoring treatment with this drug than it is with phenelzine (Giller and Lieb, 1980).

The therapeutic dose of isocarboxazid has also not been well studied, but 20 to 30 mg a day has been proposed. A recent study has indicated that 80 percent inhibition in platelet MAO activity correlates with clinical response to this drug (Riddle et al., 1980).

The timing of clinical response to MAOIs probably parallels the response time for tricyclics. At least the two major recent studies comparing adequate dosages of phenelzine and amitriptyline showed no significant differences in the course of response (Ravaris et al., 1980; Rowan et al., 1982). The authors, however, have seen patients, particularly patients who cannot tolerate high dosages of MAOIs, respond more slowly, requiring four to six weeks of therapy.

There are four studies, two of them well controlled, which support the value of adding L-tryptophan to a MAOI to increase the likelihood of short-term response. This combination has not been generally used clinically, and the drug's FDA-approved labeling notes that L-tryptophan is a drug *not* to be used with MAOIs (Cole et al., 1980). Since L-tryptophan presumably raises brain serotonin, this potentiation of MAOI effect in depression supports the conclusion of an important study by Gershon's group (Shopsin et al., 1976). They showed that blocking noradrenaline synthesis did not alter clinical response to tranylcypromine, while blocking serotonin synthesis in MAOI responders made depression return. In the authors' experience, however, adding L-tryptophan to the regimen of patients who fail to respond to MAOIs has not yielded much clinical benefit.

Clinical impressions suggest that tranylcypromine is more often stimulant, perhaps because of its chemical similarity to amphetamine, while phenelzine may be more sedative. Isocarboxazid may be even more sedative. However, no studies comparing these drugs have been carried out.

As noted above, phenelzine and probably other MAOIs may be more useful in reducing anxiety symptoms than amitriptyline. These drugs have been studied in Britain as adjuncts to behavioral approaches to treating anxiety states, and there is some evidence for their efficacy (Tyrer, 1976).

Although imipramine has been clearly shown to be effective in patients with recurrent panic states and associated agoraphobia, a recent well-designed study by Sheehan et al. (1980) showed that phenelzine was at least as effective. Most patients originally enrolled in the placebo-controlled study and assigned to imipramine are reported over time to have chosen to shift to phenelzine because the phenelzine patients were judged to be doing better in psychosocial adjustment.

Side Effects

The hypertensive crisis generally brought on by the ingestion of tyramine-containing foods or by the administration of sympathomimetic drugs constitutes the most worrisome side effect of MAOI therapy. The blood pressure can increase to levels as high as 220/140, and this is often accompanied by a very painful splitting headache, often with neck pain as well. It comes on ten to thirty minutes after the patient ingests the offending substance, and untreated it lasts for one or two hours. Some patients have lesser degrees of residual head pain for several days. It can be terminated by intravenous phentolamine (Regitine) in 5 to 10 mg dosage. When a headache begins, some clinicians have patients take oral antipsychotic drugs with α-adrenergic-blocking properties (e.g., chlorpromazine). The effectiveness of this tactic is unclear, though in one experiment of nature, when a whole hospital ate "bad" chicken livers, patients on tranylcypromine alone had hypertensive crises, while those on trifluoperazine as well did not. As a way of attempting to modify a crisis, oral phentolamine (50 to 100 mg) might work as well. Although hypertensive crises usually are without sequelae, cases of cerebrovascular accident or hemorrhage from an unsuspected carotid aneurysm have occurred.

Appendix 1 contains the list of food and drug instructions that the authors give to patients in their clinic (see Appendix 1). The list is deliberately overinclusive and may require modifications in accordance with patients' reliability and food preferences and more recent literature. The most recent and detailed review is by McCabe and Tsuang (1982). The substances which the authors know have caused patients to get a severe headache are cheddar cheese, chicken livers, Chianti wine, beef stroganoff, and Dimetapp Extentabs. A list of the tyramine contents of a variety of foods and drugs is available from the manufacturer and can also be found in the *Physicians' Desk Reference*.

The authors suspect that some patients can sometimes eat "forbidden" foods or drugs with impunity and then sometime later experience a hypertensive crisis. Attempts to elicit headaches in patients on MAOIs have sometimes failed; blood pressure would be elevated, but no head pain would occur. No frequency data on hypertensive crises are available, but an estimate is that 1 to 2 percent of patients on MAOIs actually experience such adverse effects. Presumably, careful patients will avoid them by adhering to food and drug restrictions, but the authors have heard of patients on MAOIs who had "spontaneous" hypertensive-crisis headaches unrelated to food or drugs. They have also heard of one patient who sustained a stroke when shifted abruptly from phenelzine to tranylcypromine. Stimulant drugs like D-amphetamine can presumably also produce crises, and some clinicians have noted hypertensive crises in patients who, in the course of dental treatment, were administered a local anesthetic that contained a sympathomimetic drug. On the other hand, cautious social drinking of hard liquor (particularly vodka) or white wine appears to be well tolerated, and several patients to date have with impunity used topical nasal sprays for severe nasal congestion.

Otherwise, MAOIs are often well tolerated. Sympathomimetic effects—dry mouth, blurred vision, constipation, urinary retention—

can occur, but they are less common than with the tricyclics. Some degree of postural hypotension can occur. Some patients feel fatigued or sedated on MAOIs, some feel stimulated, and some have relief of depression without either effect. Persistent insomnia that resists even double doses of hypnotics is occasionally a serious problem in patients who have otherwise had a good mood response. Increased appetite with weight gain is sometimes a problem. Impotence can occur in males, or in females an absence of orgasm can occur despite normal sexual arousal.

Except for postural hypotension, effects on the cardiovascular system appear to be benign. Perhaps the MAOIs are "safer" than tricyclics in patients with heart disease.

Combined MAOI-Tricyclic Use

Although a combined MAOI-tricyclic treatment appears to be used widely in Britain, there is no clear evidence that the combination is superior to adequate dosages of either drug used alone (White and Simpson, 1981). The combination is forbidden by current drug labeling in this country and should be tried only after trials on single drugs of each class have clearly failed and after a thorough review of the available literature. It appears that phenelzine-amitriptyline combinations may be safer than those involving either imipramine or tranylcypromine.

Serious adverse effects of the combination have occurred only when a tricyclic was added, usually in a somewhat high dose, in patients already on a MAOI. The authors therefore suggest waiting two weeks when going from a MAOI to a tricyclic. When going from a tricyclic to a MAOI, intervals of only a few days have ordinarily been allowed without adverse effects to date.

NEWER DRUGS

In recent years a number of nontricyclic antidepressants have been introduced into the United States (maprotiline, amoxapine, and trazodone). Several may be near to receiving approval for use with depressed patients (e.g., alprazolam and buproprion). Still others are being tested here and abroad (e.g., oxaprotiline, deprenyl, etc.). Structures for some of the recently released agents are depicted in Figure 3.

Research on the newer drugs has followed two major lines. For one, considerable effort has been expended to develop new drugs which act similarly to the tricyclic antidepressants or MAOIs but which act faster, produce fewer side effects, and enjoy wider margins of safety in overdoses. Although this effort is obviously of great use, it has a major pitfall. Using animal models to see if a new drug exerts a particular biological action similar to the existing antidepressants, such an approach risks creating only newer versions of old models or "me-too drugs."

The other tack in drug development has been to synthesize drugs that work in novel ways. This approach could lead to drugs that are not only better tolerated and safer, but that are also potential alternative treatments for those depressed patients who fail on traditional drugs. In addition, such agents may provide further tiers in the "psychopharmacologic bridge" and thus widen our understanding of the underlying biochemical processes. For example, some new drugs

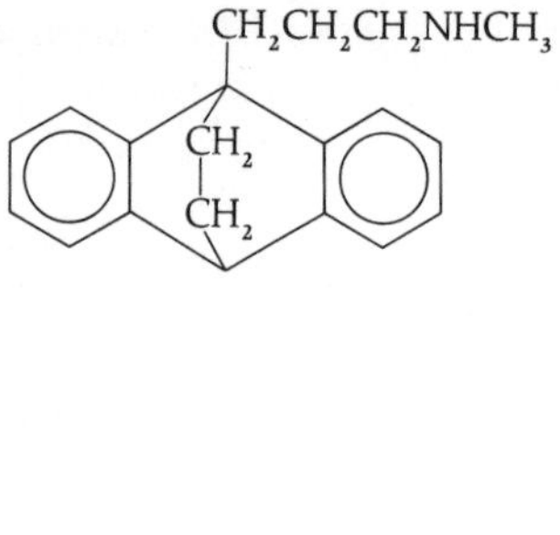

Maprotiline

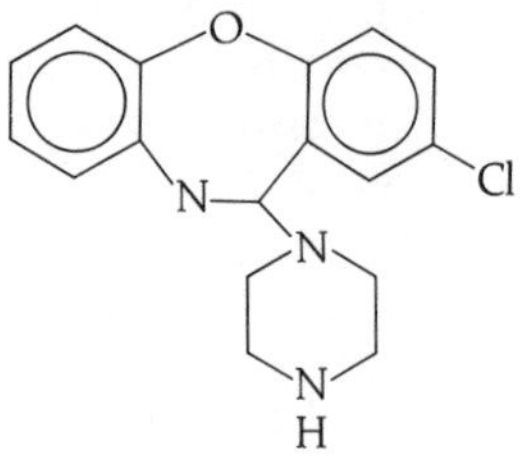

Amoxapine

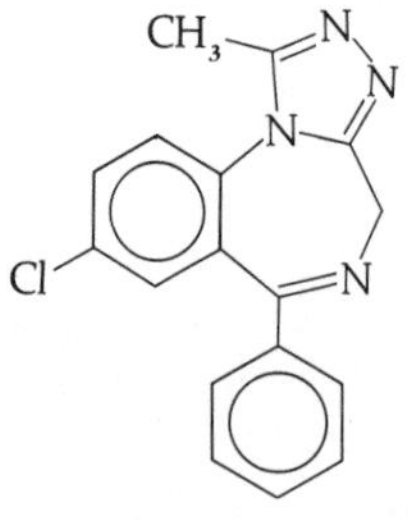

Alprazolam

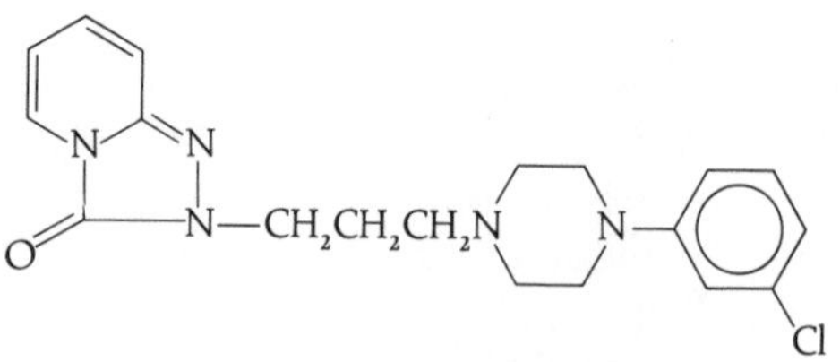

Trazodone

Figure 3. Recently released compounds

may act directly on pre- and postsynaptic receptors rather than by blocking reuptake, while others may work via other neurotransmitter systems.

Maprotiline (Ludiomil)

This tetracyclic, now available in the United States, has been in use in Europe for about ten years and is alleged to outsell all other antidepressants in Germany. In structure maprotiline is essentially a tricyclic with an extra loop connecting the top and bottom of the middle ring. Pharmacologically, it resembles existing tricyclics in its properties. It falls somewhere near desipramine in its effects but in the authors' experience is slightly more sedative (Cole, 1982; Pinder et al., 1977). Maprotiline is relatively low in anticholinergic effects and probably has less direct effect on cardiac function, as overdose is characterized by convulsions and overstimulation rather than by cardiac arrhythmias. It is clearly effective, and in about a quarter of the numerous available studies comparing maprotiline with imipramine or amitriptyline, maprotiline is either a bit faster in onset of antidepressant effect or lower in side effects. As noted earlier, it is particularly rapid in onset and effective in patients with low 24-hour MHPG excretion (in one study). Effective plasma levels are probably in the 200 to 400 ng/ml range. The only problem the authors have noted with maprotiline is that epileptic seizures occur in patients with prior seizure history or in patients pushed to dosages over 250 mg a day. Clinicians who generally tend to go over the package insert dosages with tricyclics in nonresponding patients would be well advised to proceed more cautiously with maprotiline. Although one would think that the noradrenergic tricyclics would be interchangeable in depressed patients, the authors have seen patients who had intolerable side effects on desipramine but tolerated maprotiline nicely, and vice versa. Given that the animal data show that maprotiline is effective in reducing hostile behavior, perhaps it will be useful in depressions with associated hostility.

Amoxapine (Asendin)

This new antidepressant serves to underline the truism that both neuroleptics and antidepressants are "tricyclic." Amoxapine is a demethylated metabolite of loxapine, a potent antipsychotic. It is as effective in the usual four- to six-week controlled clinical trials as an antidepressant. Its dosage is probably about twice that of a standard TCA (Ayd, 1980; Cole, 1982). Amoxapine allegedly has more rapid onset and fewer anticholinergic side effects than standard TCAs. Although there is some argument about the rapidity of onset (Lydiard, 1982), the authors have treated a few patients who achieved dramatic relief after a few hours or a couple of days, with an almost amphetaminelike stimulatory response. Clinically, amoxapine seems remarkably variable in its effects, stimulating in some patients and quite sedative in others. Some of the authors' patients who have responded to amoxapine have failed on several other tricyclics. Unfortunately, a number of the best responders to amoxapine showed a gradual flagging of response over one to three months, and varying the dose up or down failed to help. Since these patients were mainly treatment failures on other antidepressants and since waning of clinical response can also certainly occur with standard TCAs, these observations should not be taken as gospel. Perhaps it was the occasionally remarkable improvement seen initially in amoxapine patients that made their return to baseline more painful and noteworthy.

One untested and possibly untestable hypothesis is that early in treatment amoxapine's antidepressant effects dominate, while later its neuroleptic effects come to the fore. Certainly the drug is a neuroleptic which is itself as potent as a dopamine-receptor blocker as is loxapine in vitro and which is possessed of a 7-hydroxy metabolite as potent as haloperidol (Cohen et al., 1982). It is therefore not remarkable that parkinsonism, akathisia, galactorrhea, and elevated blood prolactin levels all occur with amoxapine. Extrapyramidal side effects, however, were not commonly reported during the published controlled clinical trials.

Amoxapine's mixed TCA-neuroleptic status could have good and bad consequences, neither proven. Amoxapine might be particularly effective in patients with psychotic depressions or depressed schizophrenics. It may well also put patients at risk for eventual tardive dyskinesia.

In overdose amoxapine tends to produce seizures and overstimulation but not major cardiac toxicity. In ordinary doses, if given at twice the dose of imipramine or amitriptyline, it can produce comparable levels of sedation, anticholinergic effects, and hypotension.

Trazodone (Desyrel)

This is the first "really nontricyclic" new antidepressant to become available in the United States (Ayd, 1979). It is a triazolopyridine derivative possessing an elongated complex structure. The pharmacological properties of trazodone are quite different from those of a tricyclic. It has no measurable anticholinergic effects on biological systems, being α-adrenergic and serotonergic (Riblet and Taylor, 1981). Dosage is about twice that of a standard TCA. The major side effect of trazodone is sedation, with dizziness and headache also occurring. Despite the drug's lack of direct anticholinergic activity, dry mouth, constipation, dysuria, and so forth can occur, probably an adrenergic effect; but these side effects happen less commonly than with amitriptyline or imipramine (Gershon and Newton, 1980). In the authors' experience, a reasonable proportion of tricyclic-intolerant or unresponsive patients have improved on trazodone: about a quarter do very well, and another quarter show some improvement (Cole et al., 1981; Gershon et al., 1981).

Trazodone does not cause the persistent orthostatic hypotension seen with TCAs, but patients can become hypotensive during peak blood level about an hour after they take a dose on an empty stomach. Otherwise, the drug has to date shown no clear cardiac effects, and it seems to be a good deal safer in overdose than other currently available antidepressants. Reportedly, trazodone does not lower convulsive threshold in experimental animals, probably a unique property among currently available antidepressants.

Alprazolam (Xanax)

This is a benzodiazepine with a triazolo group added (a chemical unit also occurring in trazodone). Alprazolam has recently been marketed for use in anxiety in doses up to 3 mg a day. However, during its antianxiety trials, the data indicated that it was superior to diazepam in patients labeled as having "mixed anxiety and depression," and subsequent studies have suggested some antidepressant activity in doses between 2 and 8 mg a day (Cole, 1982). Sheehan, in an open study, (David Sheehan, personal communication, 1982), and Chouinard et al. (1982), in a controlled study, have shown that alprazolam has some efficacy in patients with panic agoraphobia, a condition in which antidepressants are effective and benzodiazepines generally are not. The authors' experience with alprazolam in highly treatment-resistant depressions has been mixed. A few patients have had a dramatic and impressive relief from depression, verging occasionally on hypomania, while most of these rather atypical patients have not improved. Sedation has been the main side effect. If the drug proves effective in less resistant depressions, alprazolam would have the added advantage of causing no appreciable anticholinergic or autonomic side effects. However, it could have the problem of physical dependence if large doses were taken for prolonged periods. The authors' few but excellent results in a very heterogeneous group of depressed patients are encouraging.

Of particular interest is the fact that alprazolam appears to have more potent antidepressant properties than do the other benzodiazepines, which exert relatively little effect on core endogenous depressive symptoms such as psychomotor retardation, anergia, and so forth (Schatzberg and Cole, 1978). The biochemical actions of alprazolam that account for its antidepressant effects are unclear. Sethy (1982), however, has recently found that alprazolam causes down regulation of postsynaptic receptors in rats pretreated with reserpine, a monoamine depleter.

FUTURE DRUGS

A host of new drugs are currently under investigation here and abroad, and many of these have distinct structures and act in rather unusual ways. For example, some newly developed drugs act by blocking the presynaptic α_2 receptors which serve as thermostats controlling the production and release of norepinephrine. Several years ago, Crews and Smith (1978) found that the desensitization of these presynaptic receptors did not occur in animal models until two weeks or more of tricyclic treatment, suggesting that this step determined the lag between reuptake blockade (which occurs almost immediately with TCAs) and clinical response. Further, some investigators have begun to argue that elevated α_2-receptor activity may play a primary role in the pathophysiology of depression. Figure 4 shows the structures of selected promising new agents.

Considerable attention has been paid recently to mianserin, a tetracyclic antihistaminic drug that blocks the reuptake of serotonin and exerts a potent effect on presynaptic α_2 receptors. This drug has been in general use in Great Britain and Holland for several years but may not be marketed in the United States because its patent is running out. Another more potent α_2-receptor blocker, synaptamine, is just beginning early clinical trials in this country. These drugs appear to be safe and have few side effects. Some have suggested that combining tricyclics with α_2-receptor blockers could speed up antidepressant responses.

Two specific serotonin-reuptake blockers have received attention. Zimelidine was developed in Sweden and is now in advanced clinical trials here. It not only is a potent blocker of serotonin reuptake but also has a weak effect on blocking the reuptake of norepinephrine. Zimelidine does cause subsensitive β-adrenergic receptors, but unlike the tricyclics it has little effect on reducing β-adrenergic-receptor density. Fluoxetine, a drug developed here, does not block norepinephrine

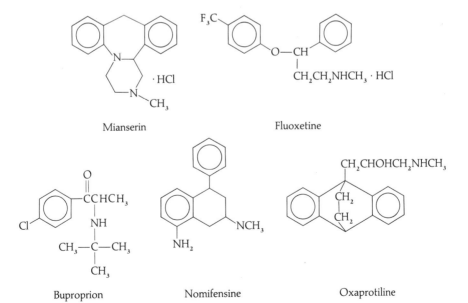

Mianserin

Fluoxetine

Buproprion

Nomifensine

Oxaprotiline

Figure 4. Selected promising new agents

reuptake, and in contrast to zimelidine, it appears to exert no effect on adrenergic receptors (Sulser, 1980). Should fluoxetine prove particularly effective in tricyclic nonresponders, it could tell us much about the possible biochemical mechanisms that underlie subtypes of depressive disorders (Schatzberg et al., 1982).

Two of the new drugs, nomifensine and buproprion, exert some effect on blocking dopamine reuptake. Nomifensine inhibits both dopamine and norepinephrine reuptake, has been extensively studied here and abroad, and may be close to release in the United States (Brogden et al., 1979; Cole, 1982). Buproprion is a unicyclic antidepressant which is currently having its New Drug Application reviewed by the FDA. It is nonsedative, nonanticholinergic, nonantihistaminic, and nonhypotensive, and it may even promote weight loss. Its biochemical action is in debate. It does not block the reuptake of either norepinephrine or serotonin but may exert an effect on dopaminergic systems (Ferris, 1982; Zung, 1982). This is still moot, since its dopamine-reuptake-blocking effect in animals occurs at doses and drug concentrations that are higher than those used in humans.

Finally, oxaprotiline is a maprotiline analogue which is in advanced clinical trial. It appears to have fewer side effects than maprotiline but to enjoy overall equal efficacy. Roffman and Gould (1982) have recently presented data which indicate that oxaprotiline is particularly effective with patients who have MHPG levels that in other studies have been associated with nonresponse to maprotiline (Schatzberg et al., 1981). These data suggest that although oxaprotiline is a maprotiline analogue, it may act via alternative mechanisms and be even more effective than maprotiline in some patients.

In short, a plethora of new drugs is emerging on the horizon. Clinicians will face the challenge of integrating these new compounds, while gaining further skill and experience with the older antidepressant agents (e.g., in the application of plasma levels). Researchers may find that comparisons of the new and old agents and study of their biochemical actions assist in unraveling the biochemical processes that underlie the depressive disorders.

APPENDIX 1.
PRECAUTIONS FOR PEOPLE TAKING
MONOAMINE OXIDASE INHIBITORS

Monoamine oxidase inhibitors (MAOIs) affect the body's reaction to most other medications. No other medication should be taken in addition to a MAOI unless its use is discussed with your physician. All physicians involved in your treatment should be told that you are on a MAOI.

It is especially important if you have to undergo surgery or dental work that you tell your doctor or dentist that you are on a MAOI as MAOIs markedly affect the body's reaction to anesthetics. Local anesthetics especially often contain a substance (epinephrine) which should not be taken by people on MAOIs.

Over-the-counter or nonprescription medications should also be avoided when one is on a MAOI. Especially dangerous are medications sold for the treatment of colds and hay fever, nasal decongestants and cough suppressants, inhalation products, and preparations used for weight reduction.

Many foods have been implicated in causing serious or dangerous reactions in people taking MAOIs. While some of the foods listed below may be safe, especially if taken in small amounts, all should be avoided.

Foods to be avoided while you are taking a MAOI include the following:*

Cheese—especially strong or aged cheese (Cream cheese, cottage cheese, ricotta, and American cheese are probably safe to eat.)

Alcoholic beverages—especially wine and beer (Chianti and sherry are particularly dangerous.)

Yogurt

Sour cream

Caffeine in large amounts

Chocolate

Cream in large amounts

Liver or foods supplemented with liver, and especially chicken liver

Yeast extracts—Marmite, Bovril

Snails

Pickled herring, canned sardines, anchovies, or lox

Citrus fruits—probably only in large amounts

Bananas or avocados—especially if overripe

Raisins

Canned figs

Papaya products—sometimes used in meat tenderizers

Broad beans, fava beans, and possibly Chinese pea pods

Sauerkraut

Pickles

Soy sauce

The most common serious reaction to eating such foods is severe headache. The development of a headache while on a MAOI and/or the occurrence of heart palpitations, neck stiffness or soreness, nausea, vomiting, excessive sweating, fever, or chest pain should be reported to your doctor immediately, and/or you should immediately go to a hospital emergency ward.

Chapter 29 Tricyclic Antidepressant Plasma Levels, Pharmacokinetics, and Clinical Outcome†

by James M. Perel, Ph.D.

INTRODUCTION

Pronounced interindividual variations have been demonstrated in the steady-state plasma level of tricyclic antidepressants, while difficulties

*Small amounts of several of these foods are probably safe in patients receiving MAOIs (e.g., small amounts of cream and bananas that are not overripe). Clinicians should refer in addition to the most recent comprehensive review of this subject: McCabe B., Tsuang M.: Dietary consideration on MAO inhibitor regimens. Journal of Clinical Psychiatry 43:178−181, 1982.

†This chapter is based in part on research supported by grants from the Foundations' Fund for Research in Psychiatry, Grant No. 77-612, and the National Institute of Mental Health, Grant No. CRC 30915.

surround attempts to make precise dosage adjustments on the basis of therapeutic effects or side effects alone. Together, these facts indicate that the plasma-level monitoring of these drugs should be a valuable aid in the treatment of depressive disorders.

The delayed introduction of routine plasma-level monitoring is due partly to the peculiar difficulties that practicing psychiatrists encounter in the treatment of depressed patients, First, they encounter the problem of making an accurate diagnosis, although the diagnostic criteria have become more standardized with DSM-III (American Psychiatric Association, 1980). A second problem is choosing an antidepressant, given the clinical response and lag between initiating the chosen pharmacotherapy. Third, clinicians must individualize the dose in the face of pharmacokinetic, age, physical-illness, and other confounding factors. Finally, it is still not certain whether the observed degree of improvement is related to the amount of drug or, even if plasma levels are measured, whether improvement is due to the parent compounds and/or metabolites. The author here attempts to expand on available clinical pharmacokinetic data, with the goal of presenting an integrated approach that makes use of pharmacokinetics, plasma level, and response parameters and that may be useful in rational pharmacotherapeutic decisions. The chapter also draws upon several recent and appropriate reviews (Gram et al., 1982; Kragh-Sorensen, 1980; Amsterdam et al., 1980; DeVane, 1980; Hrdina et al., 1982; Glassman and Perel, 1978).

CLINICAL PHARMACOKINETICS

Definitions

Pharmacokinetics can be defined as the mathematical modeling of the time course of drug absorption, distribution, metabolism, and excretion. Pharmacokinetic studies include experiments aimed at estimating the values of the various parameters which characterize these processes for individual drugs, applications of pharmacokinetic information to the design of patient treatment regimens or to the design of experiments aimed at evaluating a drug's effect, and investigations of fundamental mechanisms of drug disposition (Rowland and Tozer, 1980).

Interpretation of pharmacokinetic data depends upon understanding fundamental parameters such as half-life, volume of distribution, and clearance. The *half-life* ($t\frac{1}{2}$) of a drug in the body is the time necessary for the concentration of drug in the blood to decrease by half after absorption and distribution are complete. Elimination half-life is associated with the terminal slope of a semilogarithmic concentration-time curve. It is a function of drug binding to tissue other than plasma or blood constituents and the clearance of the free (unbound) drug, which for tricyclics takes place in the hepatic system. The apparent *volume of distribution* (V_D) is the fluid volume throughout which a drug seems to be distributed. This may include several functional compartments in the body, such as plasma water, extracellular fluid, and intracellular fluid. The distribution of a drug may depend on its degree of protein binding, its ionization, and its lipophilicity. *Total body clearance* (CL) of a drug is defined as the apparent volume of body fluids containing the amount of drug eliminated per unit time. Physiologically, CL is a product of the blood flow through the elimination organ and the fraction of the entering concentration eliminated in a single pass through the organ. Variations in $t\frac{1}{2}$, V_D, and CL due to genetic factors, age, disease

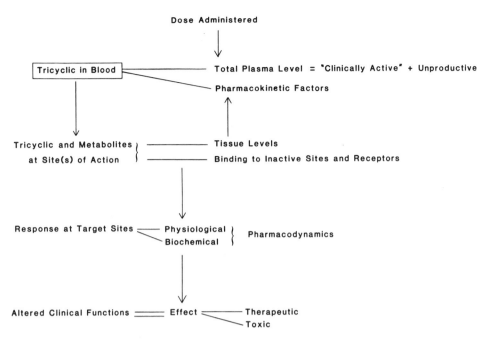

Figure 1. Interrelationships among plasma levels, clinical effects and pharmacokinetics.

states, and drug interactions cause alterations in plasma levels of psychotropic drugs. Knowledge of these pharmacokinetic changes is necessary in designing patient treatment regimens (Greenblatt and Koch-Weser, 1975; Rowland, 1978).

As with most drugs, the action of the tricyclic antidepressants depends on the concentration available for pharmacologic action and, in turn, is reflected by the level of drug circulating free (unbound) in plasma. Plasma and tissue concentrations of a drug depend not only on the amount ingested, i.e., the dose, but also on its bioavailability (distribution throughout the body) and on its biotransformation and excretion. Variations in these factors can affect the actual availability of the drug at its site of action and therefore the response to treatment. The interplay among pharmacodynamic and pharmacokinetic parameters is illustrated in Figure 1.

Metabolism and Active Metabolites

The tricyclic antidepressants are divided into two broad groups according to their chemical structures. The tertiary group includes imipramine, amitriptyline, and doxepin, and the secondary group includes desmethylimipramine, nortriptyline, and protriptyline.* The tertiary tricyclics are demethylated in the liver to their corresponding secondary methylamines, and all these compounds are subsequently eliminated via hydroxylation and glucuronidation (see Figure 2). Consequently, patients treated with tertiary tricyclics such as imipramine, amitriptyline, and doxepin also will be exposed to their corresponding secondary

*Preceptor's note: In Figure 1 of their chapter, Cole and Schatzberg display the chemical structures of the tricyclic antidepressants.

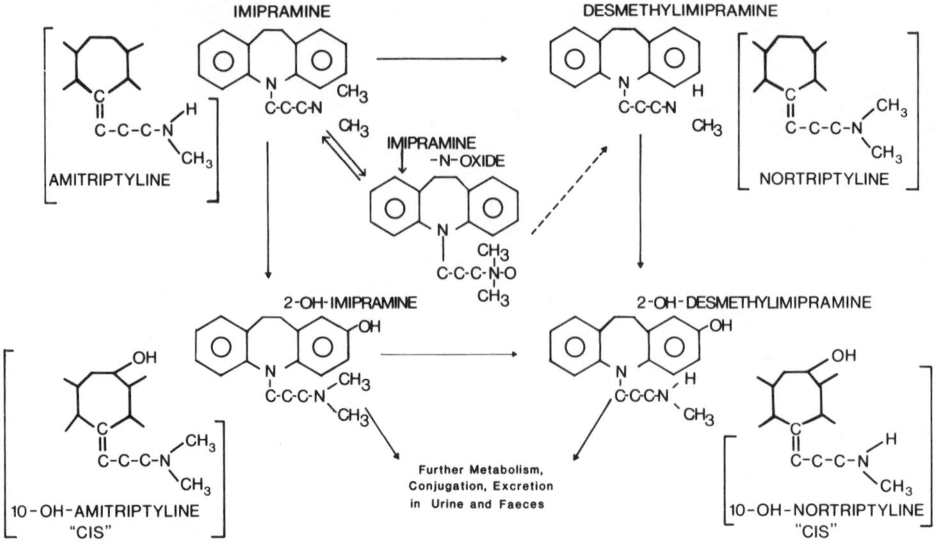

Figure 2. Pathways of imipramine and desmethylimipramine. Metabolism with comparisons to amitriptyline and nortriptyline.

amine metabolites, desmethylimipramine, nortriptyline, and desmethyl-doxepin, respectively. In some subjects, the extent of these conversions is so great that the predominant pharmacologically active compound present will be the secondary metabolite. The ratio of amitriptyline to its metabolite nortriptyline varies from less than 0.25 to more than 3.0, with a mean of about 1.0, whereas for imipramine the ratio changes from 0.1 to 3.0, with a mean of about 1.4 (Perel et al., 1978a; 1978b). Since the demethylation reaction is almost certainly not reversible, patients treated with the secondary tricyclics are exposed only to these and not to the corresponding tertiary antidepressant.

The hydroxy metabolites of tricyclics (i.e., 2-OH-imipramine, 2-OH-desmethylimipramine, 10-OH-amitriptyline, 10-OH-nortriptyline) cross the blood-brain barrier, are effective reuptake inhibitors of 5-hydroxy-tryptamine and norepinephrine, and may therefore be therapeutically active. They are present in significant concentrations in plasma, urine, and cerebrospinal fluid, unconjugated (free) or reversibly bound to glucuronic acid, the conjugate being present in two- to fourfold excess (Javaid et al., 1979; Potter et al., 1979; DeVane et al., 1981). They are not routinely measured by most laboratories, and their contribution to the therapeutic effect of the tricyclics is presently unknown but subject to current research. Some of these are highly cardioactive, and their presence may explain why some patients develop cardiac side effects at relatively low serum levels of parent compound, or alternatively why some patients with apparently unusually high levels of parent drugs but negligible conversion to hydroxy metabolites seem to tolerate tricyclic therapy (Jandhyala et al., 1977; DeVane et al., 1981).

Pharmacokinetic Aspects

Following oral administration, tricyclics are absorbed quite rapidly, with peak plasma levels usually occurring within two to six hours. Although absorption of tricyclic antidepressants from the gastrointestinal tract is complete, their bioavailability is much less than complete because the amount of available tricyclic is influenced by the "first-pass" effect: a fraction of the absorbed drug is bound and metabolized by the liver before reaching the systemic circulation. For tricyclics this effect depends mainly on hepatic blood flow (Nies et al., 1976; Wilkinson and Shand, 1975). There is considerable intersubject and interdrug variability in the first-pass effect and therefore in the amount of "available" drug. For the tertiary antidepressants, the "excess" N-demethylation observed between oral and parenteral pharmacokinetics accounts for most of the "first-pass" effect. The amount of tricyclic actually available has been shown to vary between 13 and 90 percent among subjects (Gram and Frederickson-Overø, 1975; Gram and Christiansen, 1975; Ziegler et al., 1978a; 1978b). The range of these values for a particular tricyclic indicates that the first-pass effect may be of major importance for determining the magnitude of the steady-state drug concentrations, as well as the dosage necessary for optimal clinical response (see Table 1).

It is only in the past few years that plasma levels of tricyclic antidepressants have been available to aid practicing psychiatrists in the treatment of depression. Up to a 49-fold interindividual variation was found in plasma levels in patients on identical doses of medication. It should be noted that pharmacokinetic data obtained from healthy volunteers may be different from those in depressed subjects. In the depressed subjects, altered physiological factors such as loss of appetite or reduced food intake cause a decrease in hepatic blood flow, leading to decreased hepatic clearance of these drugs (Braithwaite et al., 1978). The tertiary amine tricyclic antidepressants and the secondary amine derivatives have half-lives ranging from 4 to 58 hours, except for protriptyline which may have a half-life as long as 198 hours (mean about 100 hours) and hence may take longer to reach steady-state conditions. The secondary antidepressants have longer elimination half-lives than the corresponding tertiary (parent) drugs. For the newer antidepressants or experimental drugs such as amoxapine or zimelidine or the tetracyclic compounds such as maprotiline and mianserin, half-lives are not as firmly established as they are for the tricyclics.

The mean intraindividual steady-state plasma levels of tricyclic antidepressants are linearly related to dose in the adult patient population. However, the intersubject variation in steady-state levels is very large, with greater than thirtyfold variations being reported. While this value may represent an extreme, variations of five- to tenfold are commonly found among smaller patient populations.

Tricyclics are extensively bound to plasma proteins such as albumin and α_1-acid glycoprotein and in some cases to lipoproteins (Piafsky and Borga, 1977; Bertilsson et al., 1979; Pike and Skuterud, 1982). To date, studies examining the relationship between tricyclic plasma levels and clinical response have measured the "total" (protein bound plus "free" unbound) levels of drug in plasma. It is the free drug, rather than the total plasma concentration, that is theoretically in equilibrium with tissue levels and that should represent the pharmacologically active portion of the drug. If protein binding were to vary widely among individuals, this would decrease the usefulness of measuring total drug concentrations and make it necessary to measure only the free level of the drug, which would also vary among patients. Several groups of workers have investigated the binding of tricyclics to plasma proteins. Most have found the tricyclics to be highly bound to plasma proteins, with two- to fourfold variations in the free fraction among individuals (Glassman

Table 1. Pharmacokinetic Parameters of Tricyclic Antidepressants in Adults[1]

Drugs	Percent Bioavailability	$t_\frac{1}{2}$ (hr)	V_D (l/kg)	CL (l/hr)	Fraction Bound[2]
Imipramine	44 (29–71)	11.8 (4– 31)	14.8 (9.3–22.0)	4.2–227.0	0.63–0.96
Desipramine	(33–51)[3]	21.7 (12– 34)	37.9 (24.0–60.0)	78.0–204.0	0.73–0.92
Amitriptyline	40 (30–60)	24.5 (17– 47)	21.0 (6.4–36.0)	18.0–204.0	0.92–0.97
Nortriptyline	51 (41–70)	30.0 (18– 58)	19.1 (15.0–23.0)	17.4– 84.0	0.87–0.93
Doxepin[4]	(13–45)[3]	16.8 (8– 25)	20.2 (9.0–33.0)	41.4– 61.2	—
Protriptyline	(75–90)[3]	76.4 (54–198)	22.5 (15.0–31.0)	8.4– 30.6	0.90–0.94
Nortriptyline (17 depressed patients)	—	46.4 (21.5–88.1)	24.1 (13.8–38.2)	8.3– 55.5	—

[1]Value ranges are enclosed in parentheses.
[2]Fraction bound to human plasma proteins
[3]Calculated using an average hepatic blood flow
[4]$t_\frac{1}{2}$ for desmethyldoxepin is 51.3 (33.2–80.7).

et al., 1973; Kragh-Sorensen and Larsen, 1980). While for most patients the total plasma concentrations appear to be adequate, there probably are a small number who would benefit from "free"-level measurements as demonstrated for anticonvulsant therapeutic monitoring with diphenylhydantoin.

Repetitive administration of a constant dose of tricyclic leads to an increase in the plasma concentrations until steady-state plasma levels are reached, generally within 7 to 21 days, although protriptyline with its longer half-life requires more than 25 days. At steady state, the daily elimination of drug equals the amount of drug ingested, and plasma and tissue concentrations are approximately the same at similar times on successive days. The importance of steady-state plasma levels (or more accurately the steady-state "free" plasma levels) lies in the fact that they reflect the amount of drug available for biological action. They give a far better indication of drug availability at the receptor site than does the oral dose. The rate and magnitude of buildup to steady state are determined by the elimination half-life; the longer this value, the longer (four to five half-lives) it takes for higher steady-state levels to be achieved. It should be noted, however, that although it may take one to two weeks to reach steady-state levels, appreciable levels of tricyclics are often built up rapidly, and side effects from these drugs are common within the first few days of starting dosage. The wide differences in the steady-state plasma levels are due mainly to differences in the metabolism of the drug by liver microsomal enzymes. Although this activity appears to be largely genetically determined, certain drugs can cause changes in the activity of these enzymes. While the clinical relevance of these effects has not been demonstrated conclusively, it would be expected that drugs which inhibit metabolism of the tricyclics would decrease the dose needed for beneficial therapeutic effect, while the converse is true for drugs which stimulate tricyclic metabolism.

Another factor which to date has not received much attention is the influence of somatic illnesses, in particular inflammatory diseases, on plasma concentrations of tricyclic antidepressants. Recently Piafsky and Borga (1977) showed that the free fraction of imipramine is strongly correlated to the concentration of α_1-acid glycoprotein in plasma. The concentration of this protein is increased in certain inflammatory diseases, and the investigators have shown that the pharmacokinetics of such agents as chlorpromazine may be influenced in patients with different somatic illnesses combined with high concentrations of α_1-acid glycoprotein (Piafsky et al., 1978). The clinical significance of this problem has not yet been evaluated, but Kragh-Sorensen and Larsen (1980) have shown that changes in plasma nortriptyline concentration during inflammatory diseases can possibly have relevance for therapeutic outcome.

Effects in Children and the Elderly*

Both the young and old seem more sensitive than adults to the effects of psychotropic medication. The age-related changes in the pharmacokinetics and pharmacodynamics of psychotropic drugs are summarized

*Editor's Note: In Part III of Psychiatry 1982 (Psychiatry Update: Volume I), Dr. Joaquim Puig-Antich discusses plasma levels and therapeutic responses of depressed children treated with imipramine (pages 291–292). The particular issues of treating elderly people with tricyclic antidepressants are discussed by Friedel in Part II of this volume and by Cole and Schatzberg in the previous chapter.

Table 2. Age-Related Pharmacologic Changes in the Elderly

Pharmacologic Factor	Age-Related Changes
Absorption	Altered due to decrease with actively transported drugs, but probably not clinically significant
Distribution	Increase in V_D due to increased fat-muscle ratio
	Lower serum albumin-globulin ratio with increased free drug due to decrease in protein binding
Hepatic Metabolism	Decreased liver blood flow and enzyme activity, leading to a prolongation of elimination half-life and a reduction of total drug clearance
Excretion	Decreased renal blood flow, glomerular filtration rate, and tubular secretory function, leading to decreased elimination
Receptor-Site Sensitivity	Decreased CNS cholinergic functioning, decrease in nigrostriatal dopamine, increased sensitivity to the CNS effects of drugs

Source: Hicks et al. (1981).

in Table 2. Elderly people may also have concurrent medical illnesses (cardiovascular, hepatic, or renal) that further alter the pharmacokinetics, and they are generally victims of polypharmacy, which makes them more susceptible to possible adverse drug interactions.

Since elderly people have diminished hepatic enzyme activity and reduced hepatic blood flow, they will have higher steady-state plasma levels of tricyclic antidepressant at "therapeutic" doses (Hrdina et al., 1982; Dawling et al., 1980). This appears to be the case with imipramine, desipramine, doxepin, and nortriptyline. A markedly reduced clearance and a longer elimination half-life of imipramine in elderly persons is well documented. Due to delayed elimination by the kidney, the elderly also have an increased concentration of the hydroxy metabolites of tricyclics (Kitanaka et al., 1982). Older people also appear to be more sensitive to the cardiac effects of the tricyclics at therapeutic plasma levels. They more frequently develop orthostatic hypotension and conduction disturbances in the EKG, and they are at risk for developing congestive heart failure because of the myocardium-depressant activity of the tricyclics. This age group is also more sensitive to the anticholinergic effects of the antidepressants.

The pharmacokinetics of imipramine and nortriptyline are also altered in children. A decreased fat-to-muscle ratio leads to a small V_D in children, and they are therefore not protected from excessive dosage situations by the large "sink" of fatty tissue. Children also have larger hepatic mass (percent of hepatic occupancy) relative to body size and hence tend to metabolize drugs at a faster rate. Like the elderly, children have diminished protein binding of drugs due to lower plasma albumin levels. Thus, for the tricyclic antidepressants, $t_{\frac{1}{2}}$ is usually shorter in children because of the faster hepatic metabolism; $t_{\frac{1}{2}}$ for imipramine is 5 to 13 hours, and for nortriptyline 11 to 24 hours (Geller et al., 1982a; Perel et al., unpublished data).

Prediction from Single-Dose Kinetics

Clinical applications of drug-level monitoring require that the information obtained about the drug concentration in plasma be usable for proper dose adjustment. The calculation of an appropriate dose in order to obtain a therapeutic drug level can be based on measurements of drug concentrations at steady state or on early measurements after single or multiple doses. Pharmacokinetic data can be applied to predict the dosing regimen most likely to achieve targeted steady-state plasma concentrations in individual patients. At least three approaches are possible: (1) empirically adjusting dosage based on random plasma concentrations, (2) dosing based on total body clearance determined from a single-dose study, and (3) dosing based on a plasma concentration obtained after the first dose.

The conventional technique of adjusting dosages involves a delay of two weeks or longer until steady-state conditions are assumed and plasma concentrations can be determined. For example, consider a patient taking 150 mg of oral imipramine per day, who at the end of two weeks of continuous treatment achieves a combined imipramine plus desipramine plasma concentration of 150 ng/ml. An upward dosage adjustment is desirable, either immediately or after four weeks if the patient remains nonresponsive, to increase the steady state to within the presumed therapeutic range of 225 ng/ml or greater. Thus, we divide the patient's steady-state level (150 ng/ml) by his or her daily dosage (150 mg) to determine the ng/ml plasma concentrations produced by each mg of drug administered per day. We then divide this quotient (1.0 ng/mg · ml) into the desired steady-state concentration (225 ng/ml), which gives us the target dosage, which in this example is 225 mg per day. This simple approach to adjusting dosages makes several assumptions. First, it assumes that the systemic availability remains constant. Second, it assumes that enzyme stimulation or inhibition does not occur between the first steady-state plasma level and subsequent determinations. And finally, it assumes that metabolism remains linear over the dosage range employed.

These assumptions cannot frequently be validated. For example, in geriatric patients nonlinearity appears upon imipramine administration, evidenced by an exaggerated increase due to disproportionate increases of desmethylimipramine plasma levels with increasing dose (Thayssen et al., 1981). Although some deviation from the predicted steady state often occurs, this method remains the simplest pharmacokinetic approach to adjustment of dosing without making additional assumptions of individual pharmacokinetic parameters based on population means. For the tricyclics, this would be a tenuous generalization, given their variable metabolism. Therefore, to achieve 225 ng/ml with the patient in the foregoing example, it would be wiser to increase the dosage in gradual steps of 25 mg per day on each of three days and to allow a two- or three-day interval between the increments.

A second pharmacokinetic approach to predicting dosage at the outset of therapy is to determine the total body clearance from a single dose (Braithwaite et al., 1982; Potter et al., 1980). This requires that precisely timed, multiple blood samples be obtained during the concentration-time course of a single dose covering 48 to 72 hours or longer. Many pharmacokinetic parameters can be determined from these data, and these parameters can be used to predict the dose needed to yield a desired steady-state level. This approach has been successfully used by investigators working with imipramine, nortriptyline, and desipramine. A now classical study (Alexanderson, 1972) found that the pharmacokinetics of nortriptyline allowed accurate prediction of desipramine plasma concentrations in the same normal subjects. The same paired relationship was demonstrated with amitriptyline-chlorimipramine in depressed patients (Mellstrom et al., 1979). Conversely, the pharmacokinetics of doxepin and protriptyline were not found to be correlated in the same subjects (Ziegler et al., 1978a; 1978b). This inconsistency in findings may be related to differences in the metabolism of the individual drugs or to differences in the study subjects, but it suggests some problems in predicting concentrations of one tricyclic on the basis of the pharmacokinetics of another. Since the metabolism among different tricyclics may be strikingly different in a given patient, tolerance and/or therapeutic benefit with one tricyclic may not occur with another.

A disadvantage of determining clearance from a single dose is the three to five days required for study. Moreover, the pharmacokinetic workups are expensive, usually require institutionalization, and may delay initiation of treatment. Still, under certain conditions the determination of clearance in this manner will be valuable. Depression tends to be a recurring illness, and the information gained from the study should allow efficient dosing for years to come. By determining plasma concentrations at steady state and calculating clearances, the knowledge gained from a protracted single-dose study is available for future use, while the need for future studies may be obviated.

A third approach to pharmacokinetic dosing has been reported for nortriptyline, imipramine, desipramine, and amitriptyline. In these investigations, a single oral dose of tricyclic is administered, and one or two plasma concentrations are obtained before constant maintenance therapy. The single-dose plasma values are then correlated with steady-state levels (Cooper and Simpson, 1978; Brunswick et al., 1979; Montgomery et al., 1979; Slattery et al., 1980). The concentration at 48 hours has correlated best with the steady-state values in all reports and has been used to formulate dosage tables that predict maintenance doses from a single plasma concentration following a test dose. Twenty-four-hour values also had adequate but not outstanding predictability.

One should be cognizant of several limitations to predicting dosage in this manner. First of all, dosage predictions outside the range experimentally tested should not be made, lest a disproportionate degree of tricyclic accumulation occur. Furthermore, each clinical site must be evaluated or calibrated for precision of analytical and clinical procedures. The timing of the plasma sample should be about 1.5 times the population half-life of the tricyclic in question (Unadkat and Rowland, 1982). Reliance on correlation coefficient (r) for predictability should be limited because it provides misleadingly higher reliability than the data warrant. Other statistical methods provide more realistic predictions for dosage adjustment. Even these precautions may not be sufficient to ensure that the approach constitutes a clinically useful tool. For example, the correlation between plasma levels of mianserin after a single dose and repeated administration has been found rather poor (r = 0.60) (Hrdina and LaPierre, unpublished data).

ASSAY METHODS

Since initial studies demonstrated the clinical applicability of monitoring tricyclic antidepressants, numerous analytical methods have been described (Scoggins et al., 1980; Perel et al., 1978b). Under therapeutic conditions, the concentration of tricyclics is very low, in the 20 to 350 ng/ml range. In choosing a method, several requirements need to be considered. The method must be specific; that is, it must be able to measure parent drugs and metabolites individually without interference. It must also be sensitive enough to measure steady-state concentrations as low as 10 ng/ml in 1- to 2-ml plasma samples, and for single-dose kinetics, the sensitivity must be increased further to 1 to 5 ng/ml. The assay should have a routine intraassay and interassay precision of not higher than 10 percent expressed as coefficients of variation, and the procedure should be sufficiently rapid to provide results within 24 hours after specimens are received. No single assay is best for all purposes, and it might be necessary to use at least two different techniques to provide the full range of analyses with maximum cost-effectiveness. The accompanying Table 3 summarizes some of the characteristics, advantages, and disadvantages of methods in current use.

For identification of compounds in research, the combination of a mass spectrometer with gas chromatography (GC-MS) is unsurpassed. This method is highly reliable, but it requires access and time on very expensive equipment. Although GC-MS is regarded as the standard with which other methods should be compared for specificity, it is doubtful whether using GC-MS in community hospitals is feasible. The most widely used methods today are gas chromatographic (GC) techniques with several different detection systems for quantitation of tricyclics. An alkali flame ionization detector, sometimes called a nitrogen detector, has the selectivity and sensitivity for research use and is not as difficult to operate as GC-MS. Electron capture is another detection system for GC and is more sensitive than nitrogen detection; however, its operation requires more technical skill, and poor specificity is a drawback.

High performance liquid chromatography (HPLC) is an increasingly popular analytical technique offering tremendous separation capability, but it has not yet been applied to measurements of all the available tricyclics. When coupled with a fluorescence detector, it is a highly sensitive and specific assay. While moderately expensive, HPLC is a good compromise for research and clinical monitoring due to its ease of operation. HPLC also proves to be more suitable for concurrent analyses of the hydroxylated metabolites if these are also being measured.

A promising method is radioimmunoassay, which has high sensitivity, requires only a small quantity of sample, and does not involve the extensive sample preparation inherent in most other methods. Specificity, however, may be a problem due to cross-reaction of antibodies with metabolites and compounds of similar structure. Ultimately, this method may become widely used in hospitals which presently own a scintillation counter, owing to its ease of operation and low cost after initial setup.

Likewise, the immunoassay techniques which have proven to be so convenient and cost-effective with anticonvulsants, antiarrhythmics, and so forth may eventually be suitable for tricyclic analyses, but antibodies of higher specificity need to be researched.

Specimen Collection

Reports in the literature have documented the effects of Vacutainer tubes (Becton-Dickinson) on the determination of tricyclics (Bailey and Jatlow, 1976; Brunswick and Mendels, 1977). This interference was

Table 3. Methods for Determination of Tricyclic Antidepressants

Method (Sample size in ml)	Sensitivity in ng/ml	Specificity	Speed of Analysis	Skill Required	Comments
Gas Chromatography-Mass Spectrometry, Electron Impact Ionization Detector (1.0–3.0)	5–20	excellent	fair	high	Requires deuterated internal standards for best results. Complex equipment required
Gas Chromatography-Mass Spectrometry, Chemical Ionization Detector (1.0–2.0)	1–10	excellent	fair	high	Requires deuterated internal standards for best results. Complex equipment required
Gas Chromatography, Nitrogen Detector (1.0–3.0)	5–10	excellent	good	moderate	Does not usually require derivatization
Gas Chromatography, Electron Capture Detector (1.0–3.0)	1–5	poor	good	moderate	Does not always distinguish secondary and tertiary compounds. Requires derivatization
High Performance Liquid Chromatography (0.5–3.0)	25–50	good	fair	moderate-low	Subject to interference by other drugs. Detectors are not specific. Still under development
Radioimmunoassay (0.01–0.10)	1–5	poor	excellent	low	Does not distinguish metabolites from parent compound unless preextraction and/or derivatization is used
Immunoassay (Enzyme; Fluorescence)	5–20 (estimated)	poor	excellent	low	Under development, not currently available. Would be convenient, rapid

shown to be due to the presence of the plasticizer Tris(2-butoxyethyl) phosphate (TBEP) in the rubber stoppers used in the older Vacutainer tubes. This plasticizer displaces basic drugs bound to α_1-acid glycoproteins in plasma, leading to migration of free drug into red blood cells through reequilibration. Thus, after separation, plasma tricyclic concentrations yield false low values by as much as 40 percent. Furthermore, an extraneous interference peak has been noted in the nitrogen GC analyses of selected tricyclics.

More recently, selected Vacutainer tubes have not used the TBEP in the rubber-stopper formulations. The author and his colleagues have tested these (only with anticoagulants) extensively and found that plasma concentrations of tricyclics obtained with blood specimens collected under standard procedures with these tubes did not differ from samples collected with glass syringes or siliconized tubes without stoppers (Stiller et al., 1980; Perel et al., 1981).

Venojet tubes (Kimble-Terumo) have been shown to be free from this interference and thus are suitable (Veith et al., 1978). However, tubes containing gel separators, e.g., Corvac (Corning) and SST (Becton-Dickinson), are not suitable because of reduced tricyclic levels, although this lowering is not as great as that seen with the older Vacutainers.

After prompt centrifugation and separation of plasma samples, tricyclic antidepressants are stable up to one year in frozen plasma, even longer at $-15°$ C, and they are stable up to five days at ambient temperature. There is no significant difference between plasma and serum analyses in split-sample studies.

Standardization of sampling time is important for the comparison of plasma values to therapeutic ranges. Since kinetic distribution of tricyclics is complete within 3 to 11 hours after oral ingestion, it can generally be recommended that the optimal time for collection of steady-state plasma samples should be between 10 to 15 hours after the last dose of medication for patients taking antidepressants once a day, and just before the morning dose for patients on a divided-dose schedule. Whenever possible, plasma-concentration monitoring should be carried out in the morning because day-to-day variations in steady-state levels have been shown to be less pronounced in the morning than at other times (Kragh-Sorensen, 1980).

PLASMA LEVEL AND EFFECT RELATIONSHIPS

Since the introduction of imipramine by Kuhn in 1957, tricyclic antidepressants have become the treatment of choice for most types of depressive illness. Although these drugs show greater efficacy in patients suffering endogenous affective disease, other good evidence indicates that patients with neurotic or reactive depression are also responsive. It has also been recognized that tricyclics have a delayed onset of therapeutic effects and that about 30 percent of patients treated do not benefit. Efforts to hasten the onset of beneficial effects and to increase therapeutic efficacy have included concomitant administration of thyroid hormones and methylphenidate, once-daily therapy, high-dose therapy, intramuscular therapy, and now plasma-concentration monitoring.

In order to use drug-level monitoring in practical therapy, relationships among drug levels and therapeutic effects have to be established in controlled studies so that data can subsequently be used clinically.

Thus, significant treatment variables other than the drug levels must also be identified. The diagnostic classification of patients appears to be important in this context, and consistent relationships between plasma level and effect have so far been established only in endogenously depressed patients. Despite the extensive clinical use of tricyclics, the number of well-controlled and statistically valid studies which attempt to relate plasma concentration to clinical effects is limited, and most of them concern adult patients.

Criteria for Clinical Studies

Some of the problems inherent in the design and methodology for studies of plasma level and therapeutic response have been extensively discussed by DeVane (1980). For the present discussion, six salient points are summarized.

(1)   The homogeneity of the patient sample should be assured by using rating scales with high interrater reliability to assess the intensity of depression and to follow change in symptomatology. It is important that these scales have international relevance to allow comparisons, since most of the data on antidepressants originate outside the United States.

(2)   In addition to an initial drug washout period (usually one week), a placebo week is necessary in order to exclude spontaneous responders whose data would otherwise obscure possible correlations. Placebo response is about 20 to 22 percent in the first two weeks and increases slightly in subsequent weeks.

(3)   The selection and dosage of patients should be such that, on the basis of prior clinical experience, response rate will be held down to 50 to 60 percent. Although a major consideration in studies of plasma level and effect is to define the concentration range at which patients will respond, the design must allow sufficient variance to obtain statistically significant correlations. Too high a response rate (higher than 80 percent) or too low a response rate (less than 20 percent) will invalidate these objectives.

(4)   Constant dosage, preferably weight adjusted, is needed to define the therapeutic range and to provide the wide range of plasma concentrations for evaluating response. Random dosage changes produce biased clinical effects and often narrow the band of plasma levels.

(5)   Since compliance is a critical issue, initial studies should involve inpatients despite their high cost. Plasma levels are useful only in detecting complete noncompliance, and partial noncompliance is best avoided with institutionalized patients.

(6)   The time required to achieve meaningful steady-state conditions (elimination equals daily intake) is four to five half-lives. Only under these conditions will plasma concentrations reflect a pseudoequilibrium between "free" or unbound drugs in plasma and at the site of action. Therefore, in order to include slow metabolizers, a minimum of 7 to 21 days is needed to assure steady-state plasma levels in all the study patients. Since the development of full antidepressant effects is further delayed *after* achievement of steady state, a minimum of four weeks should elapse before calculating the correlation between patients' plasma concentrations and responses. The author and his colleagues have found that with imipramine an average minimum of 5 days is needed to observe stable responses after achievement of steady state (Perel et al., 1978a; Glassman et al., 1977).

Findings

IMIPRAMINE Two large independent studies of imipramine show nearly identical results concerning the relationship between the level of imipramine plus desmethylimipramine and therapeutic effect. Total levels below 150 ng/ml were much less effective, whereas the therapeutic effect became gradually better with higher drug levels: the therapeutic effect was maximal at total levels above 225 to 240 ng/ml (Reisby et al., 1977; Glassman et al., 1977). There was no indication of poor therapeutic effect in patients with particularly high levels, and the upper recommendable plasma level will be mainly determined by the occurrence of side effects. In terms of the individual components, the critical lower limits for antidepressant response were determined to be 45 ng/ml or greater for imipramine *plus* 75 ng/ml or greater for desmethylimipramine. Data from the study by Glassman et al. (1977) indicated in addition that 24 percent of nonresponding patients improved when plasma concentrations exceeded 200 ng/ml at the conclusion of the study.

Two smaller studies, although not convincing by themselves because of sample size and methodological problems (Olivier-Martin et al., 1975; Simpson et al., 1982), are nevertheless in agreement with the two larger studies. Furthermore, the developmental constancy of the therapeutic range has been demonstrated by the findings of Puig-Antich et al. (1979; 1983) with prepubertal major depressive disorders. In summary, these studies of imipramine agree (1) that interindividual metabolic differences do influence outcome, (2) that the percentage of patients responding favorably increases as blood levels are increased up to 200 to 250 ng/ml (although some patients show very favorable clinical response at lower blood levels), and (3) that higher levels (greater than 250 ng/ml) can produce more side effects but no decrease in antidepressant response.

NORTRIPTYLINE For nortriptyline, the majority of studies report a curvilinear relationship between plasma concentration and effect, with a "therapeutic window" between 50 and 150 ng/ml (reviewed by Gram, 1980). Plasma levels below 50 ng/ml are associated with poor response due to insufficient drug availability, whereas levels greater than 150 ng/ml not only show poor response, but also show exacerbation of selected symptom clusters. The reasons for this "window" effect are still unclear, but it is not related to toxicity. About 65 percent of patients maintained on 150 mg/day fall within the window, and most of the others have elevated plasma levels. It appears that response is extended to about 80 to 85 percent of the patients upon readjustment of dosages (Sorensen et al., 1978). Once clinical response is achieved, maintenance at that concentration should be continued for optimal prophylactic effect. As with imipramine, children with depression have been shown to respond to nortriptyline at the same "therapeutic window" as adults, but in contrast to imipramine, there are minimal cardiovascular effects in either children or adults (Geller et al., 1982a; 1982b; Giardina et al., 1981; Vohra et al., 1975a; 1975b).

AMITRIPTYLINE Amitriptyline has been studied in several larger studies involving a total of more than 300 patients. The results are less consistent than for imipramine and nortriptyline, and some groups have failed to show any relationship whatsoever between plasma level and effect. Altogether, the studies seem to indicate a lower effective total level (amitriptyline plus nortriptyline) of 80 to 120 ng/ml. An upper plasma-level limit, above which the therapeutic effect is poor, has been suggested in some studies but not others. Combining the results of the studies supporting a linear response, the concentration for most responders falls between 80 and 210 ng/ml total level, and there is no evidence of decreased response above 220 ng/ml (Kupfer et al., 1977; Ziegler et al., 1976). The studies supporting a curvilinear response allocate an upper limit of 220 to 250 ng/ml (Montgomery et al., 1979). The two largest amitriptyline studies found no useful relationship between concentration and effect. One, the World Health Organization study (Coppen et al., 1978), has been criticized because only one third of the patients responded, while the other, reported by Robinson et al. (1979), found a weak positive correlation which could increase when endogenous criteria are factored. It can be concluded that although the majority of studies indicate a linear relationship, there is still sufficient uncertainty to warrant additional studies of higher quality.

OTHER ANTIDEPRESSANTS   Plasma level and effect relationships for protriptyline, doxepin, and desipramine have not been thoroughly studied. For protriptyline, the study of Biggs and Ziegler (1977) supports a plasma concentration range of greater than 70 ng/ml. One additional protriptyline study (Whyte et al., 1976) found a curvilinear response, with a range of 165 to 240 ng/ml for responders, but due to insufficient length of protocol, steady-state plasma levels were not achieved in most of the patients.

For doxepin, Friedel and Raskind (1975) reported that improvement was related to levels greater than 110 ng/ml in an uncontrolled study of 15 patients. Kline et al. (1976) reported that improvement correlated with desmethyldoxepin concentration and not with doxepin in a study of 12 outpatients. A more recent study with doxepin (Ward et al., 1982) indicated an optimal therapeutic range between 125 and 250 ng/ml of doxepin plus desmethyldoxepin and found that higher and lower plasma levels were associated with lesser response. Due to methodological flaws, including variable dosing, failure to achieve steady-state levels, use of both outpatient and inpatient samples, and the possibility of "carry-over" effects due to short intervals between dose changes, the conclusions of this study cannot be extrapolated.

Desipramine concentrations have been reported in relation to clinical response in three studies, but steady-state conditions were not assured in any of these. Twenty-six outpatients were studied in a larger desipramine study, and improvement was related to concentrations of up to 160 ng/ml. Although the data suggested a decline in therapeutic response at plasma concentrations above 160 ng/ml, the study's lack of a drug-free period and/or placebo control vitiates these findings, since nondrug responders might also have been included (Friedel et al., 1979). A more recent study with only seven inpatients, after a washout placebo period of five to seven days prior to active treatment, appeared to suggest a curvilinear relationship, the optimum being 80 to 175 ng/ml, but verification will be necessary (Hrdina and LaPierre, 1981). The largest and most definitive study included thirty nondelusional unipolar depressed inpatients who met DSM-III criteria for Major Depressive Episode with Melancholia (Nelson et al., 1982). The data indicated an

Table 4. Present Status of Knowledge Concerning Tricyclic Antidepressant Plasma Concentrations and Clinical Response

Drug	Total Patients Studied	Usual Dosage Range (mg/day)	Type of Correlation	Therapeutic Range (ng/ml)
Imipramine	259	75–300	Linear	$\geq 225-240^1$
Nortriptyline	414	30–150	Curvilinear	50–150
Amitriptyline	321	75–300	Uncertain	$120-250^1$
Desipramine	63	75–300	Probably linear	≥ 125
Doxepin	42	75–300	Uncertain	$110-250^1$
Protriptyline	49	15–60	Probably curvilinear	70–250
		Data for Prepubertal Major Depression		
Imipramine	30	Avg: 4.3 mg/kg/day	Linear	155–284
Nortriptyline	10 (ongoing)	0.5–1.6 mg/kg/day	Curvilinear	45–130 (tentative)

[1]Parent drug plus N-desmethyl metabolite

overall linear plasma level and effect relationship, with optimal antidepressant effectiveness occurring at 125 ng/ml or greater and the ultimate overall response being about 84 percent. Although the proportion of the sample above 300 ng/ml was meager, the study found no evidence of decreased therapeutic effectiveness at relatively high levels.

In summary, the most evidence for a defined therapeutic plasma-level range exists for imipramine and nortriptyline. A therapeutic range for amitriptyline is also probably operational, but there has been some difficulty in defining its limits, due perhaps to the heterogeneity and possible noncompliance of the patients studied. Therapeutic ranges for protriptyline, doxepin, and desipramine await confirmation. Kragh-Sorensen (1980) has described two of his studies which indicated that plasma concentrations should be maintained in the same range for continuation therapy as for the treatment of active depression. A summary of current knowledge regarding presumed therapeutic plasma concentrations of tricyclics is provided in Table 4.

PLASMA LEVELS IN CLINICAL MANAGEMENT

Preconditions for Plasma-Level Monitoring
Plasma levels of drugs are widely used in medical practice to improve pharmacotherapeutic management of disease and to reduce drug toxicity. Sheiner and Tozer (1978) have outlined the specific preconditions for the rational use of plasma-level data. These include:

(1) *Difficulty in accurate measurements or assessments of a specific "target effect" or definitive treatment end points.* Tricyclics readily meet these criteria. With tricyclic antidepressants, the therapeutic effect is not immediately observable, and there is a lack of definite intermediate effect measurement. It is difficult to measure objectively many of the target symptoms of depression, although symptoms are used to assess treatment response. Their imprecision as measures is further influenced by their sensitivity to multiple psychosocial and/or biologic factors.

(2) *A wide interindividual variability in pharmacokinetics and little intra-individual variability.* Neither plasma levels nor therapeutic response can be uniformly predicted for tricyclics by administering a normal oral dosage or by weight adjustments.

(3) *A narrow therapeutic plasma level and/or relatively close therapeutic and toxic plasma levels.* It appears that the tricyclic toxic plasma level is two to four times the therapeutic level, and slow metabolizers may reach potentially toxic plasma levels while taking relatively "standard" dosages.

(4) *Established relationships between plasma drug concentrations and therapeutic effects.* For nortriptyline and imipramine, plasma levels correlate with therapeutics.

(5) *A need to sustain the effect of the drug and its plasma level over a relatively prolonged period.*

(6) *Validated assay procedures.*

(7) *Clinical pharmacokinetic parameters that have been elucidated with patients.*

(8) *Evidence of compliance problems.*

Appropriate tricyclic dosage can be determined through clinical judgment without using plasma levels in about two thirds of the patients. The cost of each plasma-level determination ($25 to $50) further inhibits routine use. Plasma levels therefore should be considered in special clinical situations involving nonresponders, placebo responders, polypharmacy, and patients at risk.

Clinical Indications

NONRESPONDERS Plasma-level determinations are helpful in the management of patients who are not responding to pharmacotherapeutic treatment. Failure to respond may result from any of the following four circumstances. (1) There may be insufficient and/or excessive concentration of tricyclic at sites of action. (2) The patient may be failing to take the drug as prescribed. (3) The tricyclic selected may be incorrect. If nonresponse continues in the face of adequate plasma levels, changing to a different tricyclic may be appropriate. For example, biochemically different types of depression may respond preferentially, i.e., tertiary drugs are predominantly serotonin potentiating, whereas secondary drugs are primarily norepinephrine activating. (4) The tricyclics may have been prescribed for a disorder unlikely to respond at therapeutic concentrations, e.g., delusional depression. If the plasma level has been adequate without clinical response, then the diagnosis should be re-evaluated prior to the application of other treatments.

PLACEBO RESPONDERS A significant decrease in depressive symptomatology during the first week of tricyclic administration may indicate a placebo response or a sedative side effect. Very low plasma levels could help to identify the placebo responder and suggest the advisability of discontinuing tricyclics and using another equally effective treatment that has fewer potential side effects.

POLYPHARMACY Alcohol, barbiturates, tobacco smoking, and co-administration of many other drugs appear to lead to an increase in tricyclic metabolism, i.e., an increase in intrinsic clearance with a decrease in plasma levels (Perel et al., 1976; 1978b; Ciraulo et al., 1982). A baseline plasma level during a period of good response serves as a reference point against which subsequent values may be checked in case clinical decompensation results from alterations in drug metabolic parameters. As a corollary of the above rationale, some experts have advocated measuring plasma levels in every patient treated with any antidepressant when they respond, so that a record is kept on the level at which the individual patient responds. Such data may be useful to assess compliance in patients who relapse during maintenance drug treatment and may assist the clinician with patients who have recurrent depressive episodes. Other experts question the potential usefulness of applying such records, and prospective cost-effectiveness studies would help to settle this issue.

PATIENTS AT RISK   Older patients develop higher steady-state plasma levels than younger patients treated with equivalent dosage because of their reduced hepatic metabolism. Since these patients are more vulnerable to side effects and toxicity, plasma levels would ensure that geriatric patients receive adequate and precise amounts of tricyclic, usually one third to one half the amounts recommended for younger patients.

Patients affected with prepubertal depression (in the age range of 6 to 13) metabolize tricyclic much faster than adults (Puig-Antich et al., 1983). Since clinical and diagnostic variables lack predictive power in regard to total imipramine plasma levels, and since no pharmacologic parameter besides plasma level is associated with clinical response, plasma levels will probably be quite helpful to the practicing pediatric psychiatrist. Similar considerations seem to be derived from preliminary studies with nortriptyline, where the "therapeutic window" for nonpsychotic unremitting depression seems to be similar for children and adults. Since the presence of hallucinations and/or delusions requires much higher plasma levels for response (Puig-Antich et al., 1983; Spiker et al., unpublished data), it would seem that whenever psychotic symptoms are present, the clinician would want to determine a target plasma level, titrate dose, and monitor side effects until such level is achieved.

Patients with physical illness constitute another risk group where plasma levels would be helpful. Patients with hepatic and/or renal dysfunction would tend to have abnormally high accumulations of tricyclics and their hydroxy metabolites. Inflammatory disease also seems to cause a dramatic increase in tricyclic plasma levels in association with a rise of plasma α_1-acid glycoprotein. It is speculated that the increase in observed total (free and bound) concentration represents only the increase in drug bound to the protein, and through compensatory equilibrium the free or active concentration form of drug remains the same. This could lead to an overestimation such that the clinician might then reduce the dosage, leading to subtherapeutic concentrations at the site of action. These effects are presently being investigated. Patients with cardiovascular disorders also appear to metabolize tricyclics to a slower extent, probably because of reduced hepatic blood flow.

All these patients could be treated with tricyclics more precisely and confidently if dosage were controlled for a targeted therapeutic level. For nortriptyline, therapeutic levels are attainable in elderly patients without major cardiovascular effects, except for moderate impairment in myocardial contractility. The use of imipramine, however, is limited by orthostatic hypotension at subtherapeutic plasma levels, such that a majority of elderly patients do not reach therapeutic plasma levels.

Nonetheless, while nortriptyline is not associated with severe orthostatic hypotension at therapeutic blood levels, the influence of nortriptyline on cardiac performance does indicate cautious treatment and careful monitoring of its plasma levels in elderly or cardiovascular patients, especially in cases of latent cardiac failure (Giardina et al., 1981; Thayssen et al., 1981). It also would appear that patients on nortriptyline maintenance treatment (three to six months) and prophylactic treatment (years) are candidates for plasma-level monitoring, and there is evidence that relapse rates are thereby demonstrably reduced and new episodes in depressive disease prevented (Kragh-Sorensen, 1980).

Finally, as with any endeavor, a number of additional research topics involving tricyclic plasma levels still need elucidation. These topics include: the interaction of antidepressants in different types of depression; the significance of active hydroxy metabolites; the individual contribution of secondary metabolites to the overall activity of parent tertiary drugs; the chronopharmacokinetics of tricyclics and clinical response; the time lag in the onset of antidepressant action; neurochemical and pharmacokinetic factors; the significance of plasma protein-binding variability; and the clinical pharmacodynamics of tricyclic therapy.

Summary

The schematic diagram in Figure 3 was adapted from the approach by Sjoqvist (1971) and updated by DeVane (1980) and illustrates a

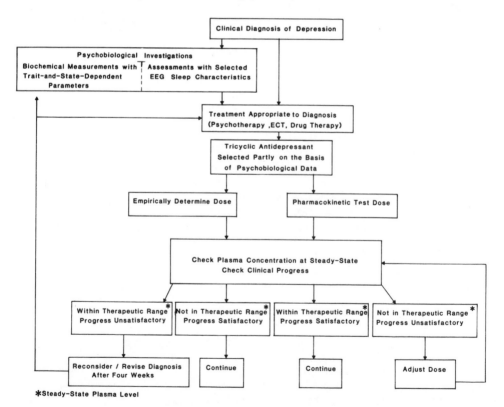

Figure 3. An integrated pharmacokinetic and psychobiological approach to the treatment of depression (based on Sjoqvist, 1981; DeVane, 1980).

decision-tree system for applying tricyclic plasma-concentration data in the treatment of depression. Once the clinical diagnosis of depression is made, appropriate treatment may include tricyclics. Ongoing and future research developments in biochemical, neuroendocrine, and polysomnographic correlates of depression may help to determine which tricyclic is specifically indicated for an individual patient.* Dosage may be selected empirically or by using the information in the pharmacokinetic and clinical response tables, beginning with a small single dose and following with stepwise increments to reach a maintenance dose determined by one of the prediction methods previously discussed. For any of the selected tricyclics, measurements of plasma concentration at the expected steady state (four to five half-lives) are useful to assess absorption and compliance and to identify individuals who achieve excessive plasma concentrations. Excessive levels should especially be avoided in the elderly and in those patients with preexisting physical conditions. Chemotherapeutic precision is markedly increased when the selected tricyclic is imipramine or nortriptyline, since therapeutic ranges appear to be well established for these agents.

When patient progress is satisfactory and unacceptable side effects are absent, no adjustment in dose is necessary unless plasma concentrations are excessive. When patient progress is unsatisfactory, the dosage may need to be adjusted, as described in the earlier example of using a conventional technique of dosage adjustment, in order to increase or decrease the plasma concentration to therapeutic range. Upon achievement of therapeutic concentrations, at least four weeks should elapse with continuous dosing to allow for the usual lag in full efficacy before reconsidering diagnosis or changing therapy. If a switch to another tricyclic is made, dosage should be titrated in the same manner as before. With patients on maintenance therapy, one should attend to physiological and polypharmaceutical factors through periodic monitoring as needed and when symptoms or unexpected side effects occur. This overall approach should result in better pharmacotherapeutic precision by minimizing the contributing pharmacokinetic "noise" which has been shown to decrease tricyclic antidepressant effectiveness.

Chapter *30* Psychotherapies for Depression†
by Maria Kovacs, Ph.D.

INTRODUCTION

The conditions currently known as major depressive disorders have been acknowledged for thousands of years. The Book of Job, for instance, contains a clear and moving account of the sufferer's despair, anhedonia, social isolation, sense of worthlessness, and profound sleep disturbance. An Egyptian papyrus from 2000 B.C. that relates a dispute over suicide conveys a painfully precise picture of a despondent man's hopelessness, nihilism, inability to go through the daily business of

*Preceptor's note: In their earlier chapter in this Part, Schildkraut, Schatzberg, Mooney, and Orsulak discuss some of these developments and the clinical implications.
†Preparation of this chapter was supported by National Institute of Mental Health Grant No. MH 33990.

living, and desire to die (Thomas, 1958). The later clinical descriptions of depression or melancholia by the Greeks and the Romans (Zilboorg, 1941), by Burton (1628), and by Kraepelin (1921) provide stunning proof of the omnipresence of this ancient malady of mankind. In our time, depressive disorders represent the most common psychiatric disturbance (Secunda et al., 1973). In terms of mental health dollars, loss of economic productivity, and reduced effectiveness in the family, their cost is enormous and far-reaching. It is therefore not surprising that in the last few decades there has been an explosion of research on the characteristics, treatment responsivity, and course of depressive disorders.

Substantial knowledge has accumulated on the tricyclic antidepressants and monoamine oxidase inhibitors in the treatment of depressions (for a review, see Morris and Beck, 1974; and Cole and Schatzberg's chapter in this volume). Impressive gains have been made in psychobiological studies including neurotransmitter, neuroendocrine, and sleep functions in depression (for overviews, see Essman and Valzelli, 1979; Mendels and Amsterdam, 1980; and the chapter by Schildkraut et al. in this volume). Controversy continues regarding the best ways to classify the depressions and regarding the relative importance of putative etiology, psychobiological correlates, family history, and treatment response (for an overview, see Rush, 1982). At the same time, operational diagnostic criteria are helping to identify target populations and to enable clearer communication among professionals (American Psychiatric Association, 1980; Feighner et al., 1972; Spitzer et al., 1978).

And yet in the choice of treatments one is faced with a dilemma. The effectiveness of pharmacotherapy notwithstanding, the data are beginning to suggest that even after good initial response and adequate maintenance, a notable portion of patients remain psychosocially impaired and chronically symptomatic (Weissman et al., 1976). Up to one third may develop a *new* depression within one year of recovery from the index episode (Keller and Shapiro, 1982). Moreover, some patients cannot be maintained on pharmacological agents because of severe side effects, and others are nonresponsive to drug therapy. For still others pharmacotherapy is medically contraindicated. And some patients decline it in the first place, while others are poor pharmacotherapy candidates because of noncompliance. Thus, there are probably substantial numbers of depressed individuals for whom psychotherapy alone or in combination with pharmacotherapy is clearly warranted.

The purpose of this chapter is to review several major psychotherapeutic approaches, with a focus on their rationales, salient strategies, and apparent effectiveness. Parloff (1976) has estimated that there are more than one hundred different psychotherapies. Clearly, the confines of this chapter prevent a summary of even the dozen or so most prominent systems or even a detailed discussion of every facet of one particular psychotherapy. The review therefore reflects several selection criteria.

Since depressive disorders tend to be phasic and time limited (for an overview, see Beck, 1972), an effective symptom-oriented psychosocial intervention needs to be able to accomplish its goals in a relatively short time. Thus, the only potentially "testable" therapies are those that can be applied with maximum fidelity over a span of less than six to nine months, the estimated average duration of depressive episodes. One criterion for selecting treatment modalities for this review was therefore that they be short-term and, in one way or another, aimed at overt symptom remission. Another criterion was that the modalities have been tested specifically for the treatment of depression and through randomized clinical trials. In clinical trials, effectiveness is typically defined as decreased symptomatology or remission. Cognitive therapy, one form of behavior therapy, and interpersonal psychotherapy have been subjected to such tests. While the efficacy of psychodynamic psychotherapy for depression has been examined in one study, the study viewed it as a control or comparison treatment, and it may not have been given a fair trial. Nonetheless, psychodynamic psychotherapy is reviewed here because it is probably the most common form of psychological treatment.

Each of the reviews begins with a short statement as to the modality's apparent origins. Next, the theoretical assumptions and postulates of the treatment approach are summarized since they influence or determine the therapeutic tactics. Finally, each system is described in terms of its general stance, its therapeutic strategies, and its effectiveness in the amelioration of depression.

COGNITIVE THERAPY

As developed and described by Aaron T. Beck, cognitive therapy is historically rooted in the work of Adler (1927), George Kelly (1955), and Horney (1950). Its explanatory paradigm has been influenced by theoretical and laboratory work on problem solving and cognitive processes and the cognitive approach to the emotions. A number of its therapeutic tactics were derived from behavior modification. Detailed overviews of the basis of cognitive therapy and extended discussions of the areas covered below may be found in Beck (1972) and Beck et al. (1979) and in the 1979 chapter by the author and Beck (Kovacs and Beck, 1979). Succinct summaries may be found in an article by the author (Kovacs, 1980a) and in Young and Beck (1982).

Theoretical Assumptions

The cognitive view of behavior assumes that one *assigns* meaning and value to one's perceptions and experiences. The nature of the consequent emotions and behaviors are presumed to be in harmony with one's evaluations, opinions, and notions. Thus, the cognitive approach focuses on man's ability to think: to size up, evaluate, and make sense out of internal and external events. Cognition therefore refers both to the processes of thinking, evaluating, judging, imaging, daydreaming, and the like, and to the products of such processes (solutions, decisions, attitudes, opinions, and so forth).

Consistencies in behavior are explained with reference to stable constructs called cognitive schemata. Cognitive schemata are presumed to act like templates or filters. They are organized representations of prior experience that help a person to screen, encode, and categorize perceptions. Since different aspects of experience are organized via different schemata, these constructs also help to explain unevenness across behavioral realms. For example, one may have a complex and detailed set of categories and systems that process work-related stimuli and yet be unable to interpret and respond to the nonverbal communication of a young child.

THE CONCEPT OF DEPRESSION   In line with the above, the cognitive view assumes that a depressed person's emotional distress and functional impairment are best understood and ameliorated by an exposition and correction of his or her relevant cognitions and schemata. Thus, with the depressed person, the distorted, maladaptive, and exaggeratedly negative views of oneself and the world represent the core psychological problem.

Depressed patients interpret trivial issues as substantial, read disparagement into harmless comments by others, and devalue themselves. They see events in a globally negative and highly self-referential fashion. They minimize prior positive experiences but exaggerate current or anticipated failures. Moreover, they abstract those isolated elements from situations that are most consistent with their bleak and hopeless outlook.

In the depressions, cognitive content generally revolves around themes of personal loss: losses of achievement, interpersonal acceptance, possessions, values, ideals, and the like. Thus, the depressive schemata are assumed to be specific to situations that represent subtractions from the patient's personal domain. While such schemata were probably developed to organize an earlier set of specific experiences, they may eventually be reactivated by stimuli that are only remotely similar to the historically etiologic context. When such earlier schemata are used to handle a current situation, their results become evident in misinterpretations and biased information processing. The profusion of distorted negative cognitions inevitably leads to dysphoria, depressed mood, reduced desire to provide for one's pleasure and needs, increased passivity, and concomitant vegetative alterations. Anhedonia, fatigue, and other symptoms are then *reconstrued* by the patient as additional proof of his or her worthlessness. Thus, the depressive cycle of symptoms and signs is in full swing.

Format and Strategies

Cognitive therapy is present oriented, structured, and collaborative. It requires that the patient and the therapist work together to identify and to reach various goals. The patient's active participation serves to minimize "resistance," increase self-confidence, enhance a sense of control and responsibility, and assure acceptance of therapeutic tactics. The overall goal is to identify and correct the patient's distorted negative cognitions, to elucidate and challenge the underlying cognitive schemata, and to increase the patient's adaptive problem-solving repertoire. As noted above, while negative evaluations of events are assumed to be the first link in the chain of depressive symptoms, any depressive symptom or sign may be targeted for initial modification.

SALIENT TACTICS   During cognitive therapy, the clinician uses several categories of intervention tactics.

(1)   *Didactic techniques* entail explanations of the cognitive paradigm, including the relationship between depressive symptomatology and thinking, affect, and behavior. The didactics are illustrated with examples from the patient's daily life and are provided in an educational spirit. Within the therapy, new intervention strategies are accompanied by explanations to clarify their rationales.

(2) *Behavioral techniques* help the patient to monitor his or her daily functioning and to control and modify selected depressive symptoms. Behavioral tasks and homework assignments actively engage the patient and directly break into the depressive cycle. They are most helpful in the beginning of treatment when the patient's cognitions may be so pervasive that some respite from them is of definite value. The behavioral assignments selected must be meaningful to the patient and must be ones that the patient is likely to complete, such as keeping a daily record of activities. Success in a behavioral task, no matter how simple, reflects functional competence, provides the therapist with data to challenge the patient's distorted notions, and facilitates the learning of specific skills that can be used independently.

(3) *Semantic techniques* require that the depressed person first learn to monitor (be aware of, observe, report on, record) his or her cognitions. Negative maladaptive cognitions are identified by inductive questioning or by asking the patient to image or role play a distressing scenario and to verbalize the accompanying thoughts. Eventually, the patient is asked to write down (record) negative cognitions at the time they occur and to bring the records to the sessions.

Through a number of strategies, the patient learns to examine and modify maladaptive notions or beliefs. For example, in *questioning the evidence*, the patient lists all supporting and contradicting information relevant to a particular cognition (e.g., "I am a terrible mother"). Each bit of evidence is then further examined to assess whether it represents a reasonable stance or mirrors cognitive distortions. The patient can be also asked to provide *alternate explanations* of a given negative interpretation (e.g., "John must be tired of me since he didn't call for two days"). The therapist him- or herself may offer various perspectives, and the patient can be encouraged to ask friends how *they* would react to or view a similar incident. *Reattribution* is a tactic most useful in the modification of unrealistic self-blame. Together, the therapist and the patient review the issue at hand and attempt to identify factors and variables that, in addition to the patient's own behavior, may be viable causal explanations.

The successful use of semantic techniques requires that the therapist elicit the patient's own interpretation of a particular word or concept and that constructs be defined in fairly concrete terms. For example, a depressed person may use the word lazy when the concept that he or she has in mind is anhedonia. Similarly, the statement "I am a failure" cannot be challenged unless it is first reduced to concrete terms and applied to specific events.

Throughout the treatment process, the therapist modifies, checks, and rechecks various formulations of the patient's basic assumptions and their underlying schemata. The therapist infers these formulations from repeated themes that run across different situations in the patient's life, stereotypical patterns of interpretations and variations on a theme that emerge in dissimilar scenarios.

In the later stages of treatment, the therapist presents his or her hypotheses about the patient's underlying assumptions and cognitive schemata so that the patient can "try them on for size." The patient then actively examines the validity and usefulness of those hypotheses in his or her current daily life. Elucidating and correcting the patient's relevant assumptions and schemata are assumed to be necessary for the maintenance of recovery and the prevention of relapse.

GENERAL CHARACTERISTICS In summary, cognitive therapy has three sets of fundamental characteristics: (1) a truly collaborative therapist-patient relationship that includes joint selection of target problems, mutual feedback, and active and significant input from the patient; (2) structured treatment sessions that focus on the present rather than on the past, that emphasize target issues rather than diffuse concerns, and that end with a wrap-up, the assignment of homework, or the resolution of a specific issue; and (3) an emphasis on teaching skills that the patient can take away from the therapy and apply on his or her own in order to assure a continuity of adaptive functioning.

BEHAVIOR THERAPY

As described and elaborated on by Lewinsohn, McLean, and Rehm, the historical antecedents of behavior therapy of depression (at times also referred to as cognitive-behavior therapy) are threefold: Skinner's operant learning theory, the laboratory and clinical single-case applications of Skinner's theory, and Ferster's (1973) seminal paper on the operant approach to depression. For more detailed overviews of the basis of behavior therapy and extended discussions of the areas that are covered below, see McLean (1982), Rehm and Kornblith (1979), and Lewinsohn et al. (1982). A historical account of behavior modification may be found in Kazdin (1978). In addition, the author has published elsewhere a succinct summary of behavioral treatments of depression (Kovacs, 1980b).

Theoretical Assumptions

The behaviorist approach focuses on repeatable, verifiable, and observable events. It assumes that all behavioral classes are learned (acquired) and maintained in accordance with some basic principles of reinforcement. Behaviorists thus view man in the context of specific stimulus situations. While behavior entails identifiable sets of changing and interrelated actions, it is also complex. And to bring some order into this complexity, one must study limited and circumscribed areas (Green, 1962).

The basic units of behavior consist of time-ordered stimulus-response chains within which a given response may also function as a stimulus in the chain. A behavioral unit is changed by means of appropriate contingencies or reinforcers. By definition, a reinforcer is anything that strengthens or maintains a response. Concomitantly, a previously reinforced behavior will decrease in strength if the reinforcement is no longer forthcoming. Among the various categories of reinforcers, the class of generalized reinforcers (reinforcers that are effective over a wide range of different conditions) are most relevant to social behavior. Within this paradigm, reinforcement follows a response or behavioral unit in time but does not cause it. Thus, operant learning may take place in and subsume numerous conditions, such as learning by trial and error, instrumental or verbal conditioning, concept formation, and so forth.

Although some time ago behavioral approaches focused only on overt variables, more recent theorists have addressed private, covert, or "cognitive" events. This cognitive revolution in behaviorism (Mahoney, 1977) assumes that thinking obeys the same laws of acquisition and maintenance as other more overt behavior classes. Thus, McLean (1982) argues that the word *cognitive* in cognitive-behavior therapy is unnecessary and redundant.

THE CONCEPT OF DEPRESSION The behaviorist approach to psychopathology assumes that a person's symptomatology and impairment are best understood and ameliorated by an exposition and alteration of his or her reinforcement field and personal behavior. Such a targeted approach is assumed to be the most effective way of changing associated affect and thinking.

According to McLean (1982), the currently active behavioral models of depression propose that altered rates of reinforcement account for the development and maintenance of depressions. The model which Lewinsohn et al. (1982) have based on operant learning theory assumes that depressive symptomatology results from a decreased rate of response-contingent positive reinforcement. That is, adaptive behavior is no longer positively reinforced, while depressive behavior is maintained through the empathic, supportive reactions of others. The low rate of positive reinforcement may be a function of the unavailability of potentially satisfying personal events and activities, the unavailablity of environmental reinforcers, and personal-social skills that are insufficient for eliciting reinforcement.

Rehm's self-control behavior therapy (Rehm, 1977; Rehm and Kornblith, 1979) puts more emphasis on covert processes that are presumably necessary to maintain behavior in the absence of immediate external reinforcement. Here it is assumed that the inability to tolerate reinforcement loss is due to failure in self-control processes and shows as faulty self-monitoring, deficient self-evaluation, and poor self-reinforcement. In the social-interaction behavioral model, however, the focus is on social events as reinforcers of behavior. As McLean (1982) notes, entries into, exits from, and interactions with others in one's social field are assumed to be the key reinforcing mechanisms that account for the development and maintenance of depressive behaviors.

Format and Strategies

All behavioral approaches focus on units of the depressed patient's behavior, aim at specific goal attainment, emphasize and utilize the principles of reinforcement, highlight successful performance as the most viable intervention, and require active participation in the form of self-monitoring and rehearsal. The overall thrust is to teach specific goal-relevant skills and thereby facilitate the patient's adaptive coping with vicissitudes in his or her reinforcement field.

Self-monitoring and behavioral tasks teach skills by doing. Successful task completion is enhanced by careful, gradual, and systematic use of positive reinforcers. Whether the intervention is in the traditional operational mold or what McLean (1982) calls multicomponent behavioral treatment, the therapist has a choice of reinforcement classes with which to work. Some reinforcers are delivered by oneself (e.g., compliments, getting a date), and some are part of the environment (e.g., cultural events, getting a raise).

SALIENT TACTICS Lewinsohn's social skills therapy, McLean's multicomponent behavioral treatment, and Rehm's self-control training program share a common pool of behavioral strategies. Because Lewinsohn's model is the most extensively documented and space is limited here, only his intervention will be described.

In social skills therapy, it is of utmost importance to identify and pinpoint the specific person-environment interactions that are related to the patient's depression. The self-rated Pleasant Events and Unpleasant Events Schedules both sample a variety of person-environment situations and furnish information on the patient's recent social behaviors and on social conditions that are potentially enjoyable (reinforcing) and potentially aversive. The information is used to formulate treatment goals. For example, low positive reinforcement in the marital situation may be targeted for modification. Reduction in highly aversive work interactions could also be an initial target.

During the course of social skills training, the therapist uses four sets of intervention tactics.

(1) *Self-monitoring* revolves around behaviors and situations that the patient rated as most pleasant and as most aversive. Based on these ratings, a personal activity schedule is constructed, and the patient uses the schedule to monitor his or her daily interactions. This strategy supplies immediate feedback to the patient about progress with increasing reinforcing interactions and decreasing aversive ones. Self-ratings of mood provide additional information to identify patterns of mood and social interaction that may be maintaining the passive or unassertive social behaviors characteristic of the patient.

(2) *Environment or contingency management techniques* are used to implement specific treatment goals. If the low rate of positively reinforcing events is a function of a barren or aversive environment, the depressed patient may be assisted to shift his or her circumstances, for instance by moving. Alternatively, significant others may be called upon and taught to reinforce positively (praise, pay attention to) the patient's adaptive behaviors.

(3) *Social learning techniques* are desirable if the patient's depression is related to poor social skills, that is, ineffectiveness in eliciting reinforcers. The training may encompass self-change tactics and modification of interpersonal behaviors. These entail didactic explanations of the skill to be learned, modeling and coaching of the behavior by the therapist, repeated practice by the patient within and outside the treatment sessions, and systematic applications of the behavior in the daily business of living. Self-change or self-management can include learning self-reinforcement. After a particular adaptive behavior, the patient may give him- or herself credit or actually reward him- or herself with a desirable event like going shopping. Changes in interpersonal behaviors may be achieved through assertiveness training (using covert modeling, rehearsal, and therapist feedback) or through improved interpersonal skills such as learning to respond to others with positive interest.

(4) *Cognitive self-management* strategies, such as thought stopping, self-rewarding cognitions, self-talk, or disputing irrational thoughts, are employed to alter the patient's thinking about "reality" and to maintain his or her adaptive behaviors.

Throughout the treatment process, the emphasis is on increasing the patient's social activities and on the acquisition of adaptive social skills and their consistent use in the actual business of living.

GENERAL CHARACTERISTICS The foregoing discussion of tactics is based on Lewinsohn's model, which shares with all the behavioral approaches to depression four basic elements: (1) a collaborative therapist-patient relationship that includes mutual agreement on target problems, active patient involvement, and consistent practice of targeted behaviors; (2) individual treatment goals based on a functional analysis of the patient's situation; (3) structured therapy sessions that involve feedback, rehearsal, goal attainment scaling, and a present orientation; and (4) a consistent emphasis on reinforcement and successful behavioral performance.

INTERPERSONAL PSYCHOTHERAPY

As described and elaborated by Klerman, Weissman, and their associates, interpersonal therapy builds on Adolf Meyer's psychobiological approach to psychiatric illness, Sullivan's theory of interpersonal relations and subsequent work from the Washington School of Psychiatry, and more recent analytic expositions of the interpersonal components of depressive disorders. Its explanatory paradigm has been influenced by Bowlby's (1960) seminal work on the consequences of disrupted attachment bonds. Intervention tactics derive from psychoanalytic psychotherapy, social skills and communication training, and cognitive-behavior modification. For extensive discussions of the basis and strategies of interpersonal psychotherapy and of the areas to be covered below, see Klerman and Weissman (1982), Rounsaville and Chevron (1982), and Klerman et al. (1979).

Theoretical Assumptions

The interpersonal approach to human behavior assumes that a person is an integrated whole and can be understood only in the context of his or her interpersonal milieu. Within this paradigm, the major constructs are nurturant social bonds, proper and adequate communications, self-definition based on feedback from others, and one's own integrated and self-perceived experiences of events. Interpersonal psychotherapy presumes that man's behavior is directed toward collaborative and mutually satisfying intimate relationships (Sullivan, 1953). Thus, both normal and deviant behaviors represent adaptations to the social environment and ways of coping with interpersonal situations.

THE CONCEPT OF DEPRESSION Depressive episodes may become manifest subsequent to biological derangement, shifts in developmental, social, or economic roles, or psychological factors, and they may be potentiated by genetic or developmentally acquired vulnerabilities. Within this treatment paradigm, depression is therefore a disorder that involves a symptom complex, a social and interpersonal matrix in which it is embedded, and enduring traits that may predispose to a breakdown in normal adaptation. However, since interpersonal psychotherapy postulates an intimate connection between psychopathology and human relations, it highlights those social and interpersonal problems that are typically associated with the onset of depressive symptomatology. The patient's interpersonal situation is not viewed as the sole etiologic agent, although an interpersonal treatment focus is assumed to be critical for symptom remission.

Within this broad theoretical framework, interpersonal psychotherapy focuses on four classes of psychosocial problems that are prominent in depression: grief, interpersonal role disputes, social or familial role transitions, and interpersonal deficits. Symptom formation is presumed to represent inadequate coping in the context of grief, nonreciprocal relationships, normal life changes and transitions, and inadequate and unfulfilled personal histories. Hence, the patient's interpersonal context, including his or her expectations, needs to be clarified and renegotiated.

Format and Strategies

Interpersonal psychotherapy is a time-limited intervention that seeks to relieve the patient's depressive symptoms and to develop his or her social and interpersonal problem-solving skills. The overall thrust is to elucidate, renegotiate, and improve the social-personal context that is associated with the onset of the patient's symptomatology. While problematic relationship patterns are assumed to have developmental antecedents, the focus is on the here and now and on current situations. Moreover, the intervention is targeted at problem resolution at the conscious and preconscious levels rather than the unconscious level. Although altered interpersonal relationships are the ultimate therapeutic goal, symptom reduction may be the initial target.

SALIENT TACTICS   The interpersonal psychotherapist uses various tactics that can be grouped into six classes.

(1)   *Didactics* or verbal explanations focus on the phenomenology of depressive disorders, their phasic, time-limited nature, and their treatment responsivity. This initial educational effort seeks to provide the patient with a coherent conceptual understanding of how his or her symptoms fit together and to instill hopeful expectations about recovery.

(2)   *Environmental management* entails diverse strategies for manipulating contingencies, circumstances, and problem situations in order to mitigate the depressive symptoms. For example, if the presence of certain individuals exacerbates the patient's symptoms, the therapist may help to find ways to reduce or avoid contacts with these people. Similarly, if the patient's mood worsens when he or she is alone, the therapist may explore active ways of reducing social isolation.

While the above two classes of techniques are primarily designed to manage overt depressive symptoms, the remaining four are best suited to the exposition and amelioration of the interpersonal issues involved in abnormal grief reactions, role disputes, role transitions, and interpersonal deficits.

(3)   *Supportive techniques* include the nonjudgmental exploration of the problem that is felt to be pressing, the exposition and discussion of associated feelings, and reassurance. These techniques facilitate affective expression and the reconstruction and working through of particular dilemmas. Patients also benefit from realistic feedback about such unreasonable concerns as the fear of losing control or the alleged inappropriateness of their symptoms. In the treatment of abnormal grief reactions, a reconstruction of the patient's relationship with the deceased person and the expression of negative feelings are seen as

especially helpful. The resolution and acceptance of role transitions also require appropriate affective expression.

(4) *Insight-oriented techniques* can be applied to various interpersonal problems. In abnormal grief reactions, awareness of one's positive and negative feelings toward the deceased may facilitate a healthier way of formulating the terminated relationship. Similarly, when the depressed patient is faced with a role transition (a life change, such as divorce, that is perceived as constituting some type of loss), the patient needs to understand the connection between the event's meaning and his or her dysphoria and reduced self-esteem. In a parallel vein, to resolve an interpersonal role dispute, the patient first needs to arrive at a valid identification of the issue (e.g., "My husband does not pay attention to me") and then identify its emotional importance (e.g., "He no longer finds me attractive. Maybe he is thinking about leaving me"). Recognition of how the patient's own personality or interactional style may feed into or exacerbate such conflicts is also important.

(5) *Social-skills-related strategies* may take several forms. For some depressed patients, interpersonal role disputes may be related to maladaptive communication patterns. Thus, the therapist may resort to couples counseling, with an emphasis on highlighting and altering ambiguous and diffuse communication styles.* On the other hand, the depressed patient with a history of interpersonal deficits such as chronic isolation will probably need to learn basic communication skills. The depressed patient who faces a role transition may have to build up a new repertoire of social skills. For example, a divorced woman who suddenly needs to take care of all her business affairs may be a candidate for role playing so she can learn assertive and independent behaviors.

(6) *Behavioral change tactics* are used to resolve issues that require a new class of active behaviors. For example, a widow may be encouraged to find areas of interest that allow her to develop new social contacts. The interpersonally inadequate patient may be assisted to undertake volunteer work to reduce social isolation. The depressed person whose role transition may have entailed losing the old social support network might be helped to develop new sources of support.

GENERAL CHARACTERISTICS Interpersonal psychotherapy entails four basic elements: (1) a supportive therapeutic relationship that facilitates emotional expression, the development of insight, and patient acceptance of the treatment's interpersonal focus; (2) flexible goal setting and variable intervention tactics depending on the nature of the patient's interpersonal problem and his or her readiness to address the key issues; (3) an emphasis on current disputes and conflicts; and (4) the facilitation of sound interpersonal problem-solving approaches that can help the patient to function more effectively in the future.

PSYCHODYNAMIC PSYCHOTHERAPY

Psychodynamic psychotherapy is probably the most widely used psychological intervention for ambulatory, nonpsychotic patients. While the author therefore believed it should be included in this chapter,

---

*Editor's note: In Part III Berman discusses and illustrates with a case example various techniques of couples therapy.

some special problems arose in trying to summarize its application to the treatment of depression. Not the least of these problems was whether dynamically oriented therapists would consider short-term therapy warranted or valid. An additional concern was which form of psychodynamic therapy ought to be described. Finally, one must consider the fact that in spite of their hallowed origins, the psychodynamically oriented schools have made no recent contributions to the symptomatic treatment of major depressive disorders (Strupp et al., 1982).

Theoretical Assumptions

Psychodynamically oriented treatments of depressed patients are rooted in the conceptualizations and approaches of Rado, Abraham, and Freud (for a concise summary, see Gaylin, 1968). Within this historical stream, more recent theoretical formulations have focused on the dynamics of depression in light of autonomous ego functions such as the patient's opinions, self-evaluations, and his or her awareness of painful discrepancies (Arieti and Bemporad, 1978; Bibring, 1953).

Since brief psychodynamic psychotherapies are grounded in classical, neoclassical and ego-analytic principles, depression is viewed from a longitudinal and dynamic framework and not seen as a specific disorder that warrants unique interventions (Strupp et al., 1982). Rather, depression is seen as one manifestation of a failure in adaptive functioning. For a succinct summary of the various dynamically oriented conceptualizations of depression, see Arieti and Bemporad (1978). A more detailed exposition of the integrated review below can be found in Strupp et al. (1982).

THE CONCEPT OF DEPRESSION According to recent analytic views, the breakdown in adaptive functioning that occurs in depression is evidence of inner conflicts that the patient does not fully understand. That is, although the depressive symptomatology is subjectively real and overtly manifest, its supporting substrata are partially or totally unconscious. Viewed within the context of a current important relationship, the functional breakdown is typically related to a lack of harmony between the intrapsychic processes that maintain self-esteem and the interpersonal transactions that are needed to continue the intimacy. In the context of loss, such as the failure of a relationship, the death of a significant other, or the inability to attain a goal, the salient conflict is typically between the patient's current self-view as inadequate, helpless, and the like and his or her aspirations and ego ideals. Psychodynamic psychotherapists assume that the patient's depression reflects dysfunctional early childhood experiences with significant others, experiences that continue to exert an influence on his or her life. Thus, a conscious or unconscious preceding ideology prepares the ground for depression by determining the meaning that the patient will see in particular stressful events and by influencing his or her responses (Arieti and Bemporad, 1978). In essence depression, along with its original etiologic context, is basically a problem of disturbed interpersonal relationships.

Given the putative etiologic factors in depression and other disorders and the traditional focus on the interpretation of the transference neurosis and on structural personality change, many analytically oriented therapists would debate the wisdom of short-term psychodynamic psychotherapy. Nonetheless, brief intensive approaches have been proposed in recent years (see, for example, Sifneos, 1979). While these approaches use different labels and more planning, Strupp et al. (1982) point out that the basic psychoanalytic techniques are still employed.

Format and Strategies

The most detailed recent descriptions of focused, short-term dynamic therapy have been provided by Sifneos (1979) and Malan (1979). However, as Strupp et al. (1982) note, in most reports or outcome studies of psychodynamically treated depressed patients, the descriptions are so brief as to preclude determination of precisely what sort of therapy was practiced. The following summary, therefore, is based on the synthesis which Strupp et al. (1982) have written on the key elements of short-term psychodynamic psychotherapy.

In view of the time limits, the critical elements of the therapeutic format become the establishment of an effective therapeutic alliance, the maintenance of an active and directive stance on the part of the therapist, and the setting of a therapeutic focus. The basic thrust is to modify aspects of the patient's personality structure, that is, to bring about an alteration in learned and habitually practiced maladaptive interpersonal coping patterns. The therapeutic techniques are therefore designed to elucidate and to alter the patient's neurotic maneuvers, to strengthen his or her adaptive capacities, and in the process to gratify in some part the patient's need for an understanding and supportive relationship.

SALIENT TACTICS To reach the above goals, the psychodynamic therapist uses three sets of maneuvers.

(1) *Active interpretation of the transference* is the crucial tactic. The rationale is that the patient's historically persistent and conflicted relationship patterns can be corrected only through the use of a current interpersonal relationship. Whether the patient experiences the therapeutic encounter as reminiscent of earlier relationships or as quite different from them, the quality of his or her relatedness provides the therapist with interpretative material. Transference interpretation entails clarifying the patient's defense mechanisms, including his or her resistance to change and to impending termination, his or her neurotic interpersonal and intrapsychic strategies and their goals, and the manner in which such strategies are woven across past and present relationships. As the patient fully appreciates his or her present motives and behaviors, the resultant insight is used to prepare for more adaptive functioning.*

(2) *Evocative and direct questioning or confrontation* as a facilitator of short-term dynamic therapy is mentioned by both Strupp et al. (1982) and Zaiden (1982). These tactics focus the patient on critical treatment issues, facilitate his or her transition from a passive-helpless stance to a more active interactional style, and mobilize and highlight relevant neurotic defenses.

*Editor's note: In his chapter in Part I, Michels presents a thoughtful and systematic formulation of the function and process of interpretation within the framework of contemporary psychoanalytic theory.

(3) *An empathic, understanding, and supportive stance*, when used properly, provides the patient with some succorance and nurturance and also communicates that he or she is a worthwhile human being.

GENERAL CHARACTERISTICS In summary, short-term psychodynamic psychotherapy is distinguished by its use of time as a dynamic process variable, by the therapist's active and vigilantly interpretative stance, and by its targeted approach. Since the transference interpretation is central to problem resolution, the speedy establishment of therapeutic alliance is crucial. Finally, the overall thrust is to provide the patient with a corrective interpersonal experience. Through this experience maladaptive characterological patterns are elucidated, understood, and modified in order to enhance adaptive functioning.

DISCUSSION AND CONCLUSIONS

The field of psychotherapy is in crisis. Practitioners are under increasing pressure to demonstrate the efficacy of their interventions. Concomitantly, in psychosocial treatment research the emphasis on randomized clinical trials is mounting. Diagnostically homogeneous study samples and treatment manuals that facilitate standardized therapist behaviors are seen as critical to such research efforts.

Treatment Outcome Data and Their Implications

With respect to the treatment of depressions, the literature now suggests that certain psychosocial interventions are clinically useful for symptom management and are potentiators of, equal to, or better than pharmacotherapeutic agents. Case studies of traditional behavior therapy which have used repeated-measures designs reveal that contingency management is clearly successful in the short-term control of isolated depressive symptoms and signs and inappropriate behavior. Reports on Lewinsohn's social skills treatment suggest that improved interpersonal skills and increased pleasant activities are associated with decrements in self-rated depressive symptomatology (for detailed reviews of the above, see Kovacs, 1980b; Rehm and Kornblith, 1979). Studies of depressed female volunteers found that self-control training is significantly more likely to produce symptom remission than nondirective therapy or waiting-list status and leads to greater improvement than social skills training (Fuchs and Rehm, 1977; Rehm et al., 1979). Among depressed university health service clients, cognitive therapy was more effective in symptom reduction than social skills treatment, nondirective therapy, or waiting-list status, whether assessed by self-report or clinician ratings (Shaw, 1977).

Three sets of studies on carefully diagnosed depressed psychiatric outpatients attest further to the usefulness of time-limited interventions for the amelioration of depressive disorders. In one project (McLean and Hakstian, 1979), multimodal social-skills-related behavior therapy was associated with the lowest dropout rate and had more favorable outcome ratings than dynamically oriented psychotherapy, tricyclic pharmacotherapy, or progressive muscle relaxation (treatment control). The work of the Boston-New Haven group indicates that in the maintenance treatment of remitted depressed female patients, weekly interpersonally oriented psychotherapy was just as effective as amitriptyline or the combination of the two (Klerman et al., 1974). Subsequently, the group found that for acutely depressed outpatients,

interpersonal psychotherapy, amitriptyline, and their combined administration were equally efficacious in producing and maintaining symptom
remission. Furthermore, all the active interventions were more effective
in preventing symptomatic failure than nonscheduled contact (control)
(Weissman et al., 1979). In a comparison of Beck's cognitive therapy
and an imipramine regimen for nonpsychotic depressed outpatients,
cognitive therapy produced greater symptomatic improvement on self-
report, clinician-completed, and therapist-rated measures and a considerably lower dropout rate (Rush et al., 1977). However, according to
two follow-up studies, the initial outcome differences wash out, and a
sizable portion of the patients develop a chronically symptomatic course
(Kovacs et al., 1981; Weissman et al., 1976).

Notwithstanding the generally positive results of the treatments that
have been tested, the data cannot be generalized to other psychosocial
interventions. Thus, not much is known about the effectiveness of
short-term psychodynamic therapy with depression. Uncontrolled clinical reports are not scientifically acceptable (for a review, see Strupp
et al., 1982). While in McLean and Hakstian's (1979) comparative
treatment study psychodynamic psychotherapy did not fare as well as
the other interventions, it could be argued that it was not given a
proper trial. Since the focus of psychodynamic psychotherapy is different from that of behavior therapy or pharmacotherapy, the symptomatic outcome measures may have obscured other improvements.

Future research must therefore address the appropriateness of comparing psychosocial treatments which have dissimilar targets. In turn,
psychotherapists will have to agree on outcomes that are socially and
economically acceptable and clinically meaningful. Some justifiably
argue that symptom remission is a poor index of therapeutic efficacy.
However, improvement in psychological areas that do not lend themselves to quantification or reliable assessment, such as reduced neurotic
conflicts or characterological changes, may be unacceptable as treatment
indices to third-party insurers.

The field must also come to terms with the fact that some therapies
may not lend themselves to operational definitions and the construction of step-by-step how-to manuals and that adherents of certain
approaches may reject clinical trials. Some have argued that the clinical
trial that became popular in the course of testing pharmacological
agents is inappropriate to investigations of psychotherapeutic efficacy.
Concern has been also expressed that the current trend to standardize
therapists' behaviors may distort and maim individual differences and
other variables that may be critical to successful treatment (Ryle, 1982).
Such concerns and arguments cannot be dismissed lightly. Some dialogue between research-oriented and clinically oriented psychotherapists may be necessary to effect a rapprochement between opposing
viewpoints.

Theories, Tactics, and Etiology

Another crisis in the field of psychotherapy concerns the relationship
between an intervention, its strategies, and competing theories on the
development of depression. For example, according to McLean (1982),
the effectiveness of cognitive therapy for depression cannot be specifically credited to the cognitive manipulations. Since cognitive therapy
uses behavioral tactics, outcome does not shed any light on the validity
of the cognitive paradigm. It can also be argued, however, that behavior

therapies rely on cognitive techniques just as much as the other way around, that interpersonal psychotherapy entails traditional behaviorist tactics, or that psychodynamically oriented therapy incorporates client-centered strategies. Undeniably, the modalities reviewed share a common pool of techniques. Indeed, since all psychosocial treatments derive from a limited number of schools of thought that have over time become intertwined, some strategic overlap is probably inevitable. Therefore, a great deal of research is needed to resolve whether an intervention's effectiveness can be specifically credited to presumably unique and theoretically consistent strategies.

Furthermore, certain tactics in the common pool of therapeutic interventions have no evident relationship to a particular theoretical paradigm. For example, direct questioning and confrontation are not clear derivatives of the psychoanalytic view of depression. The cognitive theory in itself does not explain why the patient should keep a daily log. Environmental manipulation does not logically follow from the basic tenets of interpersonal psychotherapy.

One rebuttal is that the strategies alone do not distinguish the therapies. What distinguishes the therapies is the use to which the strategies are put and their fit with the intervention's goals and cosmology. An intriguing and potentially testable question is whether it is the treatment's theoretical stance and explanation of depression or the use of a particular set of interrelated strategies that is critical to the amelioration of the patient's distress.

The least valid concern is the various therapeutic systems' inabilities to account fully for the development and phenomenology of depression. By definition, psychosocial interventions are based on psychological, behavioral, or social explanations of psychopathology. Neither do they claim to explain nor can they be expected to explain the development and maintenance of all depressive symptoms. Rather, the theories re-order manifest phenomena in their own unique ways, highlighting different facets of the disabling condition and providing alternate approaches to its amelioration. In line with George Kelly's (1955) thinking, it is therefore best to view the various psychotherapeutic and pharmacotherapeutic systems as alternate constructions of human experience, no one of which really negates the others.

The Choice of a Psychotherapy

According to Strupp (1978) and others, the question of which therapy will work best for what sort of patient is central in psychotherapy research. The question implies that a system ought to exist for matching an intervention with presumably relevant patient characteristics. Indeed, there are several empirically validated "matching rules." For example, barring medical contraindications, tricyclics for uncomplicated depression and major tranquilizers for schizophrenia constitute two good sets of matches. Furthermore, tricyclics are generally a better choice for endogenous or melancholic depressions than for depressions without such features.* Similarly, substantial data support the advisability of behavior therapies for phobic disorders.

*Preceptor's note: Cole and Schatzberg, in the section of their chapter on indications for tricyclics, present some new data suggesting that the tricyclics may have a wider therapeutic efficacy than previously thought.

As already noted, though, less than a handful of psychotherapies have been tested with respect to their specificity for or efficacy in the amelioration of particular depressive disorders, and even fewer have been compared with each other. For example, it has been proposed that endogenously depressed patients are better candidates for medication than for psychotherapy (Rush, 1982), and practitioners generally believe that for a suicidal depressed patient drugs rather than psychosocial intervention should be the primary choice. In both cases, unequivocal supporting data are lacking.

SUGGESTED GUIDELINES In the absence of validated or uniformly accepted guidelines on which psychotherapy is best for a particular type of depression, Rush (1982) calls attention to three general principles. He recommends that treatment objectives be matched with a therapy that targets the desired goals and that entails relevant strategies. Whether the patient can actively participate in the treatment should be the second consideration. Finally, treatment choice should be guided by some evidence that the disorder is responsive to the intervention. Rehm et al. (1979) imply that ultimately the nature of the observed deficits should guide the choice of intervention. Thus, if the depressed patient is most impaired in social functioning, he or she should receive social skills training. If the disorder's most prominent impact is on the person's thinking, cognitive therapy would be indicated.

The above recommendations are sensible. Nonetheless, some of the suggestions may be of limited practical significance to the clinician. The clinician may lack training in a potentially warranted therapy or be theoretically committed to a particular psychotherapy. Or the clinician may not have access to other professionals who have different expertise and could be consulted or treat the patient. In light of these realities, some "bottom-line" criteria may be helpful in selecting depressed patients for psychosocial treatments.

BOTTOM-LINE CRITERIA All traditional forms of psychotherapy entail oral communication. It is assumed that the patient can share with the therapist the culturally accepted connotations and denotations of spoken words, can follow verbal explanations and instructions, and can ask and respond to questions. It is also assumed that the patient can conceptualize problems orally, can accept psychotherapy (including verbal, emotional, and behavioral examinations of and solutions to problems) as relevant to his or her distress, and can be responsible for some of the contractual aspects of therapy. Demographic variables and the psychotic-nonpsychotic dimension are therefore fundamentally relevant. A severely mentally retarded individual, a person who is mute, or a person who does not speak the therapist's language is not a viable candidate for psychotherapy. The depressed patient who is delusional or hallucinating or both is also unlikely to meet the basic demands of most psychotherapies. Consequently, decisions about psychotherapeutic candidacy should be preceded by a careful and thorough diagnostic workup.

Regardless of what intervention is being considered, what the therapist eventually does and what the patient is asked to do communicate an explanation of psychopathology. For example, the administration of antidepressant drugs, with little if any discussion of other issues, communicates that the disorder is biologically based. In such a case, the therapeutic cosmology highlights relatively autonomous bodily processes. In contrast, social skills training implies that both one's behavior and the environment need to be altered. The disorder is thus conceptualized as a person-environment problem in which the patient has control over the resolution. Consequently, the patient's manner of looking at the world and at physical and emotional illness can either accommodate or counter the therapeutic system's cosmology. Prior to the initiation of therapy, it may therefore be useful to explain the what, how, and why of the intervention and to ascertain that the patient does not find the explanation to be totally alien, repugnant, or bizarre. Many of the so-called noncompliant or resistant patients may well be those to whom the intervention's explanatory system makes no sense.

From a psychological perspective, the latter recommendation is entirely predictable. Psychological and psychosocial approaches view both normalcy and deviance as person variables. In contrast, the more medically based orientations focus on disorders per se rather than on disordered persons (American Psychiatric Association, 1980). In testing the psychotherapies, it remains to be seen whether the medically based clinical-trial format, which highlights the treatment of disorders, can or should accommodate the potentially relevant psychological and person variables.

References for the Introduction

Carroll B.J.: Clinical applications of the dexamethasone suppression test for endogenous depression. Pharmacopsychiatria 15:19−24, 1982.

Kupfer D.J., Foster F.G., Reich L., et al.: EEG sleep changes as predictors in depression. Am. J. Psychiatry 133:622, 1976.

References for Chapter 22

The Nosology and Diagnosis of Depressive Disorders

Akiskal H.S., Djenderedjian A.H., Rosenthal R.H., et al.: Cyclothymic disorder: validating criteria for inclusion in the bipolar affective group. Am. J. Psychiatry 134:1227, 1977.

American Psychiatric Association: Diagnostic and Statistical Manual of Mental Disorders, 3rd ed. Washington, D.C., American Psychiatric Association, 1980.

Astrup C., Fossum A., Homboe R.: A follow-up study of 270 patients with acute affective psychoses. Acta Psychiat. et Neurol. Scand. Suppl. 135 34:1−65, 1959.

Avery D., Winokur G.: Mortality in depressed patients treated with electroconvulsive therapy and antidepressants. Arch. Gen. Psychiatry 33:1029, 1976.

Barrett J., Hurst M.N., DiSalla C., et al.: Prevalence of depression over a 12-month period in a nonpatient population. Arch. Gen. Psychiatry 35:741, 1978.

Beck A.T.: Depression: Causes and Treatment. Philadelphia, University of Pennsylvania Press, 1972.

Bleuler E.: Textbook of Psychiatry. New York, Dover, 1951.

Bratfos O., Haug J.O.: The course of manic-depressive psychosis. A follow-up investigation of 215 patients. Acta Psychiatr. Scand. 44:89−112, 1968.

Chodoff P.: The depressive personality. Arch. Gen. Psychiatry 27:666, 1972.

Cohen M.B., Baker G., Cohen R.A., et al.: An intensive study of twelve cases of manic-depressive psychosis. Psychiatry 17:103, 1954.

Feighner J.P., Robins E., Guze S.B., et al.: Diagnostic criteria for use in psychiatric research. Arch. Gen. Psychiatry 26:57−63, 1972.

Fenichel O.: The Psychoanalytical Theory of Neurosis. New York, W.W. Norton & Co., 1945.

Freedman D.X.: Introduction, in· Depression: Biology, Psychodynamics, and Treatment. Edited by Cole J.O., Schatzberg A.F., Frazier S.H. New York, Plenum Press, 1978.

Gershon E.S.: The search for genetic markers in affective disorders, in Psychopharmacology: A Generation of Progress. Edited by Lipton M.A., DiMascio A., Killam K.F. New York, Raven Press, 1978.

Griest J., Griest T.: Antidepressant Treatment. Baltimore, Williams & Wilkins, 1979.

Hirschfeld R.M.A., Klerman G.L.: Personality attributes and affective disorders. Am. J. Psychiatry 136:67, 1979.

Hornstra R.K., Klassen D.: The course of depression. Compr. Psychiatry 18:119, 1977.

Huston P.E., Locher L.M.: Involutional psychosis. Course when untreated and when treated with electric shock. Arch. Neurol. Psychiatry 59:385−394, 1948a.

Huston P.E., Locher L.M.: Manic-depressive psychosis. Course when treated and untreated with electric shock. Arch. Neurol. Psychiatry 60:37−48, 1948b.

Jacobs T.J., Gogelson S., Charles E.: Depression ratings in hypochondria. N.Y. State J. Med. 68:3119, 1968.

Jacobson E.: Depression. New York, International Universities Press, 1971.

Kahn E.: The depressive character. Folia. Psychiatr. Neurol. Jpn. 29:292, 1975.

Kasanin J.: Acute schizoaffective psychoses. Am. J. Psychiatry 90:97, 1933.

Kielholz P.: Masked Depression. Bern, Hans Huber, 1973.

Kiloh L., Garside R.: The independence of neurotic depression and endogenous depression. Br. J. Psychiatry 109:451, 1963.

Klerman G.L., Barrett J.: Clinical and epidemiologic aspects of affective disorders, in Lithium: Its Role in Psychiatric Research and Treatment. Edited by Gershon E.S., Shopsin B. New York, Plenum Press, 1973.

Klerman G.L., Endicott J., Hirschfeld R.M.A.: Neurotic depression. Am. J. Psychiatry 136:57, 1979.

Klerman G.L., Hirschfeld R.M.A.: Treatment of depression in the elderly. Geriatrics 34:51, 1979.

Kraepelin E.: Manic Depressive Insanity and Paranoia. Edinburgh, E&S Livingstone, 1921.

Krauthammer C., Klerman G.L.: Secondary mania. Arch. Gen. Psychiatry 35:1333−1339, 1978.

Kuhn R.: Über die Behandlung depressiver Zustände mit einem Iminodibenzylderivat (G22355). Schweizer Medizinische Wochenschrift. J. Suisse de Médecine 87:1135−1140, 1957.

Leonhard K.: Aufteilung der endogenen Psychosen. Berlin, Akademie Verlag, 1957.

Lesse S.: Psychotherapy in combination with antidepressant drugs in patients with severe masked depressions. Am. J. Psychiatry 31:185, 1977.

Lewinsohn P.: A behavioral approach to depression, in The Psychology of Depression: Contemporary Theory and Research. Edited by Friedman R., Katz M. New York, John Wiley & Sons, 1974.

Lipsitt D.R.: Medical and psychological characteristics of "crocks." Psychiatry Med. 1:15, 1970.

Lundquist G.: Prognosis and course in manic-depressive psychoses. A follow-up study of 319 first admissions. Acta Psychiat. et Neurol. Suppl. 35:1−96, 1945.

Mendels J., Cochrane C.: The nosology of depression: the endogenous-reactive concept. Am. J. Psychiatry 124:1, 1968.

Morrison J., Winokur G., Crowe R.: The Iowa 500: the first follow-up. Arch. Gen. Psychiatry 39:678, 1973.

Murphy G.E., Woodruff R.A. Jr., Herjanic M., et al.: Variability of the clinical course of primary affective disorder. Arch. Gen. Psychiatry 30:757, 1974.

Paykel E.S., Klerman G.L., Prusoff B.A.: Prognosis of depression and the endogenous-neurotic distinction. Psychol. Med. 4:57, 1974.

Paykel E.S., Weissman M.M.: Social adjustment and depression: a longitudinal study. Arch. Gen. Psychiatry 28:650, 1973.

Perris C.: A study of bipolar (manic-depressive) and unipolar recurrent psychoses. Acta Psychiatr. Scand. Suppl. 194:1, 1966.

Pottenger M., McKernon J., Patrie L.E., et al.: The frequency and persistence of depressive symptoms in the alcohol abuser. J. Nerv. Ment. Dis. 166:562, 1978.

Prien R.F., Klett C.J., Caffey E.M.: A comparison of lithium carbonate and imipramine in the prevention of affective disorders in recurrent affective illness, in Cooperative Studies in Psychiatry. Prepublication report #94. Perry Point, MD, Veterans Administration, 1973.

Robins E., Guze S.: Classification of affective disorders: the primary-secondary, and the endogenous, and the neurotic-psychotic concepts, in Recent Advances in the Psychobiology of Depressive Illness. Edited by Williams T.A., Katz M.M., Shield J.A. Washington, D.C., Department of Health Education and Welfare, 1972.

Seligman M.: Depression and learned helplessness, in The Psychology of Depression: Contemporary Theory and Research. Edited by Friedman R., Katz M.M. New York, John Wiley & Sons, 1974.

Schou M.: Lithium in psychiatric therapy and prophylaxis. J. Psychiatr. Res. 6:67, 1968.

Stenstedt A.: A study in manic-depressive psychosis. Clinical, social and genetic investigations. Acta Psychiat. et Neurol. Scand. Suppl. 79:1–111, 1952.

Tellenbach H.: Psychopathologie der Cyclothymie. Nervenarzt 48:335, 1977.

Van Valkenburg C., Lowry M., Winokur G., et al.: Depression spectrum disease versus pure depressive disease. J. Nerv. Ment. Dis. 165:341, 1977.

Watts C.A.H.: The incidence and prognosis of endogenous depression. Br. Med. J. 1:1392–1397, 1956.

Weissman M.M., Klerman G.L.: The chronic depressive in the community: unrecognized and poorly treated. Compr. Psychiatry 18:523, 1977.

Weissman M.M., Myers J.K.: Clinical depression in alcoholism. Am. J. Psychiatry 137:372–373, 1980.

Weissman M.M., Paykel E.S.: The Depressed Woman: A Study of Social Relationships. Chicago, University of Chicago Press, 1974.

Winokur G.: Unipolar depression: is it divisible into autonomous subtypes? Arch. Gen. Psychiatry 36:47, 1979.

Winokur G., Behar D., Van Valkenburg C., et al.: Is a familial definition of depression both feasible and valid? J. Nerv. Ment. Dis. 166:764, 1978.

References for Chapter 23

Personality, Life Events, and Social Factors in Depression

Abraham K.: Selected Papers on Psychoanalysis. London, Hogarth Press, 1948.

Altman J.H., Wittenborn J.R.: Depression-prone personality in women. J. Abnorm. Psychol. 89:303–308, 1980.

Bech P., Shapiro R.W., Sihm F., et al.: Personality in unipolar and bipolar manic-melancholic patients. Acta Psychiat. Scand. 62:245–257, 1980.

Benjaminsen S.: Primary non-endogenous depression and features attributed to reactive depression. J. Affective Disord. 3:245–259, 1981a.

Benjaminsen S.: Stressful life events preceding the onset of neurotic depression. Psychol. Med. 11:369–378, 1981b.

Bowlby J.: Attachment. New York, Basic Books, 1969.

Brown G.W., Harris T.: The Social Origins of Depression. London, Tavistock, 1978.

Brown G.W., NiBhrolchain M., Harris T.O.: Social class and psychiatric disturbance among women in an urban population. Sociology 9:225–254, 1975.

Brown G.W., NiBhrolchain M., Harris T.O.: Psychotic and neurotic depression: Part 3. Aetiological and background factors. J. Affective Disord. 1:195–211, 1979.

Brown G.W., Prudo R.: Psychiatric disorder in a rural and an urban population: I. Aetiology of depression. Psychol. Med. 11:581–599, 1981.

Brown G.W., Sklair F., Harris T.O., et al.: Life events and psychiatric disorders: Part I. Some methodological issues. Psychol. Med. 3:74–87, 1973.

Chodoff P.: The depressive personality. Arch. Gen. Psychiatry 27:666–673, 1972.

Cofer D.H., Wittenborn J.R.: Personality characteristics of formerly depressed women. J. Abnorm. Psychol. 89:309–314, 1980.

Cohen M.B., Baker G., Cohen R.A., et al.: An intensive study of twelve cases of manic-depressive psychosis. Psychiatry 17:103–137, 1954.

Costello C.G.: Social factors associated with depression: a retrospective community study. Psychol. Med. 12:329–339, 1982.

Crook T., Eliot J.: Parental death during childhood and adult depression: a critical review of the literature. Psychol. Bull. 82:252–259, 1980.

Donnelly E.F., Murphy D.C., Goodwin F.K.: Cross-sectional and longitudinal comparisons of bipolar and unipolar depressed groups on the MMPI. J. Consult. Clin. Psychol. 44:233–237, 1976.

Fava G.A., Munari F., Pavan L., et al.: Life events and depression: a replication. J. Affective Disord. 3:159–165, 1981.

Finlay-Jones R., Brown G.W.: Types of stressful life events and the onset of anxiety and depressive disorders. Psychol. Med. 11:803–815, 1981.

Freud S.: Mourning and melancholia (1917), in Complete Psychological Works, standard ed., vol. 14. London, Hogarth Press, 1957.

Gershon E.S., Mark A., Cohen N., et al.: Transmitted factors in the morbid risk of affective disorders: a controlled study. J. Psychiatr. Res. 12:283–299, 1975.

Hirschfeld R.M.A.: Situational depression: validity of the concept. Br. J. Psychiatry 139:297–305, 1981.

Hirschfeld R.M.A., Cross C.K.: Epidemiology of affective disorders: psychosocial risk factors. Arch. Gen. Psychiatry 39:35–46, 1982.

Hirschfeld R.M.A., Klerman G.L.: Personality attributes and affective disorders. Am. J. Psychiatry 136:67–70, 1979.

Hirschfeld R.M.A., Klerman G.L., Clayton P.J., et al.: Assessing personality: effects of depressive state on trait measurement. Am. J. Psychiatry, in press, 1983.

Holmes T.H., Rahe R.H.: The social readjustment rating scale. J. Psychosom. Res. 11:213–218, 1967.

Hudgens R.W., Robins E., DeLong W.B.: The reporting of recent stress in the lives of psychiatric patients. Br. J. Psychiatry 117:635–643, 1970.

Jacobs S.C., Prusoff B.A., Paykel E.S.: Recent life events in schizophrenia and depression. Psychol. Med. 4:444–453, 1974.

Klerman G.L., Barrett J.E.: The affective disorders: clinical and epidemiological aspects, in Lithium: Its Role in Psychiatric Research and Treatment. Edited by Gershon E.S., Shopsin B. New York, Plenum Press, 1973.

Kraepelin E.: Manic-Depressive Illness and Paranoia. Edinburgh, E&S Livingstone, 1921.

Kretschmer E.: Physique and Character. Translated by Miller E. London, Kegan, Paul, Trench, Trubner & Co., 1936.

Lewinsohn P.: A behavioral approach to depression, in The Psychology of Depression: Contemporary Theory and Research. New York, John Wiley & Sons, 1974.

Liebowitz M.R., Stallone F., Dunner D.L., et al.: Personality features of patients with affective disorder. Acta Psychiat. Scand. 60:214–224, 1979.

Lloyd C.: Life events and depressive disorders reviewed: I. Events as predisposing factors. Arch. Gen. Psychiatry 37:529–535, 1980a.

Lloyd C.: Life events and depressive disorders reviewed: II. Events as precipitating factors. Arch. Gen. Psychiatry 37:541–548, 1980b.

Lloyd C., Zisook S., Click M., et al.: Life events and response to antidepressants. J. Human. Stress 7:2–15, 1981.

Mattussek P., Neuner R.: Loss events preceding endogenous and neurotic depressions. Acta Psychiat. Scand. 64:340–350, 1981.

Murray H.A.: Explorations in Personality. New York, Oxford University Press, 1938.

Murray L.G., Blackburn I.M.: Personality differences in patients with depressive illness and anxiety neurosis. Acta Psychiat. Scand. 50:183–191, 1974.

Myers J.K., Lindenthal J.J., Pepper M.P.: Life events and psychiatric impairment. J. Nerv. Ment. Dis. 152: 149–157, 1971.

Myers J.K., Lindenthal J.J., Pepper M.P.: Life events and mental status: a longitudinal study. J. Health Soc. Behav. 13:398–406, 1972.

Orvaschel H., Weissman M.M., Kidd K.K.: The children of depressed parents; the childhood of depressed patients; depression in childhood. J. Affective Disord. 2:1–16, 1980.

Patrick V., Dunner D.L., Fieve R.F.: Life events and primary affective illness. Acta Psychiat. Scand. 58:48–55, 1978.

Paykel E.S., Klerman G.L., Prusoff B.A.: Personality and symptom pattern in depression. Br. J. Psychiatry 129:327–334, 1976.

Paykel E.S., Myers J.K., Dienelt M.N., et al.: Life events and depression: a controlled study. Arch. Gen. Psychiatry 21:753–760, 1969.

Rahe R.H., Meyer M., Smith M., et al.: Social status and illness onset. J. Psychosom. Res. 8:35–44, 1964.

Roy A.: Risk factors and depression in Canadian women. J. Affective Disord. 3:65–70, 1981a.

Roy A.: Specificity of risk factors for depression. Am. J. Psychiatry 138:959–961, 1981c.

Roy A.: Vulnerability factors and depression in men. Br. J. Psychiatry 138:75–77, 1981b.

Schneider K.: Psychopathic Personalities. Translated by Hamilton M.W. London, Cassell, 1958.

Seligman M.E.P.: Helpless: On Depression, Development, and Death. San Francisco, W.H. Freeman & Co., 1975.

Snaith R.P., McGuire R.J., Fox K.: Aspects of personality and depression. Psychol. Med. 1:239–246, 1971.

Solomon A., Bromet E.: The role of social factors in affective disorder: an assessment of the vulnerability model of Brown and his colleagues. Psychol. Med. 12:123–130, 1982.

Tennant C., Bebbington P., Hurry J.: Parental death in childhood and risk of adult depressive disorders: a review. Psychol. Med. 10:289–299, 1980.

Thomson K.C., Hendrie H.C.: Environmental stress in primary depressive illness. Arch. Gen. Psychiatry 26: 130–132, 1972.

Weissman M.M., Prusoff B.A., Klerman G.L.: Personality and the prediction of long-term outcome of depression. Am. J. Psychiatry 135:797–800, 1978.

Wetzel R.D., Cloninger C.R., Hong B., et al.: Personality as a subclinical expression of the affective disorders. J. Abnorm. Psychol. 89:309–314, 1980.

References for Chapter 24

The Epidemiology of Affective Disorders: Rates and Risk Factors

Adelstein A.M., Downham D.Y., Stein Z., et al.: The epidemiology of mental illness in an English city. Soc. Psychiatry 3:47–59, 1968.

American Psychiatric Association: Diagnostic and Statistical Manual of Mental Disorders, 3rd ed. Washington, D.C., American Psychiatric Association, 1980.

Angst J.: Zur Ätiologie und Nosologie endogener depressiver Psychosen. Berlin, Springer Verlag, 1966. Reprinted in Foreign Psychiatry 2:1–108, 1973.

Bagley C.: Occupational status and symptoms of depression. Soc. Sci. Med. 7:327–339, 1969.

Bash K.W., Bash-Liechti J.: Studies on the epidemiology of neuropsychiatric disorders among the rural population of the province of Khuzestran, Iran. Soc. Psychiatry 4:137–143, 1969.

Bash K.W., Bash-Liechti J.: Studies on the epidemiology of neuropsychiatric disorders among the population of the city of Shiraz, Iran. Soc. Psychiatry 9:163–171, 1974.

Bebbington P.E.: The epidemiology of depressive disorder. Cult. Med. Psychiatry 2:297–341, 1978.

Boyd J.H., Weissman M.M.: The epidemiology of psychiatric disorders of middle age: depression, alcoholism, and suicide, in Modern Perspectives in the Psychiatry of Middle Age. Edited by Howells J.G. New York, Brunner/Mazel, 1981.

Blumenthal M.D.: Measuring depressive symptomatology in a general population. Arch. Gen. Psychiatry 32:971–978, 1975.

Bratfos O., Haug J.O.: The course of manic depressive psychosis: a follow-up investigation of 215 patients. Acta Psychiatr. Scand. 44:89–112, 1968.

Brown G.W., Davidson S., Harris T., et al.: Psychiatric disorder in London and North Uist. Soc. Sci. Med. 11:367–377, 1977.

Brown G.W., Harris T.: Social Origins of Depression. London, Tavistock, 1978.

Chodoff P.: The depressive personality: a critical review. Int. J. Psychiatry Med. 27:196–217, 1972.

Cohen M.B., Baker G., Cohen R.A., et al.: An intensive study of twelve cases of manic depressive psychosis. Psychiatry 17:103–137, 1954.

Comstock G.W., Helsing K.J.: Symptoms of depression in two communities. Psychol. Med. 6:551–563, 1976.

Crocetti G.M., Lemkau P.V., Kulcar Z., et al.: Selected aspects of the epidemiology of psychoses in Croatia, Yugoslavia. Am. J. Epidemiol. 94:126–134, 1971.

Dube K.C., Kumar N.: An epidemiological study of manic depressive psychosis. Acta Psychiatr. Scand. 49: 691–697, 1973.

Duncan-Jones P., Henderson S.: The use of a two-phase design in a prevalence survey. Soc. Psychiatry 13: 231–237, 1978.

Eaton W.W., Regier D.A., Locke B.Z., et al.: The epidemiologic catchment area program of the National Institute of Mental Health. Public Health Rep. 96: 319–323, 1981.

Endicott J., Spitzer R.L.: Use of the research diagnostic criteria and the schedule for affective disorders and schizophrenia to study affective disorders. Am. J. Psychiatry 136:52–59, 1979.

Essen-Möller E., Hagnell O.: The frequency and risk of depression within a rural population group in Scania. Acta Psychiatr. Scand. 162:28–32, 1961.

Faris R.E.L., Dunham H.W.: Mental Disorders in Urban Areas: An Ecological Study of Schizophrenia and Other Psychoses. Chicago, Il., University of Chicago Press, 1939.

Feighner J.P., Robins E., Guze S.B., et al.: Diagnostic criteria for use in psychiatric research. Arch. Gen. Psychiatry 26:57–63, 1972.

Gibson R.W.: The family background and early life experience of the manic-depressive patient: A comparison with the schizophrenic patient. Psychiatry 21: 71–90, 1958.

grad de Alarcón J., Sainsbury P., Costain W.R.: Incidence of referred mental illness in Chinchester and Salisbury. Psychol. Med. 5:32–54, 1975.

Hällström T.: Mental Disorder and Sexuality in the Climacteric. Goteborg, Orsadius Boktryckeri, 1973.

Helgason T.: Frequency of depressive states within geographically delimited population groups: the frequency of depressive states in Iceland as compared with the other Scandinavian countries. Acta Psychiatr. Scand. 162:81–90, 1961.

Helgason T.: Psychiatric services and mental illness in Iceland: incidence study (1966–1967) with 6–7 year follow-up. Acta Psychiatr. Scand. Suppl. 268:1–140, 1977.

Hirschfeld R.M.A., Klerman G.L.: Personality attributes and affective disorders. Am. J. Psychiatry 136:67–70, 1979.

Hirschfeld R.M., Cross C.K.: The epidemiology of affective disorders: psychosocial risk factors. Arch. Gen. Psychiatry 39:35–46, 1982.

Husaini B.A., Neff J.R., Harrington J.B., et al.: Depression in rural communities: establishing CES-D cutting points. Health Research Projects. Nashville, TN., Tennessee State University, 1979.

Ilfeld F.W.: Current social stressors and symptoms of depression. Am. J. Psychiatry 134:161–166, 1977.

James N.M., Chapman C.J.: A genetic study of bipolar affective disorder. Br. J. Psychiatry 126:449–456, 1975.

Juel-Nielsen N., Bille M., Flygenring J., et al.: Frequency of depressive states within geographically delimited population groups: incidence (the Aarhus County investigation). Acta Psychiatr. Scand. 162:69–80, 1961.

Katsrup M., Nakane Y., Dupong A., et al.: Psychiatric treatment in a delimited population—with reference to outpatients: a demographic study. Acta Psychiatr. Scand. 53:35–50, 1976.

Kidd K.K., Weissman M.M.: Why we do not yet understand the genetics of affective disorders, in Depression: Biology, Psychodynamics, and Treatment. Edited by Cole J.O., Schatzberg A.F., Frazier S.H. New York, Plenum Press, 1978.

Klerman G.L.: Overview of affective disorders, in Comprehensive Textbook of Psychiatry, 3rd ed. Edited by

Kaplan H.J., Freedman A.M., Sadock B.J. Baltimore, Williams & Wilkins, 1980.

Klerman G.L., Barrett J.E.: The affective disorders: clinical and epidemiologic aspects, in Lithium: Its Role in Psychiatric Research and Treatment. Edited by Gershon E.S., Shopsin B. New York, Plenum Press, 1973.

Kraepelin E.: Manic Depressive Insanity and Paranoia. Edinburgh, E&S Livingstone, 1921.

Kramer M.: Cross-national study of diagnosis of the mental disorders: origins of the problem. Am. J. Psychiatry Suppl. 125:1–11, 1969.

Krauthammer C., Klerman G.L.: The epidemiology of mania, in Manic Illness. Edited by Shopsin B. New York, Raven Press, 1979.

Kulcar Z., Crocetti G.M., Lemkau P.V. et al. Selected aspects of the epidemiology of psychoses in Croatia, Yugoslavia. Am. J. Epidemiol. 94:118–125, 1971.

Lehmann H.E.: The epidemiology of depressive disorders, in Depression in the 70s. Edited by Fieve R.R. The Hague, Excerpta Medica, 1971.

Leighton D.C., Harding J.A., Macklin D.B., et al.: Psychiatric findings of the Stirling County study. Am. J. Psychiatry 119:1021–1026, 1963.

Leonhard K: Aufteilung der Endogenen Psychosen. Berlin, Akademie-Verlag, 1957.

MacMahon B., Pugh T.F.: Epidemiology—Principles and Methods. Boston, Little, Brown & Company, 1970.

Martin F.M., Brotherston J.H.F., Chave S.P.W.: Incidence of neurosis in a new housing estate. Br. J. Prev. Soc. Med. 11:196–202, 1957.

Mayer-Gross W.: A mental health survey in a rural area. Eugenics Review 40:140–148, 1948.

Mellinger G.D., Balter M.B., Parry H.J. et al.: An overview of psychotherapeutic drug use in the United States, in Drug Use: Epidemiological and Sociological Approaches. Edited by Josephson E., Carrol E.E. New York, Hemisphere Publishing Corp., 1974.

Monnelly E.P., Woodruff R.A., Robins L.N.: Manic depressive illness and social achievement in a public hospital sample. Acta Psychiatr. Scand. 50:318–325, 1974.

Myers J.K., Weissman M.M.: Use of a self-report symptom scale to detect depression in a community sample. Am. J. Psychiatry 137:1081–1089, 1980.

Nielsen J.: The Samsø project from 1957 to 1974. Acta Psychiatr. Scand. 54:198–222, 1976.

Nielsen J., Nielsen J.A.: Treatment prevalence in a community mental health service with special regard to depressive disorders. Compr. Psychiatry 20:67–77, 1979.

Orley J., Blitt D.M., Wing J.K.: Psychiatric disorders in two African villages. Arch. Gen. Psychiatry 36:513–520, 1979.

Orvaschel H., Weissman M.M., Kidd K.K.: Children and depression: the children of depressed parents; the childhood of depressed patients; depression in children. J. Affective Disord. 2:1–16, 1980.

Paffenbarger R.S., McCabe L.J.: The effect of obstetric and perinatal events on risk of mental illness in women of childbearing age. Am. J. Public Health 56:400–407, 1966.

Parsons P.L.: Mental health of Swansea's old folk. Br. J. Prev. Soc. Med. 19:43–47, 1965.

Paykel E.S., Emms E.M., Fletcher J., et al.: Life events and social support in puerperal depression. Br. J. Psychiatry 136:339–346, 1980.

Pederson A.M., Barry D.J., Babigian H.M.: Epidemiological considerations of psychotic depression. Arch. Gen. Psychiatry 27:193–197, 1972.

Perris C.: A study of bipolar (manic-depressive) and unipolar recurrent depressive psychoses. Acta Psychiatr. Scand. Suppl. 194:1–189, 1966.

Perris C.: Frequency and hereditary aspects of depression, in Depression: Behavioral, Biochemical, Diagnostic and Treatment Concepts. Edited by Gallant D.M., Simpson G.M. New York, Spectrum Publications, 1976.

Pope H.G., Lipinski J.F.: Diagnosis in schizophrenia and manic-depressive illness. Arch. Gen. Psychiatry 35:811–828, 1978.

Pugh T.F., Jerath B.K., Schmidt W.M., et al.: Rates of mental disease related to childbearing. N. Engl. J. Med. 268:1224–1228, 1963.

Radloff L.S.: Sex differences in depression: the effects of occupation and marital status. Sex Roles 1:249–265, 1975.

Robins L.N., Helzer J., Croughan J.: Renard Diagnostic Interview. St. Louis MO., Washington University Medical School, 1977.

Robins L.N., Helzer J., Croughan J., et al.: NIMH Diagnostic Interview Schedule: Version Two. Rockville, MD, Center for Epidemiologic Studies, National Institute of Mental Health, 1980.

Robins L.N., Helzer J.E., Croughan J., et al.: National Institute of Mental Health Diagnostic Interview Schedule: its history, characteristics and validity. Arch. Gen. Psychiatry 38:381–389, 1981.

Roth W.F., Luton F.H.: Mental health program in Tennessee. Am. J. Psychiatry 99:662–675, 1943.

Silverman C.: The Epidemiology of Depression. Baltimore. Johns Hopkins University Press, 1968.

Spicer C.C., Hare E.H., Slater E.: Neurotic and psychotic forms of depressive illness: evidence from age incidence in a national sample. Br. J. Psychiatry 123:535–541, 1973.

Spitzer R.L., Endicott J., Robins E.: Clinical criteria for psychiatric diagnosis and DSM-III. Am. J. Psychiatry 132:1187–1192, 1975.

Spitzer R.L., Endicott J., Robins E.: Research Diagnostic Criteria (RDC). New York, New York State Psychiatric Institute, Biometrics Research, 1978a.

Spitzer R.L., Endicott J., Robins E.: Research diagnostic criteria: rationale and reliability. Arch. Gen. Psychiatry 35:773–782, 1978b.

Spitzer R.L., Endicott J.: Schedule for Affective Disorders and Schizophrenia. New York, Biometrics Research, Evaluation Section, New York State Psychiatric Institute, 1978c.

Sørensen A., Strömgren E.: Frequency of depressive states within geographically delimited population groups: prevalence (the Samsø investigation). Acta Psychiatr. Scand. 162:62–68, 1961.

Stevens B.: Marriage and Fertility of Women Suffering from Schizophrenia or Affective Disorders. Maudsley Monograph 19. London, University of Oxford Press, 1969.

Thacore U.R., Gupta S.C., Suraiya M.: Psychiatric morbidity in a north Indian community. Br. J. Psychiatry 126:364–369, 1975.

Turns D.: The epidemiology of major affective disorders. Am. J. Psychiatry 32:5–19, 1978.

Warheit G.J., Holzer C.E. III, Schwab J.J.: An analysis of social class and racial differences in depressive symptomatology: a community study. J. Health Soc. Behav. 14:291–299, 1973.

Watts C.H., Cowte E.C., Kuensberg E.V.: Survey of mental illness in general practice. Br. Med. J. 2:1351–1359, 1964.

Weeke A., Bille M., Videbech T., et al.: Incidence of depressive syndromes in a Danish county. Acta Psychiatr. Scand. 51:28–41, 1975.

Weissman M.M.: The myth of involutional melancholia. JAMA 242:742–744, 1979.

Weissman M.M., Klerman G.L.: Sex differences in the epidemiology of depression. Arch. Gen. Psychiatry 34:98–111, 1977.

Weissman M.M., Klerman G.L.: Epidemiology of mental disorders: emerging trends in the U.S. Arch. Gen. Psychiatry 35:705–712, 1978.

Weissman M.M., Myers J.K.: Affective disorders in a U.S. urban community. Arch. Gen. Psychiatry 35:1304–1311, 1978a.

Weissman M.M., Myers J.K.: Rates and risks of depressive symptoms in a United States urban community. Acta Psychiatr. Scand. 57:219–231, 1978b.

Weissman M.M., Myers J.K., Thompson W.D.: Depression and its treatment in a U.S. urban community, 1975–76. Arch. Gen. Psychiatry 38:417–421, 1981.

Weissman M.M., Myers J.K., Tischler G.L., et al.: The Yale Epidemiology Catchment Area Study. Paper read at the Scientific Program of the Montreal W.H.O. Collaborating Centre for Research and Training in Mental Health. Montreal, March 1982.

Wing J.K., Mann S.A., Leff J.P., et al.: The concept of a 'case' in psychiatric population surveys. Psychol. Med. 8:203–217, 1978.

Winokur G.: Depression in the menopause. Am. J. Psychiatry 130:92–93, 1973a.

Winokur G.: The types of affective disorders. J. Nerv. Ment. Dis. 156:82–96, 1973b.

Winokur G.: Unipolar depression: is it divisible into autonomous subtypes? Arch. Gen. Psychiatry 36:47–52, 1979.

Winokur G., Morrison J.: The Iowa 500: follow-up of 225 depressives. Br. J. Psychiatry 123:543–548, 1973.

Woodruff R.A., Robins L.N., Winokur G., et al.: Manic depressive illness and social achievement. Acta Psychiatr. Scand. 47:237–249, 1971.

Zubin J.: Cross-national study of diagnosis of the mental disorders: methodology and planning. Am. J. Psychiatry Suppl. 125:12–20, 1969.

References for Chapter 25

Epidemiologic and Risk Factors in Suicide

Avery D., Winokur G.: Mortality in depressed patients treated with electroconvulsive therapy and antidepressants. Arch. Gen. Psychiatry 33:1029–1037, 1976.

Barraclough B., Bunch J., Nelson B., et al.: A hundred cases of suicide: clinical aspects. Br. J. Psychiatry 125:355–373, 1974.

Beck A.: Thinking and depression. Arch. Gen. Psychiatry 9:324–333, 1963.

Blath R.A., McClure J.N., Wetzel R.D.: Familial factors in suicide. Dis. Nerv. Sys. 34:90–93, 1973.

Brown J.: Suicide in Britain. Arch. Gen. Psychiatry 36:1119–1124, 1979.

Brown J.: Is suicide ever rational? (Ltr. to ed.). Lancet 1:660–661, 1981.

Carlson G.A., Miller D.C.: Suicide, affective disorder, and women physicians. Am. J. Psychiatry 138:10, 1981.

Clayton P.J.: A further look at secondary depression, in Treatment of Depression: Old Controversies and New Approaches. Edited by Clayton P.J., Barrett J. New York, Raven Press, 1983.

Clayton P.J.: Schizoaffective disorders. J. Nerv. Ment. Dis. 170:646–650, 1982.

Clayton P.J., Marten S., Davis M., et al.: Mood disorder in women professionals. J. Affective Disord. 2:37–46, 1980.

Coryell W., Noyes R., Clancy J.: Excess mortality in panic disorder. Arch. Gen. Psychiatry 39:701–703, 1982.

Dabbagh F.: Family suicide. Br. J. Psychiatry 130:159–161, 1977.

Dorpat T.L., Ripley H.S.: A study of suicide in the Seattle area. Compr. Psychiatry 1:349–359, 1960.

Dorpat T., Boswell J.: An evaluation of suicidal intent in suicide attempts. Compr. Psychiatry 4:117–125, 1963.

Grove O., Lynge J.: Suicide and attempted suicide in Greenland. A controlled study in Nuuk (Godthaab). Acta Psychiatr. Scand. 60:375–391, 1979.

Guze S.B., Robins E.: Suicide and primary affective disorders. Br. J. Psychiatry 117:437–438, 1970.

Hellon C., Solomon M.: Suicide and age in Alberta, Canada, 1951–1977. Arch. Gen. Psychiatry 37:505–510, 1980.

Juel-Nielsen J., Videbech T.: A twin study of suicide. Acta Genet. Med. Gemellol. 19:307–310, 1970.

Kety S.: Disorders of the human brain. Sci. Am. 241:202–214, 1979.

Khin-Maung-Zaw: A suicidal family. Br. J. Psychiatry 139:68–69, 1981.

Kreitman N.: Parasuicide. New York, John Wiley & Sons, 1977.

Liberman R.P., Eckman T.: Behavior therapy vs. insight-oriented therapy for repeated suicide attempters. Arch. Gen. Psychiatry 38:1126–1130, 1981.

Minkoff K., Bergman E., Beck A., et al., Hopelessness, depression, and attempted suicide. Am. J. Psychiatry 130:455–459, 1973.

Montgomery S.A., Montgomery D.B.: Psychopharmacology and suicidal behavior, in The Affective Disorders. Edited by Davis J.M., Maas J.W. Washington, D.C. American Psychiatric Press, Inc, 1983.

Murphy G.E.: Clinical identification of suicidal risk. Arch. Gen. Psychiatry 27:356–359, 1972.

Murphy G.E.: Editorial, Suicide and the right to die. Am. J. Psychiatry 130:4, 1973.

Murphy G.E.: The physician's responsibility for suicide. I. An error of omission. Ann. Intern. Med. 82:301–304, 1975a.

Murphy G.E.: The physician's responsibility for suicide. II. Errors of omission. Ann. Intern. Med. 82:305–309, 1975b.

Murphy G.E.: Suicide and attempted suicide. Hosp. Pract. 12:73–81, Nov., 1977.

Murphy G.E., Armstrong J., Hermele S., et al.: Suicide and alcoholism. Arch. Gen. Psychiatry 36:65–69, 1979.

Murphy G.E., Wetzel R.: Suicide risk by birth cohort in the United States, 1949 to 1974. Arch. Gen. Psychiatry 37:519–523, 1980.

Murphy G.E., Wetzel R.D., Swallow C.S., et al.: Who calls the suicide prevention center: a study of 55 persons calling on their own behalf. Am. J. Psychiatry 126:314–324, 1969.

Oliver R., Hetzel B.: Rise and fall of suicide rates in Australia: relation to sedative availability. Med. J. Aust. 2:919–923, 1972.

Pallis D.J., Barraclough B.M.: Seriousness of suicide attempt and future risk of suicide: a comment on Card's paper. Omega 8:141–149, 1977.

Pallis D.J., Birtchnell J.: Seriousness of suicide attempt in relation to personality. Br. J. Psychiatry 130:253–259, 1977.

Plath S.: The Bell Jar. London, Faber & Faber, 1963.

Resnik H.L.P.: Suicidal Behaviors. Boston, Little, Brown & Co., 1968.

Rich C.L., Pitts F.N. Jr.: Suicide by male physicians during a five-year period. Am. J. Psychiatry 136:1089–1090, 1979.

Robins E., Gassner S., Kayes J., et al.: The communication of suicidal intent: a study of 135 consecutive cases of successful (completed) suicide. Am. J. Psychiatry 115:724–733, 1959.

Robins E., Murphy G., Wilkinson R., et al.: Some clinical considerations in the prevention of suicide based on a study of 134 successful suicides. Am. J. Public Health 49:888–899, 1959.

Robins E., Schmidt E.H., O'Neal P.: Some interrelations of social factors and clinical diagnosis in attempted suicide: a study of 109 patients. Am. J. Psychiatry 114:221–231, 1957.

Sainsbury P.: Suicide: opinions and facts. Proc. R. Soc. Med. 66:579–587, 1973.

Schmidt E.H., O'Neal P., Robins E.: Evaluation of suicide attempts as guide to therapy. JAMA 155:549–557, 1954.

Schulsinger F., Kety S.S., Rosenthal D., et al.: A family study of suicide, in Origin, Prevention and Treatment of Affective Disorders. Edited by Schou M., Strömgren E. New York, Academic Press, 1979.

Stengel E.: Suicide and Attempted Suicide, Bristol, MacGibbon and Kee, 1965.

Traskman L., Asberg M., Bertilsson L., et al.: Monoamine metabolites in CSF and suicidal behavior. Arch. Gen. Psychiatry 38:631–636, 1981.

Tsuang M.T.: Suicide in schizophrenics, manic depressives, and surgical controls. Arch. Gen. Psychiatry 35:153–155, 1978.

Tsuang M.T., Dempsey G.M., Fleming J.A.: Can ECT prevent premature death and suicide in 'schizoaffective' patients? J. Affective Disord. 1:167–171, 1979.

References for Chapter 26

The Genetics of Affective Disorders

Ablon S.L., Davenport Y.B., Gershon E.S., et al.: The married manic. Am. J. Orthopsychiatry 45:854–866, 1975.

Abrams R., Taylor M.A.: Mania and schizoaffective disorder, manic type—a comparison. Am. J. Psychiatry 133:1445–1447, 1976.

Akiskal H.S., Djenderedjian A.H., Rosenthal R.H.: Cyclothymic disorder: validating criteria for inclusion in the bipolar affective group. Am. J. Psychiatry 134:1227–1233, 1977.

Akiskal H.S., Khan M.K., Scott-Strauss A.: Cyclothymic temperamental disorders. Psychiatr. Clin. North Am. 2:527–554, 1979.

Andreasen N.C., Grove W.M., Shapiro R.W., et al.: Reliability of lifetime diagnosis. Arch. Gen. Psychiatry 38:400–405, 1981.

Angst J.: Clinical subgroups of bipolar affective disorders—results of a genetic study. Presented at the Third World Congress on Biological Psychiatry, Stockholm, Sweden, July 1981.

Angst J.: Zur Ätiologie und Nosologie endogener depressiver Psychosen, in Monographien aus dem Gesamtgebiete der Neurologie and Psychiatrie. Berlin, Springer Verlag, 1966.

Angst J., Felder W., Lohmeyer B: Schizoaffective disorders: results of a genetic investigation, I. J. Affective Disord. 1:139−153, 1979.

Angst J., Frey R., Lohmeyer B., et al.: Bipolar manic-depressive psychoses: results of a genetic investigation. Hum. Genet. 55:237−254, 1980.

Asano N.: Clinico-genetic study of manic-depressive psychoses, in Clinical Genetics in Psychiatry. Edited by Mitsuda H. Osaka-Takatsuki, Osaka Medical College, 1967.

Asberg M., Thoren P., Traskman L., et al.: Serotonin depression—a biochemical subgroup within the affective disorders? Science 191:478−480, 1976.

Baron M.: Linkage between an X-chromosome marker (deutan color blindness) and bipolar affective illness. Arch. Gen. Psychiatry 34:721−725, 1977.

Baron M., Klotz J., Mendlewicz J., et al.: Multiple threshold transmission of affective disorders. Arch. Gen. Psychiatry 38:79−88, 1981a.

Baron M., Rainer J.D., Risch N.: X-linkage in bipolar affective illness. Perspective on genetic heterogeneity, pedigree analysis and the X-chromosome map. J. Affective Disord. 3:141−157, 1981b.

Beckman G., Beckman L., Cedergen B., et al.: Genetic markers in cycloid psychosis. Neuropsychobiology 4:276−282, 1978.

Bennahum D.A., Troup G.M., Rada R.T., et al.: The histocompatibility antigens of schizophrenic and manic-depressive patients. Unpublished data.

Bennahum D.A., Troup G.M., Rada R.T., et al.: Human leukocyte antigens (HLA) in psychiatric illness. Clin. Res. 23:260A, 1975.

Bertelsen A.: Origin, Prevention and Treatment of Affective Disorders. Edited by Schou M., Strömgren E. London, Academic Press, 1979.

Bertelsen A., Harvald B., Hauge M.: A Danish twin study of manic-depressive disorders. Br. J. Psychiatry 130:330−351, 1977.

Brodie H.K.H., Leff M.J.: Bipolar depression: a comparative study of patient characteristics. Am. J. Psychiatry 127:1086−1090, 1971.

Bucher K.D.: The genetics of manic depressive illness: a pedigree and linkage study. Ph.D. Thesis for Department of Biostatistics, Institute of Statistics, Mimeo Series 1141. Chapel Hill, University of North Carolina, 1977.

Bucher K.D., Elston R.C.: The transmission of manic depressive illness. I. Theory, description of the model and summary of results. J. Psychiatr. Res. 16:53−63, 1981.

Bucher K.D., Elston R.C., Green R., et al.: The transmission of manic depressive illness. II. Segregation analysis of three sets of family data. J. Psychiatr. Res. 16:65−78, 1981.

Cantwell D.P., Sturzenberger S., Burroughs J., et al.: Anorexia nervosa: an affective disorder. Arch. Gen. Psychiatry 34:1087−1093, 1977.

Carroll B.J., Feinberg M.P.: Intracellular lithium. Neuropharmacol. 16:527 (abstract), 1977.

Childs B.: Contemporary medical genetics. Neurosci. Res. Program Bull. 14:13−18, 1976.

Clayton P.J., Rodin L., Winokur G.: Family history studies, Part 3 (schizoaffective disorder, clinical and genetic factors including a one to two year follow-up). Compr. Psychiatry 9:31−49, 1968.

Cohen S.M., Allen M.G., Pollin W., et al.: Relationship of schizoaffective psychosis to manic-depressive psychosis and schizophrenia. Arch. Gen. Psychiatry 26:539−551, 1972.

Collins G.S., Sandler M.: Human blood platelet monoamine oxidase. Biochem. Pharmacol. 20:389−396, 1971.

Comings D.E.: Application of two-dimensional gel electrophoresis, recombinant DNA, and tissue culture techniques to the major psychoses, in Genetic Research Strategies for Psychobiology and Psychiatry. Edited by Matthysse S., Breakfield X.O., Ciaranello R.D. Pacific Grove, CA, Boxwood Press, 1981.

Comings D.E.: Pc 1 Duarte, a common polymorphism of a human brain protein, and its relationship to depressive disease and multiple sclerosis. Nature 277:28−32, 1979.

Coryell W., Winokur G., Andreasen N.: The effect of case definition on affective disorder rates. Am. J. Psychiatry 138:1106−1109, 1981.

Crowe R.R., Namboodiri K.K., Ashby H.B., et al.: Segregation and linkage analysis of a large kindred of unipolar depression. Neuropsychobiology 7:20−25, 1981.

Donnelly C.H., Murphy D.L.: Substrate and inhibition related characteristics of human platelet monoamine oxidase. Biochem. Pharmacol. 26:853−858, 1976.

Dorus E., Pandey G.N., Davis J.M.: Genetic determinant of lithium ion distribution. An in vitro and in vivo monzygotic-dizygotic twin study. Arch. Gen. Psychiatry 32:1097−1102, 1975.

Dorus E., Pandey G.N., Frazer A., et al.: Genetic determinant of lithium ion distribution: I. An in vitro monozygotic-dizygotic twin study. Arch. Gen. Psychiatry 31:463−465, 1974.

Dorus E., Pandey G.N., Shaughnessey R., et al.: Lithium transport across the red cell membrane: a cell membrane abnormality in manic-depressive illness. Science 205:932−934, 1979b.

Dorus E., Pandey G.N., Shaughnessey R., et al.: Lithium transport across the red cell membrane: a study of genetic factors. Arch. Gen. Psychiatry, in press.

Dorus E., Pandey G.N., Shaughnessey R., et al.: Low platelet monoamine oxidase activity, high red blood cell lithium ratio, and affective disorders: a multivariate assessment of genetic vulnerability to affective disorders. Biol. Psychiatry 14:989−994, 1979a.

Dunner D.L., Dwyer T., Fieve R.R.: Depressive symptoms in patients with unipolar and bipolar affective disorder. Compr. Psychiatry 17:447−451, 1976.

Dunner D.L., Meltzer H.L., Fieve R.R.: Clinical correlates of the lithium pump. Am. J. Psychiatry 135:1062−1064, 1978.

Dustman R.E., Beck E.C.: The visually evoked potential in twins. Electroencephalogr. Clin. Neurophysiol. 19:570−575, 1965.

Dyson W.L., Barcai A.: Treatment of children of lithium-responding parents. Curr. Ther. Res. 12:286−290, 1970.

Edwards D.J., Chang S.: Multiple forms of monoamine oxidase in rabbit platelets. Life Sci. 17:1127−1134, 1975.

Edwards D.J., Spiker D.G., Kupfer D.J., et al.: Platelet monoamine oxidase in affective disorders. Arch. Gen. Psychiatry 35:1443−1446, 1978.

Egeland J.A.: Affective disorders among the Amish: 1976−1980. Presented at the Annual Meeting of the American College of Neuropsychopharmacology, Puerto Rico, December, 1980.

Elston R.C.: Ascertainment and age of onset in pedigree analysis. Hum. Hered. 23:105−112, 1973.

Elston R.C.: Segregation analysis, in Current Developments in Anthropological Genetics. Edited by Mielke J.H., Crawford M.H. New York, Plenum Press, 1980.

Elston R.C., Sobel E.: Sampling considerations in the gathering and analysis of pedigree data. Am. J. Hum. Genet. 31:62−69, 1979.

Elston R.C., Stewart J.: A general method for the genetic analysis of pedigree data. Hum. Hered. 21:523–542, 1971.

Elston R.C., Yelverton K.C.: General models for segregation analysis. Am. J. Hum. Genet. 27:31–45, 1975.

Elston R.C., Namboodiri K.K., Hames C.G.: Segregation and linkage analysis of dopamine-β-hydroxylase activity. Hum. Hered. 29:284–292, 1979.

Essen-Möller E.: Twin research and psychiatry. Acta Psychiatr. Scand. 39:65–77, 1963.

Felder W.: Katamnestische und genetische Untersuchung über 85 Patienten mit schizoaffektiver Mischpsychose. Med. Diss., Zurich, 1977.

Fischer M., Harvald B., Hauge M.: A Danish twin study of schizophrenia. Br. J. Psychiatry 115:981–990, 1969.

Gardos G.: Agoraphobia—a type of affective disorder. Presented at the meeting of the American Psychopathological Association, Washington, D.C., March 1980.

Gershon E.S.: Genetics of the affective disorders. Hosp. Practice 14:117–122, 1979.

Gershon E.S., Bunney W.E. Jr.: The question of X-linkage in manic-depressive illness. J. Psychiatr. Res. 13:99–117, 1976.

Gershon E.S., Hamovit J.: Genetic methods and preventive psychiatry. Prog. Neuropsychopharmacol. 3:565–573, 1979.

Gershon E.S., Jonas W.: A clinical and genetic study of erythrocyte soluble catechol-O-methyltransferase activity in primary affective disorder. Arch. Gen. Psychiatry 32:135–136, 1975.

Gershon E.S., Liebowitz J.H.: Sociocultural and demographic correlates of affective disorders in Jerusalem. J. Psychiatr. Res. 12:37–50, 1975.

Gershon E.S., Baron M., Leckman J.F.: Genetic models of the transmission of affective disorders. J. Psychiatr. Res. 12:301–317, 1975a.

Gershon E.S., Lake C.R., Leckman J.F.: Reduced erythrocyte COMT and plasma DBH activities not associated with affective disorders in patients and relatives, in Catecholamines: Basic and Clinical Frontiers. Edited by Usdin E., Kopin I., Barchas J.D. New York, Pergamon Press. 1979a.

Gershon E.S., Belmaker R.H., Ebstein R., et al.: Plasma monoamine oxidase activity unrelated to genetic vulnerability to primary affective illness. Arch. Gen. Psychiatry 34:731–734, 1977a.

Gershon E.S., Bunney W.E. Jr., Leckman J.F., et al.: The inheritance of affective disorders: a review of data and of hypotheses. Behav. Genet. 6:227–261, 1976.

Gershon E.S., Goldin L.R., Lake C.R., et al.: Genetics of plasma dopamine-β-hydroxylase (DBH), erythrocyte catechol-O-methyltransferase (COMT), and platelet monoamine oxidase (MAO) in pedigrees of patients with affective disorders, in Enzymes and Neurotransmitters in Mental Disease. Edited by Usdin E., Sourkes P., Youdim M.B.H. London, Wiley Interscience, 1980.

Gershon E.S., Goldin L.R., Weissman M.M., et al.: Family and genetic studies of affective disorders in the Eastern United States: a provisional summary. Presented at the Third World Congress on Biological Psychiatry, Stockholm, Sweden, July 1981.

Gershon E.S., Hamovit J.R., Guroff J.J., et al.: A family study of schizoaffective, bipolar I, bipolar II, unipolar and normal control probands. Arch. Gen. Psychiatry 39:1157–1167, 1982.

Gershon E.S., Hamovit J.R., Schreiber J.L., et al.: Anorexia nervosa and major affective disorders associated in families: a preliminary report, in Childhood Psychopathology and Development. Edited by Guze J.B., Earls F. J., Barrett J.E. New York, Raven Press, 1983.

Gershon E.S., Mark A., Cohen N., et al.: Transmitted factors in the morbidity of affective disorders: a controlled study. J. Psychiatr. Res. 12:283–299, 1975b.

Gershon E.S., Targum S.D., Kessler L.R., et al.: Genetic studies and biologic strategies in the affective disorders, in Progress in Medical Genetics, vol. 2. Philadelphia, W.B. Saunders Co., 1977b.

Gershon E.S., Targum S.D., Leckman J.F., et al.: Platelet monoamine oxidase (MAO) activity and genetic vulnerability to bipolar (BP) affective illness. Psychopharmacol. Bull. 15:27–30, 1979b.

Gershon E.S., Targum S.D., Matthysse S., et al.: Color blindness not closely linked to bipolar illness. Arch. Gen. Psychiatry 36:1423–1434, 1979c.

Goetzl V., Green R., Whybrow P., et al.: X-linkage revisited: a further family study of manic depressive illness. Arch. Gen. Psychiatry 31:665–673, 1974.

Goldin L.R., Gershon E.S., Lake C.R., et al.: Segregation and linkage studies of plasma dopamine-β-hydroxylase (DBH), erythrocyte catechol-O-methyltransferase (COMT) and platelet monoamine oxidase (MAO): possible linkage between the ABO locus and a gene controlling DBH activity. Am. J. Hum. Genet. 34:250–262, 1982.

Goldin L.R., Gershon E.S., Targum S.D., et al.: Segregation and linkage analyses in families of patients with bipolar, unipolar and schizoaffective mood disorders. Am. J. Hum. Genet., in press, 1983.

Groshong R., Baldessarini R.J., Gibson D.A., et al.: Activities of types A and B MAO and catechol-O-methyltransferase in blood cells and skin fibroblasts of normal and chronic schizophrenia subjects. Arch. Gen. Psychiatry 35:1198–1208, 1978.

Groshong R., Gibson D.A., Baldessarini R.J.: Monoamine activity in cultured human skin fibroblasts. Clin. Chim. Acta 80:113–120, 1977.

Hauger M., Harvald B., Fischer M., et al.: The Danish twin register. Acta Genet. Med. Gemellol. 17:319–332, 1968.

Helzer J.E., Winokur G.: A family interview study of male manic depressives. Arch. Gen. Psychiatry 31:73–77, 1974.

Hokin-Neaverson M., Spiegel D.A., Lewis W.C.: Deficiency of erythrocyte sodium pump activity in bipolar manic-depressive psychosis. Life Sci. 15:1739–1748, 1974.

James N.M., Chapman C.J.: A genetic study of bipolar affective disorder. Br. J. Psychiatry 126:449–456, 1975.

Johnson G.F.S., Leeman M.M.: Analysis of familial factors in bipolar affective illness. Arch. Gen. Psychiatry 34:1074–1083, 1977.

Kety S.S.: Disorders of the human brain. Sci. Am. 241:202–218, 1979.

Kringlen E.: Heredity and Environment in the Functional Psychoses. London, Heinemann, 1967.

Kupfer D.J., Pickar D., Himmelhoch J., et al.: Are there two types of unipolar depression? Arch. Gen. Psychiatry 32:866–871, 1975.

Leckman J.F., Gershon E.S., McGinniss M.H., et al.: New data do not suggest linkage between the Xg blood group and bipolar illness. Arch. Gen. Psychiatry 36:1435–1441, 1979.

Levitt M., Mendlewicz J.: A genetic study of plasma dopamine-β-hydroxylase in affective disorder. Mod. Probl. Pharmacopsychiatry 10:89–98, 1975.

Levitt M., Dunner D.L., Mendlewicz J. et al.: Plasma

dopamine-β-hydroxylase activity in affective disorders. Psychopharmacologia 46:205–210, 1976.

Mazure C.M., Gershon E.S.: Blindness and reliability in lifetime psychiatric diagnosis. Arch. Gen. Psychiatry 36:521–525, 1979.

McCabe M.S.: Reactive psychoses. Acta Psychiatr. Scand. Suppl. 259, 37:1–133, 1975.

McCabe M.S., Cadoret R.J.: Genetic investigations of atypical psychoses, Part 1 (morbidity in parents and siblings). Compr. Psychiatry 17:347–352, 1976.

Meltzer H.Y., Cho H.W., Carroll B.J., et al.: Serum dopamine-β-hydroxylase activity in the affective psychoses and schizophrenia. Arch. Gen. Psychiatry 33:585–591, 1976.

Mendels J., Frazer A.: Intracellular lithium concentration and clinical response: towards a membrane theory of depression. J. Psychiatr. Res. 10:9–18, 1973.

Mendlewicz J.: Genetic studies in schizoaffective illness, in The Impact of Biology on Modern Psychiatry. Edited by Gershon E.S., Belmaker R.H. Kety S.S., Rosenbaum M. New York, Plenum Publishing Corp., 1976.

Mendlewicz J.: X-chromosome markers in bipolar illness (ltr. to ed.). Arch. Gen. Psychiatry 38:719, 1981.

Mendlewicz J., Fleiss J.L.: Linkage studies with X-chromosome markers in bipolar (manic-depressive) and unipolar (depressive) illnesses. Biol. Psychiatry 9:261–294, 1974.

Mendlewicz J., Rainer J.D.: Adoption study supporting genetic transmission in manic-depressive illness. Nature 268:327–329, 1977.

Mendlewicz J., Rainer J.D.: Morbidity risk and genetic transmission in manic-depressive illness. Am. J. Hum. Genet. 26:692–701, 1974.

Mendlewicz J., Fleiss J.L., Fieve R.R.: Evidence for X-linkage in the transmission of manic-depressive illness. JAMA 222:1624–1627, 1972.

Mendlewicz J., Fleiss J.L.,Fieve R.R.: Linkage studies in affective disorders: the Xg blood group and manic-depressive illness, in Genetics and Psychopathology. Edited by Fieve R.R., Rosenthal D., Brill H. Baltimore, Johns Hopkins University Press, 1975.

Mendlewicz J., Linkowski P., Guroff J.J., et al.: Color blindness linkage to bipolar manic-depressive illness. Arch. Gen. Psychiatry 36:1442–1449, 1979.

Mendlewicz J., Linkowski P., Wilmette J.: Linkage between glucose-6-phosphate dehydrogenase deficiency and manic-depressive psychosis. Br. J. Psychiatry 137:337–342, 1980a.

Mendlewicz J., Linkowski P., Wilmette J.: Relationship between schizoaffective illness and affective disorders or schizophrenia-morbidity risk and genetic transmission. J. Affective Disord. 2:289–302, 1980b.

Morrison J.R.: The family histories of manic depressive patients with and without alcoholism. J. Nerv, Ment. Dis. 160:227–229, 1975.

Murphy D.L., Redmond D.E. Jr., Garrick N., et al.: Brain region distribution and some characteristics of monoamine oxidase type A and B activities in the vervet monkey. Neurochem. Res. 4:53–62, 1979.

Negri F., Melica A.M., Zuliani R., et al.: Assortative mating and affective disorders. J. Affective Disord. 1:247–253, 1979.

Nies A., Robinson O.S., Harris L.S., et al.: Comparison of monoamine oxidase substrate activities in twins, schizophrenics, depressives and controls. Adv. Biochem. Psychopharmacol. 12:57–70, 1974.

Nurnberger J.I. Jr., Gershon E.S., Simmon S., et al.: Behavioral, biochemical and neuroendocrine responses to amphetamine in normal twins and "well state" bipolar patients. Psychoneuroendocrinology, in press, 1982.

Nurnberger J.I. Jr., Pandey G.N., Gershon E.S.: Lithium ratios in psychiatric patients: a caveat. Presented at the Annual Meeting of the American Psychiatric Association, Toronto, May 1982.

Pandey G.N., Dorus E., Davis J.M., et al.: Lithium transport in human red blood cells. Arch. Gen. Psychiatry 36:902–908, 1979a.

Pandey G.N., Dorus E., Schumacher R., et al.: Genetically determined reduction of platelet MAO and vulnerability to psychiatric disorders. Presented at the Annual Convention and Scientific Meeting of the Society of Biological Psychiatry, Chicago, May 1979b.

Pandey B.N., Ostrow, D.C., Haas M., et al.: Abnormal lithium and sodium transport in erythrocytes of a manic patient and some members of his family. Proceedings of the National Academy of Sciences, USA. 74:3607–3611, 1977.

Perris C.: A study of bipolar (manic-depressive) and unipolar recurrent depressive psychoses. Acta Psychiatr. Scand. Suppl. 194:15–44, 1966.

Perris C.: A study of cycloid psychoses. Acta Psychiatr. Scand. Suppl. 253:1–77, 1974.

Persico M.G., Toniolo D., Nobile C., et al.: cDNA sequences of human glucose-6-phosphate dehydrogenase cloned in pBR322. Nature 294:778–780, 1981.

Pettersen U.: Manic-depressive illness: a clinical, social and genetic study. Acta Psychiatr. Scand. Suppl. 269:1–93, 1977.

Price J.: The genetics of depressive behavior, in Recent Developments in Affective Disorders. Edited by Coppen A., Walk A. Br. J. Psychiatry Special Publication No. 2, 37–54, 1968.

Reich T., Clayton P.J., Winokur G.: Family history studies. V. The genetics of mania. Am. J. Psychiatry 125:1358–1369, 1969.

Reich T., James J.W., Morris C.A.: The use of multiple thresholds in determining the mode of transmission of semi-continuous traits. Ann. Hum. Genet. 36:163–184, 1972.

Rieder R., Gershon E.S.: Genetic strategies in biological psychiatry. Arch. Gen. Psychiatry 35:866–873, 1978.

Rinieris P.M., Stefanis C.N., Lykouras E.P., et al.: Affective disorders and ABO blood types. Acta Psychiatr. Scand. 60:272, 278, 1979.

Rosenthal N.E., Davenport Y., Cowdry R.W., et al.: Monoamine metabolites in cerebrospinal fluid of depressive subgroups. Psychiatry Res. 2:113–119, 1980.

Rosenthal T.L., Akiskal H.S., Scott-Strauss A., et al.: Familial and developmental factors in characterological depressions. J. Affective Disord. 3:183–192, 1981.

Ross S.B., Wetterberg L., Myrhed M.: Genetic control of plasma dopamine-β-hydroxylase. Life Sci. 12:529–532, 1973.

Ruddle F.H.: A new era in mammalian gene mapping: somatic cell genetics and recombinant DNA methodologies. Nature 294:115–120, 1981.

Rybakowski J.: Pharmacogenetic aspect of red blood cell lithium index in manic-depressive psychosis. Biol. Psychiatry 12:425–429, 1977.

Schuckit M.A., Rayses V.: Ethanol ingestion: differences in blood acetaldehyde concentrations in relatives of alcoholics and controls. Science 203:54, 1979.

Schulsinger F., Kety S.S., Rosenthal D., et al.: A family study of suicide, in Origin, Prevention and Treatment of Affective Disorders. Edited by Schou M., Strömgren E. London, Academic Press, 1979.

Sedvall G., Fyro B., Gullberg B., et al.: Relationships in healthy volunteers between concentrations of mono-amine metabolites in cerebrospinal fluid and family history of psychiatric morbidity. Br. J. Psychiatry 136:366–374, 1980.

Shapiro R.W., Bock E., Rafaelsen O.J., et al.: Histocompatibility antigen and manic-depressive disorder. Arch. Gen. Psychiatry 33:823–825, 1976.

Shopsin B., Mendlewicz J., Suslak L., et al.: Genetics of affective disorders, Part 2, (morbidity risk and genetic transmission). Neuropsychobiology 2:28–36, 1976.

Smeraldi E., Negri F., Heimbuch R.C., et al.: Familial patterns and possible modes of inheritance of primary affective disorder. J. Affective Disord. 3:173–182, 1981.

Smeraldi E., Negri F., Melica A.M.: A genetic study of affective disorder. Acta Psychiatr. Scand. 56:382–398, 1977.

Smeraldi E., Negri F., Melica A.M., et al.: HLA system and affective disorders: a sibship genetic study. Tissue Antigens 12:270–274. 1978a.

Smeraldi E., Negri F., Melica A.M., et al.: HLA typing and affective disorders: a study in the Italian population. Neuropsychobiology 4:344–352, 1978b.

Stember R.H., Fieve R.R.: Histocompatibility antigens in affective disorders. Clin. Immunol. Immunopathol. 7:10–14, 1977.

Stenstedt A.: A study in manic-depressive psychosis. Acta Psychiatr. Neurol. Scand. Suppl. 79:1952.

Stewart J., Elston R.C.: Biometrical genetics with one or two loci: the inheritance of physiological characters in mice. Genetics 73:675–693, 1973.

Suslak L., Shopsin B., Silbey E., et al: Genetics of affective disorders, Part 1 (familial incidence study of bipolar, unipolar and schizoaffective illnesses). Neuropsychobiology 2:18–27, 1976.

Takahashi S.: Monoamine oxidase activity in blood platelets from manic and depressed patients. Folia Psychiatr. Neurol. Jpn. 31:37–48, 1977.

Tanna V.L., Winokur G., Elston R.C., et al.: A linkage study of depression spectrum disease. The use of the sib pair method. Neuropsychobiology 2:52–62, 1976.

Targum S.D., Gershon E.S.: Genetic counseling for affective illness, in Mania: An Evolving Concept. Edited by Belmaker R.H., Van Praag H.M. Jamaica, N.Y., Spectrum Publications, 1980.

Targum S.D., Dibble E.D., Davenport Y.B., et al.: The family attitude questionnaire: patients and spouses view bipolar illness. Arch. Gen. Psychiatry 38:562–568, 1981.

Targum S.D., Gershon E.S., Van Eerdewegh M., et al.: Human leukocyte antigen (HLA) system not closely linked to and associated with bipolar manic-depressive illness. Biol. Psychiatry 14:615–636, 1979.

Taylor M.A., Abrams R.: Early onset and late onset bipolar illness. Arch. Gen. Psychiatry 38:58–61, 1981.

Taylor M.A., Abrams R., Hayman M.A.: The classification of affective disorders: a reassessment of the bipolar-unipolar dichotomy. J. Affective Disord 2:95–109, 1980.

Temple H., Dupont B., Shopsin B.: HLA antigen and affective disorders: a report and critical assessment of histocompatibility studies. Neuropsychobiology 5:50–58, 1979.

Tienari P.: Psychiatric illnesses in identical twins. Acta Psychiatr. Scand. Suppl. 171, 1963.

Tsuang M.T.: Schizoaffective disorder—dead or alive? Arch. Gen. Psychiatry 36:633–634, 1979.

Tsuang M.T., Dempsey G.M., Dvoredsky A., et al.: A family history study of schizoaffective disorder. Biol. Psychiatry 12:331–338, 1977.

Tsuang M.T., Dempsey G.M., Rauscher F.: A study of "atypical schizophrenia"—comparison with schizophrenia and affective disorder by sex, age of admission, precipitant, outcome, and family history. Arch. Gen. Psychiatry 33:1157–1160, 1976.

Tsuang M.T., Winokur G., Crowe R.R.: Morbidity risks of schizophrenia and affective disorders among first degree relatives of patients with schizophrenia, mania, depression and surgical conditions. Br. J. Psychiatry 37:497–504, 1980.

Turner W.J., King S.: Two genetically distinct forms of bipolar affective disorder. Biol. Psychiatry 16:417–439, 1981.

Van Eerdewegh M.M., Gershon E.S., Van Eerdewegh P.M.: X-chromosome threshold models of bipolar manic-depressive illness. J. Psychiatr. Res. 15:215–238, 1980.

Van Praag H.M., de Haan S.: Central serotonin metabolism and frequency of depression. Psychiatry Res. 1:219–224, 1979.

Van Praag H.M., de Haan S.: Depression vulnerability and 5-hydroxytryptophan prophylaxis. Psychiatr. Res. 3:75–83, 1980.

Van Praag H.M., Korff J.: Endogenous depressions with and without disturbances in the 5-hydroxytryptamine metabolism: a biochemical classification? Psychopharmacologia 19:148, 1971.

Weinshilboum R.H.: Serum dopamine-β-hydroxylase. Pharmacol. Rev. 30:133–166, 1979.

Weissman M.M., Myers J.K.: Affective disorder in a U.S. urban community. Arch. Gen. Psychiatry 35:1304–1309, 1978.

Weissman M.M., Gershon E.S., Kidd K.K., et al.: Psychiatric disorders in the relatives of probands with affective disorders: the Yale-NIMH collaborative family study. In preparation.

Weissman M.M., Kidd K.K., Prusoff B.A.: Affective illness in relatives of severe and mild nonbipolar depressives and normal controls. Abstracts 2, F514, Third World Congress of Biological Psychiatry, Stockholm, Sweden, July 1981.

Weitkamp L.R., Pardue L.H., Huntzinger R.S.: Genetic marker studies in a family with unipolar depression. Arch. Gen. Psychiatry 37:1187–1192, 1980.

Weitkamp L.R., Stancer H.C., Persad E., et al.: Depressive disorders and HLA: a gene on chromosome 6 that can affect behavior. New Engl. J. Med. 305:1301–1306, 1981.

Winokur A., March V., Mendels J.: Primary affective disorder in relatives of patients with anorexia nervosa. Am. J. Psychiatry 137:695–698, 1980.

Winokur G., Clayton P.: Recent Advances in Biological Psychiatry, vol. 9. Edited by Wortis J. New York, Plenum Press, 1967.

Winokur G., Tanna V.L.: Possible role of X-linked dominant factor in manic-depressive disease. Dis. Nerv. Syst. 30:87–94, 1969.

Winokur G., Clayton P., Reich T.: Manic-Depressive Illness. St. Louis, C.V. Mosby, 1969.

Winter H., Herschel M., Propping P., et al.: A twin study on three enzymes (DBH, COMT, MAO) of catecholamine metabolism: correlations with MMPI. Psychopharmacology 57:63–69, 1978.

References for Chapter 27

Depressive Disorders and the Emerging Field of Psychiatric Chemistry

Adler S.A., Gottesman I.I., Platz Kizuka P.A., et al.: Platelet MAO activity in psychiatric patients: relationship to clinical and psychometric variables. Schizophr. Bull. 6:227–231, 1980.

Beckmann H., Goodwin F.K.: Antidepressant response to tricyclics and urinary MHPG in unipolar patients. Arch. Gen. Psychiatry 32:17–21, 1975.

Beckmann H., Goodwin F.K.: Urinary MHPG in subgroups of depressed patients and normal controls. Neuropsychobiology 6:91–100, 1980.

Belmaker R.H., Ebbesen K., Ebstein R., et al.: Platelet monoamine oxidase in schizophrenia and manic-depressive illness. Br. J. Psychiatry 129:227–232, 1976.

Blombery P.A., Kopin I.J., Gordon E.K., et al.: Conversion of MHPG to vanillylmandelic acid. Arch. Gen. Psychiatry 37:1095–1098, 1980.

Bond P.A., Jenner F.A., Sampson G.A.: Daily variations of the urine content of 3-methoxy-4-hydroxyphenylglycol in two manic-depressive patients. Psychol. Med. 2:81–85, 1972.

Bond P.A., Dimitrakoudi M., Howlett D.R., et al.: Urinary excretion of the sulfate and glucuronide of 3-methoxy-4-hydroxyphenylethyleneglycol in a manic-depressive patient. Psychol. Med. 5:279–285, 1975.

Briley M.S., Raisman R., Langer S.A.: Human platelets possess high-affinity binding sites for ^{3}H-imipramine. Eur. J. Pharmacol. 58:347–348, 1979.

Briley M.S., Langer S.Z., Raisman R., et al.: Tritiated imipramine binding sites are decreased in platelets of untreated depressed patients. Science 209:303–305, 1980.

Bunney W.E., Murphy D.L.: Strategies for the systematic study of neurotransmitter receptor function in man, in Pre- and Postsynaptic Receptors. Edited by Usdin E., Bunney W.E. New York, Marcel Dekker, 1975.

Bunney W.E., Post R.M., Andersen A.E., et al.: A neuronal receptor sensitivity mechanism in affective illness (a review of evidence). Commun. Psychopharmacol. 1:393–405, 1977.

Carroll B.J., Greden J.F., Haskett R., et al.: Neurotransmitter studies of neuroendocrine pathology in depression. Acta Psychiatr. Scand. 61:183–199, 1980.

Carroll B.J., Feinberg M., Greden J.F., et al.: A specific laboratory test for the diagnosis of melancholia. Arch. Gen. Psychiatry 38:15–22, 1981.

Casper R.C., Davis J.M., Pandey G.N., et al.: Neuroendocrine and amine studies in affective illness. Psychoneuroendocrinology 2:105–113, 1977.

Charney D.S., Menkes D.B., Heninger G.R.: Receptor sensitivity and the mechanisms of action of antidepressant treatment. Arch. Gen. Psychiatry 38:1160–1180, 1981.

Cobbin D.M., Requin-Blow B., Williams L.R., et al.: Urinary MHPG levels and tricyclic antidepressant drug selection. Arch. Gen. Psychiatry 36:1111–1115, 1979.

Cobbin D.M., Cairncross K.D., Jurd S., et al.: Urinary MHPG levels and the dexamethasone test predict clinical response to the antidepressant drug mianserin. Neuroendocrine Letters 3:133–138, 1981.

Cohen R.M., Campbell I.C., Cohen M.R., et al.: Presynaptic noradrenergic regulation during depressions and antidepressant drug treatment. Psychiatry Res. 3:93–105, 1980.

Coppen A., Swade C., Wood K.: Platelet 5-hydroxytryptamine accumulation in depressive illness. Clin. Chim. Acta 87:165–168, 1978.

Coppen A., Rama Rao V.A., Ruthven C.R.J., et al.: Urinary 4-hydroxy-3-methoxyphenylglycol is not a predictor for clinical response to amitriptyline in depressive illness. Psychopharmacology 64:95–97, 1979.

Davidson J.R., McLeod M.N., Turnbull C.D., et al.: Platelet monoamine oxidase activity and the classification of depression. Arch. Gen. Psychiatry 37:771–773, 1980.

Davis K.L., Hollister L.E., Goodwin F.K., et al.: Neurotransmitter metabolites in cerebrospinal fluid of man following physostigmine. Life Sci. 21:933–936, 1977.

DeLeon-Jones F.D., Maas J.W., Dekirmenjian H., et al.: Urinary catecholamine metabolites during behavioral changes in a patient with manic-depressive cycles. Science 179:300–302, 1973.

DeLeon-Jones F., Maas J.W., Dekirmenjian H., et al.: Diagnostic subgroups of affective disorders and their urinary excretion of catecholamine metabolites. Am. J. Psychiatry 132:1141–1148, 1975.

Edwards D.J., Spiker D.G., Kupfer D.J., et al.: Platelet monoamine oxidase in affective disorders. Arch. Gen. Psychiatry 35:1443–1446, 1978.

Edwards D.J., Spiker D.G., Neil J.F., et al.: MHPG excretion in depression. Psychiatry Res. 2:295–305, 1980.

Enna S.J., Kendall D.A.: Interactions of antidepressants with brain neurotransmitter receptors. J. Clin. Psychopharmacol. Suppl. 1:125–175, 1981.

Extein I., Tallman J., Smith C.C., et al.: Changes in lymphocyte β-adrenergic receptors in depression and mania. Psychiatry Res. 1:191–197, 1979.

Fain J.H., Garcia-Sainz J.A.: Role of phosphatidylinositol turnover in α_1 and of adenylate cyclase in α_2 effects of catecholamines. Life Sci. 26:1183–1194, 1980.

Fieve R.R., Kumbaraci T., Kassir S., et al.: Platelet monoamine oxidase activity in affective disorders. Biol. Psychiatry 15:473–478, 1980.

Gaertner H.J., Kreuter F., Scharek G., et al.: Do urinary MHPG and plasma drug levels correlate with response to amitriptyline therapy? Psychopharmacology 76:236–239, 1982.

Garcia-Sevilla J.A., Zis A.P., Hollingsworth P.J., et al.: Platelet α_2-adrenoreceptors in major depressive disorders (MDD). The Pharmacologist 23:216 (abstract 536), 1981a.

Garcia-Sevilla J.A., Zis A.P., Hollingsworth P.J., et al.: Platelet α_2-adrenergic receptors in major depressive disorders. Arch. Gen. Psychiatry 38:1327–1333, 1981b.

Garcia-Sevilla J.A., Zis A.P., Zelnick T.C., et al.: Tricyclic antidepressant drug treatment decreases α_2-adrenoreceptors on human platelet membranes. Eur. J. Pharmacol. 69:121–123, 1981c.

Garfinkel P.E., Warsh J.J., Stancer H.C.: CNS monoamine metabolism in bipolar affective disorders. Arch. Gen. Psychiatry 34:735–739, 1977.

Garfinkel P.E., Warsh J.J., Stancer H.C.: Depression: new evidence in support of biological differentiation. Am. J. Psychiatry 136:535–539, 1979.

Garver D.L., Davis J.M.: Biogenic amine hypothesis of affective disorders. Life Sci. 24:383–394, 1979.

Gattaz W.F., Beckmann H.: Platelet MAO activity and personality characteristics: a study in schizophrenic patients and normal individuals. Acta Psychiatr. Scand. 63:479–485, 1981.

Gold M.S., Pottash A.L.C., Extein I: Hypothyroidism and depression evidence from complete thyroid function evaluation. JAMA 245:1919–1922, 1981.

Goodwin F.K., Post R.M.: Studies of amine metabolites in affective illness and in schizophrenia: a comparative analysis, in Biology of Major Psychoses. Edited by Freedman D.X. New York, Raven Press, 1975.

Goodwin F.K., Potter W.Z.: Norepinephrine metabolite studies in affective illness, in. Catecholamines: Basic and Clinical Frontiers, vol. 2. Edited by Usdin E., Kopin I., Barchas J. New York, Pergamon Press, 1979.

Gottfries C.G., von Knorring L., Oreland L.: Platelet monoamine oxidase activity in mental disorders: 2. affective psychoses and suicidal behavior. Prog. Neuropsychopharmacol. 4:185–192, 1980.

Greenspan K., Schildkraut J.J., Gordon E.K., et al.: Catecholamine metabolism in affective disorders III. MHPG and other catecholamine metabolites in patients treated with lithium carbonate. J. Psychiatr. Res. 7:171–183, 1970.

Gudeman J.E., Schatzberg A.F., Samson J.A., et al.: Toward a biochemical classification of depressive disorders VI: platelet MAO activity and clinical symptoms in depressed patients. Am. J. Psychiatry 139:630–633, 1982.

Hoffman B.B., Delean A., Wood C.L., et al.: α-adrenergic receptor subtypes: quantitative assessement by ligand binding. Life Sci. 24:1739–1746, 1979.

Hollister L.E., Davis K.L., Berger P.A.: Subtypes of depression based on excretion of MHPG and response to nortriptyline. Arch. Gen. Psychiatry 37:1107–1110, 1980.

Hollister L.E., Davis K.L., Overall J.E., et al.: Excretion of MHPG in normal subjects. Implications for biological classification of affective disorders. Arch. Gen. Psychiatry 35:1410–1415, 1978.

Honecker H., Fahndrich E., Coper H., et al.: Serum DBH and platelet MAO in patients with depressive disorders. Pharmacopsychiatria 14:10–14, 1981.

Janowsky D.S., El-Yousef M., Davis J.M., et al.: A cholinergic-adrenergic hypothesis of mania and depression. Lancet II:632–635. 1972.

Kafka M.S., vanKammen D.P., Kleinman J.E., et al.: α-adrenergic receptor function in schizophrenia, affective disorders, and some neurological diseases. Commun. Psychopharmacol. 4:477–486, 1980.

Kasper S., Moises H.W., Beckmann H.: The anticholinergic biperiden in depressive disorders. Pharmacopsychiatria 14:195–198, 1981.

Kirkegaard C.: The thyrotropin response to thyrotropin-releasing hormone in endogenous depression. Psychoneuroendocrinology 6:189–212, 1981.

Landowski J., Lysiak W., Angielski S.: Monoamine oxidase activity in blood platelets from patients with cyclophrenic depressive syndromes. Biochem. Med. 14:347–354, 1975.

Langer S.Z., Moret C., Raisman R., et al.: High affinity (^{3}H)-imipramine binding in rat hypothalamus: association with uptake of serotonin but not of norepinephrine. Science 210:1133–1135, 1980.

Langer S.Z., Zarifian E., Briley M., et al.: High-affinity binding of ^{3}H-imipramine in brain and platelets and its relevance to the biochemistry of affective disorders. Life Sci. 29:211–220, 1981.

Leckman J.F., Gershon E.S., Nichols A.S.: Reduced MAO activity in first degree relatives of individuals with bipolar affective disorders: a preliminary report. Arch. Gen. Psychiatry 34:601–606, 1977.

Lecrubier Y., Puech A.J., Jouvent R., et al.: A β-adrenergic stimulant (salbutamol) versus clomipramine in depression: a controlled study. Br. J. Psychiatry 136:354–358, 1980.

Lefkowitz R.F.: Identification and regulation of α- and β-adrenergic receptors. Fed. Proc. 37:123–129, 1978.

Linnoila M., Karoum F., Potter W.Z.: High correlation of norepinephrine and its major metabolite excretion rates. Arch. Gen. Psychiatry 39:521–523, 1982.

Maas J.W.: Biogenic amines and depression: biochemical and pharmacological separation of two types of depression. Arch. Gen. Psychiatry 32:1357–1361, 1975.

Maas J.W.: Clinical and biochemical heterogeneity of depressive disorders. Ann. Intern. Med. 88:556–663, 1978.

Maas J.W., Landis D.H.: In vivo studies of metabolism of norepinephrine in central nervous system. J. Pharmacol. Exp. Ther. 163:147–162, 1968.

Maas J.W., Dekirmenjian H., DeLeon-Jones F.: The identification of depressed patients who have a disorder of norepinephrine metabolism and/or disposition, in Frontiers in Catecholamine Research—Third International Catecholamine Symposium. Edited by Usdin E., Snyder S. New York, Pergamon Press, 1973.

Maas J.W., Fawcett J.A., Dekirmenjian H.: Catecholamine metabolism, depressive illness and drug response. Arch. Gen. Psychiatry 26:252–262, 1972.

Maas J.W., Fawcett J.A., Dekirmenjian H.: 3-Methoxy-4-hydroxyphenylglycol (MHPG) excretion in depressive states. Arch. Gen. Psychiatry 19:129–134, 1968.

Maas J.W., Hattox S.E., Greene N.M., et al.: 3-Methoxy-4-hydroxyphenethyleneglycol production by human brain in vivo. Science 205:1025–1027, 1979.

Maas J.W., Kocsis J.H., Bowden C.L., et al.: Pretreatment neurotransmitter metabolites and response to imipramine or amitriptyline treatment. Psychol. Med. 12:37–43, 1982.

Maggi A., U'Pritchard D.C., Enna S.J.: Differential effects of antidepressant treatment on brain monoaminergic receptors. Eur. J. Pharmacol. 61:91–98, 1980.

Mann J.: Altered platelet monoamine oxidase activity in affective disorders. Psychol. Med. 9:729–736, 1979.

Mardh G., Sjoquist B., Anggard E.: Norepinephrine metabolism in man using deuterium labelling: the conversion of 4-hydroxy-3-methoxyphenylglycol to 4-hydroxy-3-methoxymandelic acid. J. Neurochem 36:1181–1185, 1981.

Meltzer H.Y., Arora R.C., Baber R., et al.: Serotonin uptake in blood platelets of psychiatric patients. Arch. Gen. Psychiatry 38:1322–1326, 1981.

Modai I., Apter A., Golomb M., et al.: Response to amitriptyline and urinary MHPG in bipolar depressive patients. Neuropsychobiology 5:181–184, 1979.

Murphy D.L., Weiss R.: Reduced monoamine oxidase activity in blood platelets from bipolar depressed patients. Am. J. Psychiatry 128:1351–1357, 1972.

Murphy D.L., Donnelly C., Moskowitz J.: Inhibition by lithium of prostaglandin E$_1$ and norepinephrine effects on cyclic adenosine monophosphate production in human platelets. Clin. Pharmacol. Ther. 14:810–814, 1973.

Nies A., Robinson D.S., Harris L.S., et al.: Comparison of monoamine oxidase substrate activities in twins, schizophrenics, depressives and controls, in Neuropsychopharmacology of Monoamines and Their Regulatory Enzymes. Edited by Usdin E. New York, Raven Press, 1974.

Nies A., Robinson D.S., Ravaris C.L., et al.: Amines and monoamine oxidase in relation to aging and depression in man. Psychosom. Med. 33:470, 1971.

Orsulak P.J., Schildkraut J.J., Schatzberg A.F., et al.: Differences in platelet monoamine oxidase activity in subgroups of schizophrenia and depressive disorders Biol. Psychiatry 13:637–647, 1978.

Pandey G.N., Dysken M.W., Garver D.L., et al.: β-adrenergic receptor function in affective illness. Am. J. Psychiatry 136:675–678, 1979.

Paul S.M., Rehavi M., Rice X.C., et al.: Does high affinity (^{3}H)-imipramine binding label serotonin reuptake sites in brain and platelet? Life Sci. 28:2753–2760, 1981a.

Paul S.M., Rehavi M., Skolnich P., et al.: Depressed patients have decreased binding of tritiated imipramine to platelet serotonin "transporter". Arch. Gen. Psychiatry 38:1315–1317, 1981b.

Paul S.M., Rehavi M., Skolnich P., et al.: Demonstration of specific "high affinity" binding sites for (^{3}H)-imipramine on human platelets. Life Sci. 26:953–959, 1980.

Peroutka S.J., Snyder S.H.: Longterm antidepressant treatment decreases spiroperidol-labeled serotonin receptor binding. Science 210:88–90, 1980.

Post R.M., Stoddard F.J., Gillin C., et al.: Alterations in motor activity, sleep and biochemistry in a cycling manic-depressive patient. Arch. Gen. Psychiatry 34:470–477, 1977.

Rehavi M., Paul S.M., Skolnich P., et al.: Demonstration of specific high affinity binding sites for (^{3}H)-imipramine in human brain. Life Sci. 26:2273–2279, 1980.

Reveley M.A., Glover V., Sandler M., et al.: Increased platelet monoamine oxidase activity in affective disorders. Psychopharmacology 73:257–260, 1981.

Risch S.C., Cohen R.M., Janowsky D.S., et al.: Mood and behavioral effects of physostigmine on humans are accompanied by elevations in plasma β-endorphin and cortisol. Science 209:1545–1546, 1980.

Risch S.C., Kalin N.H., Janowsky D.S.: Cholinergic challenges in affective illness: behavioral and neuroendocrine correlates. J. Clin. Psychopharmacol. 1:186–192, 1981a.

Risch S.C., Kalin N.H., Murphy D.L.: Neurochemical mechanisms in the affective disorders and neurochemical correlates. J. Clin. Psychopharmacol. 1:180–185, 1981b.

Risch S.C., Kalin N.H., Murphy D.L.: Pharmacological challenge strategies: implications for neurochemical mechanisms in affective disorders and treatment approaches. J. Clin. Psychopharmacol. 1:238–243, 1981c.

Roffman M., Gould E.E., and the Oxaprotiline Study Group (Research Department, CIBA-GEIGY Corp.): Comparison of oxaprotiline to amitriptyline and placebo in depressed patients: relationship to MHPG. Presented at 13th Congress of the Collegium Internationale Neuropsychopharmacologicum, Jerusalem, Israel, June 1982.

Rosenbaum A.H., Maruta T., Schatzberg A.F.: Urinary free cortisol and MHPG levels in anxious patients and normal controls. Abstract No. 78, p. 106. Presented at Society of Biological Psychiatry Annual Meeting, New Orleans, May 1981.

Rosenbaum A.H., Maruta T., Schatzberg A.F., et al.: Toward a biochemical classification of depressive disorders VII: Urinary free cortisol and urinary MHPG in depressions. Am. J. Psychiatry, in press, 1983.

Rosenbaum A.H., Schatzberg A., Maruta T., et al.: MHPG as a predictor of antidepressant response to imipramine and maprotiline. Am. J. Psychiatry 137:1090–1092, 1980.

Rubin R.T., Marder S.R.: Biological markers in affective and schizophrenic disorders: a review of contemporary research, in Affective and Schizophrenic Disorders: New Approaches to the Diagnosis and Treatment. Edited by Zales M.R. New York, Brunner/Mazel, 1983.

Sacchetti E., Allaria E., Negri F., et al.: 3-Methoxy-4-hydroxyphenylglycol and primary depression: clinical and pharmacological considerations. Biol. Psychiatry 14:473–484, 1979.

Sandler M., Reveley M.A., Glover V.: Human platelet monoamine oxidase activity in health and disease: a review. J. Clin. Pathol. 34:292–302, 1981.

Schanberg S.M., Breese G.R., Schildkraut J.J., et al.: 3-methoxy-4-hydroxyphenylglycol sulfate in brain and cerebrospinal fluid. Biochem. Pharmacol. 17:2006–2008, 1968a.

Schanberg S.M., Schildkraut J.J., Breese G.R., et al.: Metabolism of normetanephrine-H^3 in rat brain-identification

of conjugated 3-methoxy-4-hydroxyphenylglycol as major metabolite. Biochem. Pharmacol. 17:247–254, 1968b.

Schatzberg A.F., Orsulak P.J., Rosenbaum A.H., et al.: Toward a biochemical classification of depressive disorders IV: pretreatment urinary MHPG levels as predictors of antidepressant response to imipramine. Commun. Psychopharmacol. 4:441–445, 1980–1981.

Schatzberg A.F., Orsulak P.J., Rosenbaum A.H., Toward a biochemical classification of depressive disorders V: heterogeneity of unipolar depressions. Am. J. Psychiatry 139:471–475, 1982.

Schatzberg A.F., Rosenbaum A.H., Orsulak P.J., et al.: Toward a biochemical classification of depressive disorders III: pretreatment of urinary MHPG levels as predictors of response to treatment with maprotiline. Psychopharmacology 75:34–38, 1981.

Schildkraut J.J.: The catecholamine hypothesis of affective disorders: a review of supporting evidence. Am. J. Psychiatry 122:509–522, 1965.

Schildkraut J.J.: Neuropsychopharmacology and the Affective Disorders. Boston, Little, Brown & Co. 1970.

Schildkraut J.J.: Norepinephrine metabolites as biochemical criteria for classifying depressive disorders and predicting responses to treatment: preliminary findings. Am. J. Psychiatry 130:696–699, 1973.

Schildkraut J.J., Keeler B.A., Grab E.L., et al.: MHPG excretion and clinical classification in depressive disorders. Lancet I:1251–1252, 1973a.

Schildkraut J.J., Keeler B.A., Papousek M., et al.: MHPG excretion in depressive disorders: relation to clinical subtypes and desynchronized sleep. Science 181:762–764, 1973b.

Schildkraut J.J., Keeler B.A., Rogers M.P., et al.: Catecholamine metabolism in affective disorders: a longitudinal study of a patient treated with amitriptyline and ECT. Psychosom. Med. 34:470, 1972 (plus erratum Psychosom. Med. 35:274, 1973).

Schildkraut J.J., Orsulak P.J., LaBrie R.A., et al: Toward a biochemical classification of depressive disorders II: application of multivariate discriminant function analysis to data on urinary catecholamines and metabolites. Arch. Gen. Psychiatry 35:1436–1439, 1978a.

Schildkraut J.J., Orsulak P.J., Schatzberg A.F., et al.: Elevated platelet monoamine oxidase (MAO) activity in schizophrenia-related depressive disorders. Am. J. Psychiatry 135:110–112, 1978b.

Schildkraut J.J., Orsulak, P.J., Schatzberg A.F., et al.: Biochemical discrimination of subgroups of depressive disorders based on differences in catecholamine metabolism, in Biological Markers in Psychiatry and Neurology. Edited by Hanin I., Usdin E. New York, Pergamon Press, 1982.

Schildkraut J.J., Orsulak P.J., Schatzberg A.F., et al.: Possible pathophysiological mechanisms in subtypes of unipolar depressive disorders based on differences in urinary MHPG levels. Psychopharmacol. Bull. 17:90–91, 1981.

Schildkraut J.J., Orsulak P.J., Schatzberg A.F., et al.: Toward a biochemical classification of depressive disorders I: differences in urinary MHPG and other catecholamine metabolites in clinically defined subtypes of depressions. Arch. Gen. Psychiatry 35:1427–1433, 1978c.

Schildkraut J.J., Watson R., Draskoczy P.R., et al.: Amphetamine withdrawal: depression and MHPG excretion. Lancet II: 485–486, 1971.

Scott R.E.: Effects of prostaglandins, epinephrine and NaF on human leukocyte, platelet and liver adenylcyclase. Blood 35:514–516, 1970.

Scott M., Reading H.W., Ludon J.B.: Studies on human blood platelets in affective disorders. Psychopharmacology 60:131–135, 1979.

Segawa T., Mizuta T., Nomura Z.: Modification of central 5-hydroxytryptamine binding sites in synaptic membranes from rat brain after long term administration of tricyclic antidepressants. Eur. J. Pharmacol. 58:75–83, 1979.

Siever L., Insel T., Uhde T.: Noradrenergic challenges in the affective disorders. J. Clin. Psychopharmcol 1:193–206, 1981.

Sitaram N., Gillin C.: Development and use of pharmacological probes of the CNS in man: evidence of cholinergic abnormality in primary affective illness. Biol. Psychiatry 15:925–955, 1980.

Spiker D.G., Edwards D., Hanin I., et al.: Urinary MHPG and clinical response to amitriptyline in depressed patients. Am. J. Psychiatry 137:1183–1187, 1980.

Spitzer R.L., Endicott J., Robins E.: Research diagnostic criteria. Rationale and reliability. Arch. Gen. Psychiatry 35:773–782, 1978.

Steinbook R.M., Jacobson A.F., Weiss B.L., et al.: Amoxapine, imipramine and placebo: a double-blind study with pretherapy urinary 3-methoxy-4-hydroxyphenylglycol levels. Curr. Ther. Res. 26:490–496, 1979.

Sullivan J.L., Cavenar J.O., Maltbie A., et al: Platelet monoamine oxidase activity predicts response to lithium in manic-depressive illness. Lancet II:1325–1327, 1977.

Sulser F., Vetulani J., Mobley P.K.: Mode of action of antidepressant drugs. Biochem. Pharmacol. 27:257–261, 1978.

Takahashi S., Karasawa T.: A sensitive nonisotopic assay for monoamine oxidase activity in human blood platelets. Clin. Chim. Acta 62:383–400, 1975.

Talvenheimo J., Nelson P.J., Rudnick G.: Mechanism of imipramine inhibition of platelet 5-hydroxytryptamine transport. J. Biol. Chem. 254:4631–4635, 1979.

Taube S.L., Kirstein L.S., Sweeney D.R., et. al.: Urinary 3-methoxy-4-hydroxyphenylglycol and psychiatric diagnosis. Am. J. Psychiatry 135:78–82, 1978.

Tuomisto J., Tukiainen E., Ahlfors U.G.: Decreased uptake of 5-hydroxy-tryptamine in blood platelets from patients with endogenous depression. Psychopharmacology 65:141–147, 1979.

Tyrer P. Towards rational therapy with monoamine oxidase inhibitors. Brit. J. Psychiat. 128:354–360, 1976.

U'Pritchard D.C., Daiguji M., Tong C., et al.: α_2-adrenergic receptors: comparative biochemistry of neural and nonneural receptors, and in vitro analysis of psychiatric patients, in Biological Markers in Psychiatry and Neurology. Edited by Usdin E., Hanin I. New York, Pergamon Press, 1982.

Waldmeier P.C.: Noradrenergic transmission in depression: under- or overfunction? Pharmacopsychiatria 14:3–9, 1981.

Wang Y.C., Pandey G.N., Mendels J., et al.: Platelet adenylate cyclase responses in depression: implications for a receptor defect. Psychopharmacologia (Berl.) 36:291–300, 1974.

Watson R., Hartmann E., Schildkraut J.J.: Amphetamine withdrawal: affective state, sleep patterns and MHPG excretion. Am. J. Psychiatry 129:263–269, 1972.

White K., Shih J., Fong T., et al.: Elevated platelet monoamine oxidase activity in patients with nonendogenous depression. Am. J. Psychiatry 137:1258–1259, 1980.

Whybrow P.C., Prange A.J.: A hypothesis of thyroid-catecholamine interaction. Arch. Gen. Psychiatry 38:106–113, 1981.

Williams L.T., Snyderman R., Lefkowitz R.J.: Identification of β-adrenergic receptors in human lymphocytes by (-) (^{3}H) alprenolol binding. J. Clin. Invest 57:149–155, 1976.

Wood C.L., Arnett C.D., Clarke W.R., et al.: Subclassification of α-adrenergic receptors by direct binding studies. Biochem. Pharmacol. 28:1277–1282, 1979.

References for Chapter 28

Antidepressant Drug Therapy

American Psychiatric Association: Diagnostic and Statistical Manual of Mental Disorders, 3rd ed. Washington, D.C., American Psychiatric Association, 1980.

Asberg M., Cronholm B., Sjoquist F.B., et al.: Relationship between plasma level and therapeutic effect of nortriptyline. Br. Med. J. 3:331–334, 1971.

Ayd F: A unique broad spectrum antidepressant. International Drug Ther. Newsltr. 14:33–40, 1979.

Ayd F.: Amoxapine: a new tricyclic antidepressant. International Drug Ther. Newsltr. 15:33–40, 1980.

Baldessarini R.J.: Overview of recent advances in antipressant pharmacology: Part II. McLean Hosp. J. 7:1–27, 1982.

Baldessarini R.J., Willmuth R.L.: Psychotic reactions during amitriptyline therapy. Can. Psychiatr. Assoc. J. 13:571–573, 1968.

Beckmann H., Goodwin F.K.: Antidepressant response to trycyclics and urinary MHPG in unipolar patients. Arch. Gen. Psychiatry 32:17–21, 1975.

Branconnier R., DeVitt D., Cole J.O., et al.: Amitriptyline selectively disrupts verbal recall from secondary memory of the normal aged. Neurobiol. Aging 3:55–59, 1982.

Brogden R., Heel R., Speight T., et al.: Nominfensine: a review of its pharmacological properties and therapeutic efficacy in depressive illness. Drugs 18:1–24, 1979.

Chouinard G., Annable L., Fontaine R., et al.: Alprazolam in the treatment of anxiety and panic disorders: a double-blind placebo-controlled study. Psychopharmacology, in press, 1982.

Cohen B., Harris P., Altesman R., et al.: Amoxapine: a neuroleptic as well as an antidepressant. Am. J. Psychiatry, in press, 1982.

Cole J.O.: New antidepressant drugs. McLean Hosp. J., in press, 1982.

Cole J.O., Schatzberg A.F.: Memory difficulty and tricyclic antidepressants. McLean Hosp. J. 1:102–107, 1976.

Cole J.O., Sunderland P: The drug treatment of borderline patients, in Psychiatry 1982: The American Psychiatric Association Annual Review (Psychiatry Update: Volume I). Edited by Grinspoon L. Washington, D.C., American Psychiatric Press, Inc, 1982.

Cole J.O., Hartmann E., Brigham P.: L-tryptophan: clinical studies, in Psychopharmacology Update. Edited by Cole J.O. Lexington, MA., Collamore Press, 1980.

Cole J.O., Schatzberg A.F., Griffin C., et al.: Trazodone in treatment-resistant depression: an open study. J. Clin. Psychopharmacol. Suppl. 6, 1:49S–54S, 1981.

Crane G.E.: Iproniazid (marsilid) phosphate: a therapeutic agent for mental disorders and debilitating diseases. Psychiatr. Res. Reports 8:142–152, 1957.

Crews F.T., Smith C.B.: Presynaptic α-receptor subsensitivity after long-term antidepressant treatment. Science 202:322–324, 1978.

Davis J.: Overview: maintenance therapy in psychiatry: II. Affective disorders. Am. J. Psychiatry 133:1–13, 1976.

de Montigny C., Grunberg F., Mayer A., et al.: Lithium induces rapid relief of depression in tricyclic antidepressant drug non-responders. Br. J. Psychiatry 138: 252–255, 1981.

Donlon P., Biertuemphel H., Willenbring M.: Amoxapine and amitriptyline in the outpatient treatment of endogenous depression. J. Clin. Psychiatry 42:11–15, 1981.

Everett H.C.: The use of bethanechol chloride with tricyclic antidepressants. Am. J. Psychiatry 132:1202–1206, 1976.

Fawcett J., Maas J.W., Dekirmenjian H.: Depression and MHPG excretion: response to dextroamphetamine and tricyclic antidepressant. Arch. Gen. Psychiatry 26: 246–251, 1972.

Fawcett J., Sabelli H., Javaid J., et al.: Methylphenidate test differentiates between desipramine responder (type A) and nortriptyline responder (type B) depressions. Am. J. Psychiatry, in press, 1982.

Ferris R.: The mode of action of buproprion. J. Clin. Psychiatry, in press, 1982.

Gelenberg A: Effects of tricyclic antidepressant on cardiac function. Mass. Gen. Hosp. Biol. Ther. Psychiatry 5: 9–10, 1982a.

Gelenberg A: T$_3$ to augment tricyclics. Mass. Gen. Hosp. Biol. Ther. Psychiatry 5:11–12, 1982b.

Gershon E.S., Newton R.E.: Lack of anticholinergic side effects with a new antidepressant—trazodone. J. Clin. Psychiatry Suppl. 3, 41:100–104, 1980.

Gershon E.S., Mann J., Newton R.E., et al.: Evaluation of trazodone in the treatment of endogenous depression: results of a multicenter double-blind study. J. Clin. Psychopharmacol. Suppl. 6, 1:139–44, 1981.

Giardana R., Bigger J., Johnson L.: The effect of imipramine and nortriptyline on ventricular premature depolarizations and left ventricular function. Meeting Abstract, circulation 64 S-Y:316, 1981.

Giller E., Lieb J.: MAO inhibitors and platelet MAO inhibition. Presented at the Annual Meeting of the American Psychiatric Association, San Francisco, May 1980.

Glass B., Uhlenhuth E., Hartel F., et al.: Cognitive dysfunction and imipramine in outpatient depressives. Arch. Gen. Psychiatry 38:1048–1052, 1981.

Glassman A.H., Bigger J., Giardina E.: Clinical characteristics of imipramine-induced orthostatic hypotension. Lancet 1:468–472, 1979.

Glassman A.H., Kantor S.J., Shostak M.: Depression, delusions, and drug response. Am. J. Psychiatry 132: 716–719, 1975.

Glassman A.H., Perel J.M., Shostak M., et al.: Clinical implications of imipramine plasma levels for depressive illness. Arch. Gen. Psychiatry 34:197–204, 1977.

Goodwin F.K., Prange A., Post R., et al.: L-triiodothyronine converts tricyclic antidepressant non-responders to responders. Am. J. Psychiatry 139:34–38, 1982.

Granacher R.P., Baldessarini R.J.: Physostigmine: its use in acute anticholinergic syndrome with antidepressant and antiparkinson drugs. Arch Gen. Psychiatry 23:375–380, 1975.

Hollister L.E., Davis K.L., Berger P.A.: Subtypes of depression based on excretion of MHPG and response to nortriptyline. Arch. Gen. Psychiatry 37:1107–1110, 1980.

Johnston E.C., Marsh W.: Acetylator status and response to phenelzine in depressed patients. Lancet 1:567–570, 1973.

Kahn R., McNair D., Covi L., et al.: Effects of psychotropic agents in high anxiety subjects. Psychopharmacol. Bull. 17:97–100, 1981.

Kiloh L.G., Ball J.R.B., Garside R.D.: Prognostic factors in treatment of depressive states with imipramine. Br. Med. J. 1:1225–1227, 1962.

Klerman G.L., DiMascio A., Weissman M.M., et al.: Treatment of depression by drugs and psychotherapy. Am. J. Psychiatry 131:186–191, 1974.

Kline N.S.: Clinical experience with iproniazid (marsilid). J. Clin. Exp. Psychopathol. 19:72–78, 1958.

Kuhn R.: Über die Behandlung depressiver Zustände mit einem Iminodibenzylderivat (G22355). Schweizer Medizinische Wochenschrift. Journal Suisse de Médecine 87:1135–1140, 1957.

Lydiard R.B.: Amoxapine. Biol. Ther. Psychiatry 5: 21–22, 1982.

Maas R.: Biogenic amines and depression. Biochemical and pharmacological separation of two types of depression. Arch. Gen. Psychiatry 32:1357–1361, 1975.

Maas R., Fawcett J.A., Dekirmenjian H.: Catecholamine metabolism, depressive illness and drug response. Arch. Gen. Psychiatry 26:252–262, 1972.

McCabe B., Tsuang M.: Dietary consideration on MAO inhibitor regimens. J. Clin. Psychiatry 43:178–181, 1982.

Minter R.D., Mandel N.: A prospective study of the treatment of psychotic depression. Am. J. Psychiatry 153:1470–1472, 1979.

Mirin S.M., Schatzberg A.F., Creasey D.E.: Hypomania and mania after tricyclic withdrawal. Am. J. Psychiatry 138:87–89, 1981.

Modai I., Apter M., Golomb M., et al.: Response to amitriptyline and urinary MHPG in bipolar depressive patients. Neuropsychobiology 5:181–184, 1979.

Nelson J.C., Bowers M.B.: Delusional unipolar depression: description and drug response. Arch. Gen. Psychiatry 35:1321–1328, 1978.

Pinder R., Brogden R., Speight T., et al.: Maprotiline: a review of its pharmacological properties and therapeutic efficacy in mental depressive states. Drugs 13:321–387, 1977.

Pollack M., Klein D.F., Willner A., et al.: Imipramine-induced behavioral disorganization in schizophrenic patients: physiological and psychological correlates, in Recent Advances in Biology and Psychiatry. Edited by Wortis J. New York, Plenum Press, 1965.

Preskorn S., Irwin H.: Toxicity of tricyclic antidepressants—kinetics, mechanisms, intervention: a review. J. Clin. Psychiatry 43:151–156, 1982.

Prien R.: Maintenance drug therapy in depression: current status and strategies. Paper presented at the New Clinical Drug Evaluation Unit Meeting, Key Biscayne, Florida, May 1981.

Prien R., Caffey E., Klett J.: Lithium carbonate and imipramine in prevention of affective disorders. Arch. Gen. Psychiatry 29:420–425, 1973.

Quitkin F., Rifkin A., Klein D.: Prophylaxis of affective disorders. Arch. Gen. Psychiatry 33:337–341, 1976.

Ravaris C.L., Nies A., Robinson D.S., et al.: A multiple-dose controlled study of phenelzine in depression-anxiety states. Arch. Gen. Psychiatry 33:347–350, 1976.

Ravaris C.L., Robinson D.S., Ives J.O., et al.: Phenelzine and amitriptyline in the treatment of depression. Arch. Gen. Psychiatry 37:1075–1080, 1980.

Riblet L.A., Taylor D.P.: Pharmacology and neurochemistry of trazodone. J. Clin. Psychopharmacol. Suppl. 6 1:17–22, 1981.

Richelson E.: Tricyclic antidepressants. Interactions with histamine and muscarinic acetylcholine receptors, in Antidepressants: Neurochemical, Behavioral and Clinical Perspectives. Edited by Enna S.J., Malick J.B., Richelson E. New York, Raven Press, 1981.

Riddle M., Giller E., Bialos D., et al.: MAO inhibition responsive atypical depression. New Res. Abstr. NR 12. Presented at the Annual Meeting of the American Psychiatric Association, San Francisco, May 1980.

Roffman M., Gould E.E., and the Oxaprotiline Study Group (Research Department, CIBA-GEIGY Corp.): Comparison of oxaprotiline to amitriptyline and placebo in depressed patients: relationship to MHPG. Presented at the 13th Congress of the Collegium Internationale Neuropsychopharmacologicum, Jerusalem, Israel, June 1982.

Roose S., Glassman A.H., Bruno R.: Tricyclic antidepressant induced postural hypotension: comparative studies. New Res. Abstr. 33. Presented at the Annual Meeting of the American Psychiatric Association, San Francisco, May 1980.

Rosenbaum A.H., Schatzberg A.F., Maruta T., et al.: MHPG as a predictor of antidepressant response to imipramine and maprotiline. Am. J. Psychiatry 137:1090–1092, 1980.

Rowan P., Paykel E., Parker R.: Phenelzine and amitriptyline: effects on symptoms of neurotic depression. Br. J. Psychiatry 140:475–483, 1982.

Schatzberg A.F., Cole J.O.: Benzodiazepines in depressive disorders. Arch. Gen. Psychiatry 35:1359–1365, 1978.

Schatzberg A.F., Cole J.O., Blumer D.P.: Speech blockage: a tricyclic side effect. Am. J. Psychiatry 135:600–601, 1978.

Schatzberg A.F., Orsulak P.J., Rosenbaum A.H., et al.: Toward a biochemical classification of depressive disorders IV: pretreatment urinary MHPG levels as predictors of antidepressant response to imipramine. Commun. Psychopharmacol. 4:441–445, 1980.

Schatzberg A.F., Orsulak P.J., Rosenbaum A.H., et al.: Toward a biochemical classification of depressive disorders V: heterogeneity of unipolar depressions. Am. J. Psychiatry 139:471–475, 1982.

Schatzberg A.F., Rosenbaum A.H., Orsulak P.J., et al.: Toward a biochemical classification of depressive disorders III: pretreatment urinary MHPG levels as predictors of response to treatment with maprotiline. Psychopharmacology 75:34–38, 1981.

Schildkraut J.J.: Norepinephrine metabolites as biochemical criteria for classifying depressive disorders and predicting responses to treatment: preliminary findings. Am. J. Psychiatry 130:695–699, 1973.

Sethy V.H.: A possible mode of antidepressant activity of alprazolam. The pharmacology of benzodiazepines. Presented at the National Institutes of Health Conference, April 1982.

Sheehan D.V., Ballenger J., Jacobsen G.: Treatment of endogenous anxiety with phobic, hysterical and hypochondriacal symptoms. Arch. Gen. Psychiatry 37:51–59, 1980.

Shopsin B., Friedman E., Gershon E.S.: Parachlorophenylalanine reversal of tranylcypromine effects in depressed patients. Arch. Gen. Psychiatry 33:811–819, 1976.

Spiker D.G., Edwards D., Hanin E., et al.: Urinary MHPG and clinical response to amitriptyline in depressed patients. Am. J. Psychiatry 137:1183–1187, 1980.

Spiker D.G., Hanin I., Cofsky J., et al.: Pharmacological treatment of delusional depressives. Psychopharmacol. Bull. 17:201–202, 1981.

Steinbook R.M., Jacobsen A.F., Weiss B.L., et al.: Amoxapine, imipramine and placebo: a double-blind study with pretherapy urinary 3-methoxy-4-hydroxyphenylglycol levels. Curr. Ther. Res. 26:490–496, 1979.

Stewart J., Quitkin F., Fyer A., et al.: Effect of desipramine in endogenomorphically depressed patients. J. Affective Disord. 2:165–176, 1980.

Stewart J., Quitkin F., Liebowitz M., et al.: Efficacy of desipramine in mildly depressed patients: a double-blind placebo-controlled trial. Psychopharmacol. Bull. 17:136–138, 1981.

Sulser F.: Review of the mode of action of antidepressant drugs. J. Clin. Psychiatry, in press, 1982.

Sulser F.: Pharmacology: current antidepressants. Psychiatric Annals. 10:528–533, 1980.

Thayssen P., Bjerre M., Kragh-Sorenson P., et al.: Cardiovascular effects of imipramine and nortriptyline in elderly patients. Psychopharmacology 74:360–364, 1981.

Tyrer P.: Towards rational therapy with monoamine oxidase inhibitors. Br. J. Psychiatry 128:354–360, 1976.

Veith R., Raskind M., Caldwell J., et al.: Cardiovascular effects of tricyclic antidepressants in depressed patients with chronic heart disease. New Engl. J. Med. 306:954–959, 1982.

Wharton R.N., Perel J.M., Dayton P.G., et al.: A potential clinical use for methylphenidate with tricyclic antidepressants. Am. J. Psychiatry 127:1619–1625, 1971.

White K., Simpson G.: Combined MAOI tricyclic antidepressant treatment: a reevaluation. J. Clin. Psychopharmacol. 1:264–282, 1981.

Zung W.: Placebo-controlled trials with buproprion. J. Clin. Psychiatry, in press, 1982.

References for Chapter 29

Tricyclic Antidepressant Plasma Levels, Pharmacokinetics, and Clinical Outcome

Alexanderson B.: Pharmacokinetics of desmethylimipramine and nortriptyline in man after single and multiple oral doses—a cross-over study. Eur. J. Clin. Pharmacol. 5:1–10, 1972.

American Psychiatric Association: Diagnostic and Statistical Manual of Mental Disorders, 3rd ed. Washington, D.C., American Psychiatric Association, 1980.

Amsterdam J., Brunswick D., Mendels J.: The clinical application of tricyclic antidepressant pharmacokinetics and plasma levels. Am. J. Psychiatry 137:653–662, 1980.

Bailey D.N., Jatlow P.I.: Gas chromatographic analysis for therapeutic concentration of imipramine and desipramine in plasma with use of a nitrogen detector. Clin. Chem. 22:1697–1701, 1976.

Bertilsson L., Braithwaite R., Tybring R., et al.: Techniques for plasma protein binding of demethylchlorimipramine. Clin. Pharmacol. Ther. 26:265–271, 1979.

Biggs J.T., Ziegler V.E.: Protriptyline plasma levels and antidepressant response. Clin. Pharmacol. Ther. 22:269–273, 1977.

Braithwaite R., Dawling S., Montgomery S.A.: Prediction of steady-state plasma concentrations and individual dosage regimens of tricyclic antidepressants from a single test dose. Ther. Drug. Monit. 4:27–31, 1982.

Braithwaite R., Montgomery S.A., Dawling S.: Nortriptyline in depressed patients with high plasma level II. Clin. Pharmacol. Ther. 23:303–308, 1978.

Brunswick D.J., Amsterdam J.D., Mendels J., et al.: Prediction of steady-state imipramine and desmethylimipramine plasma concentrations from single-dose data. Clin. Pharmacol. Ther. 25:605–610, 1979.

Brunswick D.J., Mendels J.: Reduced levels of tricyclic antidepressants in plasma from vacutainers. Commun. Psychopharmacol. 1:131–134, 1977.

Ciraulo D.A., Alderson L. M., Chapron D.J., et al.: Imipramine disposition in alcoholics. J. Clin. Psychopharmacol. 2:2–7, 1982.

Cooper T.B., Simpson G.M.: Prediction of individual dosage of nortriptyline. Am. J. Psychiatry 135:333–335, 1978.

Coppen A., Ghose K., Montgomery S.A., et al.: Amitriptyline plasma-concentration and clinical effect. World Health Organization Collaborative Study. Lancet 1:63–66, 1978.

Dawling S., Crome P., Braithwaite R.: Pharmacokinetics of single oral doses of nortriptyline in depressed elderly hospital patients and young healthy volunteers. Clin. Pharmacokinet. 5:399–401, 1980.

DeVane C.L.: Tricyclic antidepressants, in Applied Pharmacokinetics. Edited by Evans W.E., Schentag J.J., Jusko W. J. San Francisco, Applied Therapeutics, Inc., 1980.

DeVane C.L., Jusko W.J.: Plasma concentration monitoring of hydroxylated metabolites of imipramine and desipramine. Drug Intell. Clin. Pharm. 15:263–266, 1981.

DeVane C.L., Wolin R.E., Rovere R.A., et al.: Excessive plasma concentrations of tricyclic antidepressants resulting from usual doses: a report of six cases. J. Clin. Psychiatry 42:143–147, 1981.

Friedel R.O., Raskind M.A.: Relationship of blood levels of sinequan to clinical effects in the treatment of depression in aged patients, in Sinequan (Doxepine HCl), A Monograph of Recent Clinical Studies, Exerpta Medica, 1975.

Friedel R.O., Veith R.C., Bloom V., et al.: Desipramine plasma levels and clinical response in depressed outpatients. Commun. Psychopharmacol. 3:81–87, 1979.

Geller B., Perel J.M., Knitter E.F., et al.: Nortriptyline in major depressive disorder in children. Presented at the NIMH, New and Clinical Drug Evaluation Unit Annual Meeting. Key Biscayne, FL, June 1982b.

Geller B., Perel J.M., Knitter E.F., et al.: Pilot study of nortriptyline in major depressive illness in children aged 6–11, with monitoring of plasma levels and prediction of steady-state plasma levels from 48-hour single dose kinetics. Read at the Annual Meeting of the American Academy of Child Psychiatry, 1982a.

Giardina E.G., Bigger J.T., Glassman A.H., et al.: Cardiovascular effects of tricyclic antidepressants. Primary Cardiol. 7:132–144, 1981.

Glassman A.H., Perel J.M.: Tricyclic blood levels and clinical outcome: a review of the art, in Psychopharmacology: A Generation of Progress. Edited by Lipton M., DiMascio A., Killiam K.F. New York, Raven Press, 1978.

Glassman A.H., Hurwic M.J., Perel J.M.: Plasma binding of imipramine and clinical outcome. Am. J. Psychiatry 130:1367–1369, 1973.

Glassman A.H., Perel J.M., Shostak M., et al: Clinical implications of imipramine plasma levels for depressive illness. Arch. Gen. Psychiatry 34:197–204, 1977.

Gram L.F.: Pharmacokinetics and clinical response to tricyclic antidepressants. Acta Psychiatr. Scand. Suppl. 280, 61:169–180, 1980.

Gram L.F., Christiansen J.: First-pass metabolism of imipramine in man. Clin. Pharmacol. Ther. 17:555–563, 1975.

Gram L.F., Fredrickson-Overø K.: First-pass metabolism of nortriptyline in man. Clin. Pharmacol. Ther. 18:305–413, 1975.

Gram L.F., Pedersen O. L., Kristensen C. B., et al.: Drug level monitoring in psychopharmacology: usefulness and clinical problems, with special reference to tricyclic antidepressants. Ther. Drug Monit. 4:17–25, 1982.

Greenblatt D.J., Koch-Weser J.: Clinical pharmacokinetics. New Engl. J. Med. 293:702–705 and 964–970, 1975.

Hicks R., Dysken M. W., Davis J. M., et al.: The pharmacokinetics of psychotropic medication in the elderly: a review. J. Clin. Psychiatry 42:374–385, 1981.

Hrdina P.D., LaPierre Y.D.: Clinical response, plasma levels and pharmacokinetics of desipramine in depressed inpatients. Prog. Neuropsychopharmacol. 4:591–600, 1981.

Hrdina P.D., Hutchinson L.J., LaPierre Y.D., et al.: Pharmacokinetics of psychotropics: what can it tell us? Prog. Neuropsychopharmacol., in press, 1982.

Jandhyala B.S., Steenberg M.L., Perel J.M., et al.: Effects of several tricyclic antidepressants on the hemodynamics and myocardial contractility of anestheticzed dogs. Eur. J. Pharmacol. 42:403–410, 1977.

Javaid J.L., Perel J.M., Davis J.M.: Inhibition of biogenic amine uptake by imipramine, desipramine, 2-OH-imipramine and 2-OH-desipramine in rat brain. Life Sci. 24:21–28, 1979.

Kitanaka I., Ross R., Cutler N., et al.: Altered hydroxy-desipramine concentrations in elderly depressed patients. Clin. Pharmacol. Ther. 31:51–55, 1982.

Kline N.S., Cooper T.B., Johnson B.: Doxepin and desmethyldoxepin serum levels and clinical response, in Pharmacokinetics of Psychoactive Drugs—Blood Levels and Clinical Response. Edited by Gottschalk L.A., Merlis S. New York, John Wiley and Sons, 1976.

Kragh-Sorensen P.: The use of clinical kinetic data in treatment with antidepressant drugs. Acta Psychiatr. Scand. Suppl. 280, 61:157–166, 1980.

Kragh-Sorensen P., Larsen N.E.: Factors influencing nortriptyline steady-state kinetics: plasma and saliva levels. Clin. Pharmacol. Ther. 28:796–803, 1980.

Kuhn R.: Über die Behandlung depressiver Zustände mit einem Iminodibenzylderivat (G22355). Schweizer Medizinische Wochenschrift. Journal Suisse de Médecine 87:1135–1140, 1957.

Kupfer D.J., Hanin I., Spiker D.G., et al.: Amitriptyline plasma levels and clinical response in primary depression. Clin. Pharmacol. Ther. 22:904–911, 1977.

Mellstrom B., Bertilsson L., Traskman L., et al.: Intraindividual similarity in the metabolism of amitriptyline and chlorimipramine in depressed patients. Pharmacology 19:282–287, 1979.

Montgomery S.A., McAuley R., Montgomery D.B., et al.: Dosage adjustment from simple nortriptyline spot level predictor tests in depressed patients. Clin. Pharmacokinet. 4:129–136, 1979.

Nelson J.C., Jatlow P.: Desipramine plasma concentration and antidepressant response. Arch. Gen. Psychiatry 39:1419–1422, 1982.

Nies A.S., Shand D.G., Wilkinson G.R.: Altered hepatic blood flow and drug disposition. Clin. Pharmacokinet. 1:135–155, 1976.

Olivier-Martin R., Marzin D., Buschenschutz E., et al.: Concentrations plasmatiques de l'imipramine et de la desmethylimipramine et effet anti-dépresseur au cours d'un traitement contrôlé. Psychopharmacologie 41:187–196, 1975.

Perel J.M., Irani F., Hurwic M., et al.: Tricyclic antidepressants: relationships among pharmacokinetics, metabolism and clinical outcome, in Depressive Disorders. Edited by Garrattini S., Lindenlaub E. Stuttgart-New York, F.K. Schattauer Verlag, 1978a.

Perel J.M., Shostak M., Gann E., et al.: Pharmacodynamics of imipramine and clinical outcome in depressed patients, in Pharmacokinetics of Psychoactive Drugs: Blood Levels and Clinical Response. Edited by Gottschalk L.A., Merlis S. New York, John Wiley and Sons, 1976.

Perel J.M., Stiller R.L., Glassman A.H.: Studies on Plasma level/effect relationships in imipramine therapy. Commun. Psychopharmacol. 2:429–439, 1978b.

Perel J.M., Stiller R.L., Lin F.C., et al.: Effect of blood collection systems on the analysis of neuroleptic drugs. Abstract, Clin. Chem. 27:1102–1103, 1981.

Piafsky K.M., Borga O.: Plasma protein binding of basic drugs II. Importance of α_1-acid glycoprotein for individual variation. Clin. Pharmacol. Ther. 22:545–549, 1977.

Piafsky K.M., Borga O., Odar-Cederlof I., et al.: Increased plasma protein binding of propanolol and chlorpromazine mediated by disease-induced elevations of plasma α_1-acid glycoprotein. New Engl. J. Med. 299:1435–1439, 1978.

Pike E., Skuterud B.: Plasma binding variations of amitriptyline and nortriptyline. Clin. Pharmacol. Ther. 32:228–234, 1982.

Potter W.Z., Calil H.M., Manian A.A., et al.: Hydroxylated metabolites of tricyclic antidepressants: preclinical assessment of activity. Biol. Psychiatry 14:601–613, 1979.

Potter W.Z., Zavadil A.P., Kopin I. J., et al.: Single-dose kinetics predict steady-state concentrations of imipramine and desipramine. Arch. Gen. Psychiatry 37:314–320, 1980.

Puig-Antich J., Perel J.M., Lupatkin W., et al.: Imipramine effectiveness in prepubertal major depressive disorders. I. Relationship of plasma levels to clinical response of the depressive syndrome. Arch. Gen. Psychiatry, in press, 1983.

Puig-Antich J., Perel J.M., Lupatkin W., et al.: Plasma levels of imipramine and desmethylimipramine in clinical response to prepubertal major depressive disorder J. Am. Acad. Child Psychiatry 18:616–627, 1979.

Reisby N., Gram L.F., Bech P., et al.: Imipramine: clinical effects and pharmacokinetic variability. Psychopharmacology 54:263–272, 1977.

Robinson D.S., Cooper T.B., Rovaris C.L., et al.: Plasma tricyclic drug levels in amitriptyline-treated depressed patients. Psychopharmacology 63:223–231, 1979.

Rowland M.: Drug administration and regimens, in Clinical Pharmacology, 2nd ed. Edited by Melman K.L., Morelli H.F. New York, MacMillan Publishing Co., 1978.

Rowland M., Tozer T.N.: Clinical Pharmacokinetics: Principles and Applications. Philadelphia, Lea & Febiger, 1980.

Scoggins B.A., Maguirre K.P., Norman T.R., et al.: Measurements of tricyclic antidepressants. Part I: a review of methodology. Part II: applications of methodology. Clin. Chem. 26:5–17 and 805–815, 1980.

Sheiner L.B., Tozer T.N.: Clinical pharmacokinetics: the use of plasma concentrations of drugs, in Clinical Pharmacology, 2nd ed. Edited by Melman K.L., Morelli, H.F. New York, MacMillan Publishing Co., 1978.

Simpson G.M., White K.L., Boyd J.L., et al.: Relationship between plasma antidepressant levels and clinical outcome for inpatients receiving imipramine. Am. J. Psychiatry 139:358–369, 1982.

Slattery J.T., Gibaldi M, Koup J.R.: Prediction of maintenance dose required to attain a desired drug concentration at steady-state from a single determination of concentrations after an initial dose. Clin. Pharmacokinet. 5:377–385, 1980.

Sjoqvist F.: A pharmacokinetic approach to the treatment of depression. Int. Pharamacopsychiatry 6:147–169, 1971.

Sorensen B., Kragh-Sorensen P., Larsen N.E., et al., The practical significance of nortriptyline plasma control. A prospective evaluation under routine conditions in endogenous depression. Psychopharmacology 59:35–39, 1978.

Stiller R.L., Perel J.M., Lin F.C., et al.: A comparative study of serum plasma for tricyclic antidepressant drugs. Clin. Chem. 26:1000–1002, 1980.

Thayssen P., Bjerre M., Kragh-Sorensen P., et al., Cardiovascular effects of imipramine and nortriptyline in elderly patients. Psychopharmacology 74:360–364, 1981.

Unadkat J.D., Rowland M.: Further considerations of the single-point, single-dose method to estimate individual maintenance dosage requirements. Ther. Drug Monit. 4:201–208, 1982.

Veith R.C., Raisys V.A., Perera C.: The clinical impact of blood collection methods on tricyclic antidepressants as measured by GC/MS-SIM. Commun. Psychopharmacol. 2:491–494, 1978,

Vohra J., Burrows G.D., Hunt D., et al.: The effect of toxic and therapeutic doses of tricyclic antidepressant drug on intracardiac conduction. Eur. J. Cardiol. 3:219–227, 1975a.

Vohra J., Burrows G.D., Sloman G.: Assessment of cardiovascular side effects in therapeutic doses of tricyclic anti-depressant drugs. Aust. NZ J. Med. 5:7–11, 1975b.

Ward N.G., Bloom V.L., Wilson L., et al.: Doxepin plasma levels and therapeutic response in depression: preliminary findings. J. Clin. Psychopharmacol. 2:126–128, 1982.

Whyte S.F., MacDonald A.J., Naylor G.L., et al.: Plasma concentrations of protriptyline and clinical effects in depressed women. Br. J. Psychiatry 128:384–390, 1976.

Wilkinson G.R., Shand D.A.: A physiologic approach to hepatic drug clearance. Clin. Pharmacol. Ther. 18:377–390, 1975.

Ziegler V.E., Biggs J.T., Wylie L.T., et al.: Doxepin kinetics. Clin. Pharmacol. Ther. 23:573–579, 1978b.

Ziegler V.E., Biggs J.T., Wylie L.T., et al.: Protriptyline kinetics. Clin. Pharmacol. Ther. 25:580–584, 1978a.

Ziegler V.E., Co B.T., Taylor J.R., et al.: Amitriptyline plasma levels and therapeutic response. Clin. Pharmacol. Ther. 19:795–801, 1976.

References for Chapter 30

Psychotherapies for Depression

Adler A.: Understanding Human Nature. New York, Greenberg, 1927.

American Psychiatric Association: Diagnostic and Statistical Manual of Mental Disorders, 3rd ed. Washington, D.C., American Psychiatric Association, 1980.

Arieti S., Bemporad J.: Severe and Mild Depression: The Psychotherapeutic Approach. New York, Basic Books, 1978.

Beck A.T.: Depression: Causes and Treatment. Philadelphia, University of Pennsylvania Press, 1972.

Beck A.T., Rush A.J., Shaw B.F., et al.: Cognitive Therapy of Depression. New York, Guilford Press, 1979.

Bibring E.: The mechanism of depression, in Affective Disorders. Edited by Greenacre P. New York, International Universities Press, 1953.

Bowlby J.: Grief and mourning in infancy and early childhood. Psychoanal. Study Child 15:9–52, 1960.

Burton R.: The Anatomy of Melancholy (1628). Edited by Jackson H. New York, Vintage Books, 1977.

Essman W. B., Valzelli L. (eds.): Current Developments in Psychopharmacology. New York, SP Medical & Scientific Books, 1979.

Feighner J.P., Robins E., Guze S.B., et al.: Diagnostic criteria for use in psychiatric research. Arch. Gen. Psychiatry 26:57–63, 1972.

Ferster C.B.: A functional analysis of depression. Am. Psychol. 28:857–870, 1973.

Fuchs C.Z., Rehm L.P.: A self-control behavior therapy program for depression. J. Consult Clin. Psychol. 45:206–215, 1977.

Gaylin W. (ed.): Psychoanalytic Contributions to the Understanding of Depression. New York, Science House, 1968.

Green E.J.: The Learning Process and Programmed Instruction. New York, Holt, Rinehart & Winston, 1962.

Horney K.: Neurosis and Human Growth. The Struggle Toward Self-realization. New York, W.W. Norton & Co., 1950.

Kazdin A.E.: History of Behavior Modification: Experimental Foundation of Contemporary Research. Baltimore, University Park Press, 1978.

Keller M.B., Shapiro R.W.: Double depression: Superimposition of acute depressive episodes on chronic depressive disorders. Am. J. Psychiatry 139:438–442, 1982.

Kelly G.A.: The Psychology of Personal Constructs. New York, W.W. Norton & Co., 1955.

Klerman G.L., DiMascio A., Weissman M.M., et al., Treatment of depression by drugs and psychotherapy. Am. J. Psychiatry 131:186–191, 1974.

Klerman G.L., Rounsaville B., Chevron E., et al., Manual for Short-Term Interpersonal Psychotherapy (IPT) of Depression. Unpublished manuscript, 1979.

Klerman G.L., Weissman M.M.: Interpersonal psychotherapy: theory and research, in Short-Term Psychotherapies for Depression. Edited by Rush A.J. New York, Guilford Press, 1982.

Kovacs M.: Cognitive therapy in depression. J. Am. Acad. Psychoanal. 8:127–144, 1980a.

Kovacs M.: The efficacy of cognitive and behavior therapies for depression. Am. J. Psychiatry 137:1495–1501, 1980b.

Kovacs M., Beck A.T.: Cognitive-affective processes in depression, in Emotions in Personality and Psychopathology. Edited by Izard C.E. New York, Plenum Press, 1979.

Kovacs M., Beck A.T.: Maladaptive cognitive structures in depression. Am. J. Psychiatry 135:525–533, 1978.

Kovacs M., Rush A.J., Beck A.T., et al: Depressed outpatients treated with cognitive therapy or pharmacotherapy. A one-year follow-up. Arch. Gen. Psychiatry 38:33–39, 1981.

Kraepelin E.: Manic-Depressive Insanity and Paranoia. Translated by Barclay R.M. Edited by Robertson G.M. Edinburgh, E. & S. Livingstone, 1921.

Lewinsohn P.M., Sullivan J.M., Grosscup S.J.: Behavioral therapy: clinical applications, in Short-Term Psychotherapies for Depression. Edited by Rush A.J. New York, Guilford Press, 1982.

Mahoney M.J.: Reflections on the cognitive-learning trend in psychotherapy. Am. Psychol. 32:5–13, 1977.

Malan D.H.: Individual Psychotherapy and the Science of Psychodynamics. London, Butterworth, 1979.

McLean P.D.: Behavioral therapy: theory and research, in Short-term Psychotherapies for Depression. Edited by Rush A.J. New York, Guilford Press, 1982.

McLean P.D., Hakstian A.R.: Clinical depression: comparative efficacy of outpatient treatments. J. Consult. Clin. Psycho. 47:818–836, 1979.

Mendels J., Amsterdam J.D. (eds.): The Psychobiology of Affective Disorders. New York, S. Karger, 1980.

Morris J.B., Beck A.T.: The efficacy of antidepressant drugs: a review of research (1958 to 1972). Arch. Gen. Psychiatry 30:667–674, 1974.

Parloff M.B.: Shopping for the right therapy. Saturday Review 3:14–20, February 21, 1976.

Rehm L.P.: A self-control model of depression. Behav. Ther. 8:787–804, 1977.

Rehm L.P., Fuchs C.Z., Roth D.M., et al.: A comparison of self-control and social skills treatments of depression. Behav. Ther. 10:429–442, 1979.

Rehm L.P., Kornblith S.J.: Behavior therapy for depression: a review of recent developments, in Progress in Behavior Modification, vol 7. Edited by Hersen M., Eisler R.M, Miller P.M. New York, Academic Press, 1979.

Rounsaville B.J., Chevron E.: Interpersonal psychotherapy: clinical applications, in Short-Term Psychotherapies for Depression. Edited by Rush A.J. New York, Guilford Press, 1982.

Rush A.J.: Diagnosing depressions, in Short-Term Psychotherapies for Depression. Edited by Rush A.J. New York, Guilford Press, 1982.

Rush A.J., Beck A.T., Kovacs M., et al.: Comparative efficacy of cognitive therapy and pharmacotherapy in the treatment of depressed outpatients. Cog. Ther. Res. 1:17–37, 1977.

Rush A.J., Beck A.T., Kovacs M., et al.: Comparison of the effects of cognitive therapy and pharmacotherapy on hopelessness and self-concept. Am. J. Psychiatry 139:862–866, 1982.

Ryle A.: The focus in brief psychotherapy: a cross-fertilization between research and practice, in Short-Term Psychotherapies for Depression. Edited by Rush A.J. New York, Guilford Press, 1982.

Secunda S.K., Katz M.M., Friedman R.J., et al.: The Depressive Disorders, DHEW Publication 73–9157. Washington, D.C., U.S. Government Printing Office, 1973.

Shaw B.F.: Comparison of cognitive therapy and behavior therapy in the treatment of depression. J. Consult. Clin. Psychol. 45:543–551, 1977.

Sifneos P.E.: Short-Term Psychotherapy: Evaluation and Technique. New York, Plenum Press, 1979.

Spitzer R.L., Endicott J.: Schedule for Affective Disorders and Schizophrenia—Life-Time Version (SADS-L), 3rd ed. New York, New York State Psychiatric Institute, Biometrics Research, 1977.

Spitzer R.L., Endicott J., Robins E.: Research diagnostic criteria. Rationale and reliability. Arch. Gen. Psychiatry 35:773–782, 1978.

Strupp H.H.: Psychotherapy research and practice: an overview, in Handbook of Psychotherapy and Behavior Changes: An Empirical Analysis, 2nd ed. Edited by Garfield S.L., Bergin A.E. New York, John Wiley & Sons, 1978.

Strupp H.H., Sandell J.A., Waterhouse G.J., et al. Psycho-dynamic therapy: theory and research, in Short-Term Psychotherapies for Depression. Edited by Rush A.J. New York, Guilford Press, 1982.

Sullivan H.S.: The Interpersonal Theory of Psychiatry. New York, W.W. Norton & Co., 1953.

Thomas D.W.: Documents from Old Testament Times. New York, Harper & Row, 1958.

Weissman M.M., Kasl S.V., Klerman G.L.: Follow-up of depressed women after maintenance treatment. Am. J. Psychiatry 133:757–760, 1976.

Weissman M.M., Prusoff B.A., DiMascio A., et al.: The efficacy of drugs and psychotherapy in the treatment of acute depressive episodes. Am. J. Psychiatry 136:555–558, 1979.

Young J.E., Beck A.T.: Cognitive therapy: clinical applications, in Short-Term Psychotherapies for Depression. Edited by Rush A.J. New York, Guilford Press, 1982.

Zaiden J.: Psychodynamic therapy: clinical approaches, in Short-Term Psychotherapies for Depression. Edited by Rush A.J. New York, Guilford Press, 1982.

Zilboorg G.: A History of Medical Psychology. New York, W.W. Norton & Co., 1941.

Index

and self-perception (changes in), **83:**216
and sex therapy, **82:**25
and sleep, *see* Sleep disorders
and suicide, **83:**433
and tardive dyskinesia, **82:**147
See also Aging
Age Discrimination Act in Employment (1967), **83:**106
Aggression: erotized and nonerotized, **82:**30–32
mob manifestation of, **83:**22, 23, 24–25
narcissism and, **82:**511, 513, 514–16
pregenital and oral, **82:**473
primary and secondary, **82:**31
Aging: and adjustment to retirement, **83:**106
biologic changes and theories of, **83:**97–100
cross-linkage or eversion theory, **83:**98–99
and epidemiology of psychiatric disorder, **83:**87–93
physiological changes in, **83:**99, 113, 140–51 (*see also* Metabolism)
psychosocial theories of and approaches to, **83:**105–06
primary and secondary, **83:**96
and sexuality, **82:**7, 8, 42, 45–47; **83:**147–51
societies and agencies concerned with, **83:**84–86
as term, **83:**96
See also Age; Late-life psychiatric disorders
Agnoli, A., et al., **82:**200
Agoraphobia, **82:**440, 457, 468; **83:**443
drug therapy for, **82:**465, 467; **83:**483, 488
See also Panic disorders
Ahlfors, U. G., et al., **83:**310, 311
Akiskal, Hagop S., **82:**436, 437, 442, 443; **83:**270–84 passim, 288–90 passim, 442; et al., **82:**440–41, 444, 453, 454; **83:**271–92 passim, 374, 375
A. K. Rice Group Relations Conferences, **83:**32
Albert, N., **82:**282
Albrecht, P., et al., **82:**121
Alcohol, Drug Abuse, and Mental Administration, U.S., **83:**406n, 409
Alcoholism: alcoholic hallucinosis (distinguished from schizophrenia), **83:**289, 290
in bipolar illness, **83:**279, 281, 282, 286, 320, 442, 453
borderline disorders and, **82:**438, 441, 442, 454
and depression, **83:**365, 373–81 passim, 420, 422, 432
the family and, **83:**178
family therapy for, **83:**189
and Korsakoff's syndrome, **83:**115
late-life, **83:**94, 109, 115
MAO activity decrease in, **82:**126; **83:**452
as "mental illness" or disease, **82:**337; **83:**286, 442
morbidity risk for, **82:**290
police and, **82:**385
studies of, **83:**174
and suicide, **83:**429, 430, 431, 432
Aldrich, R. F., **82:**332
Alexander, A. A., et al., **83:**139
Alexander, F., **83:**55
Alexander, G. J., **82:**351
Alexander, J. F., **83:**190
Alexander, P. E., et al., **82:**210

Alexanderson, B., **83:**499
Alfredsson, G., et al., **82:**200
Alfrey, A. C., et al., **83:**111
Alignment with potential states of being: mother-infant relationships and, **83:**20–21. *See also* Empathy; Mother-child relationship
Allen, Edward B., Award, **83:**85
Allen, Frederick, **82:**264
Allergies: decreased prevalence of, **82:**118. *See also* Immune system
Althusser, L., **83:**34
Altman, J. H., **83:**387, 389, 392
Altruism, pathological: and sexual dysfunction, **82:**30
Aluminum concentration: and Alzheimer's disease, **83:**101, 111
Alzheimer's disease, *see* Dementia, Primary Degenerative
Amarasingham, L. R., **83:**173
Ambelas, A., **83:**277
American Association of Sex Educators, Counselors and Therapists (AASECT), **82:**7
American Board of Medical Specialties, **83:**86
American Board of Psychiatry and Neurology, **83:**86
American Geriatrics Society, **83:**85
American Law Institute (ALI) Rule, **82:**391, 392
American Law Reports, **82:**328
American Medical Association, **82:**7, 329
American Psychiatric Association (APA), **82:**425, 449
cited, **82:**143, 209, 339nn16, 18, 450; **83:**84, 89, 90, 106–08 passim, 118–20 passim, 131, 140, 272, 277, 290–94 passim, 357, 367–70 passim, 408, 479, 492, 512, 528 (*see also* DSM-III)
and confidentiality issue, **82:**330, 331–32, 334
Council(s)
on Aging, **83:**84
on Government Policy and the Law, **82:**326
on Research, **83:**85
and criterion of dangerousness, **82:**339
and legislation, **82:**323, 330
Principles of Medical Ethics, **82:**329
Task Force(s)
on geriatric psychiatry, aging, dying, **83:**85
on psychiatric participation in sentencing, **82:**395
on Vitamin Therapy, **82:**143
Amish population: affective disorders among, **83:**271, 448
Amkraut, A., et al., **82:**115
Amnesia: as criterion for incompetence, **82:**388
infantile, **83:**17–18
late-life, **83:**109
amnestic syndrome, **83:**115
secondary, in manic psychosis, **83:**328
See also Memory
Amphetamine, **82:**131, 132, 462; **83:**127, 480, 483
affective disorders produced by, **83:**365, 374, 379, 461, 484
and paranoid psychosis, **82:**137, 138, 197; **83:**290
-PEA model of schizophrenia, **82:**137, 148, 152
stereotyped behavior induced by, **82:**137, 144

classification of/criteria for, **83**:119, 271–75 passim, 295, 296, 354, 367, 368, 371, 410, 423, 427

definition of, **83**:422–23

dementia praecox separated from, **82**:82; **83**:269

depressive phase, **83**:126, 279–80, 328, 332, 367, 386, 420 (*see also* Depression)

diagnosis of, **83**:122, 271, 278–79, 407, 410
  childhood, **83**:283
  differential, **83**:125, 285, 287–90, 293, 295, 465–66
  DST in, *see* DST (dexamethasone suppression test)
  and misdiagnosis, **83**:280, 281, 284

drug therapy for, *see* Bipolar (manic-depressive) Disorder, treatment of, *below*; Lithium therapy

epidemiology/prevalence rate of, **83**:270–71, 275, 283, 407, 415, 420–27 passim, 435, 439, 447, 455

etiology of, **83**:249, 285, 319, 320

and the family (impact on), **83**:249, 279, 302, 305, 329

family therapy for, **83**:249–52

genetics/family history and, **82**:265; **83**:271–78 passim, 282–83, 287, 289, 329, 427, 435–57

Kraepelin's concept of, *see* Kraepelin, Emil

late-life, **83**:125–26, 285

manic state, *see* Manic state (bipolar I)

MAO activity in, **83**:467–68

mixed states in, **83**:280–81, 367

mood changes and discrimination in, **83**:281, 286, 326–30 passim, 334, 374

personality and, **83**:384, 386–92, 426

prevention of, **83**:454–57

prognosis for, **83**:250–51, 282
  recurrence and fears of, **83**:285, 304, 305–07, 311–16 passim, 327–35 passim, 425

psychoanalytic view of (pre-lithium), **83**:319

rapid-cycling, **83**:303, 312, 318

related to borderline disorders, **82**:439, 442, 448, 454

risk factors in, **83**:423, 438–45 passim, 454–56 (*see also* genetics/family history and, *above*)

social implications of, **83**:285–86, 297, 303, 320, 331, 423

subgroups of, **83**:367, 410, 439

and suicide, **83**:286–87, 320, 329, 330, 334, 429, 430

symptoms of, **83**:280, 281–82, 320

unipolar compared to/distinguished from/related to, *see* Unipolar/nonbipolar depression

urinary MHPG and VMA levels in, **83**:272–73, 460–66, 468–69

validation of typology of, **83**:282–83

See also Cyclothymic Disorder; Dysthymic Disorder; Major Depression; Schizoaffective Disorder

Bipolar (manic-depressive) Disorder, treatment of:
  drug therapy, **83**:250, 276, 303–18, 368
  compliance/noncompliance with, **83**:251, 301, 315–18 passim, 321–37 passim
  conditions requiring, **83**:305–07
  dosage, **83**:126, 316–17
  duration of, **83**:315
  family approach to, **83**:249–52, 305
  imipramine/TCA, **83**:307, 311, 312, 371, 380, 480
  lithium, *see* Lithium therapy
  long-term vs. continuation, **83**:304
  other drugs, **83**:126, 312, 318, 370
  psychotherapy combined with, **83**:316, 320–37
  UCLA-Columbia study of, **83**:322, 332–37 passim

ECT, **83**:126, 302

family or marital therapy, **83**:189, 249–52

hospitalization, **83**:125, 249, 275, 293–97 passim, 303, 306, 318, 320, 326, 330, 334, 423, 424, 438, 439

outpatient, **83**:271, 297–98, 303, 326

psychoanalysis, **83**:319–20, 329

psychotherapeutic issues in, **83**:319–37

Bipolar self, *see* Self

Bird, E. D., **82**:138; et al., **82**:132, 133

Birkett, D. P., **83**:114

Birleson, P., **82**:287

Birley, J. L. T., **82**:102, 172; **83**:174, 242

Birnbaum, Morton, **82**:361–62

Birren, J. E., **83**:108

Birtchnell, J., **83**:431

Birth control, **82**:7

Bisexuality, **82**:55. *See also* Sexuality

Bishop, M. P., **82**:180, 181, 184

Black, A. L., **83**:114

Blackburn, I. M., **83**:279, 387, 389

Blacks: bipolar illness among, **83**:270, 290, 426
  depressive symptoms among, **83**:413, 420
  in elderly population, **83**:88
  schizophrenia among, **82**:102; **83**:270, 290

Blackwell, B., **83**:304

Blanchard, M., **83**:277

Bland, R. C., **82**:100

Blath, R. A., et al., **83**:432

Blazer, Dan G., **83**:87, 90–95 passim, 132

Bleuler, Eugen P., **82**:82–88 passim, 112–13, 149, 166, 197, 444; **83**:289, 357–58, 359

Bleuler, M., **82**:88, 161

Bloch, Donald A., **83**:171, 172

Blombery, P. A., et al., **83**:461

Blood glucose levels, **82**:293

Blood pressure: antidepressant effect on, **82**:291–92; **83**:469, 477–78, 484–85
  during orgasm, **82**:12
  penile, **82**:46
  See also Drug side effect(s); Hypertension

Blood type O, **83**:450

Bloom, L., **83**:20

Blum, H. P., **83**:44, 46, 62

Blum, J. E., **83**:129

Blumenthal, M. D., **83**:123, 412, 413

Bohannon, P., **83**:227

Boklage, C., **82**:124

Bolen, D. W., **83**:189

Bond, P. A., et al., **83:**461
Bondareff, W., et al., **83:**110, 117
Böök, J. A., et al., **82:**126, 127
Bookhammer, R. S., **82:**158; et al., **82:**217–18
Borderline Personality Disorder, **82:**491
  characteristics of, **82:**417, 452–54, 464–66, 468, 512–13
    vs. institutionalization symptoms, **82:**456
    MBD, **82:**441–42, 454
    in psychotherapeutic situation, **82:**472–76
    transference patterns, **82:**489 (*see also* Transference)
  coexistence of, with other disorders, **82:**466
  as definable/discrete syndrome, **82:**416, 417, 424, 425, 433–37 passim, 454, 455, 456
  epidemiology/prevalence rate of, **82:**415, 455
  etiology of, **82:**438, 452–56
  and gender disturbance, **82:**48, 52, 56
  genetic factors in, **82:**437–56
    biologic markers, **82:**452–56
  morbidity in, **82:**416
  prognosis for, **82:**486–87
  and psychosexual dysfunctions, **82:**19
  regression in, **82:**473
  schizophrenia compared to/discriminated from/related to, **82:**416, 436, 439–43 passim, 444–57 passim
  treatment of
    drug therapy, **82:**444, 456–67, 469–70, 484; **83:**480
    and effect on nursing staff, **83:**28–29
    goals of, **82:**482–83, 485
    hospital, **82:**424, 450, 470–74 passim, 482
    problems in, **82:**415
    psychoanalytic, **82:**471
    psychotherapeutic, **82:**425, 467, 470–87
Borderline Personality Disorder, diagnosis of, **82:**465
  in adoptive studies, **82:**446–48
  criteria for, **82:**424–28, 436, 441, 443, 444, 457
    Borderline Personality Scale (BPS) II, **82:**431–34 passim
    Diagnostic Interview for Borderlines (DIB), **82:**417, 423, 424, 428–35 passim, 439–40, 456, 466
    DMS-III, **82:**428–36 passim, 440–43 passim, 448, 449–51, 454–66 passim, 470; **83:**288
    Gund-R scale, **82:**429, 430
    Research Diagnostic Criteria (RDC), **82:**423, 434
    Schedule for Affective Disorders and Schizophrenia (SADS), **82:**432
    Schedule for Interviewing Borderlines (SIB), **82:**429, 430, 432, 433, 452
    Schedule for Schizotypal Personalities (SSP), **82:**432
    Spitzer et al. (17) Item List, **82:**424–25, 429–34 passim
    Structural Interview (Kernberg), **82:**431, 432, 433, 438, 440, 454
    Symptom Scale for Borderline Schizophrenia, **82:**448
  and cyclothymic personality, **82:**444; **83:**288
  diagnostic schemes compared, **82:**433–35

differential, **83:**288
empirical studies and, **82:**415–37, 448
Borderline Personality Scale, *see* BPS
Borga, O., **83:**495, 497
Borison, R. L., et al., **82:**137
Bornstein, M. H., **83:**12
Borowski, T., **82:**171
Borton, R. W., **83:**12
Boscolo, L., **83:**247
Boston University Center for Law and Health Sciences, **82:**364
Boswell, J., **83:**430
Boszormenyi-Nagy, Ivan, **83:**170, 187, 194, 199, 219, 223, 236
Bowden, C., **83:**274
Bowen, D. M., **83:**109; et al., **83:**109, 110
Bowen, Murray, **83:**170, 194, 222, 223, 234, 235, 242
Bower, G., **83:**16, 17
Bowers, M. B., **82:**133, 140; **83:**480
Bowlby, J., **82:**266, 275; **83:**360, 404, 519
Boyd, Jeffrey H., **83:**270, 355, 406, 406n, 438
Boyd, W. H., **83:**189
BPRS (Brief Psychiatric Rating Scale), **82:**199
BPS (Borderline Personality Scale): I, **82:**432; II, **82:**432–33, 434
Braden, G., et al., **83:**314
Braden, W., et al., **83:**289
Bradley, C., **82:**263
Bradley, J., **83:**144
Bradley, S. J., **82:**434
Brain, the: aging effects on, **83:**99–101
  damage to, as drug side effect, **83:**305
  neurobiology of, **83:**458
  trauma, and borderline disorders, **82:**442
  See also Catecholamines; Neurotransmitters; Protein factors
Brain disorders, *see* Organic brain disorders; Stroke
Braithwaite, R., et al., **83:**495, 499
Branchley, M. H., et al., **83:**114, 137
Branconnier, R., et al., **83:**476
Brandeis, L. D., **82:**328
Brant, R., **82:**57
Bratfos, O., **83:**286, 372
Braunschweig, D., **83:**33
Braverman, E., **82:**144
Brazelton, T. B., **83:**9; et al., **83:**10
Breast, the: cancer of, **82:**40, 202
Brennan, Justice William, **82:**323n5
Brenner, M. H., **82:**100, 103
Breskin Rigidity Test, **83:**336
Bretherton, I., **83:**19
Brethren, The (Woodward and Armstrong), **82:**363
Bridge, T. P., **83:**131, 132, 139; et al., **83:**131
Brief Psychiatric Rating Scale (BPRS), **82:**199
Briley, M. S., et al., **83:**470
Brinkley, J., et al., **82:**457, 460, 464
Brinkman, S. D., et al., **83:**113
British Medical Journal, **83:**114
Brockington, I. F., **82:**102
Brockington, L., et al., **82:**209
Brodie, H. K. H., **83:**100, 286, 456

Brody, J. E., **82:**26
Brogden, R., et al., **83:**490
Bromet, E., **83:**401, 403, 404
Bronx Municipal Hospital Center, **82:**423
Brook, Mary Potter, **83:**170
Brooks, A., **82:**391
Brooks, G. W., **82:**88
Brotman, Judge, **82:**383
Brotman, R. K., et al., **82:**188
Broverman, I. K., et al., **83:**38
Brown, George W., **82:**102, 172; **83:**94, 395, 396, 400–04 passim, 421–22; et al., **82:**88, 109; **83:**94, 174, 242, 244, 385, 394–400 passim, 414, 416
Brown, G. M., **82:**293; et al., **82:**200
Brown, J., **83:**431, 433, 434
Brown, S. L., **83:**230, 236
Brown, W. A., **82:**135, 200, 203
Brown, W. T., **83:**316
Brownmiller, S., **82:**58
Bruch, Hilde, **82:**155
Bruner, J. S., **83:**13
Brunswick, D. J., **83:**501; et al., **83:**500
Bucher, K. D., **83:**446; et al., **83:**446
Buchsbaum, M. S., **82:**453; et al., **82:**125, 452
Bucht, G., **83:**314
Buckman, M. T., **82:**203
Buie, D. H., **82:**480, 496
Bumberry, W., et al., **82:**270
Bunney, W. E., **83:**272, 278, 311, 448, 470; et al., **83:**298, 469
Burger, Chief Justice Warren, **82:**323, 361, 363–64, 373
Burgess, A. W., **82:**61, 62, 63
Burnet, F. M., **83:**111
Burnside, I. M., **83:**114
Burt, R., **82:**387
Burton, N., **82:**266, 267–68
Burton, Richard, **83:**512
Busch, D. A., et al., **82:**200
Busse, Ewald W., **83:**84, 86, 102, 104, 142, 143
Butler, Robert N., **83:**84, 86

C

Cade, J. F., **83:**298, 320, 328
Cadoret, R. J., **83:**440
Caffeinism, **83:**146, 280, 296
Caffey, E. M., **82:**205; **83:**316; et al., **82:**190, 192, 226
Caine, E. D., **83:**119
California Department of Mental Health, **82:**350
Campbell, J. C., **82:**288–89; **83:**279, 283
Canada: depressive disorders diagnosed in, **83:**108
lithium therapy used in, **83:**481
schizophrenia studies in, **82:**98, 145
Canadian Mental Health Association, **82:**143
Cancer: breast, **82:**40, 202
chromosome damage and, **83:**97
depressive patients and, **83:**366

schizophrenic patients and, **82:**115
surgery for, **82:**39, 40
uterine, dangers of, **83:**149
Cancro, R., **82:**83, 95, 153
Canetti, E., **83:**25
Canino, I. A., **83:**283
Canter, A., **83:**285
Cantwell, D. P., **82:**266, 268, 282, 297; et al., **83:**442
Capitalism: sexuality repressed by, **83:**34
Carcinoid syndrome: as drug side effect, **83:**128
Cardiac disorders: as drug side effect, *see* Drug side effect(s)
of elderly patients, **83:**96, 123, 498
and pacemakers, **83:**478
TCAs and, **83:**123, 477–78, 509
See also Heart rate; Physical illness; Vascular disorders
Cardozo, Justice Benjamin, **82:**350
CARE (Comprehensive Assessment and Referral Evaluation), **83:**116
Carlson, G. A., **82:**266, 268, 282, 289, 291, 294, 297; **83:**279, 284, 289, 302, 434; et al., **83:**250
Carlsson, A., **82:**132, 135, 196
Carp, R., **82:**121
Carpenter, G., **83:**10
Carpenter, L., **82:**102
Carpenter, William T., Jr., **82:**85–89 passim, 108, 109, 154–61 passim, 167, 416; **83:**130; et al., **82:**157, 170, 416, 418; **83:**279, 289
Carroll, Bernard J., **83:**283, 289, 355, 452; et al., **82:**290, 436, 452–53; **83:**121, 273, 460, 463
Carroll, P. J., **83:**114
Carskodan, M., et al., **83:**147
Carter, E. A., **83:**216
Casacchia, M., et al., **82:**200
Casey, D. E., et al., **82:**141
Casey, J. F., et al., **82:**209
Casper, R. C., et al., **83:**461
Cassano, G. B., et al., **82:**201
Castelden, C. M., **83:**114
Castration anxiety, *see* Anxiety
CAT (choline acetyltransferase): in Alzheimer's disease, **83:**109–10, 113
Cataracts, *see* Vision
Catatonic stupor or excitement: bipolar illness misdiagnosed as, **83:**280
and competency, **82:**354
Catecholamines, **82:**127, 129, 139, 144, 146, 147
and catecholamine hypothesis of affective disorders, **82:**265; **83:**380, 458–59
Catechol-O-methyltransferase (COMT), **82:**128, 131; **83:**451, 454
heightened levels of, in older males, **83:**133
urinary, **83:**464–67 (*see also* Urinary MHPG levels)
CATEGO (computer diagnosis), *see* Diagnosis
Cation transport parameters, **83:**451, 452–53. *See also* Genetic factors
Cause-effect, *see* Relationships
CDI (Children's Depression Inventory), **82:**270–71
Cebiroglu, R., **82:**291; et al., **82:**282
Cecchin, G., **83:**247

Celiac disease, **82:**145, 146. *See also* Physical illness

Census, U.S. Bureau of the, **83:**88

Central nervous system, *see* CNS

Cerebral atrophy: schizophrenia and, **82:**117, 120, 122, 148

Cerebrospinal fluid, *see* CSF

Cesarec-Marke Personality Scale, **83:**386–87

Chalmers, R. J., **82:**204

Chambers, W., et al., **82:**270

Chandler, M. J., **83:**229, 230

Chang, S. S., **83:**452; et al., **83:**299

Chapanis, Natalia, **82:**49n2

Chapman, C. J., **83:**424, 438, 446

Charalampous, K. D., et al., **82:**180, 182, 184

Charatan, F. B., **83:**114

Charles, E., **82:**423

Charney, D. S., et al., **83:**459, 460, 469

Chasin, R., **83:**186, 230, 238

Chasseguet-Smirgel, J., **83:**23, 24, 25, 35, 36

Cheadle, J., **82:**193

Cheetham, R. W. S., **82:**102

Chell, B., **82:**350

Chemotherapy, *see* Drug therapy

Chevron, E., **83:**519

Chien, C. P., et al., **82:**204

Child abuse, **83:**188, 196, 229
  and child psychosis, **83:**206
  mandatory reporting of, **82:**332
  sexual, **82:**58
  and sexual dysfunction, **82:**28, 31, 32

Childhood: "adjustment disorder" in, **82:**263
  adoption in, *see* Adoption studies
  bipolar illness in, **83:**283, 284
  and child participation in couples therapy, **83:**225
  CT scan use for ailments of, **83:**184
  deprivation during, effects of, **82:**32, 273; **83:**229
  development during, **82:**276; **83:**42
    latent stages of, **82:**277–78
    prediction of, **83:**229
  drug therapy in, **83:**283, 498, 505, 509
  encopresis in, **83:**176–77
  family therapy for disorders of, **82:**265, 307; **83:**171, 188–201 passim, 209, 228–41
  gender differentiation in, **83:**42–43
  gender dysphoria in, **82:**49–51, 53, 55
  and infant mortality, **82:**274
  memories of, Freud's view of, **83:**63
  object relations in, **83:**218
  psychoanalysis in, **83:**55, 192
  punishment for sexual behavior in, **82:**32
  and scapegoating of child, **83:**233–34, 239, 240
  schizophrenia in, **82:**89, 108, 263, 306
  seduction in, **82:**57–58 (*see also* Incest)
  selfobject in structure building in, **82:**501
  studies of disorders of, **83:**174, 176–77
  superego in, **82:**272
  withdrawal during, and later schizophrenia, **82:**89
  See also Adolescent(s); Age; Child abuse; Family, the; Infancy; Mother-child relationship; Parent(s); Parent-child relationship; Separation fears

Childhood depression: adult model for, **82:**26, 269, 270, 289–90
  vs. developmental, **82:**271–72
  definition of, **82:**267–69
  diagnosis of
    biological correlates, **82:**290, 292–95
    as clinical entity, **82:**263–72 passim, 283, 288–90
    criteria (and RDC) for, **82:**270, 288, 289–90, 293, 296–99, 304
    depressed affect and, **82:**269, 297, 305, 306
    differential, **82:**305–07
    failure in, **82:**287
    measurement techniques in, **82:**269–71
  epidemiology/prevalence rate, **82:**267, 281–88, 289
    high risk factors in, **82:**285–88, 290–91
    sociodemographic variables in, **82:**283–85
  etiology of, **82:**274, 275, 280, 285–86, 288
  prevention of, **82:**287–88
  and suicide, **82:**278, 301, 303
  symptoms of, **82:**274–78, 287
    clinical characteristics, **82:**296–305
    cluster of, **82:**268, 296
    as developmental phenomena, **82:**267, 268, 269
    at developmental stages, **82:**280
    masking (depressive equivalents), **82:**268, 272, 297
    and symptom-oriented methods for assessing, **82:**270–71
  treatment of, **82:**278, 287–88, 302, 307
    family therapy, **82:**265, 307
    imipramine/TCA, **82:**290, 291–92, 307; **83:**505, 509

Child psychiatry, **82:**263–65, 289, 305
  drug therapy in, **83:**509
  family therapy in, **82:**265, 307; **83:**228–41

Children's Depression Inventory (CDI), **82:**270–71

Children's Rights Report, **82:**352

Childs, B., **83:**450

China: age of leaders of, **83:**84

Cho, J. T., et al., **83:**303

Chodoff, P., **82:**89; **83:**364, 365, 383, 385–86, 407, 421

Chodorow, N., **83:**40, 41

Choline acetyltransferase, *see* CAT

Cholinergic agents: in dementia, **83:**113

Cholinergic system: Alzheimer's disease and, **83:**110, 111
  and depressive disorders, **83:**463
  drugs and, *see* Drug side effect(s)

Cholinesterase: aging and, **83:**96

Chouinard, G., et al., **83:**488

Christiansen, J., **83:**495

Christie, A. B., **83:**107

Christie, J. E., et al., **83:**113

Chromatography, *see* GC (gas chromatography); HPLC (high performance liquid chromatography)

Chromosome loss or damage, **83:**97, 110. *See also* Genetic factors

Chu, H. M., et al., **83:**139

and growth hormone (GH) levels, **82:**135, 136, 203–04
high-dosage, **82:**183, 187–90
and immunological abnormalities, **82:**117–18, 121
for paraphrenia, **83:**139
and PG (prostaglandin) absorption, **82:**146
psychotherapy vs. or combined with, **82:**156, 157, 160, 168–69, 178, 215, 219–25
(*see also* Lithium therapy; Schizophrenia, treatment of)
CL (total body clearance) of, **83:**113, 492, 499–500
half-life of, **83:**113, 115–16, 476, 492–500 passim, 504, 511
hallucinogens, **82:**130, 139–41; **83:**295
hypnotics, **83:**113, 116, 150, 485
judicial view of use of, **82:**381–82, 383
MAO inhibitors, *see* MAO (monoamine oxidase)
new, **82:**180–96; **83:**485–90
prolactin (PRL) response to, **82:**135–36, 200–203; **83:**487
psychotropic, **82:**175, 215, 359–60, 455; **83:**95, 121, 436, 497
rauwolfias, **83:**369, 379
reaction to, and child psychosis, **82:**306
and REM sleep, **83:**115
sedative or tranquilizing, **83:**121, 476, 480–88 passim, 526
chronic or overuse of, **83:**365, 374
for elderly, **83:**95, 115–16, 126, 141, 146, 150
for manic illness, **83:**281, 301
for schizophrenics, **82:**217
and suicide, **83:**430, 433
sensitivity to, of elderly patients, **83:**96–97, 113, 126, 498
side effects of, *see* Drug side effect(s)
steroids and corticosteroids, **82:**140; **83:**121, 123, 369, 374, 379, 478
with supportive therapy, **82:**484, 485
tricyclics (TCAs), **82:**464–67 passim; **83:**321, 359, 361, 458, 472–97, 503 (*see also* TCA [tricyclic antidepressant] response)
volume of distribution of, **83:**492
See also Drug abuse/addiction; Drugs, list of; Drug therapy; Hormone(s)
Drugs, list of: alprazolam, **83:**472, 474, 485, 488
amitriptyline, **82:**466; **83:**123, 124, 127, 312, 371, 462, 468–96 passim, 524–25
and plasma levels, **83:**500, 505–06, 507
amobarbitol, **82:**462, 464
amoxapine, **83:**124–25, 312, 472, 474, 480, 485, 487, 495
amphetamines, *see* Amphetamine
apomorphine, **82:**134–35, 136, 196, 203, 204
arecoline, **83:**113
benzodiazepines, **82:**139, 461, 464, 465; **83:**121, 141, 146, 479, 480–81, 488 (*see also* individual forms)
bethanecol, **83:**476
bromocriptine, **82:**135, 197
buproprion, **83:**312, 474, 485, 490
butaperazine, **82:**189
butyrophenones, **83:**323

carbamazepine, **83:**303, 307, 311–12, 318
carbidopa, **82:**200; **83:**461
centrophenoxine, **83:**112
chloral hydrate, **83:**115
chlordiazepoxide, **82:**465; **83:**381, 479, 480
chlorimipramine (clomipramine), **83:**480, 500
chlorpromazine (CPZ), **83:**271, 484, 497
in acute mania, **83:**298, 300–301, 302
in borderline disorders, **82:**462, 463, 464
in schizophrenia, **82:**118, 143, 178, 180, 189, 199–200, 201, 208
cimetidine, **83:**123, 475
clozapine, **82:**182, 201
cocaine, **82:**197
cyclandelate, **83:**112
deprenyl, **83:**485
desipramine, **82:**466; **83:**123, 124, 472–80 passim, 486, 487
and plasma levels, **83:**477, 498, 506, 507
prediction of response to, **83:**468, 473, 499–500
dexamethasone, **83:**121, 469 (*see also* DST [dexamethasone suppression test])
diazepam, **82:**461; **83:**115–16, 488
dihydroergotoxine, **83:**112
diphenylhydantoin, **82:**465, 467; **83:**121, 122, 497
domperidone, **82:**200
dopamine, **82:**144; **83:**122 (*see also* DBH)
doxepin, **82:**461; **83:**123, 125, 146, 472–80 passim, 493, 496
and plasma levels, **83:**124, 498, 500, 506, 507
fludrocortisone, **83:**478
fluoxetine, **83:**474, 489–90
flupenthixol decanoate, **83:**307, 311, 318
fluphenazine, **82:**463; **83:**139
in schizophrenia, **82:**178, 182, 187–88, 195–96, 204–05, 219
flurazepam, **83:**115–16
haloperidol, **83:**487
and GH response, **82:**203, 204
in mania, **83:**113, 126, 298, 300, 301
in schizophrenia, **82:**183, 195–96, 199
hydralazine, **83:**123
5-hydroxytryptophan (5-HTP), **83:**113, 312
imipramine, *see* Imipramine
iproniazid, **83:**482
isocarboxazid, **83:**472, 482, 483
isoproterenol, **83:**470
L-dopa (levodopa), **82:**131, 132, 136; **83:**113, 123, 368
L-tryptophan, **83:**312, 483
legatrile, **82:**197
limbitrol, **83:**480
lisuride, **82:**197
lithium (carbonate), *see* Lithium therapy
lorazepam, **83:**116
loxapine, **82:**180, 182, 184–86; **83:**487
LSD (lysergic acid diethylamide), **82:**130, 139, 140
maprotiline, **83:**146, 312, 468–74 passim, 478, 485–90 passim, 495
marijuana, **82:**140
melperone, **82:**201
meprobamate, **82:**461; **83:**121

mescaline, **82:**139, 140
methamphetamine, **82:**462 (*see also* Amphetamine)
methyldopa, **83:**123
methylphenidate, **82:**197, 462; **83:**480
mianserin, **83:**312, 469, 489, 495, 500
molindone, **82:**180, 181
muscimol, **82:**139
naftidrofuryl, **83:**112
naloxone, **82:**141, 209, 212–14; **83:**113
nomifensine, **83:**474, 490
nortriptyline, **83:**123, 124, 312, 468, 472–80 passim, 493–500 passim
   and plasma levels, **83:**499–500, 505–11 passim
nylidrin hydrochloride, **83:**112
oxaprotiline, **83:**462, 469, 485, 490
oxazepam, **83:**116
p-chlorophenylalenine (PCPA), **82:**130
papaverine, **83:**112
pargyline, **83:**482
pemoline, **82:**462–63
penfluridol, **82:**182, 195
perphenazine, **82:**183, 461; **83:**125
phencyclidine (PCP), **82:**139–40
phenelzine, **82:**464, 466; **83:**127–28, 471, 472, 479, 482–84, 485
phenothiazine, **82:**131, 198, 218, 220, 461, 463; **83:**139, 323, 370 (*see also individual forms*)
phentolamine, **83:**484
physostigmine, **83:**113, 463, 476
pimozide, **82:**182, 204; **83:**122
pipotiazine, **82:**195
piracetam, **83:**112
primidone, **82:**465
probenecid, **82:**133
procaine hydrochloride, **83:**112
propanolol, **82:**131–32, 152, 205, 208; **83:**123, 478
protriptyline, **83:**124, 147, 472–80 passim, 493–500 passim, 506, 507
quanethadine, **83:**123
quinidine, **83:**123, 478
reserpine, **82:**131, 196; **83:**123, 459, 488
sulperide, **82:**201
synaptamine, **83:**489
thioridazine, **82:**200–201, 203, 218, 461, 463; **83:**113, 301
thiothixene, **82:**182, 188, 200–201, 461; **83:**113, 125, 301
tranylcypromine, **82:**462; **83:**127, 472, 482–85 passim
trazodone, **83:**312, 472, 474, 475, 485, 487–88
trifluoperazine, **83:**125, 484
   in borderline disorders, **82:**461–64 passim
   in schizophrenia, **82:**178, 180, 183, 188
triiodothyronine, **83:**481
trimipramine, **83:**472–76 passim, 480 (*see also* Imipramine)
tyrosine, **83:**113
valproic acid, **83:**312
vincamine, **83:**112
zimelidine, **83:**489–90, 495
Drug side effect(s), **83:**142, 147, 323, 512
   affective disorders, **83:**287, 368, 379
   age and, **83:**123, 126, 128, 301, 321n, 477, 497–98, 509–10
   anticholinergic, **83:**113, 123, 124, 127, 302, 313, 315, 317, 332, 336, 459–60, 463, 474–80 passim, 484–88 passim, 498
   of antidepressants, **83:**142, 459–60, 463, 469
   of antipsychotics, **82:**182, 183, 196, 205, 208, 382, 464, 465; **83:**125, 126, 130, 291, 301, 302 (*see also* tardive dyskinesia, *below*)
   brain damage, **83:**301
   cardiac/cardiovascular, **83:**114, 126, 128, 314, 475, 477–78, 484–86 passim, 491, 494, 498, 505, 509, 510
   delirium, **83:**108, 475
   depression, **83:**369, 374, 379
   headache, **83:**484, 488, 491
   hepatic necrosis, **83:**482
   hypertension, **83:**482, 484
   hypomania, **82:**464; **83:**273–77 passim, 280, 368, 375, 479–80, 488
   hypotension, **83:**113–14, 123, 302, 475, 477–78, 485–88 passim, 498, 509
   as legal issue, **82:**382
   mania/manic episode, **83:**126, 277, 278, 287, 311
   of MAO inhibitors, **83:**127–28, 475, 484–85
   on memory, **83:**113, 336, 475–76
   parkinsonian, **82:**196, 205; **83:**128, 302, 478, 487
   plasma-level monitoring for, **83:**507 (*see also* Plasma factors/levels)
   psychosis, **82:**137, 138, 139–40, 197; **83:**290
   renal damage, **83:**126, 301, 314, 316
   on sex life, **82:**8, 39; **83:**150, 475, 485
   tardive dyskinesia, **82:**147–48, 152–53, 169, 193, 195; **83:**125, 480, 487
   on vision, **82:**169; **83:**475, 484
   weight gain, **83:**313, 332, 336, 475, 478, 485
   See also Extrapyramidal symptoms; Imipramine; Lithium therapy; TCA (tricyclic antidepressant) response
Drug therapy, **83:**172, 358–59
   for anxiety, **83:**479, 483, 498
   for bipolar illness, *see* Bipolar (manic-depressive) Disorder, treatment of; Lithium therapy
   for borderline disorders, **82:**444, 456–67, 469–70, 484
   chemotherapy effects in cancer treatment, **82:**39
   for children, **83:**283, 498, 505
   compliance/noncompliance with, **82:**170, 467, 470; **83:**124, 127, 139, 251, 301, 312, 315–18 passim, 321–37, 504, 508, 509, 512
   contraindicated, **83:**123, 126, 479–80, 512
   for dementia, **83:**111–12, 113–14, 137
   for depressive disorders, **82:**466; **83:**122–28, 195, 366, 370, 371, 381, 457–71, 472–91, 512
   psychotherapy vs., **83:**252, 369, 524–28 passim
   (*see also* Lithium therapy; MAO [monoamine oxidase]; TCA [tricyclic antidepressant] response)
   dosage, **83:**317, 472, 479, 482–83, 487, 488
   for elderly, **83:**112, 123–28 passim, 141, 150

mania and, **83**:279
rejection-sensitive or hysteroid, **82**:457, 463–64, 467, 468, 470
See also Depression
Dysthymic Disorder, **82**:441
as bipolar variant, **83**:275–77, 278, 281–82, 285
course and manifestations of, **83**:276–77, 281–82, 289, 365, 366, 372–73
and depression, **83**:365, 371–74
DSM-III category for, *see* DSM-III categories/criteria
late-life, **83**:91, 92, 95, 119, 128
thymoleptic-responsive, **83**:275–76, 281
variants of, **83**:373–74

E

Eastwood, P. R., **83**:320
Eastwood, R., et al., **83**:138
Eaton, W. W., **82**:100; et al., **83**:90, 408
Ebstein's anomaly, **83**:314
ECA, *see* Epidemiologic Catchment Area Program
Eckman, T., **83**:434
Eckstein, R., **82**:475
ECT (electroconvulsive therapy): consent to, **82**:357–58, 359
for depression, **83**:121, 125, 366, 369, 370, 381, 382, 480
in elderly (unilateral vs. bilateral), **83**:126
legislation regarding, **82**:332–33, 353
for manic patient, **83**:281, 302
and schizophrenia, **82**:142, 143, 209, 220
and suicide, **83**:431
Edgerton, R. B., **82**:100
Edward B. Allen Award, **83**:85
Edwards, D. J., **83**:452; et al., **83**:452, 461, 467
EE (expressed emotion): and schizophrenia relapse, **82**:103–05, 110, 111, 172–74; **83**:175, 242–49 passim, 256. *See also* Anger; Hostility; Rage
EEG (electroencephalogram), **82**:124
abnormal, **82**:118, 148, 453–54, 455, 465
delirium and, **83**:107
of elderly patient, **83**:102, 126, 145
of infant, **83**:10
of schizoaffective, **83**:291
sleep studies, **83**:122, 145, 291
Egeland, J. A., **83**:270, 271, 448
Eger, C. L., **82**:328
Ego, **82**:497, 500, 502
development of, **82**:493, 494, 501; **83**:49
and ego identity/identity diffusion, **83**:24 (*see also* Identity)
and ego states of borderline patients, **82**:472–81 passim, 486
functions, **83**:31, 370
adaptive, **82**:515
autonomous, **83**:15
deficiencies of, **82**:29–30, 35, 286
development of, **82**:501
reduction of (in mob), **83**:21, 34

impairment of, in gender dysphoria, **82**:54, 56
primitive (preoedipal) ideal, in group, **83**:23
-self distinction, Freud and, **82**:488, 489
strength, and success of therapy, **82**:33, 56, 478
-superego conflict, **82**:272
See also Narcissism; Self
Ego boundaries, **83**:31
Ego-dystonic behavior, **82**:31, 416
Ego psychology, **82**:500, 503, 516
depression as viewed by, **82**:272
development of, **82**:488; **83**:21
and narcissism, **82**:488, 490, 519
and psychoanalysis, **83**:7
See also Self psychology
Ego-syntonic behavior, **82**:29; **83**:190, 217, 280, 374
Eimas, P. D., **83**:12; et al., **83**:12
Eisdorfer, Carl, **83**:87, 133, 134, 135, 136, 150; et al., **83**:132, 136, 138
Eisenberg, T., **82**:324n8
Eissler, Kurt, **82**:476; **83**:42, 54, 60
Ejaculation, **82**:10
aging and, **82**:46
and postejaculation difficulties, **82**:16
premature, **82**:10, 15, 16, 19, 32
therapy for, **82**:22, 24, 25, 32
retarded, therapy for, **82**:21
retrograde (prostatectomy and), **82**:39
as separate from male orgasm, **82**:15
urethral surgery and, **82**:38
See also Orgasm
EKG (electrocardiogram), **82**:291–92; **83**:122, 126, 299
in monitoring TCA therapy, **83**:478, 498
Ekstein, R., **82**:444
Elderly, the, *see* Aging; Geriatric psychiatry; Late-life psychiatric disorders
Electrocardiogram, *see* EKG
Electroconvulsive therapy, *see* ECT
Electroencephalogram, *see* EEG
Eliot, J., **83**:404
Elizur, A., et al., **82**:207
Ellenberg, M., **82**:37
Ellerbook, R. C., **82**:143
Ellis, Havelock, **82**:8
Ellsworth, R. B., **82**:174; et al., **82**:175
Elston, R. C., **83**:445, 446, 450; et al., **83**:451
Emde, R. N., **83**:229, 230; et al., **83**:10
Emerson, Ralph Waldo, **83**:37
Emler, N. T., **83**:37
Emmeneger, H., **83**:112
Emotionally Unstable Character Disorder, **82**:457, 463, 467, 468, 470; **83**:288
Emotions: hierarchy of, **82**:273. *See also* Affective Disorders; Depression; Mood disorders
Empathy: during infancy, **83**:19–20
narcissism and, **82**:490–91, 495, 496–97, 513
parental or caretaker, failure of, **82**:492, 494
of patient, with projected aggression, **82**:474
of therapist, *see* Therapist, the
Emphysema, **83**:98
Emrich, H. M., et al., **82**:213
Encephalitis, **82**:121

and borderline disorders, **82**:442
herpes, lethargica, Vilyuisk, **82**:120
See also Viruses
Encopresis: childhood, studies of, **83**:176–77
Endicott, J., **82**:424; **83**:408
Endocrine system: aging and, **83**:99
antipsychotic effects on, **82**:200–204
disorders of
and mood dysfunction, **83**:379, 422, 460
and psychosexual dysfunctions, **82**:37
and TSH response, **83**:122
hypothalamic-pituitary-adrenocortical (HPA) axis, **83**:460, 463
lithium effects on, **83**:126, 303
neuroendocrine correlates with depression, **83**:512
childhood depression, **82**:290, 292–94
and sexual development, **82**:11
See also Hormone(s)
Endorphins, **82**:146
and schizophrenia, **82**:141–42
Engel, G. L., **82**:161, 274; **83**:107, 204
England, *see* Great Britain
English, O. S., **83**:319, 329
Enna, S. J., **83**:469
Ennis, B. J., **82**:339
Environmental factors: in aging process (and in treatment of older patient), **83**:105, 114, 139
in child development, **83**:229, 230
in consanguinity method studies, **82**:93
and culture shock, **83**:139
and depression, **82**:284, **83**:413, 421, 458, 518, 520, 526, 528
and manic states, **83**:278
in paranoia, **83**:137, 138, 139
in schizophrenia, **82**:88–89, 96–97, 99, 106, 155; **83**:138
See also Nurture-nature debate
Enzymatic alterations, **82**:125–29, 130–31, 138–39, 144. *See also* DBH (dopamine); MAO (monoamine oxidase)
EPI (Eysenck Personality Inventory), **83**:336, 386
Epidemiologic Catchment Area Program (ECA), **83**:406n, 408, 410, 428
Epidemiology: defined, **82**:281; **83**:406
among elderly, **83**:87–95
terms (point prevalence, morbid risk, incidence, risk factor) defined, **83**:410
See also individual disorders
Epileptic disorders, **83**:296
and borderline disorders, **82**:442, 455
as drug reaction, **83**:478, 486
as "mental illness," **82**:337
temporal lobe epilepsy, drug therapy for, **83**:311
Episodic dyscontrol, **82**:465, 467, 468
EPS (extrapyramidal symptoms), **82**:182, 195, 196, 201, 205, 208; **83**:113, 125, 487. *See also* Drug side effect(s)
Epstein, N. B., **83**:215
Equilibrium (in family systems approach), **83**:205–06, 213. *See also* Family therapy
Equus-Laingian view of madness, **83**:331
Erection: of nipples, **82**:12
penile, **82**:9, 10, 12, 23, 39, 43

age and, **82**:46; **83**:149, 151
failure of, **82**:17, 37, 39; **83**:151
Ericksen, S. E., **82**:187; et al., **82**:183, 188, 189
Erikson, Erik H., **82**:278, 490; **83**:15, 51, 83
Ervin Act, **82**:373, 374
Esman, A. H., **83**:9
Essen-Möller, E., **82**:451; **83**:415, 416, 418, 420, 441
Essman, W. B., **83**:512
Esterson, A., et al., **82**:217
Estroff, N., **83**:248
Estrogen: post-menopausal levels of, **82**:10, 11; **83**:149
risk in use of, **82**:11; **83**:149
and TSH response, **83**:122
Ethical considerations: in criminal cases, **82**:386, 393–96. *See also* Confidentiality; Values
Ethnicity: and depression or bipolar illness, **82**:284; **83**:361, 413, 420, 426
and schizophrenia, **82**:101, 102
See also Blacks
Ettig, P., et al., **82**:203
Euphoria: in bipolar illness, **83**:279, 423. *See also* Bipolar (manic-depressive) Disorder
Evans, M., **82**:26
Everett, H. C., **83**:476
Exercise (as therapy), **83**:142, 146
Exner, J., **82**:209
Expectations: cultural, *see* Cultural factors
of family members, **82**:279; **83**:196–97, 198–99, 217, 218, 426 (*see also* Family, the; Family therapy; Marital therapy)
staff, of patients, **83**:30
See also Relationships
Expressed emotion, *see* EE
Expressive psychotherapy, *see* Psychotherapy
Extein, I., et al., **83**:289, 470
Externalization, **83**:237. *See also* Defense mechanisms
Extrapyramidal symptoms, *see* EPS
Eye movement, *see* REM (rapid eye movement); SPEM (smooth pursuit eye movement)
Eysenck, H. J., **83**:387
Eysenck Personality Inventory, *see* EPI
Ezriel, H., **83**:27, 28

F

Face-Hand Test (FHT), **83**:116
Faerman, I., et al., **82**:37
Fagan, J. F., **83**:15
Fain, J. H., **83**:470
Fain, M., **83**:33
Fairbairn, W. R. D., **82**:470, 490; **83**:26, 218
Fairburn, C. G., **82**:212
Falloon, I. R. H., **82**:111; **83**:245–48 passim, 253, 256; et al., **82**:109, 110–111
Falret, Jean Pierre, **83**:269
Family, the: adolescent dependence on, **82**:279; **83**:241

bipolar illness and, **83**:249, 279, 297–98, 302, 305, 329, 374, 426, 435

child as scapegoat of, **83**:233–34, 239, 240

critical events/stress and, **83**:188, 197–98, 214–15, 216, 239

of depressive patient, **83**:364, 372, 380, 405, 414

and elderly members of, **83**:88, 114, 129, 138, 150

and family identity, **83**:177–78

and gender development, **82**:55

genogram of, **83**:199, 207, 209, 215

importance of, **83**:169–70, 364

and indigenous family culture, **83**:179–83

intergenerational family-of-origin problems in, **83**:199, 212, 222, 223, 231, 236–37, 241

lack of moral guidance by, **83**:35

life cycles of, **83**:209–12, 216 (*see also* Adolescent[s]; Aging; Childhood; Infancy; Young adults)

loyalties to, **83**:199, 219, 234

patriarchal, and capitalism, **83**:34

and physical illness, **83**:169, 193, 195, 213–14

and schizophrenia (etiology and relapse), **82**:103–06, 107, 110, 112, 163, 172–74; **83**:171, 175–76, 242–49

See also Marriage; Mother-child relationship; Parent(s); Parent-child relationship; Sibling(s)

Family Crucible, The (Napier and Whitaker), **83**:215

Family history: of affective disorders, **83**:274, 282–83, 288, 295, 380, 420–21, 434–57 (*see also* Depression)

"living" (initial interview and), **83**:208

and mania/manic episode, **83**:288, 295

of schizophrenic states, **83**:132, 283

See also Genetic factors; History-taking

Family therapy: for bipolar or unipolar disorder, **82**:265, 307; **83**:249–53

for childhood disorders, **82**:265, 307; **83**:171, 188–201 passim, 209, 228–41

choice of, **83**:187–92

combined with drug therapy, **83**:195, 243, 252

defined, **83**:185

education of family in, **82**:173; **83**:201, 243–50 passim, 253–56

family or marital evaluation, **83**:188–91, 193–95, 197, 222

"family systems theory" in, **83**:186, 194, 203–15, 217, 229, 239–40

geriatric patients and, **83**:129

group process theories and, **83**:33

importance and advantages of, **83**:169–70, 185, 234–35

vs. individual, **83**:188, 189–92, 203, 204, 239–41

and multiple family group (MFG), **83**:242, 244, 246, 247, 256

in schizophrenia, **83**:189, 252

behavioral, **83**:246–47

psychoeducational, **82**:163, 173; **83**:245–46, 253–56

and relapse, **82**:106, 110–11, 172–74; **83**:242–49 passim

studies of, **82**:217, 219, 225; **83**:170, 175, 242

strategic and systemic, **83**:247–48, 256

the therapist and, **83**:179–80, 182–85, 186

empathy of, **83**:171, 173, 194, 200, 201, 206–07, 244, 246

intervention by, **83**:187, 196–203, 211, 238–39, 241

interviews by, **83**:207–09, 231, 232, 238, 239

role assumption by, **83**:201, 223–24, 226, 238

training for, **83**:183

See also Marital therapy

Fang, V. S., **82**:135

Fann, W. E., **83**:150

Faris, R. E. L., **83**:424, 425, 426

Farkas, T., et al., **83**:117

Farley, I. J., et al., **82**:132

Farmer, P. M., et al., **83**:110

Fascism, **83**:35

Father, the: absence/rejection of, **83**:35

oedipal, Freud's view of, **83**:34–35, 36

participation of, in family therapy, **83**:194, 233n

Father image: "contamination" of (by aggession), **82**:473

Fatigue: depression and, **83**:127, 328, 480, 514

childhood depression, **82**:303–04

Fauman, M. A. and B. J., **82**:140

Fava, G. A., et al., **83**:395, 396

Fawcett, J., et al., **83**:480

Federal Organizations for Professional Women, **82**:57

Federal Trade Commission, **82**:325

Federn, P., **82**:444

Feer, H., et al., **82**:141

Feighner, J. P., et al., **82**:289, 422; **83**:272, 278, 286, 293, 294, 376, 408, 409, 512

Feinberg, I., **83**:145; et al., **83**:145

Feinberg, M. P., **83**:452

Feldberg, W., **82**:146

Felder, W., **83**:440

Female(s): anatomy of, **82**:10–11 (*see also* Genitalia)

antipsychotic prolactin levels of, **82**:202–03

bipolar illness of, **83**:304, 424, 426

depressive, **83**:373, 387, 393, 400–04, 411–14 passim, 420–22, 433, 524

"involutional," **83**:92, 412

dysthymic disorders among, **83**:373

elderly

and late-life psychiatric disorders, **83**:94, 107, 110, 132, 133, 142, 420

sexual functions of, **83**:149, 151

U.S. population figures, **83**:88

life expectancy for, **83**:89

lithium reactions of/compliance by, **83**:333, 334, 335

masturbation by, **82**:10, 11, 18, 21

pre- and postmarital sexuality of, **82**:43, 44

schizophrenia in, **82**:108

stress and, **83**:94

surgery on, **82**:39–41

in therapeutic relationship, **83**:38–40

treatment goals of, **83**:39–40

See also Female psychology; Feminist move-

hospital staff and therapeutic community models of, 83:28–30

and the mob/crowds, 83:21, 22, 24, 34, 36

object-relations approach to, 83:24–25, 31

psychoanalytic studies of, 83:7–8, 33

Group-relations conferences (England and U.S.), 83:32–33

Group therapy: in childhood depression, 82:307

couples therapy combined with, 83:195

development of, 83:26–28

family therapy difference from, 83:184

for geriatric patient, 83:130

in schizophrenia, 82:170–72, 217, 219

in sex therapy, 82:21, 24–25, 26

See also Family therapy

Grove, O., 83:434

Growe, G., et al., 82:209, 211

Growth hormone (GH), *see* Hormone(s)

Gruen, P. H., et al., 82:200, 201, 203, 290

Gruenberg, E. M., 82:281, 283, 287

Grugett, A., 82:58

Gruman, G. W., 83:83

Grunberger, B., 82:519

Grunebaum, Henry, 83:182, 186, 195, 215, 217, 230, 238; et al., 83:190, 244n

Gruzelier, J., et al., 82:208

Guam: neurofibrillary degeneration in, 83:100

Gudeman, J. E., et al., 83:467

Guilt feelings: of bipolar patient, 83:329

as depression symptom, 83:479

childhood depression, 82:302

incestuous experiences and, 82:59

of rape victims, 82:62, 63

and sexual dysfunction, 82:31, 38, 62

of spouse of ill patient, 82:36

surgery as cause of, 82:38

of therapist, 83:331

Gulliver's Travels (Swift), 83:83

Gunderson, John G., 82:88, 159, 413–19 passim, 423–30 passim, 433–56 passim, 466, 467, 468, 470; et al., 82:416, 418, 419, 428, 430, 434, 436, 466

Gund-R scale, 82:429, 430

Gunne, L. M., et al., 82:141, 212, 214

Gurevitz, H., 82:331

Gurland, B. J., 83:116; et al., 83:116

Gurman, A. S., 83:171, 185, 190, 191

Gustafson, L., et al., 83:112

Gutheil, Thomas G., 82:323, 326, 327, 330, 333, 351, 353, 361n2, 368, 379–83 passim, 384n8

Guze, S. B., 82:8, 415; 83:89, 287, 376, 379, 381, 429

H

Haase, A. T., et al., 82:122

Habot, B., 83:108

Hachinski, V. C., et al., 83:114

Haefely, W. E., 82:139

Haglund, R. M., 83:116

Hagnell, O., 83:415, 416, 418, 420

Haier, R. J., et al., 82:126

Hakstian, A. R., 83:524, 525

Haley, Jay, 83:170, 192, 220, 244, 247, 248–49

Halfway houses, 82:177

Hall, K., 83:250

Halleck, Seymour L., 82:58, 326, 327, 361, 366n12, 392

Hällström, T., 83:412, 413, 416–20 passim

Hallucinations, 82:139

antipsychotics and, 82:197, 200, 209

bipolar illness and, 83:278, 281, 312

childhood, 82:306

depressive disorders and, 83:125, 362, 370, 371, 373, 381, 527

paranoid, in geriatric patients, 83:132, 136, 137

and plasma levels, 83:509

schizophrenia and, 82:85, 86, 87, 126, 141, 148, 149, 167, 197, 200, 209; 83:130, 131, 138

See also Alcoholism

Hallucinogens, *see* Drugs

Halonen, P., et al., 82:121

Halpern, C. R., 82:387

Hamadah, K., 82:146

Hamilton Depression Rating Scale, 82:466; 83:362, 400, 467

Hammen, C. L., 82:270

Hamovit, J. R., 83:435n, 455

Hampson, J. L. and J. G., 82:55

Handicap, *see* Learning disorders; Physical handicap

Hanlon, T. E., et al., 82:204, 209

Hansen, J. C., 83:222

Hanson, L. B., et al., 82:209

Hanssen, T., et al., 82:207

Harding, C. M., 82:88

Hare, M., 83:116

Hargreaves, W. A., 82:225, 226

Harris, R., 83:189

Harris, T., 83:94, 421–22

Harrison, M. J. G., 83:109

Harroff, P. B., 83:233

Harrow, M., et al., 82:88

Hart, R. W., 83:98

Hartford, J. T., 83:99, 115

Hartford, M. E., 83:129

Hartigan, C., 83:304

Hartmann, E., 82:128

Hartmann, Heinz, 82:489

Harvard Law Review, 82:323n6, 348n66, 366, 381

"Notes," 82:365, 366–67, 368

Hastings, D., 82:55

Haug, J. O., 83:286, 372

Hauger, M., et al., 83:444

Hauser, S. T., 83:184

Havighurst, R., 83:105

Hayflick, L., 83:97

Hays, S. E., 82:200, 203, 204

Headache: as drug/food reaction, 83:484, 488, 491

Health and Human Services, U.S. Department of, 82:325

Health care system: dysthymic patients' use of, 83:372, 373

family as component of, 83:213

late-life use of, 83:94–95, 117

See also Family, the; Hospitalization; Nursing homes; Outpatient treatment; Social support networks; Therapy; Third-party payment

Hearing loss: age-related (presbycusis), 83:103–04, 133–34
conductive, 83:104, 133
family therapy in cases of, 83:189
and paranoia, 83:133–38 passim
See also Sensory deficits

Heart rate: drug side effect on, 83:478
orgasm and, 82:12
See also Cardiac disorders

Heath, R. G., 82:115, 118; et al., 82:118–19
Hedberg, D. L., et al., 82:459, 462
Heimann, P. A., 82:473, 474
Heinicke and Westheimer study (of child separation from mother), 82:275
Heinrichs, Douglas W., 82:154, 158, 160, 161
Helgason, Larus, 83:419n5, 425n5
Helgason, Tomas, 83:416, 418, 419, 423, 424, 425
Hellon, C., 83:433
Helsing, K. J., 83:412, 413
Helzer, J. E., 83:438, 442, 446; et al., 83:278
Hematoma, subdural: in delirium, 83:108
Henderson, S., 83:409, 416
Hendrickson, E., et al., 83:117
Hendrie, H. C., 83:395
Henry, W., 83:105
Henschke, P. J., et al., 83:111
Herbert, M. E., 83:132, 139
Heredity, see Family history; Genetic factors
Herjanic, M., 83:372
Herpes virus(es), 82:120, 121; 83:109. See also Virus(es)
Herrington, B. S., 82:160
Hersen, M., 82:108, 109
Hertz, A., et al., 82:213
Herz, M. I., 82:88, 226; et al., 82:226
Hestbech, J., et al., 83:314
Heston, L. L., 82:89, 95; 83:101, 110; et al., 83:110
Hetherington, E. M., et al., 83:234
Hetzel, B., 83:433
Hicks, R., 83:112; et al., 83:113, 498
Hier, D., 82:124; et al., 82:124
High performance liquid chromatography (HPLC), 83:501
Hilberman, E., 82:63
Hill, A. B., et al., 83:115
Himmelhoch, J. M., et al., 83:279, 281
Hippocrates, 82:10, 327; 83:269
Hird, F., 82:227
Hirsch, S. R., 82:172; 83:291; et al., 82:207
Hirschfeld, Robert M. A., 83:286, 355, 379, 385, 387, 388, 397, 399, 406, 413, 414, 421; et al., 83:384, 394
Hirschowitz, J., 82:136; et al., 82:211
Hispanics: in elderly population, 83:88
History-taking: in assessment and diagnosis, 83:116–17, 363, 384–85
in family therapy, 83:188, 208, 231
in genetic counseling, 83:456
See also Family history
Histrionic Personality Disorder, 82:18, 436
DSM-III criteria for, 82:470

HLA (human leukocyte antigen), see Antigens
Hoch, P., 82:444, 462
Hodge, S. E., 83:111
Hofer, M., 83:18
Hoff, L. A., 82:61
Hoffer, A., 82:143; et al., 82:142
Hoffman, B., 82:361n2
Hoffman, B. B., et al., 83:470
Hoffman, P. B., 82:349
Hogan, R. T., 83:37
Hogarty, G. E., 82:173, 190, 191, 193, 195; 83:245; et al., 82:88; 160, 173, 176, 177, 195, 219
Hokin-Neaverson, M., et al., 83:452
Holland: drug therapy in, 83:489
Hollender, M. H., 83:305
Hollingshead, A. B., 83:93, 184
Hollister, L., 83:111, 113, 116; et al., 83:462, 468, 473
Holmboe, R., 83:372
Holmes, T. H., 83:394
Holmstrom, L. L., 82:61, 62
Holzman, P., 82:188, 189, 199, 475; et al., 82:453
Holzman Thought Disorder Index, 82:199
Homeostasis: aging and, 83:99
Homophilia: gender disturbance and, 82:51
Homosexuality, 82:33–34
defensive, 82:32–33
treatment of, 82:34
family therapy for (tendency), 83:189
narcissism and, 82:488, 512, 519
and sexual identity, 82:49
Honecker, H., et al., 83:467
Hopkins, S. M., 83:112
Hormone(s): adrenocorticotrophic (ACTH), 83:113
in aging, 83:99, 102
cross-sexual, gender disturbance and, 82:53
definition of, 83:102
growth (GH)
depression and, 83:460
drug therapy and, 82:135, 136, 203–04; 83:469
response of, to insulin-induced hypoglycemia, 82:290, 292–93, 295
and memory, 83:113
and neurohormones, 83:102
postmenopausal use of, 82:11, 46; 83:149
and sexual development, 82:11
thyroid, 83:102, 303, 503
thyrotropin-releasing (TRH), 83:113
thyrotropin-releasing/thyroid-stimulating (TRH/TSH) response test, 83:121–22, 273, 289, 314
See also Endocrine system
Horn, A. S., 82:196
Horn, J. L., 83:119
Horney, Karen, 82:490; 83:42–43, 45, 47, 513
Hornstra, R. K., 83:365
Horrobin, D., 82:146
Horwitz, W. A., et al., 82:217
Hospitalization: for bipolar illness, see Bipolar (manic-depressive) Disorder, treatment of
of borderline patients, 82:424, 450, 470–74 passim, 482
for depression, see Depression

distinguished (by courts) from treatment, **82**:381
economic conditions and, **82**:103
of elderly, **83**:94, 125, 145, 150
family evaluation preceding, **83**:188
family therapy vs., **83**:191
in forensic hospital, **82**:387, 395, 396
for gender dysphoria, **82**:54
and hospital staff group reactions, **83**:28–29
as least restrictive alternative, **82**:348–49 (*see also* Civil commitment)
length of, as factor, **82**:121, 138, 177, 222, 225–27, 228
and paranoia statistics, **83**:133, 137
as rejection or punishment, **83**:326
for schizophrenia, *see* Schizophrenia, treatment of
for transference psychosis, **82**:475
See also Nursing homes; Therapy
Hospitalization of the Mentally Ill Act, **82**:373
Hostility: drug therapy for, **83**:487
illness viewed as act of, **82**:36
mania and, **83**:279
postmarital, **82**:43, 44
and sexual dysfunctions, **82**:28–31 passim
and scapegoating, **83**:233–34
toward psychiatry, **83**:40, 129
toward therapist, **82**:156–57, 474 (*see also* Therapeutic relationship)
See also EE (expressed emotion)
Hounsfield Units (HU): in senile dementia, **83**:117
Houpt, J. L., **83**:90, 91
Howell, E., **83**:42
HPLC (high performance liquid chromatography), **83**:501
Hrdina, P. D., **83**:500, 506; et al., **83**:492, 498
Huber, G., et al., **82**:88
Hudgens, R. W., et al., **83**:385
Huessey, H., et al., **82**:463
Huffine, C. L., **82**:109
Hughes, J., **82**:141; et al., **83**:112
Hullin, R. P., **83**:316
Human rights committees, **82**:358
Human Sexuality (American Medical Association), **82**:8
Huntington's chorea, **82**:121, 138; **83**:109, 366
Hurt, S. W., **82**:188, 189, 199
Hurvitz, N., **83**:190, 191
Husaini, B. A., et al., **83**:412
Huston, P. E., **83**:372
Huws, D., **82**:200
Hydinger-MacDonald, M., **82**:200
Hydrocephalus, normal-pressure, **83**:109
Hymnowitz, P., **82**:383n6
Hyperactivity, **82**:303; **83**:283, 423, 443
Hyperkinetic syndrome, **82**:462. *See also* ADD (Attentional Deficit Disorder)
Hypersexuality: in bipolar illness/manic episode; **82**:15; **83**:281
Hypersomnia, *see* Sleep disorders
Hypertension: as drug/food side effect, **83**:482, 484
drug therapy for, **83**:482
and stroke, **83**:114

Hypnotherapy: for sexual dysfunction, **82**:21, 22–23
Hypoactivity: in childhood depression, **82**:297, 303
Hypochondriasis, **82**:491
depression and, **83**:372, 373
drug therapy and, **83**:143, 480
DSM-III category for, **83**:142
late-life, **83**:91, 142–44
Hypoglycemia: insulin-induced, **82**:290, 292–93, 295
Hypomania: as bipolar (II) disorder, **83**:278, 279, 292–98 passim, 304, 423, 424, 466
and appeal or fear of hypomanic state, **83**:280, 285, 328, 331, 334, 335
biologic/genetic factors in, **83**:272–73, 439–446 passim, 453
and compliance in therapy, **83**:330, 332, 335, 337
in cyclothymic/dysthymic variants, **83**:275–77, 281
in borderline disorders, **82**:463, 464, 467
in childhood, **83**:283
depression and, **83**:288, 465
drug-induced, *see* Drug side effect(s)
as drug withdrawal effect, **83**:481
in narcissistic disorder, **82**:514
Hypotension: as drug side effect, *see* Drug side effect(s)
Hypothalamus: and aging, **83**:99
Hysteria, **83**:376. *See also* Affective Disorders

I

Iacono, W. G., **82**:453
Iatrogenic disorders: drug-induced, *see* Drug side effect(s)
Ibsen, Henrik, **83**:40
ICD-9 (*Manual of the International Classification of Diseases, Injuries, and Causes of Death, 9th rev.*, World Health Organization), **82**:14; **83**:380, 409, 410
ICH, Freud's use of, **82**:488, 489
Id, **82**:497, 500, 502; **83**:23
ID (Index of Definition), **83**:409, 427
Idealization: of leader by group, **83**:21–22, 24, 25
of parent(s) by child, **82**:491
narcissistic, *see* Narcissistic Personality Disorder
Idealizing (selfobject) transference, *see* Transference
Identification: in family therapy, **83**:200, 201
of mob with leader, **83**:21, 34
projective, *see* Projective identification
Identity: family, **83**:177–78
individual loss of, in group, **83**:21–24 passim
Ideology: defined, **83**:34
group, **83**:23, 24, 25, 30, 33
"preoedipal," **83**: 36
Ilfeld, F. W., **83**:413

Illness, *see* Mental illness; Physical illness; Psychosomatic disorders; Somatic symptoms; Surgery
Imipramine, **83:**124, 312, 486, 487, 493–94, 496
　age, and effects of, **83:**498, 499, 509
　in borderline disorders, **82:** 462, 463
　for depression, **83:**311, 361, 371, 468–69, 473–74, 479, 525
　　childhood depression, **82:**290, 291–92, 295, 307
　　vs. cognitive therapy, **83:**525
　³H-, **83:**470
　introduction of, **83:**458, 472, 503
　lithium combined with or vs., **83:**307, 311, 318, 481
　in panic states, **83:**483–84
　and plasma levels, **82:**292, 295; **83:**477, 480, 497–500 passim, 504–11 passim
　sedative vs. energizing effects of, **83:**123, 476, 480
　side effects of, **83:**368, 475–78 passim, 485, 488, 509
　See also Drugs, list of
Immune system: and aging, **83:**98
　Alzheimer's disease and, **83:**111
　and schizophrenia, **82:**114–22
Immunoassay techniques, **83:**501
Impotence, **82:**14, 15, 32
　age and, **82:**46, 151
　as drug side effect, **83:**150, 475, 485
　organic dysfunctions and, **82:**37–38, 46
　surgery and, **82:**39, 46
　therapy for, **82:**21
　　and failure rate in dual-sex therapy, **82:**25
　See also Psychosexual dysfunctions
Impulse disorders, **82:**33. *See also* Psychosexual dysfunctions
Impulsivity: in borderline patients, **82:**423, 424, 450–57 passim, 462
Incest, **82:**34, 56
　aftermath of, **82:**32, 57–61
　defined, **82:**57
　group prohibition against, **83:**25, 34
Index of Definition, *see* ID
India: schizophrenia studies in, **82:**98–104 passim, 137–38
Individuation, *see* Self
Industrial revolution, **83:**35
Infancy: "autism" in (normal), **83:**10–11
　depression in, **82:**274–75, 293; **83:**360 (*see also* Childhood depression)
　empathy during, **83:**19–20
　implications of research on, for psychoanalysis, **83:**7, 8–21
　individuation (sense of self) during, **83:**14–15, 19
　infant-object interaction in, **82:**495
　intersubjectivity in, **82:**18–19
　learning and "knowledge" in, **83:**11–15
　memory during, **83:**15–18
　selfobject in structure building in, **82:**501
　"stimulus barrier," in, **83:**9–11
　symbiotic phase of, **82:**48, 55, 56; **83:**13, 14, 35
　See also Childhood

Infantile personality, **82:**433
Infant mortality, **82:**274. *See also* Mortality rate
Infection(s): Alzheimer's disease as, **83:**111
　resistance to, **82:**115; **83:**98
　See also Immune system; Physical illness; Viruses
Informed consent, law of, *see* Law and psychiatry
Inhibited sexual response, *see* Impotence; Orgasm; Sexual response
Inouye, E., **82:**451
Insanity defense, **82:**387, 389–92. *See also* Law and psychiatry
Insight: in borderline patients, **82:**475–76
Insomnia: bipolar illness and, **83:**277, 279, 281
　depression and, **83:**373, 375
　　childhood depression, **82:**304
　as drug side effect, **83:**485
　drug therapy for, **83:**480
　dysthymia and, **83:**277, 373
　late-life, **83:**145–46
　　distinguished from sleep needs, **83:**115, 145–46
　psychosocial dwarfism and, **82:**293
　See also Sleep disorders
Institute of Medicine, **83:**146
Institute of Psychiatry (London), **82:**103
Institutionalization: of elderly, **83:**128. *See also* Civil commitment; Health care system; Hospitalization; Mental retardation
Insurance companies, *see* Third-party payment
Internal-External Locus of Control (test), **83:**336
Internalization: as defense mechanism, **83:**237
　of object relations, *see* Object relations
　of superego, **83:**34
Interpretation: in psychoanalysis and psychoanalytic psychotherapy, *see* Psychoanalysis; Psychotherapy
Intersubjectivity: in infancy, **83:**18–19
Involuntary treatment, *see* Therapy
"Involutional" melancholia, *see* Melancholia
"Iowa 500" study, **83:**421, 426
Iraq: bipolar illness in, **83:**271
Ireland: schizophrenia in, **82:**120
Irritability: depression or mania and, **82:**304; **83:**274, 279, 295, 296, 330, 380, 393, 479
Irwin, H., **83:**476, 477, 478
Isolation, *see* Social isolation; Withdrawal, social
Israel: alcoholism studies in, **83:**442
　bipolar illness in, **83:**271, 442
　schizophrenia studies in, **82:**205
Itil, T. M., et al., **82:**188

J

Jackson, Don D., **83:**170, 242
Jackson, Hughlings, **82:**167, 172
Jacob, T., **83:**174
Jacobs, S. C., **82:**103; et al., **83:**395
Jacobs, T. J., et al., **83:**373
Jacobsen, B., **82:**121

Jacobson, E., **82**:489, 493, 511; **83**:375
Jacobson, N. S., **83**:220, 223
Jacobson, R., **83**:176–77
Jacobson, S., **83**:132, 139
James, N. M., **83**:424, 438, 446
Jamison, Kay R., **83**:270, 316, 317, 319n; et al.,
   83:280, 315, 317, 323, 326, 328, 333–36 passim
Jandhyala, B. S., et al., **83**:494
Jankovic, B. D., et al., **82**:117
Janowsky, D. S., **82**:133, 187; et al., **82**:197, 213,
   214; **83**:302, 319, 330, 459, 463
Japelli, G., **82**:146
Jaques, E., **83**:30
Jarvik, L. F., **83**:97, 112
Jaspers, K., **82**:162
Jatlow, P. I., **83**:125, 501
Javaid, J. L., et al., **83**:494
Jenkins Activity Survey, **83**:336
Jenner, F. A., **83**:320
Jerram, T. C., **83**:316
Jeste, D. V., **82**:147, 148; et al., **82**:131, 137, 147,
   204
Job, Book of, **83**:511
Joffee, W. G., **82**:272–73
Johns Hopkins University, **82**:55, 465
Johnson, D. A. W., **83**:291
Johnson, F. N., **83**:320
Johnson, Judge Frank, **82**:363, 371–72, 374
Johnson, G., et al., **83**:300
Johnson, G. F. S., **83**:438
Johnson, K. M., **82**:140
Johnson, Virginia E., **82**:7–13 passim, 20–22
   passim, 25–26, 35, 46, 63; **83**:41, 148, 149, 151
Johnston, E. C., **83**:483
Johnston, M. H., **82**:199
Johnstone, E. C., **82**:117; et al., **82**:123, 135, 196
Joint Commission on Accreditation of Hospi-
   tals, **82**:325
Jonas, W., **83**:451
Jones, E., **82**:511; **83**:42, 43, 47
Jones, M., **83**:29
Judd, L., et al., **82**:203
Judd, Orrin, **82**:324n10
Juel-Nielsen, N., **83**:431; et al., **83**:418, 420
Jung, Carl G., **82**:488
Juvenile delinquency: family therapy for, **83**:190,
   191. See also Crime

K

Kaes, R., **83**:33
Kafka, M. S., et al., **82**:131; **83**:470
Kagan, J., **83**:230
Kagle, A., **82**:26, 28, 29, 35
Kahlbaum, Karl Ludwig, **83**:269, 374
Kahn, E., **83**:365
Kahn, R., et al., **83**:479
Kahn, R. L., **83**:33; et al., **83**:109, 116
Kaldor, J., **82**:128
Kales, A., et al., **83**:145
Kalin, N. H., **82**:127
Kalla, V. A., **82**:186

Kallmann, F. J., **82**:93, 94
Kamp, Van H., **82**:115
Kanas, N., et al., **82**:217
Kane, J., et al., **82**:195, 294; **83**:309, 311
Kansas City community survey (of depression),
   83:365
Kaplan, B., **83**:14
Kaplan, H. S., **83**:222n1
Kaplan, L., **82**:471
Kaplan, S., **83**:189
Kapp, F. T., **82**:61
Karacan, I., et al., **82**:46; **83**:151
Karasawa, T., **83**:467
Karasu, T. B., **82**:87; **83**:109
Kardiner, A., et al., **82**:495
Karno, M., **82**:100
Karon, B. P., **82**:158, 217
Karoum, F., et al., **82**:137, 138
Karpel, M. A., **83**:227
Karpinski, E., **82**:57
Kasanin, J., **82**:108, 152; **83**:358
Kashani, Javad, **82**:264, 282, 284; et al., **82**:284–
   88 passim
Kaslow, F., **83**:227
Kasper, S., et al., **83**:460
Kastin, A. J., et al., **83**:113
Katkin, S., et al., **82**:177
Katsrup, M., et al., **83**:417
Katz, D., **83**:33
Katz, S., **82**:58, 61
Katzman, R., **83**:109
Kaufmann, C. L., **82**:358; et al., **82**:358
Kawecky, C. A., **83**:86
Kay, D. W. K., **83**:107, 109, 132, 133, 137; et al.,
   83:91, 110
Kay, S. R., **82**:145
Kazdin, A. E., **82**:269, 270; **83**:516
Keith, D., **83**:249
Keith, Samuel J., **82**:110, 154, 170, 177; **83**:242n
Kellam, S. G., et al., **82**:174
Keller, M., **83**:276, 512
Keller-Teschke, M., **82**:128
Kelly, George A., **83**:513, 526
Kendall, D. A., **83**:469
Kendler, K. S., **83**:132; et al., **82**:89
Kennedy, P., **82**:227
Kerbikov, O. V., **82**:118
Kerenyi, C., **83**:83
Kernberg, Otto F., **82**:413, 415, 423–43 passim,
   454, 461, 470–74 passim, 480, 486, 490–97
   passim, 499n1, 511–23 passim; **83**:7–8, 24–33
   passim, 51; et al., **82**:421, 426–36 passim, 471,
   486
Kernberg, Paulina, **82**:437
Kernberg's Structural Interview, see Borderline
   Personality Disorder, diagnosis of
Kerry, R. J., **83**:331
Kessler, C., **82**:201
Kessler, D. R., **83**:188, 193
Kestenbaum, C. J., **83**:283
Kety, S. S., **82**:445n; **83**:432, 445; et al., **82**:95,
   444–55 passim
Khan, M. K., **82**:471; **83**:442
Khin-Maung-Zaw, **83**:432
Khouri, P. J., et al., **82**:448, 450, 451

Kidd, K. K., **83:**421, 427
Kiddie-SADS, **82:**270. *See also* Childhood depression; SADS (Schedule for Affective Disorders and Schizophrenia)
Kielholz, T., **83:**373; et al., **83:**311
Kiloh, L. G., **83:**107, 108, 381; et al., **82:**186; **83:**479
Kilpatrick, D. M., et al., **82:**61, 63
Kiltie, H., **82:**180, 184
Kincaid-Smith, P., **83:**314
King, J. A., **82:**175
King, S., **83:**276, 449
Kinney, D., **82:**121
Kinsey, A. C., et al., **82:**7, 20, 43, 58, 62; **83:**151
Kirk, S. A., **82:**177
Kirkegaard, C., **83:**460; et al., **82:**290
Kirschenbaum, J., **83:**233
Kisimoto, A., **83:**312
Kitanaka, I., et al., **83:**498
Kjellman, B. F., et al., **83:**315
Klassen, D., **83:**365
Klee, W. A., et al., **82:**146
Klein, Donald F., **82:**108, 413, 436, 443, 458–65 passim; **83:**288; et al., **82:**463, 464; **83:**126, 479
Klein, Joel I., **82:**321, 322, 326, 348n, 364
Klein, Melanie, **82:**474, 516; **83:**26, 218
Kleinberg, D. L., **82:**204
Kleinman, Joel E., et al., **82:**132–36 passim, 142
Klerman, Gerald L., **82:**281, 283, 284, 415–28 passim, 436, 456; **83:**47, 50, 92, 273, 277, 278, 287, 294, 296, 304, 321, 365, 372, 379–88 passim, 406, 407, 411, 412, 419–26 passim, 519; et al., **82:**161; **83:**381, 481, 519, 524
Klett, C. J., **82:**205
Kline, N. S., **83:**482; et al., **82:**141; **83:**506
Knapp, S., **83:**20
Knight, A., **83:**291; et al., **82:**227
Knight, R. P., **82:**423, 434, 444, 471, 480
Kniskern, D. P., **83:**171, 185, 190, 191
Knowledge: abstract, of infant, **83:**12–14
Kobele, S., et al., **82:**422, 423
Koch, Robert, **82:**82
Koch-Weser, J., **83:**493
Kocsis, J. R., **83:**300
Koenigsberg, H., **82:**422, 424, 428, 433
Kohn, M. L., **82:**98, 107
Kohut, Heinz, **82:**414, 437, 487, 490–505 passim, 510, 511, 512, 516, 523; **83:**20, 51, 55, 59
Kokes, R. F., et al., **82:**108
Kolakowska, T., et al., **82:**200, 202, 203
Kolb, J. E., **82:**417, 419, 423–34 passim, 438–43 passim, 448–57 passim, 467, 468
Koliaskina, G., et al., **82:**117, 119
Kopeikin, H. S., **83:**245, 250, 253; et al., **83:**243, 256
Korff, J., **83:**452
Kornblith, S. J., **83:**516, 517, 524
Korsakoff's syndrome, **83:**115
Kotin, J., **83:**281
Kovacs, Maria, **82:**268, 269, 270, 283; **83:**356, 513, 516, 524; et al., **83:**525
Kraepelin, Emil, **83:**372
   and concept of manic-depressive insanity, **83:**272–79 passim, 285, 292, 357–59, 407, 423, 512

and Kraepelinian tradition, **82:**108, 166, 197; **83:**184, 323, 360, 374, 407, 444
and nosology, **82:**82–88 passim, 112–13, 149; **83:**269, 270, 282, 392, 487
on "paraphrenia," **83:**131, 137
Krafft-Ebing, Richard von, **82:**8; **83:**269
Kragh-Sorensen, P., **83:**492, 497, 503, 507, 510
Kraines, S. H., **83:**279
Kral, V. A., **83:**107
Kramer, C. H., **83:**236
Kramer, M., **83:**130, 407
Krasner, B., **83:**187, 199
Krauthammer, C., **83:**277, 287, 294, 296, 381, 406, 419, 423–26 passim
Kreitman, N., **83:**434
Kretschmer, E., **83:**392
Kringlen, E., **82:**94, 95, 451; **83:**441
Kris, A. O., **83:**64
Kroll, J., et al., **82:**415, 420–29 passim, 433–34, 436, 437
Krupp, I. M., **82:**115, 118
Kryso, J., **82:**58
Kubanis, P., **83:**110
Kugler, J., et al., **83:**112
Kuhn, B. and R., **82:**291
Kuhn, R., **83:**472, 503
Kuhn, T. S., **83:**37
Kuipers, L., **83:**246
Kukopulos, A., et al., **83:**313
Kulcar, Z., et al., **83:**417
Kumar, N., **82:**186; **83:**417
Kuperman, S., **82:**282, 284, 289
Kupfer, D. J., **82:**290, 453; et al., **82:**290, 294; **83:**121, 273, 274, 279, 283, 289, 291, 355, 439, 506
Kuriansky, J. B., et al., **82:**86
Kurland, A. A., **82:**198; et al., **82:**212
Kuro disorder, **82:**120
Kurucz, J., et al., **83:**110

L

L-γ-aminobutyric acid, *see* GABA
L-dopa, L-tryptophan, *see* Drugs, list of
Laakman, G., **82:**290
La Barre, W., **83:**136
L'Abate, L., **83:**223
Lachmann, F., **82:**511
Laing, R. D., **82:**217
Lake, R. C., et al., **82:**132
Lal, S., **82:**201
Lamb, M. E., **83:**10
Lampl-de Groot, J., **82:**499n1
Landis, D. H., **83:**460
Landis, J. T., **82:**58
Landowski, J., et al., **83:**467
Langer, G., **82:**200; et al., **82:**200, 290
Langer, S. Z., et al., **83:**470
Langer, T. S., **83:**93
Langfeldt, G., **82:**85
Langley, G. E., **83:**125, 137

Langley Porter Psychiatric Institute, **82:**215, 226, 271
Langsley, D. G., et al., **82:**172, 225; **83:**188, 189
Language: and memory, **83:**16, 17–18, 70. See also Speech
LaPierre, Y. D., **83:**500, 506
Laplanche, J., **82:**488, 489
Lapolla, A., **82:**205
Larry, J. C., **82:**100
Larsen, N. E., **83:**497
Larsson, T., et al., **83:**110
Lasch, C., **83:**34, 35–36
Last, U., et al., **82:**461
Late-life psychiatric disorders: affective, **83:**118–130
  assessment of, **83:**116–17
  bipolar illness, **83:**125–26, 285
  depressive, see Depression
  epidemiology/prevalence rate of, **83:**87–92, 95
    historical trends in, **83:**92–93
  etiology of, **83:**90–91, 93–94, 140–51
  late-onset schizophrenia, **83:**91–92, 94–95, 130–132, 138
  manic episode of, **83:**125
  paranoia ("suspiciousness"), **83:**92, 95, 131–37
  physiological changes and, **83:**140–51
  prognosis for, **83:**116
  somatoform, **83:**119, 127, 140–45 passim
  therapy for, **83:**113, 128–30, 141–44 passim (see also Drug therapy; Psychotherapy)
  See also Aging; Anxiety; Dementia, Primary Degenerative; Drug side effect(s); Geriatric psychiatry
Latent stages of development, see Childhood
Laughren, T. P., **82:**135, 203; et al., **82:**135
Law and psychiatry, **82:**321–96
  and drug therapy, **82:**382
  and insanity defense, **82:**387, 389–92
  and law of informed consent, **82:**350–55, 396
  (see also Competency/ incompetency)
  and least restrictive alternative, see Civil commitment
  malpractice claims, **82:**326, 329
  and misdiagnosis, **83:**272
Lawrence, W. G., **83:**30
Lazare-Klerman-Amor Personality Inventory (LKA), **83:**387, 393
Leach, K. A., **82:**429
Learned helplessness: and depression, **82:**286; **83:**412
Learning: in infancy, **83:**11–14
Learning disorders: and borderline personality disorders, **82:**441, 454
  and childhood depression, **82:**277, 286, 287, 302, 306
  hemispheric asymmetry and, **82:**124
Least restrictive alternative, see Civil commitment
Leavy, S. A., **83:**63
LeBlanc, H., et al., **82:**200
Le Bon, G., **83:**22
Leckman, J. F., et al., **83:**448, 467
Lecrubier, Y., et al., **83:**470
Leeman, M. M., **83:**438

Lefave, W. R., **82:**342n31
Leff, Julian P., **82:**88, 102, 104, 105, 172, 173; **83:**174, 175; et al., **82:**102; **83:**245, 246
Leff, M. J., **83:**286, 456
Lefkowitz, M. M., **82:**266, 267–68
Lefkowitz, R. F., **83:**470
Left-handedness: and schizophrenia, **82:**124
Lehmann, H. E., **82:**143; **83:**271, 420; et al., **82:**212
Lehmann, S., **82:**107
Leighton, D. C., et al., **83:**91, 93, 412
LeLord, G., et al., **82:**291
LeMay, M., **82:**124
Lemberger, L., **82:**203
Lentz, R. J., **82:**110, 175
Leon, G. R., et al., **82:**267, 269, 272
Leonhard, K., **83:**269, 272, 275, 368, 423, 441
Lepeshinskaya, O. B., **83:**84
Lepsitt, L. P., **83:**16
Lerner, H., **83:**44
Lerner, P., et al., **82:**127
Lesse, S., **83:**373
Leukemia: Down's syndrome and, **83:**110
Levay, Alexander N., **82:**8, 26, 28, 29, 35
Levine, J., **82:**108, 188, 195; et al., **82:**191, 195
Levine, R. S., **82:**364n9, 367n14
Levine, T. M., **83:**283
Levinson, D., et al., **83:**216
Levinson, H., **83:**33
Levitt, M., **83:**451; et al., **83:**451
Lewin, Kurt, **83:**26
Lewinsohn, P. M., **83:**383, 516–19 passim, 524; et al., **83:**516, 517
Lewinsohn, R., **83:**364
Lewis, J. L., **83:**278, 311
Lewis, J. M., **83:**184, 230, 233
Libb, J. W., **83:**114
Liberman, Robert Paul, **82:**92; **83:**174n, 242n, 245–47 passim, 253, 256, 434; et al., **82:**107, 110–11
Libido theory, **82:**488–89, 490, 511, 512; **83:**15, 41, 49
Libiková, H., et al., **82:**121
Libow, L. S., **83:**108, 119
Lichtenberg, J., **83:**11
Lichtenstein, H., **82:**499n1; **83:**42, 49
Lidz, Theodore, **83:**170, 242; et al., **82:**172
Lieb, J., **83:**483
Liebman, R., et al., **83:**189
Liebowitz, J. H., **83:**271, 442
Liebowitz, M. R., **82:**415, 443, 457, 459, 463; **83:**288; et al., **83:**384, 387, 388
Liedeman, R. R., **82:**117
Lief, H. I., **83:**173, 216
Liem, J. H., **82:**155; **83:**174
Life cycles, see Family, the
Life events, see Stress
Life expectancy, **83:**89. See also Mortality rate
Lindberg, D., **82:**216; **83:**112
Lindelius, R., **82:**93
Lindstrom, L. H., **82:**207
Ling, W., et al., **82:**282, 289, 291
Linkowski, P., **83:**449
Linn, L., **82:**174
Linn, M. W., et al., **82:**175, 177, 227

Linnoila, M., et al., **82**:203; **83**:461
Lipinski, J. F., Jr., **83**:279, 424
Lipinski, T., et al., **82**:212
Lipofucsin: in aging process, **83**:97, 100, 112
Lipowski, Z. J., **83**:107
Lipsedge, M., **82**:102
Lipsitt, D. R., **83**:373
Lipton, F. R., et al., **82**:107
Lipton, R. B., et al., **82**:453
Lishman, W. A., **82**:124
Liston, E. J., Jr., **83**:107
Lithium Clinic (New York State Psychiatric Institute), **83**:296
Lithium therapy, **82**:465; **83**:269, 271, 320
   in bipolar disorder, **82**:444; **83**:126, 249–51
      passim, 272–76 passim, 281–89 passim, 299–
      304, 307–18, 320–37, 368, 375, 380, 439, 466,
      481
   (*see also* in manic states, *below*)
   in borderline disorders, **82**:444, 463–67 passim
   for children, **83**:283
   combined with antipsychotics, **82**:152, 208;
      83:126, 300–301, 302–03
   combined with psychotherapy, **83**:320–37
      clinical reports on, **83**:324–25
   combined with or vs. TCAs, **83**:126, 281, 307,
      311–12, 318, 481–82
   compliance/noncompliance with, **83**:301, 312–
      18 passim, 321–37
   dosage, **83**:126, 299–300, 303, 316–17, 318
   duration of, **83**:315, 318
   and genetic studies of affective disorders,
      83:446, 452–53
   for geriatric patient, **83**:126, 285, 321n
   and high lithium ratio, **83**:452–53
   in manic states, **82**:208, 209; **83**:295–303 pas-
      sim, 359, 453, 454–55
   monitoring of, **83**:470
   vs. placebo, **83**:298, 307, 318, 481
   in schizophrenia/schizoaffective disorders,
      82:136, 152, 208–09, 210–11; **83**:439
   side effects of, **83**:126, 299, 301–02, 313–15,
      321, 326–27, 331–33, 336
   studies of (U.S.), **83**:307, 311, 316–317, 322,
      332–37 passim, 371
   in unipolar depression, **83**:274
   See also Drug therapy
Little, M., **82**:471, 472, 475
Littlewood, R., **82**:102
Litwack, T. R., 82:339n7
Liver disease: drug therapy and, **83**:128
LKA, *see* Lazare-Klerman-Armor Personality
   Inventory
Lloyd, C., **82**:285; **83**:385, 404; et al., **83**:398, 399,
   400
Locher, L. M., **83**:372
Loevinger, Jane, **82**:279, 280
Loew, C. A., **83**:114
Loewald, H., **83**:60
Logan, J., **83**:327–28
London, W. P., **83**:288
Loo, H., et al., **83**:317
Loosen, P. T., **83**:121

LoPiccolo, J. and L., **83**:222n1
Loranger, A. W., **83**:283
Lorge, I., **83**:128
Loss: and childhood depression, **82**:272, 286, 287
   denial of, **83**:277
   and depressive disorders, **83**:395, 399, 400,
      514, 521, 522
   and geriatric paranoia/anxiety, **83**:135–41
      passim
   See also Drug side effect(s); Grief reaction;
      Sensory deficits; Separation and divorce;
      Stress
Lottman, M. S., **82**:363, 365, 366, 367nn14, 15
Lovett, L. C., et al., **82**:118
Low achievement: in borderline patients,
   82:425, 457
Lowell, R., **83**:327
Lowenthal, M. F., **83**:90, 132
Lucas, A. R., **82**:286
Luchins, Daniel J., et al., **82**:124, 145
Ludwig, A., **82**:109
Luisada, P. V., **82**:140
Lundquist, G., **83**:372
Lupus erythematosus, systemic: chlorproma-
   zine and, **82**:118
   resemblance of, to bipolar illness, **83**:287
   schizophrenia and, **82**:117
Luton, F. H., **83**:416
Lydiard, R. B., **83**:487
Lying: as contraindication for supportive psy-
   chotherapy, **82**:481
Lykken, D. T., **82**:453
Lymphocytes: and immune response, **82**:114,
   115, 117–18
   MAO activity in, **82**:147
Lymphoma: in Alzheimer's disease, **83**:110
Lynge, J., **83**:434
Lysenko, T. D., **83**:84
Lyskowski, J., **82**:461

M

Maas, J. W., **83**:459, 460, 461, 474; et al., **82**:144;
   83:459, 461, 468, 473
McAllister, T. W., **83**:107, 109
McCabe, B., **83**:484, 491n
McCabe, L. J., **83**:422
McCabe, M. S., **83**:295, 302, 440, 441
McCahill, T. W., **82**:62
McCombie, S. L., **82**:61
McConville, B. J., et al., **82**:276, 277, 282
McCranie, E. W., **82**:177
McDermott, J. R., et al., **83**:111
McDermott, J., Jr., **83**:239
Macdonald, J. M., **82**:58
McDonald, R. J., **83**:112, 316–17
McFarlane, William R., **83**:172, 220, 244, 248,
   253, 255
McGarry, A. L., et al., **82**:355, 387
McGee, T. E., **83**:115

McGeer, E. G. and P. L., **82:**139
McGhie, A., **83:**90
McGlashan, T. H., **82:**88
McGoldrick, M., **83:**216
McGrath, S. D., et al., **82:**143
McGuffin, P., **82:**121
McHugh, P. R., **83:**107, 289
Mack, J. E., **82:**415, 437
MacKain, K., et al., **83:**13
Mackay, A. V., et al., **82:**134
McKinney, W. T., Jr., **83:**272
Macklin, R., **83:**37, 38, 50
McKnew, D. H., **82:**266, 269, 287, 303; et al., **82:**285; **83:**283
McLaughlin, A. I. G., et al., **83:**111
McLean, C. S., **83:**244n
McLean, P. D., **83:**516, 517, 524, 525
McLean Hospital, **82:**226, 417, 456, 461, 466
MacMahon, B., **83:**87, 89, 94, 406
McMeekan, E. R. L., **82:**124
McNaughten Rule, **82:**391, 392
MacVane, J. R., Jr., et al., **83:**250
Madanes, C., **83:**223, 244, 247, 248–49
Maddox, G. L., **83:**95, 144, 150
Maggi, A., et al., **83:**469
Maggs, R., **83:**298
Mahler, Margaret S., **82:**275, 471, 493, 511; **83:**14, 51; et al., **82:**49, 55, 511; **83:**10, 14
Mahoney, J. J., **83:**516
Main, T. F., **83:**28, 29
Major Depression, **83:**275, 292, 365, 375
  DSM-III category for, **83:**119–20, 367–75 passim, 410, 479, 506
    and supplemental classifications, **83:**375, 379–80
    with melancholia/psychotic features, **83:**120, 121, 125, 126, 367, 370
    with melancholia and without psychotic features, **83:**122–25, 369–70, 506
    without melancholia, **83:**120, 128, 367
  neurotic forms of, **83:**371
  nonbipolar, **83:**287–88, 410
  personality and, **83:**392
  and suicide, **83:**429
  treatment of, **83:**369, 370
    TCA response in, **83:**122–25, 289, 359, 369, 370, 371, 505
  See also Depression; Melancholia; Unipolar/nonbipolar depression
Malan, D. H., **83:**523; et al., **83:**27
Male(s): anatomy of, **82:**9–10 (see also Genitalia)
  catecholamine levels in, **83:**133
  dementia (repeated or multiinfarct) in, **83:**115
  elderly, U.S. population figures, **83:**88
  life expectancy for, **83:**89
  lithium compliance by, **83:**333
  masturbation by, as therapy, **82:**24
  pre- and postmarital sexuality of, **82:**43
  schizophrenia in, **82:**108
  and suicide, **83:**431, 433
  surgery on, **82:**38–39
  See also Orgasm; Sex differentiation
Malignancy: and sexual dysfunction, **82:**37. See also Physical illness

Malih, S. C., **82:**186
Malmquist, C., **82:**58, 266, 274
Malnutrition: and geriatric disorders, **83:**93–94
  and infant depression, **82:**274
  See also Diet
Malone, Charles A., **83:**171, 172, 192, 220, 229–40 passim; et al., **83:**229
Maloney, A. J. F., **83:**109
Malpractice claims, see Law and psychiatry
Mancini, A. M., et al., **82:**201
Mandel, N., **83:**480
Manganese poisoning, **82:**144
Mania: and competency, **82:**354
  defined, **83:**269, 274–75
  drug-induced, **83:**323
  DSM-III concept of, **83:**278–79, 293–95, 296, 357
  dysphoric mood in, **83:**279
  in elderly, **83:**125–26, 285
  lithium treatment of, see Lithium therapy
  morbidity risk of, **82:**290; **83:**287–88
  postpartum, **83:**277
  precipitants of, **83:**277, 287, 311 (see also Drug side effect[s])
  reactive, **83:**277 (see also Grief reaction)
  secondary, **83:**277–78, 279, 287, 294, 296, 297, 376, 381
  See also Hypomania; Manic Episode; Manic state (bipolar I)
Manic-depressive illness, see Bipolar (manic-depressive) Disorder; Major Depression
Manic-Depressive Scale, **83:**336
Manic Episode: childhood, **83:**283
  defined, **83:**423
  diagnosis of, **83:**293–97
  drug therapy for, **83:**293–303, 337
  hypersexuality and, **82:**15
  late-life, **83:**125
  prediction of (D-type scores), **83:**465–66
  See also Bipolar (manic-depressive) Disorder; Mania; Manic state (bipolar I)
Manic state (bipolar I): classification of, **83:**304, 367, 423, 466
  course of, **83:**282, 295–96, 297
  distinguished from other manias, **83:**274, 279
  and drug compliance, **83:**332, 335
  drug-induced, **83:**323, 479–80
  the family and, **83:**250
  lithium treatment of, see Lithium therapy
  morbidity risk for, **83:**439–46 passim
  See also Bipolar (manic-depressive) Disorder; Mania; Manic Episode
Manipulation: as supportive technique, **82:**484; **83:**182
Manipulativeness: in borderline disorders, **82:**457, 464, 465, 467
Mann, D. M. A., **83:**110, 112
Mann, J., **83:**467
Manschreck, T. C., **83:**131
Manton, K. G., **83:**88, 89
Manual of the International Classification of Diseases, Injuries, and Causes of Death, 9th rev., see ICD-9
MAO (monoamine oxidase), **82:**128, 129; **83:**458

Meissner, W. W., **82**:415, 436
Melancholia, **83**:272, 278, 279; **83**:269, 272, 354, 357, 512
  DSM-III use of term, **83**:369
  DST for, **83**:121, 280
  involutional, **83**:367
    among women, **83**:92, 412
  See also Depression, Major Depression
Melick M. E., **82**:361n2
Melin, L., **83**:114
Mellinger, G. D., et al., **83**:95, 412, 413
Mellor, C. S., **83**:289; et al., **83**:289
Mellstrom, B., et al., **83**:500
Meltzer, H. Y., **82**:128–35 passim, 147; et al., **82**:126, 127, 135, 143, 201; **83**:451, 470
Meltzoff, A. N., **83**:12, 13
Memory, **83**:110
  affect, **83**:16–18
  of childhood, Freud's view of, **83**:63
  drug side effects on (impairment or improvement), **83**:113, 336, 475–76
  of geriatric patients, **83**:116, 139
  infant, **83**:15–18
  language and, **83**:16, 17–18, 70
  motor, **83**:16–18
  recall or evocative, **83**:15–16, 17
  recognition, **83**:15, 16, 17
  sleep and, **83**:18
Memory loss, *see* Amnesia
Mendelian theory, **83**:446. *See also* Genetic factors
Mendels, J., **83**:381, 442, 452, 501, 512
Mendlewicz J., **83**:277, 438, 444–51 passim; et al., **83**:440, 441, 448
Mendota State Hospital, **82**:216
Menke's syndrome, **82**:144
Menn, A., **82**:175; **83**:248
Menninger, Karl, **83**:269
Menninger Foundation: Psychotherapy Research Project, **82**:471, 480, 486
Menninger Health-Sickness Scale, **82**:220
Menopause: and depression, **83**:420
  effect of, on vagina, **82**:10
  and hormone replacement therapy, **82**:11, 46; **83**:149
Mental Disability Law Reporter, **82**:332, 348n69
  "Comment," **82**:364n9
Mental element (legal concept), **82**:390, 392. *See also* Law and psychiatry
Mental Health Clinical Research Center for the Study of Schizophrenia (Camarillo State Hospital), **82**:104
Mental Health Law Project, **82**:372–73
Mental health policies: the courts and, **82**:321–27, 335–36, 349. *See also* Law and psychiatry
Mental Health Systems Act, **82**:377
Mental illness: age and, **83**:92
  classification of, **83**:357, 358
  criteria of, **82**:337–39, 348, 349, 370
  denial of, *see* Denial of illness
  difference or deviation distinguished from, **83**:38
  the family and, **83**:173–85 (*see also* Family, the)

insanity differentiated from, **82**:390–91
  among older females, *see* Female(s)
  social factors and, **83**:407 (*see also* Stress)
Mental Patients' Liberation Movement, **83**:248
Mental retardation: and bipolar illness, **83**:289
  and mass deinstitutionalization, **82**:375
  as "mental illness," **82**:337
  treatment of, **83**:527
  and treatment facilities, **82**:378
Mental Status Questionnaire, **83**:116
Menzies, I. E. P., **83**:30
Messier, M., et al., **82**:218
Metabolic diseases: and psychosexual dysfunctions, **82**:37. *See also* Physical illness
Metabolism: aging and, **83**:96, 97, 100, 117, 128, 498
  cerebral, drug treatment of (in dementia), **83**:111–12
  depression studies of, **83**:380
  and free radicals, **83**:97–98
  tricyclics and, **83**:125, 474, 493–506, 508–10
Metals, *see* Aluminum concentration; Manganese poisoning; Zinc concentration
Methionine, **82**:140
  -enkephalin concentrations, **82**:142
Meyer, Adolf, **82**:85; **83**:170, 360, 519
Meyer, Jon K., **82**:8, 48, 52–55 passim; **83**:43n
Meyer, L. C., **82**:62
Meyer, R. E., **82**:140
MFG (multiple family group), *see* Family therapy
MHPG, *see* Urinary MHPG levels
Michaux, M. H., et al., **82**:209
Michael, S. T., **82**:93
Michels, Robert, **82**:351, 355, 483; **83**:7, 8, 65, 68
"Middle game," *see* Psychoanalysis
Midtown Manhattan Study, **83**:92
Mielke, D. H., **82**:213; et al., **82**:201, 204
Miles, A., **83**:94
Miles, C. P., **83**:286–87
Mill, John Stuart, **82**:279
Miller, A. E., et al., **83**:111
Miller, Albert, **83**:457
Miller, D. C., **83**:434
Miller, E., **83**:117
Miller, E. J., **83**:30
Millett, K., **83**:45
Mills, Mark J., **82**:323, 324, 326, 361nn2, 3, 382n5; et al., **82**:351
Milne, J. F., **83**:112
Milner, G., **82**:144
Mims, R. B., et al., **82**:204
Mindus, P., et al., **83**:112
Minerals (diet supplements), **82**:144–45. *See also* Diet
Minimal brain dysfunction, *see* MBD
Minkoff, K., et al., **83**:431
Minn, K., **82**:118
Minnesota Multiphasic Personality Inventory, *see* MMPI
Minors: rights of, **82**:352. *See also* Adolescent(s); Childhood
Minter, R. D., **83**:480

Minuchin, Salvador, **83**:179, 187, 194; et al., **83**:174, 179, 189
Mirabile, C. S., **82**:453
Mirin, S. M., et al., **83**:481
Mirror (selfobject) transference, *see* Transference
Mishler, E. G., **83**:184, 242
Miskimins, R. W., **82**:171
Misogyny: of Freud, **83**:47, 48, 50
Mitscherlich, A., **83**:35
Mizell, T. A., **82**:177
MMPI (Minnesota Multiphasic Personality Inventory): borderline disorder profile in, **82**:429
depressive profiles in, **83**:387
elderly patient scores on, **83**:91
MAO activity decrease and, **82**:126
MNTS (Marke-Nyman Temperament Scale), **83**:386–87
Mob psychology, *see* Group psychology
Modai, I., et al., **83**:468, 474
Modell, A. H., **82**:480, 519; **83**:46, 56, 59
Mohr, J., et al., **82**:57
Moja, E. A., et al., **82**:137
Molholm, H. B., **82**:115
Monahan, J., **82**:393
Money, J., et al., **82**:293; **83**:43
Money-Kryle, R. E., **82**:474
Monnelly, E. P., et al., **83**:426
Monoamine oxidase, *see* MAO
Monroe, R. B., **82**:465
Monroe, S. M., **83**:272
Montgomery, D. B., **83**:434
Montgomery, S. A., **83**:434; et al., **83**:500, 506
Mood disorders, **83**:357
drug therapy for, **82**:463; **83**:480
endocrine disorders and, **83**:379, 422
and mood swings in bipolar illness, **83**:281, 286, 326–30 passim, 334, 374
See also Affective Disorders; Bipolar (manic-depressive) Disorder; Depression; Hypomania; Irritability
Mooney, John J., **83**:356
Moore, B. E., **82**:489, 499n1
Moore, D. F., **82**:185
Moore, M. K., **83**:13
Moore, N. C., **83**:134
Moorhead, P. S., **83**:97
Moos, R. H., et al., **82**:175
Morbid ideation: in childhood depression, **82**:300
Morel, Benedict Augustin, **82**:82; **83**:269
Morgan, R., **82**:193
Morgenthau, H., **83**:37
Morris, J. B., **83**:512
Morris, J. N., **83**:88, 90
Morris, N., **82**:387
Morrison, J. R., **83**:286, 421, 442; et al., **83**:372
Morrissey, J. D., **83**:107
Mortality rate: in bipolar illness, **83**:287
decline in, **83**:88–89
depression and, **83**:366
infant mortality, **82**:274
among older females, **83**:89
psychiatric disorders and, **83**:92
Mortimer, J. A., **83**:107

Mosher, L. R., **82**:110, 159, 170, 175, 177; et al., **82**:175; **83**:248
Mother, the: preoedipal, and crowd psychology, **83**:23, 35, 36
Mother-child relationship: empathic/unempathic, **82**:491–92, 494
and gender disturbance, **82**:50–51, 52, 55
hatred (of mother by child) in, **82**:473
and infant development, **83**:20–21
and narcissism, **82**:522
and schizophrenia, **82**:172
separation in, and childhood depression, **82**:274–75, 306 (*see also* Separation fears)
and sexual dysfunction, **82**:28, 32, 34
See also Parent(s); Parent-child relationship
Motion sickness, **82**:453
Moulton, R., **83**:47
Moyano, C., **82**:184
MPI (Maudsley Personality Inventory), **83**:387, 393
Muchmore, E., **82**:118
Muller, E. E., et al., **82**:201
Multiple sclerosis: viral etiology suspected, **82**:121; **83**:453
Munetz, M. R., et al., **82**:357
Munkvad, I., **82**:137
Murillo, L., **82**:209
Murphy, D. L., **82**:125, 127, 452, 453; **83**:295, 452, 467, 470; et al., **83**:452, 470
Murphy, G. E., **83**:430, 431, 433; et al., **83**:372, 431, 433
Murphy, H. B. M., **82**:120
Murray, H. A., **83**:386
Murray, L. G., **83**:387, 389
Myers, J. K., **82**:103, 281, 283; **83**:91, 271, 275, 374, 408–26 passim; et al., **83**:394
Myerson, P., **83**:56
Myotonia: as sexual response, **82**:12

N

Naber, D., et al., **82**:131, 202
Nachman, P., **83**:16
Nadelson, Carol, **82**:9, 57, 61, 62, 63
Naeser, M., et al., **82**:124
Nair, N. P. V., **82**:144, 201
Najarian, J., **82**:274
Nammalvar, N., **83**:287
Nandy, K., **83**:112
Napier, C. A., **83**:200, 215
Narcissism: "as if" personality in, **82**:515
classification of, **82**:512, 520
concept of, **82**:487, 488–90
as "female quality" (Freud), **83**:42, 43
group ideology and, **83**:23, 24, 25, 30, 35
healthy/normal, **82**:489, 511–12, 518
and child's self-esteem, **82**:301
pathological, **82**:511–12, 518; **83**:55, 59
and sexual dysfunction, **82**:30, 54
(*see also* Narcissistic Personality Disorder)
relationship of, to current society, **83**:35

integration of part to total, **82**:476, 478, 479

internalized, **82**:472–75 passim, 479–80, 512, 513, 520; **83**:24, 49

and marriage problems, **82**:32; **83**:218–19, 251

narcissism and, **82**:488, 494, 495, 512–20 passim

and object loss, *see* Loss

pathological vs. normal, **82**:511

present and past, inability to differentiate, **82**:478

and prognosis, **82**:486, 487

splitting of "good" from "bad," **82**:479

theory of, **83**:7, 49

Object representation: in borderline disorders, **82**:473, 474–75, 479–80

and ego identity, **83**:24

in narcissistic disorder, **82**:493, 511–12, 516, 517, 518

O'Brien, C., et al., **82**:171, 218

Oedipal conflictual disorders, **82**:491

Oedipal issues: and narcissistic disorders, **82**:489, 492, 494, 511–19 passim

and normal oedipal stage, **82**:48, 501, 503, 504

oedipal father, **82**:34–35

and selfobject transferences, **82**:501–08 passim

and sexual dysfunction, **82**:32

Offer, D., **83**:191

Offit, Avodah K., **82**:8

O'Grady, P., **82**:217

Ohman, R., **82**:203; et al., **82**:203

Okuma, T., **83**:312; et al., **83**:310, 311–12

Olin, G. B. and H.S. **82**:357

Oliver, R., **83**:433

Olivier-Martin, R., et al., **83**:505

Olsen, E. J., et al., **83**:112

Onset concept, **82**:103

Op Den Velde, W., **83**:110

Oppenheimer, C., **82**:214

Orchidectomy, **82**:39

Organic Affective Disorder, *see* Affective Disorders

Organic brain disorders: late-life, **83**:91, 94–95, 96, 106–18

and sleep patterns, **83**:145

Organization(s): psychoanalytic approach to, **83**:33

systems theory of, **83**:30–32

See also Group psychology; Therapeutic community

Orgasm: decline in frequency of, **83**:151

effect of childhood sexual assault on capacity for, **82**:58

female, **82**:12, 13, 14, 63

clitoral vs. vaginal, **82**:11; **83**:41

coital, **82**:11, 44, 58; **83**:41

inhibited, **82**:16, 18, 44, 62; **83**:41, 485

multiple, **82**:15, 43

male, **82**:12, 13, 14, 15, 43

inhibited, **82**:16, 18–19

(*see also* Ejaculation)

treatment of dysfunction in, **82**:16, 25, 32

Orley, J., et al., **83**:408, 409, 416

Orlov, P., et al., **82**:205

Orn, H., **82**:100

Ornstein, A., **82**:498, 502, 503

Ornstein, Paul H., **82**:414, 498, 503

Orr, M., **82**:214

Orsulak, Paul J., **83**:356; et al., **83**:467

Ortega, S. T., **82**:100

Ortega y Gasset, J., **83**:36

Orthomolecular psychiatry, **82**:142–46

Orvaschel, H., et al., **82**:284, 285, 286; **83**:283, 404, 421

Osherson, S. E., **83**:173

Osmond, H., **82**:140, 143

Ostfeld, A., et al., **83**:112

Ostow, M., **82**:461; **83**:285

Outpatient treatment: of bipolar illness, **83**:271, 297–98, 303, 326

of depression, **83**:524–25

and diagnosis, **83**:409

of late-life psychiatric disorders, **83**:94–95

of schizophrenia, **82**:159, 162, 171, 219, 228

Ovaries, surgery on, **82**:41. *See also* Surgery

Ovesey, L., **82**:34; **83**:47

P

Pacha, W., **83**:112

Paffenbarger, R. S., **83**:422

Pair-bonding, **82**:30; **83**:39

Pairing: as basic assumption of group, **83**:22, 25, 26

Palmer, A. B., **82**:357

Pallis, D. J., **83**:431

Palmore, E., **83**:103, 105

Palmour, R. M., et al., **82**:141

Pandey, G. N., et al., **82**:136; **83**:452, 470

Panic disorders, **83**:430

atypical depression differentiated from, **83**:127

drug therapy for, **83**:483, 488

late-life, **83**:127, 140–41, 142

See also Agoraphobia

Paprocki, J., **82**:185

Papua: schizophrenia in, **82**:120

Paranoid Personality Disorder: DSM-III criteria for, **82**:470; **83**:135

Paranoid reactions: amphetamines and, **82**:137, 138, 196

in geriatric patients, **83**:92, 95, 131–40

etiology and characteristics of, **83**:132–37, 140

in narcissistic personality disorder, **82**:514, 515, 517, 521

culture shock and, **83**:139

depression and, **83**:330

depression distinguished from, **83**:374

paranoid hallucinosis, **83**:136

sensory deficits/social withdrawal and, **83**:130, 133–39 passim

suspiciousness, **83**:91, 131–39 passim

therapy for, **83**:137, 138–39, 480

Paranoid schizophrenia, *see* Schizophrenia

Paraphilia, **82**:52, 54. *See also* Perversion(s)

Paraphrenia: differentiated from paranoid schizophrenia, **83:**137
late-life, **82:**149; **83:**107, 131, 133, 137–38
See also Schizophrenia
Parent(s): of adult children, **83:**199, 211
aging, **83:**212
alliance vs. splitting of, **83:**232–33
death of, *see* Death
depression of, and child depression, **82:**285, 286
and parental imagos, **82:**501
of schizophrenics, **83:**175–76, 243, 247
-therapist relationship (in child therapy), **82:**264 (*see also* Therapeutic relationship)
See also Family, the; Family therapy; Father, the; Mother, the; Mother-child relationship; Oedipal issues; Parent-child relationship
Parent-child relationship: conflict in, **83:**218
empathy in, **83:**19–20
family therapy and, **83:**192, 210, 211–12, 241
loyalty, in, **83:**219
and prediction of child development, **83:**229–30
role reversal in, **83:**231–32
and schizophrenia, **82:**155; **83:**175, 247
See also Family, the; Mother-child relationship; Object relations
Paris, J. J., **82:**325
Parkinson's disease, **83:**101, 109, 128
parkinsonian symptoms, **82:**204–05; **83:**100
See also Drug side effect(s)
Parloff, M. B., **83:**512
Parsons, H. V., 190
Parsons, P. L., **83:**424
Parsons, Talcott, **83:**142
Pasamanick, B., et al., **82:**225
Passive-aggressive type: and sexual dysfunction, **82:**15
Passivity: as "female" quality, **83:**42, 43
Patient: compliance/noncompliance with drug therapy by, *see* Drug therapy
consent to or refusal of treatment by, *see* Therapy
responsibility of, in therapy, *see* Responsibility
role of, **82:**327 (*see also* Therapeutic relationship)
selection of, for psychoanalysis, **83:**51–52, 60
-staff relations, **83:**29–30, 139
See also Relationships
Patrick, V., et al., **83:**395
Patterson, G. R., **83:**174
Paul, G. L., **83:**110, 175; et al., **82:**169–70, 175
Paul, N. L., **83:**235
Paul, S. M., et al., **83:**470
Pauling, Linus, **82:**142, 145; et al., **82:**143
Paulson, G. W., et al., **83:**115
Pauly, Ira B., **82:**8; **83:**147n
Pausanius, **83:**83
Paykel, E. S., **82:**459, 466; **83:**365, 366; et al., **83:**372, 390, 393, 394, 395, 414
Payne, E. C., et al., **82:**61
PEA (phenylethylamine) hypothesis, *see* Schizophrenia, etiology of

Peake, G. T., **82:**203
Pearce, J., **82:**282, 289
Peckhold, J. C., et al., **82:**205
Pederson, A. M., et al., **83:**415, 417, 419
Peet, M., et al., **82:**208
Penfield, P. S., **82:**284
Penis, **82:**12, 18, 23
anatomy of, **82:**9–10
anxiety over size or absence of, **82:**9, 34
and clitoral stimulation, **82:**10–11
nocturnal tumescence (NPT) of, **82:**37–38, 46
stimulation of, in dual-sex therapy, **82:**21–22; **83:**151
See also Erection
Penis envy, **82:**55; **83:**39
changing theories regarding, **83:**40–41, 43–48
Freud's theory of, **83:**40–48 passim
Pennes, H., **82:**458, 462
Pennsylvania Mental Health Procedures Act (1976), **82:**352
Perception-behavior relationship, **83:**18
Perel, James M., **83:**356, 492; et al., **83:**494, 498–504 passim, 508
Peroutka, S. J., **83:**469
Perris, C., **83:**269, 272, 292, 368, 406, 423, 438–41 passim, 447
Perry, E. K., et al., **83:**109, 110
Perry, J. C., **82:**11, 415, 419, 420, 423, 425, 428, 431–36 passim, 456
Persad, E., **83:**303
Persico, M. G., et al., **83:**449
Person, Ethel S., **82:**34; **83:**7, 8, 37, 42, 46, 49
Personality: -depression relationship, **83:**364–65, 380, 382, 383, 385–94, 405, 421, 432–33
interpersonal phenomena and, **83:**170
Personality disorders, **82:**14, 429; **83:**354
in bipolar illness, **83:**281, 282, 286, 288–89, 312
coexisting, **82:**455
depression distinguished from, **83:**365, 403
and psychosexual dysfunctions, **82:**15, 17, 18, 19
and suicide, **83:**429
See also individual disorders
Personality Factor Questionnaire (16), **83:**387, 392
Persson, E., **82:**207
Peruzza, M., **83:**148
Perversion(s), **82:**32, 33, 34; **83:**190
as defense against psychosis, **82:**58
gender dysphoria and, **82:**56
and transsexualism, **82:**52, 54 (*see also* Transsexualism)
See also Psychosexual dysfunctions
PET (positron emission tomography), *see* CT (computed tomography) findings
Peters, J. J., **82:**58, 61, 62; et al., **82:**62
Peterson, M. R., **82:**120
Petterson, U., **83:**287, 438
Petti, T. A., **83:**284, 296
Pfeiffer, C. C., **82:**144; et al., **82:**144
Pfeiffer, Eric, **82:**46, 47; **83:**87, 116, 129–30, 141–50 passim; et al., **83:**147, 148
Phallus: symbolism of, **82:**9
Pharmacokinetics: defined, **83:**492
Pharmacotherapy, *see* Drug therapy

Phenylethylamine (PEA) hypothesis, *see* Schizophrenia, etiology of
Pheochromocytoma: as drug side effect, 83:128
Philadelphia Child Guidance Clinic, 82:264
Philips, Irving, 82:264, 265, 268, 284, 285
Phillips, L., 82:108
Phillips Premorbid Scale, 82:108
Physical examination, need for, 83:296
    of elderly patient, 83:116–17, 119, 122–23, 125, 143
    lithium therapy and, 83:299
    sex therapy and, 82:21, 37
Physical handicap: and childhood depression, 82:276, 286
Physical harm, *see* Battered wives/husbands; Child abuse; Violence
Physical illness: and affective disorder, 83:378
    aging and, 83:109
    and depression, 83:118–19, 361, 365, 366, 378–80
        childhood depression vs., 82:306–07
    the family and, 83:169, 193, 195, 213–14
    mandatory reporting of disease, 82:332
    mania precipitated by, 83:277, 287
    the psychiatrist and, 82:36, 41
    and psychosexual dysfunctions, 82:15, 35–38, 41; 83:150
    and sexual activity (as "taboo"), 82:46
    stress and, 83:381
    and TCA therapy, 83:497, 498, 509
    See also Cardiac disorders; Diet; Drug side effect(s); Endocrine system; Infection(s); Mental illness; Psychosomatic disorders; Somatic symptoms; Stroke; Surgery; Vascular disorders; Viruses
Physician: as healer, 83:173, 184. *See also* Primary care physician; Therapist, the
Physicians' Desk Reference, 83:484
Piafsky, K. M., 83:495, 497; et al., 83:497
Piaget, Jean, 82:276, 278; 83:13, 16
Pick's disease, 83:109. *See also* Dementia, Primary Degenerative
Pike, E., 83:495
Pinder, R., et al., 83:486
Pitts, F. N., Jr., 83:434
Plasma factors/levels: age and, 83:123–24, 128, 498, 499, 509–10
    clinical indications of, 83:508–11
    in depressive disorders, 83:121, 122
    in lithium therapy, 83:299, 316–17
    monitoring of, 83:123, 125, 299, 470–71, 477, 492, 498–500, 503–07
        assay methods, 83:500–503
        collection of samples, 83:501–03
        cost of, 83:508, 509
        criteria for studies, 83:504
        preconditions for, 83:507–08
    in schizophrenia etiology and treatment, 82:118–19, 126–36 passim, 141, 144, 147, 182–83, 190, 200–203
    tests of, *see* DST (dexamethasone suppression test); TRH/TSH response test
    tricyclics and, 83:123–24, 125, 477, 480, 486, 491–511

imipramine, 82:292, 295; 83:477, 480, 497–500 passim, 504–11 passim
    neuroleptics and TCAs combined, 83:125
Plath, Sylvia, 83:428–29, 434
Platman, S. B., 83:300
Platt, J. J., 82:109; et al., 82:109
Platt, S., et al., 82:227
Play, symbolic, 82:276
Plotkin, R., 82:382
Pneumoencephalography, 82:122
Pokorny, A. D., 82:198
Polatin, P., 82:444, 462; 83:326, 328, 331
Police: and civil commitment, 82:385
    depression and alcoholism among, 82:385
Pollack, M., et al., 83:479
Pollin, W., 82:451; et al., 82:94, 95, 451
Pollock, H. M., 83:293
Polvan, O., 82:291
Polydipsia, 83:302, 313
Polysomnographic studies, *see* REM (Rapid eye movement) sleep
Polyuria, 83:302, 313, 336
Ponce de Leon, Juan, 83:83
Pontalis, J. B., 82:488, 489
Pope, H. G., 83:279, 424; et al., 82:152
Porter, R., 83:133–34
Positron emission tomography (PET), *see* CT (computed tomography) findings
Posner, J. B., 83:108
Post, F., 83:108, 118, 131, 132, 136–39 passim, 285, 287
Post, R. M., 83:303, 311, 312, 461; et al., 83:461
Potkin, Steven G., et al., 82:126, 137, 146
Pottenger, M., et al., 83:374
Potter, W. Z., 83:461; et al., 83:494, 499
Pourmand, M., et al., 82:200
Powell, W. J., 82:361, 364n9
Poznanski, Elva, 82:264, 266, 267, 274, 275, 277, 284–89 passim, 294, 301; et al., 82:296–300 passim, 304, 305
Prange, A. J., 82:290; 83:121, 460
Prediction of behavior, *see* Psychiatrist, the
Pregnancy: illegitimate, incestuous relationships and, 82:58
    lithium treatment during, 83:314, 321n
Presbycusis, *see* Hearing loss
Presbyopia, *see* Vision
Present State Examination, *see* PSE
Presidential Commission on Pornography (1970s), 82:7
Preskorn, S., 82:292; 83:476, 477, 478
Preventative psychiatry, *see* Psychiatry
Price, J., 83:444
Price, T. R. P., 83:107, 109
Prien, Robert F., 82:188–94 passim; 83:270, 298, 300, 311, 312, 316, 482; et al., 82:188, 210; 83:298–302 passim, 307–13 passim, 371, 481
Prilipko, L. L., 82:117
Primary care physician: and elderly patients, 83:95
    and explanation of treatment (competency), 82:356
    and sexual adjustments, 82:47
    See also Physician

Primary Degenerative Dementia, see Dementia, Primary Degenerative
Primary self pathology, 82:414
  psychoanalytic psychotherapy of, 82:498–510, 516
  See also Narcissistic Personality Disorder
Primitive defenses, see Defense mechanisms
Prince, R. M., Jr., et al., 82:171
Principles of Medical Ethics with Annotations Especially Applicable to Psychiatry (American Psychiatric Association), 82:329
Prinz, P., et al., 83:133
Prison(s): bipolar illness in population of, 83:288
  confinement in, of manic patient, 83:297
  therapy in, 82:386, 395–96
Privacy: elderly right to, 83:150
  vs. supervision of family therapy, 83:183
  See also Confidentiality
Privacy Protection Study Commission, 82:330, 331
PRL (prolactin) response, see Drugs
Pro, J. D., 83:108
Problem of the Aged Patient in the Public Psychiatric Hospital, The (GAP report), 83:85
Problem-solving skills: schizophrenia and, 82:108, 109, 112. See also Coping capacities
Procci, W. R., 83:291
Professional Standards Review Organization, 82:332
Projective identification, 82:474; 83:22, 190, 218, 235
Prolactin response (PRL), see Drugs
Promiscuity, 82:58; 83:190
Prostate problems: drug therapy and, 83:476
  prostatectomy, 82:39
Prostitution: childhood incest or rape and, 82:58
Protein factors, 82:117, 119; 83:110
  Duarte protein, 83:451, 453
  tricyclics and, 83:495, 497
Prudo, R., 83:400, 401, 404
Prusoff, B. A., 83:372; et al., 82:209
Pruyser, P. W., 82:83
Pryce, I. G., 82:358
PSE (Present State Examination), 82:100; 83:408, 409, 427
Pseudodementia, depressive, see Dementia, Primary Degenerative
Psychiatric chemistry: and depressive disorders, 83:457–71. See also Drug therapy
Psychiatric medicine, 83:172, 183–84. See also Drug therapy
Psychiatrist, the: and competency issue, 82:351–59 passim
  as double agent, 82:393, 396
  and gender disturbance cases, 82:54
  and life-threatening illness, 82:36, 41
  -physician cooperation, 82:36, 61, 356; 83:478
  and postsurgical problems, 82:38–41 passim
  prediction of behavior by, 82:172, 385, 393, 394, 395, 396; 83:220, 229
  and psychotherapy, 82:162, 215
  in public sector, see Psychiatry
  responsibility of, toward professionals and public, 82:287, 388

role of, in criminal justice system, 82:384–96
  as specialist best suited to deal with dementia, 83:117
  standard of care for, 82:329
  See also Therapeutic relationship; Therapist, the
Psychiatry: child, see Child psychiatry
  effect on, of psychopharmacologic treatment, 83:269
  forensic, 82:326, 384–96
  geriatric, see Geriatric psychiatry
  German, influence of on nosology, 82:82
  government regulation of, 82:325–26, 353, 368
  hostility toward/distrust of, 83:40, 129
    court antipathy to, 82:322–23, 336, 339
  in jails, 82:386
  law and, 82:321–96
  open-systems theory of, 83:31
  orthomolecular, 82:142–46
  preventative, 82:281, 287–88
  and psychiatric classicism, 82:86
  and psychiatric epidemiology, see Epidemiology
  public health, 82:281
  public-sector, 82:321, 324, 368, 388, 393
  in U.S., influences on, 82:85–86
Psychiatry 1982 (*Psychiatry Update Volume I*), 83:28n, 43n, 131n, 147n, 174n, 242n, 354, 355, 497n
Psychoanalysis, 83:184, 385
  analyst's task in, 82:497; 83:55, 59–60, 65–66
  biological assumptions of, 83:47–48
  for bipolar illness, 83:319–20, 329
  and borderline disorders, 82:436–37, 471, 472, 481, 482
  changes in approach to and scope of, 83:7, 8, 40–44, 48–60, 66, 67
  childhood, 83:55, 192
  childhood depression studies influenced by, 82:266, 272
  contraindications for, 82:56, 481
  criticisms of, 83:39, 40, 46–47
  defined, 83:36, 70
  empathic point of view in, 82:493, 496–97
  female psychology and, 83:38–45, 47–50
  group psychology theories and, 83:7–8, 33
  imitation of, in supportive psychotherapy, 82:485
  infancy research implications for, 83:7, 8–21
  interpretation(s) in, 83:55–56, 59
    bias in, 83:46
    content of, 83:62–65, 68
    defined, 83:61, 67
    Freud's first use of term, 83:63
    functions of, 83:61–62, 66–67
    of past and present, 83:62–65, 66, 68–70
    and selection of what to interpret, 83:65
    and the therapeutic process, 83:61–62, 69–70
  Kohut's redefinition of, 82:495, 496
  lack of systematic verification in, 83:46–47
  as "middle (chess) game," 83:51–59 passim
  and narcissism, 82:487–98, 499, 505–10, 512–20

Q

Sager, C. J., **83:**190, 199, 217, 218, 223; et al., **83:**215

Sainsbury, P., **83:**430, 431

St. Elizabeth's Hospital case (Washington, D.C.), **82:**372–77 passim

Salapatek, P., **83:**10

Saldanha, V. F., et al., **82:**204

Salk, D., **83:**110

Salzman, C., **82:**209

Salzman, R., **83:**112

Sameroff, A. J., **83:**229, 230

Samorajski, T., **83:**99, 115

Sander, L., **83:**14, 18

Sandler, J., **82:**272–73, 503; et al., **83:**61

Sandler, M., **82:**137; **83:**452; et al., **83:**467

Sandoz Pharmaceuticals, **83:**102, 104

Sartorius, N., et al., **82:**100

Satir, V., **83:**189

Saunders, J. C., **82:**118

Scafa, G. M., **82:**146

Scandinavia: depressive symptom studies in, **83:**407, 413, 423, 426

schizophrenia studies in, **82:**94, 98, 145

Scapegoating, **83:**210, 233–34, 239, 240

Schaefer, M., **83:**40

Schafer, R., **82:**497; **83:**41, 45, 48, 63

Schaie, K. W., **83:**117

Schanberg, S. M., et al., **83:**460

Schatzberg, Alan F., **83:**321, 356, 475, 481, 488, 512; et al., **83:**459, 461, 462, 468, 473, 475, 479, 490

Schedule(s): for Affective Disorders and Schizophrenia, *see* SADS

for Interviewing Borderlines (SIB), *see* Borderline Personality Disorder, diagnosis of

for Schizotypal Personalities (SSP), **82:**432

Scheibel, M. E. and A. G., **83:**100

Schenk, G. K., et al., **82:**214

Scherl, D. S., **82:**61

Schiavone, D. J., **82:**128

Schick, J. F. E., **82:**461

Schiele, B. C., **82:**185

Schiffman, S., **83:**104

Schildkraut, Joseph J., **83:**356, 457, 459, 468, 469; et al., **82:**452; **83:**460–47 passim, 473, 474, 512

Schizoaffective Disorder, **82:**144, 438, 439; **83:**282, 283, 358

as bipolar variant, **83:**439, 441–42, 447, 457, 462, 464, 465, 480

criteria for, **82:**152; **83:**290–92, 302, 376, 441, 462

genetic studies of, **83:**439–42, 446

medication for, **82:**208, 209; **83:**439

and suicide, **83:**429, 430

Schizophrenia: American concept of, **82:**86; **83:**269

borderline personality disorder compared to, discriminated from, related to, **82:**416, 436, 439–43 passim, 444–57 passim

childhood, **82:**108, 263, 306

communication deviance in, **82:**155; **83:**242, 247, 280

"core deficit" in, **82:**173, 209

decompensation in, **82:**88, 100, 103, 106, 163, 177

definitions (cross-sectional and longitudinal clinical pictures) of, **82:**84, 85–91, 100–101, 108

depression associated with, **83:**291, 376, 379, 381, 466, 467

developmental-interactive model of, **82:**161–66

diagnosis of, **82:**83, 93, 123, 138, 162, 166–68

in adoptive studies, **82:**445–48

computerized, **82:**100

criteria for, **82:**83–91 passim, 98, 101–02, 113, 149, 167, 423, 432, 448; **83:**131, 271, 282

differential, **83:**131, 278, 282, 285, 289–92, 358–59

and misdiagnosis, **82:**101–02, 120; **83:**281, 284, 285, 290

in U.S., **82:**86; **83:**271, 293, 407

epidemiology/prevalence rate of, **82:**93, 95–96, 98, 120–21, 290, 445; **83:**271, 407

diet (gluten) and, **82:**145–46

ethnic groups and, **82:**101, 102

family history and, **83:**132, 283, 439, 441

social class and, **82:**98, 100, 101; **83:**426

(*see also* late-onset, *below*)

etiology of, *see* Schizophrenia, etiology of, *below*

genetic studies of (in twins), **82:**94–95; **83:**441

history of concept of, **82:**82–83

International Study of (WHO), **82:**100

late-onset, **83:**91–92, 94–95, 130–32, 138, 140, 144

and marital status, **83:**427

paranoid, **82:**86

biochemical factors in, **82:**115, 126, 131, 132, 137–38, 142, 148, 152, 197

blacks with, **82:**102; **83:**270

classification of, **82:**86, 149

late-life, **83:**132, 144

misdiagnosis of, **83:**281

paraphrenia differentiated from, **83:**137 (*see also* Paraphrenia)

prediction of, **82:**172; **83:**175–76

premorbid functioning and, **82:**89, 90, 98, 100, 108, 109, 122, 149, 150

prognosis for, **82:**87–89, 115, 167–68

chronicity and, **82:**177

cultural and social factors in, **82:**100, 101, 107, 108

recovery, **82:**88, 89, 90, 101, 115, 154; **83:**282

vocational rehabilitation and, **82:**109–10

(*see also* relapse in, *below*)

pseudoneurotic, **82:**444, 457, 462, 468

relapse in

avoidance of, **82:**163; **83:**171, 244, 245

EE (expressed emotion) and, **82:**103–05, 110, 111, 172, 173–74; **83:**175, 242–47 passim, 249, 256

family factors and, **82:**103–06, 107, 110, 112, 172–74; **83:**171, 175–76, 242–49

medication and, **82:**102, 104, 142–43, 168–72, 190–95

model of, **82:**99

PRL (blood prolactin) as predictor of, **82:**135

rehabilitation efforts (social pressures, so-

Schweitzer, J. W., et al., **82**:137
Schwimm, C., et al., **82**:204
Schyve, D. M., et al., **82**:202
Scoggins, B. A., et al., **83**:500
Scott, A. W., Jr., **82**:342n31
Scott, F. B., et al., **83**:151
Scott, M., et al., **83**:470
Scott, R. A., **83**:173, 184
Scott, R. E., **83**:470
Scott-Strauss, A., **83**:442
Searles, H. F., **82**:161, 472
Secrets, *see* Confidentiality
Secunda, S. K., et al., **83**:512
Sedvall, G., **82**:201; et al., **83**:452
Seeman, P. P., et al., **83**:134, 196
Segal, H., **82**:474
Segawa, T., et al., **83**:469
Self: bipolar, **82**:491–92, 494, 502–05
  concept of, **82**:490–96 passim, 502, 504, 511
  defined (Kohut), **82**:500
  -ego distinction, Freud and, **82**:488, 489
  -idealization, *see* Narcissistic Personality
    Disorder
  narcissistic, **82**:494 (*see also* Narcissism)
  -other fusion (in infancy), **83**:14
  -representation
    in borderline disorders, **82**:473, 474–75, 479
    in narcissistic disorder, **82**:493, 511–12, 516,
      517, 518
  and self pathology, **82**:504–05
  sense of (individuation)
    adolescent and young adult, **83**:192, 211
    infant, **83**:14–15, 19
  separation-individuation phase and prob-
    lems of, **82**:49, 51; **83**:35, 235–36, 247
  See also Ego
Self-destructiveness, **82**:345
  in borderline disorders, **82**:424, 450, 481, 485,
    486
  in narcissistic personality disorder, **82**:515,
    520
  See also Suicide and attempted suicide
Self-esteem: in bipolar disorder, **83**:281
  in borderline disorders, **82**:462
  in depression, **83**:364, 365, 373, 387, 392, 511,
    514–15, 517
    childhood depression, **82**:272, 276, 277– 78,
      286, 296, 301, 305
    of elderly, **83**:106, 129, 130, 141
    narcissism and, **82**:488–94 passim, 504, 515, 522
    of rape victim, **82**:66
    of schizophrenic patient, **83**:291
Selfobject, **82**:492, 496, 501–02, 509, 510
  oedipal, **82**:501, 503, 504, 505
  transference, **82**:499–508 passim
Self psychology, **82**:516
  development of, **82**:497–504; **83**:7
  See also Ego psychology
Seligman, M. E. P., **82**:267, 286; **83**:364, 383
Selman, F. B., et al., **82**:180, 186
Seltzer, B., **83**:109
Selvini-Palazzoli, M., et al., **83**:247
Semantic techniques (cognitive therapy),
  83:515
Senescence, **83**:96. *See also* Aging

Senile dementia, *see* Dementia, Primary De-
  generative
Senile macular degeneration, **83**:103. *See also*
  Vision
Senility, **83**:94, 96. *See also* Aging
Sensate focus exercises, *see* Sex therapy
Sensation-Seeking Scale, **83**:336
Sensorimotor response: of newborn, **83**:11
Sensory deficits: age-related, **83**:102–04, 133–34,
    136, 137
  and paranoia, **83**:133–34, 136, 137, 140
  smell, and taste, sense of, **83**:104
  See also Hearing loss; Vision
Sentencing, psychiatry and, **82**:392–95. *See also*
  Law and psychiatry
Separation and divorce: bipolar illness and,
    83:250, 286, 426, 456
  depression and, **83**:366
  and depressive symptoms, **83**:380, 399, 413
  effects of, on child, **82**:277
  family or couples therapy in, **83**:189, 192–93,
    226, 227–28
  and paranoia, **83**:133
  and postmarital sexuality, **82**:41–45
  psychosexual dysfunction and, **82**:36
  "six stations of divorce," **83**:227–28
  trial separation, in couples therapy, **83**:226
Separation fears: vs. childhood depression,
    82:306
  of prepubertal children, **82**:269
  of "pretranssexual" children, **82**:51
  and sexual dysfunction, **82**:32
Separation-individuation, *see* Self
Serotonin: aging and, **83**:96–97, 127
  in Alzheimer's disease, **83**:110
  drug effect on, **82**:196; **83**:474, 482, 483, 489,
    490, 508
  hypothesis (of schizophrenia), **82**:129–30
  and depressive disorders, **83**:459, 460, 474,
    482, 489
  and serotonin metabolite (5-HIAA), **83**:431,
    446, 452, 470
Seth, S., et al., **82**:185
Sethy, V. H., **83**:488
Sex: as term, **82**:49
Sex differentiation: in bipolar illness, **83**:424,
    427–28
  in dementia, **83**:107, 115
  in depression, **82**:284; **83**:411–13, 415–20, 422,
    427–28
    childhood depression, **82**:284
  in hypochondriasis, **83**:142
  in late-life sexual activity, **83**:148
  in lithium side effects/compliance, **83**:333, 334,
    335
  in schizophrenic illness (among elderly),
    83:132
  in sleep patterns, **83**:145
  in suicide rate, **83**:433
Sex Information and Education Council of the
  United States (SIECUS), **82**:7
Sexism: in psychotherapies, **83**:38–40
Sex reassignment, **82**:48, 51, 53, 55, 56
  therapist's attitude toward, **82**:54
  See also Gender identity

childhood depression, **82**:290, 293–97 passim, 304

as drug side effect, **83**:124, 485

hypersomnia, **83**:279, 281, 282, 480

sleep apnea, **83**:147

See also Insomnia

Sloane, P., **82**:57

Sloane, R. Bruce, **83**:87, 108, 116

Slovenko, R., **82**:330

Small, J., et al., **82**:209, 211

Smell, sense of, *see* Sensory deficits

Smeraldi, E., et al., **83**:273, 438, 446, 449

Smith, C. B., **83**:474, 489

Smith, C. G., **82**:175

Smith, D. E., **82**:140

Smith, J. M., **82**:147

Smith, J. S., et al., **83**:109

Smith, K., et al., **82**:209

Smith, R. C., et al., **82**:135, 183, 196, 202

Smith Kline & French Laboratories, **83**:320

Smooth pursuit eye movement, *see* SPEM

Smythies, J., **82**:129, 140

Snaith, R. P., et al., **83**:391, 393

Sneznevsky, A. V., **82**:88

Snow, C., **83**:20

Snowden, P. R., et al., **83**:110, 111

Snowdon, J., **83**:107

Snyder, K. K., **82**:98

Snyder, S. H., **82**:196; **83**:101, 469; et al., **82**:196

Sobel, D., **82**:26

Sobel, E., **83**:446

Social class: and bipolar illness, **83**:286, 425–28 passim

and depression, **82**:284–85; **83**:413, 420, 428

and paranoia, **83**:133

and schizophrenia, **82**:98, 100, 101

selection-drift phenomenon in, **82**:98, 100, 112

Social competence, *see* Coping capacities

Social Diagnosis (Richmond), **83**:169–70

Social factors, *see* Stress

Social isolation: geriatric disorders and, **83**:130, 133–40 passim. *See also* Withdrawal, social

Social Security, **83**:106

Social skills: and depression, **83**:383, 517, 520, 527

childhood depression, **82**:302

family therapy training for, **83**:246–47

learning techniques for, **83**:517–18, 521, 524

MAO activity and (introversion, extraversion), **83**:467

Social support networks: and depression, **83**:364, 414, 521

and late-life psychiatric disorders, **83**:94

and schizophrenia, **82**:106–07; **83**:244

See also Health care system; Relationships

Society for Sex Therapy and Research (SSTAR), **82**:7

Sociopathy, **82**:440

Soininen, H., et al., **83**:109

Soloff, L. A., **82**:36

Soloff, P. H., **82**:417, 421–29 passim, 443

Solomon, A, **83**:401, 403, 404

Solomon, G. F., **82**:117; et al., **82**:115

Solomon, L., **83**:195

Solomon, M., **83**:433

Somatic symptoms: childhood depression and, **82**:304–05

drug therapy and, **83**:128 (*see also* Drug therapy)

of elderly patient, **83**:119, 127, 140–45 passim

See also Physical illness; Psychosomatic disorders

Sommer, C., **82**:225

Sommer, R., **83**:114

Sørensen, A., **83**:416

Sorensen, B., et al., **83**:505

Soskis, D. A., **82**:155, 357

Soteria project, **82**:175; **83**:248

Sourcebook on Aging, **83**:88

South Africa: schizophrenia in, **82**:101

Soviet Union **83**:34, 84

immunologic and virus studies in, **82**:119, 120

Sovner, R. D., **83**:289; et al., **82**:357

Spar, J. E., **83**:117

Sparacino, J., **83**:136

Spark, G. M., **83**:199, 219, 223

Spark, R. F., **82**:37

Spaulding, E., **82**:449, 453

Speech: infant learning of sounds of, **83**:11, 12, 20

poverty of content (vagueness), **82**:123; **83**:279, 289

retardation of, childhood depression and, **82**:303

See also Language

Spelke, E. S., **83**:13

SPEM (smooth pursuit eye movement): impaired, **82**:453

Spicer, C. C., et al., **83**:285, 425

Spiegel, John, **83**:170

Spiker, Duane G., **83**:480; et al., **83**:468, 474, 509

Spiro, H. R., **82**:288; **83**:286

Spitz, René, **82**:274, 283, 293

Spitzer, R. L., **83**:408; et al., **82**:270, 289, 293, 296, 298, 305, 419–41 passim, 448–53 passim; **83**:273, 278, 407, 408, 512

Spivack, G., et al., **82**:109

Splitting, *see* Defense mechanisms (primitive)

SPMSQ (Short Portable Mental Status Questionnaire), **83**:116

Spohn, H. E., **82**:383n6; et al., **82**:199, 383n6

Spring, B., **82**:98, 103

Spring, G., et al., **83**:300

Springarn, N. D., **82**:332

Spruiell, V., **82**:489

Squire, L. R., **83**:126

Sri Lanka; schizophrenia in, **82**:101

Srole, L., **83**:92; et al., **82**:283

SSP (Schedule for Schizotypal Personalities), **82**:432

SSTAR (Society for Sex Therapy and Research), **82**:7

Stabenau, J. R., **82**:451

Stack, J. J., **82**:291

Staff, *see* Nursing staff

Stallone, F., et al., **83**:297, 307, 309

Stam, F. C., **82**:208; **83**:110

and psychosexual dysfunctions, **82**:38–41, 46; **83**:151
  as "punishment," **82**:38, 41
  sex-reassignment, **82**:7, 48, 53–56
Suskind, G. W., **83**:98
Suslak, L, et al., **83**:440
Suspiciousness, *see* Paranoid reactions
Sutherland, J. D., **83**:27, 28
Sutherland, S., **82**:61
Suzuki, S., **82**:137
Sviland, M. A., **82**:47
Swann v. Charlotte-Mecklenburg Board of Education, **82**:366
Swift, Jonathan, **83**:83
Swinburne, H., **83**:145
Switzerland: bipolar illness studies in, **83**:423
Symbiotic phase, *see* Infancy
Symbolic play, **82**:276
Symonds, M., **82**:385
Syndrome approach, **82**:82–83
Systems theory: family, *see* Family therapy
  of organizations, **83**:30–32
  and systems level concept of psychopathology, **83**:176, 177
Szasz, T. S., **82**:336, 351
Szulecka, T. K., **82**:108

T

Tabrizi, M. A., et al., **82**:292
Taiwan: schizophrenia studies in, **82**:98
Takahashi, R., et al., **83**:299, 300
Takahasi, S., **83**:452, 467; et al., **82**:290
Talvenheimo, J., et al., **83**:470
Tamminga, C. A., et al., **82**:136, 139, 141, 196, 203
Tanna, V. L., **83**:448; et al., **83**:450
Taraxein, **82**:118–19
Tardive dyskinesia: and endocrine effects, **82**:136, 203–04
  risk of, **83**:272, 480, 487
  See also Drug side effect(s)
Targum, S. D., **83**:456; et al., **83**:449, 450, 457
Tartakoff, H., **82**:511
Taste, sense of, *see* Sensory deficits
TAT (Thematic Apperception Test), **82**:216
Taube, C. A., **83**:94, 95
Taube, S. L., et al., **83**:461
Tauro, Judge Joseph, **82**:381n3, 383n6
Tavistock Clinic (Leicster, England), **83**:32
Taylor, B. M., **83**:288
Taylor, D. P., **83**:488
Taylor, L., **82**:332
Taylor, M. A., **82**:152; **83**:273, 279, 440, 443; et al., **83**:279, 438
TCA (tricyclic antidepressant) response, **83**:458–59, 472–82, 489, 526
  in bipolar illness, **83**:126, 273–81 passim, 289, 312, 317, 371, 380
  in combination with other drugs or ECT, **83**:125, 126, 382, 479, 480, 481, 485, 503

dosage and, **83**:123–26, 317, 476–77, 483, 485, 487, 495, 497, 504, 508, 509
  "first-pass" effect in, **83**:495
  poor or adverse, **83**:370, 380, 381, 399–400, 479–80, 481, 487, 503, 508 (*see also* and side effects, *below*)
lithium response vs., **83**:308, 311, 481
in nonbipolar or major depression, **83**:122–25, 289, 359, 369–71 passim, 381, 505, 512, 526
in panic disorder (in elderly), **83**:142
plasma levels in, **83**:123–24, 125, 474, 477, 480, 486, 491–511
prediction of, **83**:125, 381, 468
sedative vs. stimulating, **83**:476, 508
and side effects, **82**:467; **83**:123, 127, 474–77, 480, 485–88 passim, 497, 508
  hypomania as, **83**:273–77 passim, 280, 368, 375, 479
  mania/manic episode as, **83**:126, 311
stress and, **83**:399–400
and withdrawal effects, **83**:481
See also Drugs; Drugs, list of; Drug side effect(s); Drug therapy; Imipramine
Tellenbach, H., **83**:374
Temple, H., et al., **83**:449
Tennant, C., et al., **83**:404
Teplin, L., **82**:385
Terry, R. D., **83**:100, 109, 110
Test, M. A., **82**:110, 227
Testicular removal, **82**:39. *See also* Surgery
Testimonial privilege, **82**:330–31. *See also* Confidentiality
Testosterone, **82**:11
Thacore, U. R., et al., **83**:416
Thayssen, P., et al., **83**:477, 499, 510
Thematic Apperception Test (TAT), **82**:216
Therapeutic community, *see* Health care system; Nursing staff; Therapeutic relationship
Therapeutic relationship: in bipolar disorder, **83**:302, 323, 326, 329–31, 334
  in borderline disorders, **82**:474, 477–78, 481, 482–86 (*see also* Transference)
  caregiver-infant dyad as model of, **83**:21
  in child therapy, of parent and therapist, **82**:264
  clinical illustration of, **82**:505–10
  in cognitive or behavior therapy, **83**:514–16, 519
  and consent to or refusal of treatment, **82**:351 (*see also* Therapy)
  ethical principles of, **82**:327–38, 333–34 (*see also* Confidentiality)
  the family and, **83**:173, 179, 182–84, 194, 198, 205n, 208, 210 (*see also* Family, the; Family therapy)
  with geriatric patient, **83**:130, 138–39, 144
  in group therapy, **83**:27
  in hypnotherapy, **82**:23
  with hypochondriacal patient, **83**:144
  impact of interpretations on, **83**:61–62
  as key to psychotherapy, **82**:154
  male-female, **83**:39
  mandatory reporting and, **82**:332
  in "middle game," *see* Psychoanalysis
  in narcissistic disorder, **82**:516–23

University of Michigan, **83**:121, 274
University of North Carolina, **83**:121
University of Pittsburgh, **82**:173; **83**:122, 279, 480
University of Tennessee, **83**:275, 282, 284
U'Pritchard, D. C., et al., **83**:470
Urethral surgery: and sexual dysfunction, **82**:38–39. *See also* Surgery
Urinary free cortisol (UFC) levels, **83**:462–63
Urinary MHPG levels, **83**:272–73, 460–66
    as predictors of drug response, **83**:468–69, 473–74, 486, 490
Urinary VMA levels, **83**:461, 464–65, 466
Uterus, removal of, **82**:40–41. *See also* Surgery

V

VA (Veterans Administration): facilities of, **83**:130
    -NIMH Collaborative Study of Lithium Therapy, **83**:307, 311, 316–17, 371
    schizophrenia studies by, **82**:198, 226, 227
Vagina: aging effects on, **82**:45–46
    anatomy of, **82**:10, 12
    and vaginal orgasm, **82**:11; **83**:41
Vaginismus: as inhibition, **82**:15, 20, 32
    therapy for, **82**:21, 23
Vagueness, *see* Speech
Vaillant, G., **83**:216
Valenstein, A. F., **83**:61
Values: conflict of, in couples therapy, **83**:221–22
    relationship of, to psychoanalysis, **83**:8, 36–50
    traditional, rejection of, **83**:35
    See also Ethical considerations; Self-esteem
Valzelli, L., **83**:512
Vandalism, **83**:190
Vandenbos, G. R., **82**:158, 217
Vanderstoep, E., **83**:191
Van Der Velde, C. D., **82**:180, 184
Van der Waals, H., **82**:511
Van Eerdewegh, M. M., et al., **83**:447
van Kammen, D. P., **82**:132
Vannicelli, M., et al., **82**:226
Van Praag, H. M., **82**:195; **83**:273, 452
Van Putten, Theodore, **82**:175; **83**:317, 326, 328, 331, 335
Van Valkenburg, C., et al., **83**:380
Vartanian, M. E., et al., **82**:115, 117
Vascular disorders: cardiovascular disorders
    in bipolar illness, **83**:287
    among depressives, **83**:361, 366
    drug side effects and, **83**:477–78, 484, 485, 505, 509–10
    and metabolism, **83**:509
    and psychosexual dysfunctions, **82**:36–37
    and dementia (repeated or multiinfarct), **83**:114–15
    See also Physical illness
Vasectomy, **82**:39. *See also* Surgery
Vasocongestion: as sexual response, **82**:12

Vaughn, C. E., **82**:104, 105, 172; **83**:174, 175; et al., **82**:104
Vaughn, W. T., et al., **82**:115
Vaughter, R. M., **83**:39
Veith, R. C., et al., **83**:478, 503
Verbalization, *see* Speech
Verhoeven, W. M. A., et al., **82**:141, 213
Versiani, M., **82**:185
Verwoerdt, A., et al., **83**:147–48
Verstergaard, P., **83**:314; et al., **83**:313, 314
Veterans Administration, *see* VA
Vibrator, use of, **82**:21
Victoratos, G. C., et al., **83**:109
Videbech, T., **83**:431
Vierling, L., **82**:352
Vietnam war, **82**:371
Vilkin, M. I., **82**:458, 461
Vincent, J. P., et al., **82**:140
Violence: adolescent, **83**:190
    in bipolar illness, **83**:320
    group potential for, **83**:22, 23, 25
    toward therapist, **83**:196
    See also Aggression; Dangerousness; Rape
Viruses: and affective disorders, **83**:379, 453
    and schizophrenia, **82**:119–22
    viral etiology theorized in multiple sclerosis, Alzheimer's disease, **82**:121; **83**:111, 453
    See also Physical illness
Vision: age-related changes in, **83**:102–03, 134
    cataracts, **83**:103, 134
    color blindness, **83**:436, 448–49
    glaucoma, **83**:103, 113, 475
    drug side effects on, **82**:169; **83**:113, 302, 475
    paranoia and, **83**:134
    presbyopia, **83**:103
    senile macular degeneration, **83**:103
    See also Sensory deficits
Vital Balance, The (Menninger), **83**:269
Vitamins, **82**:142–44
VMA, *see* Urinary VMA levels
Vogel, E. F., **83**:233
Vogel, G. W., et al., **82**:290
Vogel, W. H., **82**:126, 144
Vohra, J., et al., **83**:505
Volavka, J., et al., **82**:213
Volk, W., et al., **82**:206
Volkan, V., **82**:471, 480, 519
Volkmar, F. R., et al., **83**:322, 325
Voluntary admission, **82**:347. *See also* Therapy
von Zerssen, D., **82**:207
von Zerssen Personality Scale, **83**:387
Vyas, B. K., **82**:186

W

Wachtel, E. F., **83**:216
Wahlin, A., **83**:314
WAIS (Wechsler Adult Intelligence Scale), **82**:433; **83**:301
Waldmeier, P. C., **83**:469
Walford, R. L., **83**:111
Walinder, J., **82**:211

Wallerstein, R. S., **82:**475, 497, 503
Walsh, A. C., **83:**112; et al., **83:**112
Walsh, B. H., **83:**112
Walsh, F., **83:**222
Wang, H. S., **83:**102
Wang, Y. C., et al., **83:**470
Ward, B. E., et al., **83:**110
Ward, N. G., et al., **83:**506
Warheit, G. J., et al., **83:**412, 413, 414
Warren, S. D., **83:**328
Washburn, S., et al., **82:**226
Washington University, **83:**282, 293, 376
  Department of Psychiatry, **83:**32, 408, 519
Wasserman, M. D., et al., **82:**37
Watson, J. S., **83:**14
Watson, R., et al., **83:**461
Watson, S. J., et al., **82:**212
Watt, D. C., **82:**108
Watt, N. F., **82:**89
Watts, C. A. H., **83:**372; et al., **83:**417
Waxler, N. E., **82:**101; **83:**242
Weakland, John, **83:**170
Weaver, J. L., **82:**100
Webb, W., **83:**145
Wechsler Adult Intelligence Scale, *see* WAIS
Weeke, Anita, **83:**287, 419, 425; et al., **83:**418, 426
Weeks, G., **83:**223
Weeping: in bipolar disorder, **83:**280
  childhood depression and, **82:**304
Weight gain: depression and, **83:**280
  as drug side effect, *see* Drug side effect(s)
Weight loss: depression and, **83:**127, 144, 362, 371, 373, 479
    childhood depression, **82:**297, 304
    as predictor of TCA response, **83:**122
Weinberg, J., **82:**225; **83:**86–87
Weinberg, W. A., et al., **82:**267, 282, 284, 289–98 passim
Weinberger, Daniel A., **82:**122–24, 148; et al., **82:**123
Weiner, I., **82:**57
Weingartner, H., et al., **83:**107
Weinmann, B., **82:**177
Weinshilboum, R. M., **83:**451; et al., **82:**127
Weinstein, M. R., **83:**314
Weiss, James M. A., **82:**281n
Weiss, R., **82:**452; **83:**467
Weissberg, J. H., **82:**35
Weissman, Myrna M., **82:**161, 281–85 passim; **83:**91, 92, 128, 270, 271, 275, 321, 355, 365, 366, 372, 374, 406–16 passim, 420–27 passim, 438, 519; et al., **82:**281; **83:**128, 391, 393, 398, 400, 409, 416, 420, 424, 437, 438, 512, 525
Weitkamp, L. R., et al., **83:**449
Weller, E., **82:**292; et al., **82:**307
Weller, H. P., **82:**144
Wells, C. E., **83:**90, 107, 108, 109, 117
Welner, A., et al., **83:**286, 290
Welner, Z., et al., **82:**289
Wender, P. H., **82:**454; et al., **82:**95, 444, 445, 448, 454, 455, 460, 462–63
Werble, B., **82:**416
Werner, Heinz, **83:**14
Werner's syndrome, **83:**110

Wernicke, C., **83:**269
Wertham, F. I., **83:**285
Wertheimer, N. M., **82:**117
West, E. D., **83:**119, 126
West Virginia Rehabilitation Research and Training Center, **82:**109
Wetzel, R. D., **83:**433; et al., **83:**390, 392, 393
Wexler, B., **82:**124
Whaley, K., **82:**117
Whalley, L. J., et al., **83:**111
Wharton, R. N., et al., **83:**480
Whipple, B., **82:**11
Whitaker, Carl, **83:**170, 200, 215
Whitaker, P. M., et al., **82:**130
White, B. J., et al., **83:**110
White, K., **83:**485; et al., **83:**467
White, P., et al., **83:**109
White, R. A., **82:**37
Whiteley, J. S., **83:**25
Whybrow, P. C., **83:**460
Whyte, S. F., et al., **83:**506
Widowhood: and sexuality, **82:**42–43, 44–45
Wigmore, J. H., **82:**327
Wilcox, C. B., et al., **83:**111
Wilder, J. F., et al., **82:**225
Wiles, D., et al., **82:**202
Wilkie, F., et al., **83:**133
Wilkinson, G. R., **83:**495
Will, O. A., Jr., **82:**161
Willett, A., et al., **82:**416–17, 418
Williams, C. D., **83:**90, 91
Williams, L. T., et al., **83:**470
Williams, M., **83:**115
Williams, R. L., et al., **82:**294, 295; **83:**145
Williams, T., **82:**61
Williams, T. A., **82:**287
Willmuth, R. L., **83:**475
Willowbrook (New York), **82:**375
Wilmette, J., **83:**449
Wilson, R. G., et al., **82:**202
Wilson, W., **83:**144
Wilson's disease, **82:**144
Wing, J. K., **82:**88, 102, 107, 177; **83:**174, 242; et al., **82:**100; **83:**408–09, 416
Winnicott, D. W., **82:**471, 472, 477, 486, 490, 520; **83:**14, 56
Winokur, A., et al., **83:**442
Winokur, G., **83:**271–78 passim, 282–86 passim, 311, 366, 372, 380, 412, 420–23 passim, 431, 438–48 passim; et al., **82:**438, 443; **83:**118, 269, 279, 283, 287, 293, 304, 368, 380, 446–49 passim
Winter, H., et al., **83:**451, 452
Winter, J., **83:**117
Wise, C. D., **82:**127; et al., **82:**128
Wise, T. P., **82:**331
Wisniewski, H. M., **83:**100
Wistedt, B., **82:**191
Withdrawal, social: childhood, and later schizophrenia, **82:**89
  childhood depression and, **82:**297, 302
  in emotionally unstable character disorder, **82:**463
  See also Social isolation
Wittenborn, J. R., **83:**387, 389, 392

Wode-Helgodt, B., et al., **82**:183
Wohl, J., **82**:357
Wold, P. N., **83**:281
Wolf, A., **83**:26
Wolf, E. S., **82**:504, 505, 510, 511
Wolf, G., **82**:293
Wolff, P., **83**:9
Wolin, S. J., et al., **83**:176, 177–78
Women, *see* Female(s)
Women's liberation, *see* Feminist movement
Wood, C. L., et al., **83**:470
Wood, D., et al., **82**:459, 462, 463
Woodman, D., **82**:330
Woodruff, R. A., **83**:372; et al., **83**:426
Woodward, B., **82**:363
World Health Organization (WHO), **82**:14, 100–101; **83**:409, 506
Wyatt, Richard J., **82**:92, 122–24, 125, 130, 143, 147, 148, 452; **83**:131, 132; et al., **82**:118, 119, 126–29 passim, 137, 152
Wyatt right-to-treatment cases, **82**:321, 361–73 passim
Wynne, Lyman C., **82**:172; **83**:170, 190, 191, 193, 235, 242

X

X-chromosome transmission hypothesis, *see* Genetic factors

Y

Yagi, K., **82**:137
Yale Law Review Journal: "Note," **82**:363, 366, 368
Yanchyshyn, G. W., **82**:284
Yassa, R., **82**:144
Yates, C. M., **83**:111

Yates, P. O., **83**:110
Yeazell, S. C., **82**:324n8
Yelverton, K. C., **83**:446
Yesavage, J. A., et al., **83**:112
Yorkston, N. J., et al., **82**:131, 205, 206, 207
Young, J. E., **83**:513
Young adults: affective disorders in, **83**:280, 281, 287, 329, 364, 365, 372, 456
in family therapy, **83**:169, 195, 211–12
and student rebellion (France, 1968), **83**:35
Youngerman, J., **83**:283

Z

Zabarenko, R. N. and L. M., **83**:173
Zackson, H., **82**:62
Zaiden, J., **83**:523
Zajonc, R. B., **83**:16, 17
Zaleznik, A., **83**:33
Zarit, S. N., **83**:132, 133
Zarrabi, M. H., et al., **82**:117, 118
Zeisel, S., et al., **83**:113
Zetzel, E. R., **82**:472, 480; **83**:56
Ziegler, V. E., **83**:506; et al., **83**:495, 500, 506
Zigler, E., **82**:108
Zilbach, J. J., **83**:230
Zilbergeld, B., **82**:26; **83**:222n1
Zilboorg, G., **82**:444; **83**:512
Zimbardo, P. G., **83**:134
Zimmer, R., et al., **82**:139
Zinc concentration, **83**:111
Zinner, J., **83**:218, 235
Zis, A. P., **83**:306
Zitrin, C., et al., **82**:465
Zornetzer, S. F., **83**:110
Zrull, J. P., **82**:266, 267, 274, 277, 284, 285
Zubin, J., **82**:98; **83**:407
Zuk, G. H., **83**:183
Zukin, S. R. and R. S., **82**:140
Zung, W. W. K., **83**:490; et al., **83**:112
Zung scale, **83**:362